Headache and Facial Pain

Headache and Facial Pain

Franco Mongini, M.D.

Director, Unit of Facial Pain
Department of Clinical Pathophysiology
University of Turin
Italy

654 illustrations

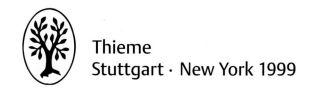

Thieme
Stuttgart · New York 1999

To Helmi, Claudia, Flavia, and Tullia

Library of Congress Cataloging-in-Publication Data

Mongini, Franco
[Le cefalee e il dolore faciale. English]
Headache and facial pain / Franco Mongini.
    p.   cm.
Includes bibliographical references and index.
ISBN 3-13-116541-3. – ISBN 0-86577-852-3
1. Headache.   2. Facial pain.   I. Title.
[DNLM: 1. Headache.   2. Facial Pain.   WL 342 M743L 1999]
RC392.M6613   1999
616.8'491 – dc21
DNLM/DLC
for Library of Congress   99-25746
                                                                CIP

Important Note: Medicine is an ever-changing science undergoing continual development. Research and clinical experience are continually expanding our knowledge, in particular our knowledge of proper treatment and drug therapy. Insofar as this book mentions any dosage or application, readers may rest assured that the authors, editors, and publishers have made every effort to ensure that such references are in accordance with the state of knowledge at the time of production of the book.

Nevertheless this does not involve, imply, or express any guarantee or responsibility on the part of the publishers in respect of any dosage instructions and forms of application stated in the book. Every user is requested to examine carefully the manufacturers' leaflets accompanying each drug and to check, if necessary in consultation with a physician or specialist, whether the dosage schedules mentioned therein or the contraindications stated by the manufacturers differ from the statements made in the present book. Such examination is particularly important with drugs that are either rarely used or have been newly released on the market. Every dosage schedule or every form of application used is entirely at the user's own risk and responsibility. The authors and publishers request every user to report to the publishers any discrepancies or inaccuracies noticed.

Title of the Italian edition:

Le cefalee e il dolore faciale
Copyright © 1998
UTET, corso Raffaello 28, 10125 Torino

© 1999 Georg Thieme Verlag, Rüdigerstraße 14,
D-70469 Stuttgart, Germany
Thieme New York, 333 Seventh Avenue,
New York, NY 10001 USA.

Typesetting and printing by Götz GmbH, Ludwigsburg
Printed in Germany

ISBN 3-13-116541-3 (GTV)
ISBN 0-86577-852-3 (TNY)   1 2 3 4 5 6

Foreword

Few disorders confound and perplex physician-scientists more than painful conditions which emanate from the head and neck. Many of these painful conditions fall within the domain of ophthalmologists, dentists, otolaryngologists, anesthesiologists, neurologists, or neurosurgeons. The most complex (and most common) among them, headache, may begin within the purview of these specialists and oftentimes confronts internists, general practitioners, psychiatrists, and obstetrician-gynecologists as well. Although physicians are now familiar with descriptions of headache syndromes, and are well along in taxonomy and nomenclature, the pathophysiological basis of headaches including migraine, episodic and chronic tension type headache, and chronic daily headache, has eluded us. To the headache sufferer who may live with the problem daily, the origins of headaches are even more perplexing as often the sufferer suspects some sinister condition of the neck, face, eye, scalp, and blood vessels. Particularly with recent onset headache, many express concern that their symptoms reflect the presence of a brain tumor. Furthermore, sufferers and specialists alike may also be confused by the odd relationship between headache onset and the occurrence of psychological stresses, allergies, foods, drugs, hormones, and even injury to the neck. Hence, there is a critical, unmet need for an integrative, comprehensive, and scholarly treatment of head pain with relation to the essential physiology and pathophysiology of tissues (e.g. nerves, muscles, bones, brain, and their integrative functions), implicated in pain syndromes collectively known as headaches.

Over the past decade, the field of headache has broadened and deepened enormously, and this book provides a timely, well-considered, and organized treatise on the most significant headache syndromes experienced in clinical practice. In this book Dr. Mongini reveals his own fascination with the subject by detailed description and explanations of basic mechanisms relevant to the clinical problem for each of the tissues noted above. The author also shares with the reader practical clinical experience, and provides information not commonly explored in standard headache texts on posture and arthrogenous pain, all with abundant reference to the literature.

The book also provides an unbiased description of therapeutic options, including biofeedback and drug treatment regimens, and is filled with case histories and illustrative figures and photos that amplify key points in the text. Hence, this book serves as a reference for students and practitioners in need of placing cephalic pain in the context of current neuroscientific thinking, and in need of a practical guide for safe and effective approaches to diagnosis and management.

Michael A. Moskowitz, M.D.
Professor of Neurology
Harvard Medical School
Charlestown, MA, USA

Preface

During my work in the field of headache and facial pain I observed many cases of patients who had received widely discordant diagnoses and treatment prescriptions following examination by a number of specialists. Likewise, a number of patients with similar problems had received varying treatment from different specialists. My belief is that this is due to two factors that complicate the assessment and management of different types of headache and facial pain: various local and systemic etiologic factors may be present in the same pain pathology, and pathologies of different types can be superimposed in the same patient. As a consequence, patients may receive a diagnosis and treatment that only take into account certain aspects of the problem, depending on the type of specialist to which they are referred. I am, therefore, convinced of the necessity of a common approach to both groups of pathologies, headache and facial pain. I also strongly believe that to study and practice this complex field of medicine sufficient information should be acquired about the impact that systemic dysfunctions, mood or personality disorders, and the dysfunction of the main craniofacial structures (in particular muscles and the temporomandibular joint) may have on the different headache and facial pain pathologies. In this book I have attempted to meet this interdisciplinary demand by taking advantage both of my experience as a neurologist — in which capacity I have been working for several years on the study and management of headache and facial pain — and of my former experience with muscular and temporomandibular joint disorders.

I have organized my work so as to first examine the classification criteria as well as the etiologic factors and pathogenetic mechanisms of different types of headache and facial pain, and second to deal with the problems related to diagnosis and choice of treatment modalities. Subsequently, individual pathologies characterized by headache and facial pain are discussed and a consistent number of clinical cases, of different degrees of severity, are described. The reader will notice that the text contains frequent cross-references with other chapters to maintain a tight relation between the theoretical and clinical aspects of the problems at hand.

I hope that I have achieved with my endeavours the target I originally set myself of making this a useful book to consult for all colleagues interested in the problem of headache and facial pain.

Franco Mongini

Acknowledgements

I would like to acknowledge gratefully the various forms of help received from the following colleagues and friends. They have contributed to this work by providing me with excellent support or material and by sharing their ideas and experiences:

Stuard W. G. Derbyshire, Hammersmith Hospital, London; Ingrid Grunert, University of Innsbruck; Karl G. Henriksson, University of Linkoping; Martin Ingvar, Karolinska Hospital, Stockholm; Barry Sessle, University of Toronto; Sara L. Shepheard, Merck Merk Sharp and Dolome Research Laboratories, Harlow, Essex; Gerhard Steinhard, Erlangen; Manfred Zimmerman, University of Heidelberg; Bruno Bergamasco, Gianni Boris Bradac, Guido Filogamo, Carlo Alberto Pagni, Giovanni Asteggiano, Paolo Benna, Flavio Mela, Roberto Romagnoli, University of Turin; Elsa Margaria, S. Anna Hospital, Turin; Carla Maccagnani, Don Gnocchi Foundation, Turin; Mario Tiengo, University of Milan; Massimo Leandri, University of Genoa; Paolo Procacci, Federigo Sicuteri, Massimo Zoppi, University of Florence; Giuseppe Nappi, Giorgio Cruccu, University of Rome; Gian Camillo Manzoni, University of Parma; Francomichele Puca, University of Bari; Luigi Alberto Pini, University of Modena; Giancarlo Carli, Anna Maria Aloisi, University of Siena; Leonardo Vecchiet, University of Chieti; Enrico Facco, University of Padua.

I owe special thanks to the professors and colleagues who taught me neurology and, in particular, to the memory of Professor Lodovico Bergamini.

My thanks also go to the staff of Thieme for the top level professional commitment they have shown.

I would also like to express my gratitude for the moral support given me by my wife, Dr. Wilhelmine Schmid, and my daughters, Claudia, Flavia, and Tullia.

Franco Mongini

Foreword to the Italian Edition

I would like to point out straight away at least three excellent features of this work. First, this is an exhaustive work representing a comprehensive guide for study and consultation. Second, the work contains a vast number of bibliographic references aiding those readers intending to take up or research a particular argument. The third notable feature is the written style. Whilst retaining a high degree of scientific precision, the work makes for very pleasant reading. Sentences and chapters flow like an account of events and episodes personally experienced by the author, as indeed they are.

Franco Mongini relates his own clinical cases, from which he gained experience and to which he applies strict scientific principles of medicine. In each case, the patients cured by Mongini do not merely represent "case studies," clearly requiring full medical treatment in complete accordance with professional ethics. Instead, the patients also present the opportunity for scientific exploration and validation, with the aim of broadening the horizons of medical science and offering unusual considerations and analyses of benefit to other scholars.

One of the greatest neurosurgeons of our time, Wilder Penfield, had the brilliant idea in 1934 of uniting neurosurgery, neurology, and neurophysiology into one department at McGill University. Unifying the individual experiences and skills from these different fields not only enabled numerous contributions to be made to the diagnosis and cure of many nervous illnesses, but also enabled great progress to be made in the physiology of human memory, language, and behaviour. To Penfield, all disciplines linked to the study of man are inseparable. Moreover, only by studying these disciplines together is it possible to achieve a multidimensional knowledge of man.

Franco Mongini is a part of this cultural tradition. He never limits himself to accurately describing "the case" in the medical sense of the term, but penetrates the problem and tries to understand the human meaning of the illness in the broadest and most intelligent way. In so doing, he extends the argument to include biology, psychology, and sociology. In a learned and attentive manner he confidently goes on to associate clinical data with the underlying principle. Therefore, in the text, general aspects and concepts of neurophysiology are cross-referenced within a logical framework and given an opportune didactic sequence. I am sure that doctors and researchers will find many of their problems, doubts, and hypotheses discussed with often new and original solutions. Consequently this work takes on an importance not only because it is a valuable clinical guide to diagnosis and therapy for — at times very complex and grave — syndromes of the face and head, but also because it proposes elements of culture and reflection increasingly experienced by the reader today.

After reading Mongini's work I was reminded of a passage from a letter in which the Nobel Prize winner Lurija wrote in the 1970s to Oliver Sachs (author of "Awakenings" and "Migraine"): "I would ask you to continue to publish your observations. They will contribute to overcoming the manner in which certain doctors confront illness and to opening the way to a deeper and more humane medicine."

Mario Tiengo

Professor Emeritus of Physiopathology and Pain Therapy
Milan University
Honorary Member, International Association for the Study of Pain

Contents

Part III   Diagnosis and Therapy of Headache

Part IV   Diagnosis and Therapy of Facial Pain

Part I Classification and Pathophysiology

1 Taxonomy of Headache and Facial Pain

General Principles. Etiological Factors and Pain Categories

The taxonomic problems of headache and facial pain are partly related to a lack of consensus concerning the etiological factors and their interplay.

There are several reasons for such controversy:
- Different etiological factors may be present in the same patient.
- The same etiological factors may lead, in different patients, to different consequences.
- Problems arising from the craniofacial structures may be complicated by the superimposition of systemic disorders.
- The disorder may be essentially systemic but, in some cases, may mimic the presence of local problems.

As a consequence, a clear distinction between the different pathologies may not always be easy: this situation is reflected in the semantic problems encountered in the definition and description of syndromes leading to headache and facial pain.

It seems reasonable, for taxonomic purposes, first to assess the etiological factors that may be present in the different headache and facial pain syndromes, drawing a preliminary distinction between local and systemic factors. Local (or segmental) factors are those that originate in the craniofacial and neck structures and whose effects are mostly or totally confined within such structures. Systemic factors are those due to alterations of the general systems that produce or reinforce the symptoms in the craniofacial area (Mongini, 1990).

Local factors may be indicated as follows:
- Local or segmental neurological disorders
- Functional disorders of the craniofacial musculature
- Alteration of head, neck and shoulder posture and/or of jaw structure

General or systemic factors are as follows:
- Alterations of the nervous system (central and/or peripheral)
- Vascular and hemodynamic alterations
- Hormonal and immune system alterations
- Psychological (psychosocial) alterations

Clearly, the interplay of the different factors is often such that some of the factors may have the consequence of producing others. Hormonal dysfunction, for example, may often lead to vascular or psychological problems. Moreover, systemic factors, and in particular psychological stress, may encourage muscle parafunction and dysfunction. Thus the latter could be regarded in these cases more as an effect than as a primary etiological factor.

In some cases, only one etiological factor is present or is the most relevant by far. However, more often, several factors may be combined in the same patient. The temporal sequence of their occurrence is also important; in some patients they may have coexisted right from the beginning of the pathogenic mechanism that led to the symptomatology; in other patients a primary factor may subsequently produce others (for instance, a relevant psychogenic factor may lead to severe chronic muscle hyperfunction and parafunction that, over time, produces jaw structure alterations).

It is also important for taxonomic and clinical purposes to consider the type of pain the patient suffers (Wilson, 1991). There are basically three putative pain categories: nociceptive, neuropathic, and psychogenic pain. *Nociceptive pain* is due to peripherally generated neuronal activity as a consequence of potentially tissue-damaging stimuli; *neuropathic pain* is related to some damage to the nervous system; *psychogenic pain* occurs in the apparent absence of either peripheral nociceptive or neural damage.

Although in some cases the patient suffers from only one type of pain, in other cases, especially when different pathologies are superimposed, two or all three of the pain categories may be represented. This is again because the etiological factors mentioned above may produce one or more than one type of pain (Fig. 1.1).

Etiological Factors

Pain	LOCAL			SYSTEMIC			
	Segmental neurological	Neuromuscular	Posture and jaw structure alterations	Neurological	Hormonal	Vascular	Psychological
Nociceptive		X	X	X	X	X	X (through the neuromuscular factor)
Neuropathic	X			X	X	X	
Psychogenic					X		X

Fig. 1.1 **The etiological factors of headache and facial pain.** An indication of tendency is given, to which exceptions may well be possible

Main Classification Systems. Similarities and Differences

The first relevant classification of headache was published by an "Ad Hoc Committee" of the American Medical Association in 1962. In more recent years two international classifications of craniofacial pain and headache syndromes have been proposed. In 1986, the Classification of Chronic Pain was published by the International Association for the Study of Pain (IASP). A second edition, extensively reviewed, of this classification was published in 1994. In this, craniofacial pain and headache are classified in a section of an extensive classification of all pain syndromes. In 1988, the Classification and Diagnostic Criteria for Headache Disorders, Cranial Neuralgias and Facial Pain was published by the International Headache Society (IHS).

Both classifications represent serious attempts to manage the problem of taxonomy of craniofacial pain and headache syndromes, based on scientific criteria and sound clinical experience. However, there are some relevant differences between the two. Some of these differences are methodological in nature, while others relate to the terminology, the systematization, and the description of the pain syndromes (Manzoni et al., 1992).

The IASP classification is based on an axial five digit coding system. The five axes (I to V) identify, respectively: the regions where pain is present, the systems involved, the temporal characteristics of pain, the patient's statement of intensity and the etiology (Table 1.1). Thus the different craniofacial pain and headache syndromes, which obviously have axis I in common, may differ on axes II to V (Table 1.2).

The IHS classification is based on a hierarchically constructed system of four different levels of sophistication. According to this system, in routine practice the diagnosis will be restricted to the first two levels, while in specialized centers it should reach for four-digit level (Table 1.3).

The items provided in the two classifications for the identification of the different pain syndromes follow different criteria. The IASP classification usually provides more extensive descriptions in which particular emphasis is given to the pathogenetic mechanisms of the disease. In the IHS classification a considerable effort is made to give precise and, as far as possible, quantitative diagnostic criteria. The way tension-type headache is described provides a good example for comparing the different characteristics of the classification systems. In the IASP classification, this disease is listed under group III: "craniofacial pain of musculoskeletal origin." Two distinct entities are described, namely "acute tension headache" and "tension headache: chronic form."

Acute tension headache (code 034.X7 a) is defined as an "acute continuous unilateral or diffuse head pain related to anxiety, depression or emotional tension." Tension headache: chronic form (code 034.X7 b) is defined as a "virtually continuous head pain, usually symmetrical, and frequently global." This headache is frequently, but not in all cases, associated with "muscle tension." The term tension is nevertheless retained; tension may also be taken to indicate stress, strain, anxiety and emotional tension. There is a frequent association between these factors, and also depressive states, and this headache. In later stages, exacerbations with a pounding headache and nausea (and, less typically, vomiting) may occasionally occur, although less typically and with less intensity then in common migraine.

The IHS classification makes a distinction between "episodic" and "chronic" tension-type headache. Episodic tension-type headache (code 2.1) is described in these terms:

Table 1.1 The five axes according to the IASP classification of chronic pain

Axis I: Regions: Record main site first; record two important regions separately. If there is more than one site of pain, separate coding will be necessary. More than three major sites can be coded, optionally, as shown.

Head, face and mouth	000
Cervical region	100
Upper shoulder and upper limbs	200
Thoracic region	300
Abdominal region	400
Lower back, lumbar spine, sacrum, and coccyx	500
Lower limbs	600
Pelvic region	700
Anal, perineal, and genital region	800
More than three major sites	900

Axis II: Systems

Nervous system (central, peripheral, and autonomic) and special senses; physical disturbance or dysfunction	00
Nervous system (psychological and social)	10
Respiratory and cardiovascular systems	20
Musculoskeletal system and connective tissue	30
Cutaneous and subcutaneous and associated glands (breast, apocrine, etc.)	40
Gastrointestinal system	50
Genitourinary system	60
Other organs or viscera (e.g. thyroid, lymphatic, hemopoietic)	70
More than one system	80
Unknown	90

Axis III: Temporal characteristics of pain: pattern of occurrence

Not recorded, not applicable, or not known	0
Single episode, limited duration (e.g., ruptured aneurysm, sprained ankle	1
Continuous or nearly continuous, nonfluctuating (e.g., low back pain, some cases)	2
Continuous or nearly continuous, fluctuation severity (e.g., ruptured intervertebral disk)	3
Recurring irregularly (e.g., headache, mixed type)	4
Recurring regularly (e.g., premenstrual pain)	5
Paroxysmal (e.g., tic douloureux)	6
Sustained with superimposed paroxysms	7
Other combinations	8
None of the above	9

Axis IV: Patient's statement of intensity: Time since onset of pain

Not recorded, not applicable, or not known	0
Mild	
1 month or less	1
1 month to 6 month	2
more than 6 month	3
Medium	
1 month or less	4
1 month to 6 month	5
more than 6 month	6
Severe	
1 month or less	7
1 month to 6 month	8
more than 6 month	9

Axis V: Etiology

Genetic or congenital disorders (e.g., congenital dislocation)	00
Trauma, operation, burns	01
Infective, parasitic	02
Inflammatory (no known infective agent), immune reactions	03
Neoplasm	04
Toxic, metabolic (e.g., alcoholic neuropathy, anoxia vascular, nutritional, endocrine), radiation	05
Degenerative, mechanical	06
Dysfunctional (including psychophysiological)	07
Unknown or other	08
Psychological origin (e.g., conversion hysteria, depressive hallucination).	09

Table 1.2 Classification of head and neck pain syndromes according to the IASP

II. Neuralgias of the head and face

1. Trigeminal neuralgia (tic douloureux)	006.X8a
2. Secondary neuralgia (trigeminal) from central nervous system lesions	006.X4 (tumor) 006.X0 (aneurysm)
Arnold–Chiaria syndrome (code only)	002.X2b (congenital)
3. Secondary trigeminal neuralgia from facial trauma	006.X1
4. Acute herpes zoster (trigeminal)	002.X2a
5. Postherpetic neuralgia (trigeminal)	003.X2b
6. Geniculate neuralgia (VIIth cranial nerve): Ramsay–Hunt syndrome	006.X2
7. Neuralgia of the nervus intermedius	006.X8c
8. Glossopharyngeal neuralgia (IXth cranial nerve)	006.X8b
9. Neuralgia of the superior laryngeal nerve (vagus nerve neuralgia)	006.X8e
10. Occipital neuralgia	004.X8 or 004.X1 (if subsequent to trauma)
11. Hypoglossal neuralgia (code only)	006.X8
12. Glossopharyngeal pain from trauma (code only)	003.X1a
13. Hypoglossal pain from trauma (code only)	003.X1b
14. Tolosa–Hunt syndrome (painful ophthalmoplegia)	002.X3a
15. SUNCT syndrome (short–lasting, unilateral, neuralgiform pain with conjunctival injection and tearing)	006.X8j
16. Raeder syndrome (Raeder paratrigeminal syndrome)	
Type I	002.X4 (tumor) 002.X1a (trauma) 002.X3b (inflammatory, etc.)
Type II	002.X8 (unknown)

III. Craniofacial pain of musculoskeletal origin

1. Acute tension headache	034.X7a
2. Tension headache: chronic form (scalp muscle contraction headache)	033.X7b
3. Temporomandibular pain and dysfunction syndrome (also called temporomandibular joint disorder)	034.X8a
4. Osteoarthritis of the temporomandibular joint (code only)	003.X6
5. Rheumatoid arthritis of the temporomandibular joint	032.X3b
6. Dystonic disorders, facial dyskinesia (code only)	003.X8
7. Crushing injury of head or face (code only)	032.X1

IV. Lesions of the ear, nose and oral cavity

1. Maxillary sinusitis	031.X2a
2. Odontalgia: Toothache 1. Due to dentinoenamel defects	034.X2b
3. Odontalgia: Toothache 2. Pulpitis	031.X2c
4. Odontalgia: Toothache 3. Periapical periodontitis and abscess	031.X2d
5. Odontalgia: 4. Tooth pain not associated with lesions (atypical odontalgia)	034.X8b
6. Glossodynia and sore mouth (also known as burning tongue or oral dysesthesia)	051.X5 (if known 051.X8 (alternative)
7. Cracked–tooth syndrome	034.X1
8. Dry socket	031.X1
9. Gingival disease, inflammatory (code only)	034.X2
10. Toothache, cause unknown (code only)	034.X8f

11. Disease of the jaw, inflammatory conditions (code only)	033.X2
12. Other and unspecified pain in jaws (code only)	03X.X8d
13. Frostbite of face (code only)	022.X1

V. Primary headache syndromes, vascular disorders, and cerebrospinal fluid syndroms

1. Classic migraine (migraine with aura)	004.X7a
2. Common migraine (migraine without aura)	004.X7b
3. Migraine variants	004.X7c
4. Carotidynia	004.X7d
5. Mixed headache	003.X7b
6. Cluster headache	004.X8a
7. Chronic paroxysmal hemicrania (CPH)	
7.1 Unremitting form or variety	006.X8k
7.2 Remitting form or variety	006.X8g
8. Chronic cluster headache	004.X8b
9. Cluster-tic syndrome	006.X8h
10. Posttraumatic headache	002.X1b
11. The syndrome of "jabs and jolts"	006.X8i
12. Temporal arteritis (giant cell arteritis)	023.X3
13. Headache associated with low cerebrospinal fluid pressure	023.X1a
14. Postdural puncture headache	023.X1b
15. Hemicrania continua	093.X8
16. Headache not otherwise specified (code only)	00X.X8f

Note: A headache crosswalk follows this group in Part II, detailed descriptions of pain syndromes.

VI. Pain of psychological origin in the head, face, and neck (code only)

1. Delusional or hallucinatory pain (code only)	01X.X9e (head or face)
2. Hysterical, conversion, or hypochondriacal pain (code only)	01X.X9f (head or face) 11X.X9f (neck)
3. Associated with depression (code only)	01X.X9g (head or face) 11X.X9g (neck)

See also: 1–16, pain of psychological origin; III-1, acute tension headache; and III-2, tension headache: chronic form

VII. Suboccipital and cervical musculoskeletal disorders

1. Stylohyoid process syndrome (Eagle syndrome)	036.X6
2. Cervicogenic headache	033.X6b
3. Superior pulmonary sulcus syndrom (Pancoast tumor)	102.X4a
4. Thoracic outlet syndrom	133.X6d or 233.X6a
5. Cervical rib or malformed first thoracic rib (see VI-4, thoracic outlet syndrome)	or 233.X6a
6. Pain of skeletal metastastic disease of the neck, arm, or shoulder girdle	233.X4 133.X4j or

Note: For cervical sprain, see IX-8, accelleration-deceleration injury of the neck (cervical sprain)

VIII. Visceral pain in the neck

1. Carcinoma of thyroid	172.X4
2. Carcinoma of larynx	122.X4
3. Tuberculosis of larynx	123.X2
4. Chronic pharyngitis (code only)	151.X5 (if known) 151.X8 (alternative)
5. Carcinoma of pharynx (code only)	153.X4

Table 1.**3** Classification of headache disorders, cranial neuralgias and facial pain according to the IHS

1. Migraine

- 1.1 Migraine without aura
- 1.2 Migraine with aura
  - 1.2.1 Migraine with typical aura
  - 1.2.2 Migraine with prolonged aura
  - 1.2.3 Familial hemiplegic migraine
  - 1.2.4 Basilar migraine
  - 1.2.5 Migraine aura without headache
  - 1.2.6 Migraine with acute onset aura
- 1.3 Ophthalmoplegic migraine
- 1.4 Retinal migraine
- 1.5 Childhood periodic syndromes that may be precursors to or associated with migraine
  - 1.5.1 Benign paroxysmal vertigo of childhood
  - 1.5.2 Alternating hemiplegia of childhood
- 1.6 Basilar migraine
  - 1.6.1 Status migrainosus
  - 1.6.2 Migrainous infarction
- 1.7 Migrainous disorder not fulfilling above criteria

2. Tension-type headache

- 2.1 Episodic tension-type headache
  - 2.1.1 Episodic tension-type headache associated with disorder of pericranial muscles
  - 2.1.2 Episodic tension-type headache unassociated with disorder of pericranial muscles
- 2.2 Chronic tension-type headache
  - 2.2.1 Chronic tension-type headache associated with disorder of pericranial muscles
  - 2.2.2 Chronic tension-type headache unassociated with disorder of pericranial muscles
  - 2.3 Headache of the tension type not fulfilling above criteria

3. Cluster headache and chronic paroxysmal hemicrania

- 3.1 Cluster headache
  - 3.1.1 Cluster headache periodicity undetemined
  - 3.1.2 Episodic cluster headache
  - 3.1.3 Chronic cluster headache
    - 3.1.3.1 Unremitting from onset
    - 3.1.3.2 Evolved from episodic
- 3.2 Chronic paroxysmal hemicrania
- 3.3 Cluster headache-like disorder not fulfilling above criteria

4. Miscellaneous headaches unassociated with structural lesion

- 4.1 Idiopathic stabbing headache
- 4.2 External compression headache
- 4.3 Cold stimulus headache
  - 4.3.1 External application of a cold stimulus
  - 4.3.2 Ingestion of a cold stimulus
- 4.4 Benign cough headache
- 4.5 Benign exertional headache
- 4.6 Headache associated with sexual activity
  - 4.6.1 Dull type
  - 4.6.2 Explosive type
  - 4.6.3 Postural type

5. Headache associated with head trauma

- 5.1 Acute posttraumatic headache
  - 5.1.1 With significant head trauma and/or confirmatory signs
  - 5.1.2 With minor head trauma and no confirmatory signs
- 5.2 Chronic posttraumatic headache
  - 5.2.1 With significant head trauma and/or confirmatory signs
  - 5.2.2 With minor head trauma and no confirmatory signs

6. Headache associated with vascular disorders

- 6.1 Acute ischemic cerebrovascular disease
  - 6.1.1 Transient ischemic attack (TIA)
  - 6.1.2 Thromboembolic stroke
- 6.2 Intracranial hematoma
  - 6.2.1 Intracerebral hematoma
  - 6.2.2 Subdural hematoma
  - 6.2.3 Epidural hematoma
- 6.3 Subarachnoid hemorrhage
- 6.4 Unruptured vascular malformation
  - 6.4.1 Arteriovenous malformation
  - 6.4.2 Saccular aneurysm
- 6.5 Arteritis
  - 6.5.1 Giant cell arteritis
  - 6.5.2 Other systemic arteritides
  - 6.5.3 Primary intracranial arteritis
- 6.6 Carotid or vertebral artery pain
  - 6.6.1 Carotid or vertebral dissection
  - 6.6.2 Carotidynia (idiopathic)
  - 6.6.3 Postendarterectomy headache
- 6.7 Venous thrombosis
- 6.8 Arterial hypertension
  - 6.8.1 Acute pressor response to exogenous agent
  - 6.8.2 Pheochromocytoma
  - 6.8.3 Malignant (accelerated) hypertension
  - 6.8.4 Preeclampsia and eclampsia
- 6.9 Headache associated with other vascular disorder

7. Headache associated with nonvascular intracranial disorder

- 7.1 High cerebrospinal fluid pressure
  - 7.1.1 Benign intracranial hypertension
  - 7.1.2 High-pressure hydrocephalus
- 7.2 Low cerebrospinal fluid pressure
  - 7.2.1 Postlumbar puncture headache
  - 7.2.2 Cerebrospinal fluid fistula headache
- 7.3 Intracranial infection
- 7.4 Intracranial sarcoidosis and other non-infectious inflammatory disease
- 7.5 Headache related to intrathecal injection
  - 7.5.1 Direct effect
  - 7.5.2 Due to chemical meningitis
- 7.6 Intracranial neoplasm
- 7.7 Headache associated with other intracranial disorder

8. Headache associated with substances or their withdrawal

- 8.1 Headache induced by acute substance use or exposure
  - 8.1.1 Nitrate/nitrite-induced headache
  - 8.1.2 Monosodium glutamate-induced headache
  - 8.1.3 Carbon monoxide-induced headache
  - 8.1.4 Alcohol-induced headache
  - 8.1.5 Other substances
- 8.2 Headache induced by chronic substance use or exposure
  - 8.2.1 Ergotamine-induced headache
  - 8.2.2 Analgesics abuse headache
  - 8.2.3 Other substances
- 8.3 Headache from substance withdrawal (acute use)
  - 8.3.1 Alcohol withdrawal headache (hangover)
  - 8.3.2 Other substances
- 8.4 Headache from substance withdrawal (chronic use)
  - 8.4.1 Ergotamine withdrawal headache
  - 8.4.2 Caffeine withdrawal headache
  - 8.4.3 Narcotics abstinence headache
  - 8.4.4 Other substances
- 8.5 Headache associated with substances but with uncertain mechanism
  - 8.5.1 Birth controll pills or estrogens
  - 8.5.2 Other substances

continued ▶

Table 1.3   (Continued)

9. Headache associated with noncephalic infection

  9.1 Viral infection
       9.1.1 Focal noncephalic
       9.1.2 Systemic
  9.2 Bacterial infection
       9.2.1 Focal noncephalic
       9.2.2 Systemic (septicemia)
  9.3 Headache related to other infections

10. Headache associated with metabolic disorder

  10.1 Hypoxia
        10.1.1 High-altitude headache
        10.1.2 Hypoxic headache
        10.1.3 Sleep apnoea headache
  10.2 Hypercapnia
  10.3 Mixed hypoxia and hypercapnia
  10.4 Hypoglycemia
  10.5 Dialysis
  10.6 Headache related to other metabolic abnormality

11. Headache or facial pain associated with disorder of cranium, neck, eyes, ears, nose, sinuses, teeth, mouth, or other facial or cranial structures

  11.1 Cranial bone
  11.2 Neck
        11.2.1 Cervical spine
        11.2.2 Retropharyngeal tendinitis
  11.3 Eyes
        11.3.1 Acute glaucoma
        11.3.2 Refractive errors
        11.3.3 Heterophoria or heterotropia
  11.4 Ears
  11.5 Nose and sinuses
        11.5.1 Acute sinus headache
        11.5.2 Other diseases of nose or sinuses
  11.6 Teeth, jaws and related structures
  11.7 Temporomandibular joint disease

12. Cranial neuralgias, nerve trunk pain and deafferentation pain

  12.1 Persistent (in contrast to tic-like) pain of cranial nerve origin
        12.1.1 Compression or distortion of cranial nerves and second or third cervical roots
        12.1.2 Demyelination of cranial nerves
                12.1.2.1 Optic neuritis (retrobulbar neuritis)
        12.1.3 Infarction of cranial nerves
                12.1.3.1 Diabetic neuritis
        12.1.4 Inflammation of cranial nerves
                12.1.4.1 Herpes zoster
                12.1.4.2 Chronic postherpetic neuralgia
        12.1.5 Tolosa–Hunt syndrome
        12.1.6 Neck–tongue syndrome
        12.1.7 Other causes of persistent pain of cranial nerve origin
  12.2 Trigeminal neuralgia
        12.2.1 Idiopathic trigeminal neuralgia
        12.2.2 Symptomatic trigeminal neuralgia
                12.2.2.1 Compression of trigeminal root or ganglion
                12.2.2.2 Central lesions
  12.3 Glossopharyngeal neuralgia
        12.3.1 Idiopathic glossopharyngeal neuralgia
        12.3.2 Symptomatic glossopharyngeal neuralgia
  12.4 Nervus intermedius neuralgia
  12.5 Superior laryngeal neuralgia
  12.6 Occipital neuralgia
  12.7 Central causes of head and facial pain other than tic douloureux
        12.7.1 Anesthesia dolorosa
        12.7.2 Thalamic pain
  12.8 Facial pain not fulfilling criteria in groups 11 or 12

13. Headache not classifiable

"Recurrent episodes of headache lasting minutes to days. The pain is typically pressing/tightening in quality, of mild or moderate intensity, bilateral or variable in location and does not worsen with physical activity. Nausea is absent, but phono or photophobia may occur." A further distinction is made between "episodic tension-type headache associated with disorders of pericranial muscles" (2.1.1) and "episodic tension-type headache unassociated with disorder of pericranial muscles" (2.1.2).

Chronic tension-type headache (2.2) is "present for more than 15 days a month during at least 6 months. The headache is usually pressing/tightening in quality, mild or moderate in severity, bilateral or of variable location, and does not worsen with physical activity." Mild nausea and photophobia occur and they may be severe on rare occasions. For chronic tension-type headache the further distinction is made between "chronic tension-type headache associated with disorders of pericranial muscles" (2.2.1) and "chronic tension-type headache unassociated with disorder of pericranial muscles" (2.2.2). Eventually, a "headache of tension-type not fulfilling above criteria" is also considered. Independently of the first three code numbers adopted, a fourth digit code number for group 2 indicates most important pathogenetic factor:

0: No identifiable pathogenetic factor
1: Multiple of the pathogenetic factors listed unter 2–9 (list in order of importance)
2: Oromandibular dysfunction
3: Psychosocial stress (DSM III-R criteria)
4: Anxiety
5: Depression
6: Other mental disorders
7: Muscular stress
8: Drug overuse for tension-type headaches
9: One of the disorders listed in groups 5–11 of the classification.

As already stated, the two systems also show differences in terminology. For example, the IASP classification makes reference to "classic migraine, common migraine and mixed headache," while in the IHS classification the terms "migraine with aura" and "migraine without aura" are used. Moreover, instead of referring to a "mixed headache" here the suggestion is to list all headache disorders diagnosed in order of importance (for instance, migraine and tension-type headache). Table 1.4 demonstrates, where possible, the correspondence between the two classifications.

A problem that is still open is that of facial pain in which the psychological factor plays the sole or predominant role. A term frequently employed to categorize this, especially by neurologists, is "atypical facial pain." In the introduction of the second edition of the IASP classification it is suggested that this term has been used by various authors to define conditions that may be better diagnosed under terms such as "temporomandibular pain syndrome," "atypical odontalgia," or "odontalgia not associated with lesions."

Alternatively, it is suggested that one may refer to a facial pain for which a diagnosis has not yet been determined. In the latest edition of the IHS classification, the term "atypical facial pain" has been dropped in favor of "facial pain which does not meet the criteria of any previous group."

For a better categorization of such pain syndromes it seems reasonable to make reference to the classification of *the Diagnostic and Statistical Manual of Mental Disorders* (DSM-IV, 4th edition; American Psychiatric Association, 1994). These syndromes may reasonably be included within the "Somatoform Disorders" of the DSM-IV. The main feature of such

Table 1.**4**   Headache and facial pain: the correspondence of the IASP classification with the IHS classification (from IASP, 1994)

	IASP		IHS
I-6	Central pain (if confined to head and face)	12.7.2	Thalamic pain
II-1	Trigeminal neuralgia (tic douloureux)	12.2.1	
II-2	Secondary neuralgia (trigeminal) from central nervous system lesions (tumor or aneurysm)	12.2.2.2	Symptomatic trigeminal neuralgia: central lesions
II-3	Secondary trigeminal neuralgia from facial trauma	12.2.2	Symptomatic trigeminal neuralgia
II-4	Acute herpes zoster (trigeminal)	12.1.4.1	Herpes zoster
II-5	Postherpetic neuralgia (trigeminal)	12.1.4.2	Chronic postherpetic neuralgia
II-6	Geniculate neuralgia (VIth cranial nerve): Ramsay–Hunt syndrome	12.1.4.1	Herpes zoster
II-8	Glossopharyngeal neuralgia (IXth cranial nerve)	12.3.1 12.3.2	Idiopathic glossopharyngeal neuralgia *Symptomatic glossopharyngeal neuralgia*
II-9	Neuralgia of the superior laryngeal nerve (vagus nerve neuralgia)	12.5	Superior laryngeal neuralgia
II-10	Occipital neuralgia	12.6	Occipital neuralgia
II-11	Hypoglossal neuralgia	12.1.7	*Other causes of persistent pain of cranial nerve origin*
II-12	Glossopharyngeal pain from trauma	12.3.2	Symptomatic glossopharyngeal neuralgia
II-13	Hypoglossal pain from trauma	12.1.7	*Other causes of persistent pain of cranial nerve origin*
II-14	Tolosa–Hunt syndrome (painful opthalmoplegia)	12.1.5	Tolosa–Hunt syndrome
III-2	Tension headache: chronic form (scalp muscle contraction headache)	2.2 2.3	Chronic tension-type headache Headache of the tension type
III-3	Temporomandibular pain and dysfunction syndrome	2.3.2	*Headache of the tension type with oromandibular dysfunction*
III-5	Rheumatoid arthritis of the temporomandibular joint	11.7	*Temporomandibular joint disease*
IV-1	Maxillary sinusitis	11.5.1	Acute sinus headache
IV-2 through IV-5	Types of odontalgia	11.6	*Headache or facial pain associated with disorder of teeth, mouth, or other facial or cranial structures*
IV-6	Glossodynia and sore mouth	11.6	*Headache or facial pain associated with disorder of teeth, mouth, or other facial or cranial structures*
IV-7	Cracked–tooth syndrome	11.6	*Headache or facial pain associated with disorder of teeth, mouth, or other facial or cranial structures*
IV-8	Dry socket	11.6	*Headache or facial pain associated with disorder of teeth, mouth, or other facial or cranial structures*
IV-9	Gingival disease, inflammatory	11.6	*Headache or facial pain associated with disorder of teeth, mouth, or other facial or cranial structures*
IV-10	Toothache, cause unknown	11.6	*Headache or facial pain associated with disorder of teeth, mouth, or other facial or cranial structures*
IV-11	Diseases of the jaw, inflammatory conditions	11.6	*Headache or facial pain associated with disorder of teeth, mouth, or other facial or cranial structures*
IV-12	Other and unspecified pain in jaw	11.6	*Headache or facial pain associated with disorder of teeth, mouth, or other facial or cranial structures*
V-1	Classic migraine (migraine with aura)	1.2.1 1.2.2 1.2.6 1.6.1	Migraine with aura
V-2	Common migraine (migraine without aura)	1.1	Migraine without aura
V-3	Migraine variants	1.2.3 1.2.4 1.3 1.4	Familial hemiplegic migraine Basilar migraine Opthalmoplegic migraine Retinal migraine
V-5	Mixed headache	1.1 2.2	Migraine without aura Chronic tension type headache

continued ▶

Table 1.**4** (Continued)

	IASP		IHS
V-6	Cluster headache	3.1.1 3.1.2	Cluster headache, periodicity undetermined Episodic cluster headache
V-7.1	Chronic paroxysmal hemicrania: unremitting form or variety	3.2	Chronic paroxysmal hemicrania
V-7.2	Chronic paroxysmal hemicrania: remitting form or variety	3.2	*Chronic paroxysmal hemicrania*
V-8	Chronic cluster headache	3.1.3	Chronic cluster headache
V-10	Posttraumatic headache	5.2.1 5.2.2	Chronic posttraumatic headache with significant head trauma or confirmatory signs Minor head trauma with no confirmatory signs
V-11	Syndrome of "jabs and jolts"	4.1	*Idiopathic stabbing headaches*
V-12	Temporal arteritis (giant cell arteritis)	6.5.1	Giant cell arteritis
V-13	Headache associated with low cerebrospinal fluid pressure	7.2.2	Cerebrospinal fluid fistula headache
V-14	Postdural puncture headache	7.2.1	Postlumbar puncture headache
V-16	Headache not otherwise specified	13.0	Headache, not classifiable
VI-2	Hysterical or hypochondriacal pain in the head, face, and neck	2.3.3	*Headache of the tension type, not fulfilling above criteria*
VI-3	Headache of psychological origin in the head, face, and neck associated with depression	2.3.3	*Headache of the tension type, not fulfilling above criteria*
VII-2	Cervicogenic headache	11.2.1	*Headache or facial pain associated with disorder of cranium, neck, etc.*
IX-1	Cervical spinal or radicular pain attributable to a fracture	11.2.1	*Headache or facial pain associated with disorder of cranium, neck, etc.*
IX-1.7	Fracture of lamina	11.2.1	*Headache or facial pain associated with disorder of cranium, neck, etc.*
IX-1.9	Fracture of the anterior arch of the atlas	11.2.1	*Headache or facial pain associated with disorder of cranium, neck, etc.*
IX-1.10	Fracture of the posterior arch of the atlas	11.2.1	*Headache or facial pain associated with disorder of cranium, neck, etc.*
IX-1.11	Burst fracture of the atlas	11.2.1	*Headache or facial pain associated with disorder of cranium, neck, etc.*

Note: Other items in the neck are not included, although they may potentially cause headache: if they do, they can be entered in the relevant section of the cervical spinal items.

| IX-8 | Acceleration-deceleration injury of the neck (cervical sprain) | 5.2.5 | *Minor head trauma with no confirmatory signs* |

disorders is "the presence of physical symptoms that suggests a general medical condition (hence the term *somatoform*) and are not fully explained by a general medical condition, by the direct effects of a substance, or by another mental disorder." In particular, these facial pain syndromes may be categorized as "pain disorder." In this, the pain is the "predominant focus of clinical attention" in which psychological factors seem "to have an important role in its onset, severity, exacerbation, or maintenance."

Critical Revisions and Validation Studies

Various critical revisions and validation studies have been conducted on the IHS classification in order to verify (a) whether some pathologies not included in the classification should be considered as independent pathologies; and (b) whether the given diagnostic criteria are valid or should be modified for some pathologies.

The first point essentially relates to two headache types that, according to several authors, should be considered independent. These are "chronic daily headache" and "cervicogenic headache."

While it is usually easy to diagnose episodic headache—*migraine or tension type headache* (TTH)—on the basis of the criteria of the IHS classification, difficulties arise as the headache frequency increases and the anamnestic and clinical characteristics of the pain syndrome become blurred (Silberstein, 1993). This applies in particular to the so-called *chronic daily headache* (CDH). In the IHS classification, CDH is not considered separately but is treated as a chronic headache of tension type (CTTH). This may lead to problems in categorization of some patients.

Solomon et al. (1992 a, b) evaluated 100 patients sent consecutively for chronic daily headache, and observed that about one-third of these patients did not meet the IHS criteria for chronic tension-type headache, owing to the frequent presence of migraine characteristics. Nevertheless, these patients could not even be classified as migraine patients, because the headache was daily and also because the characteristics of migraine were not present to a sufficient extent. These authors suggest that the IHS criteria should be modified through the inclusion of a form of headache that evolves into chronic daily headache. Manzoni et al. (1993, 1995) and Mongini et al. (1997) reached similar conclusions.

CDH is essentially defined on the basis of headache frequency: according to various authors this should be at least 6 days per week for at least 6 months. In addition, headache should be present for all or most of the day. It has been suggested that CDH evolves from migraine (Mathew et al., 1982); however, according to Silberstein (1993), it may also develop from chronic tension-type headache or may show a rapid onset.

"Cervicogenic headache" (Sjaastad et al., 1983, 1989, 1990; Fredriksen et al., 1987) is considered as an independent entity in the IASP classification of chronic pain (code VII-2) but not in the IHS classification. In the IASP classification it is described as "attacks of moderate or moderately severe headache pain without change of side, ordinarily involving the whole hemicranium usually starting in the neck or occipital areas, where the maximal pain is frequently located." The possible corresponding pathology in the IHS classification is "headache or facial pain associated with disorder of cranium, neck, etc." (code 11.2.1). Two points in particular seem to be relevant for the differential diagnosis with migraine and tension-type headache: the strictly unilateral localization and the site of pain, especially at the onset of the pain attacks (D'Amico et al., 1994; Leone at al., 1995).

Even though the criteria of the IHS classification seem to be reasonably applicable most of the time (Leone et al., 1994; Olesen, 1996), some objections were made and revisions were suggested. Iversen et al. (1990) applied the IHS criteria to 81 patients who were diagnosed as having migraine, tension headache, or both under the 1962 Ad Hoc Committee Classification of Headache criteria. They found nine cases in which, if the IHS criteria were applied, the patients could also receive a diagnosis different from the original diagnosis. They concluded that the IHS criteria might be improved with regard to accompanying symptoms. Among 410 headache sufferers, Messinger et al. (1991) found 147 (35.9%) in whom either code 1.7 of the IHS classification (migrainous disorders not fulfilling the above criteria) or code 2.3 (headache of tension type not fulfilling the above criteria) could be used. Moreover, in 79 of these 147 patients (53.7%) either code was equally valid. This was 19% of the 410 cases. The authors suggest that the various symptoms should be dealt with individually rather than being grouped as, for example, nausea, vomiting, photophobia, and phonophobia.

To achieve an optimal distinction between tension-type headache and migraine, Pfaffenrath and Isler (1993) advise that the severity of the characteristic migraine symptoms be incorporated in the diagnostic criteria. In particular, photophobia, phonophobia, and the worsening of the headache as a consequence of physical activity may be present in a light form even in tension-type headache and thus should not be considered as criteria for the exclusion of this type of headache. Michel et al. (1993) reached similar conclusions after studying the sensitivity and specificity of a self-administered screening to diagnose migraine on the basis of the IHS criteria.

One problem is that many patients have headache attacks with different characteristics. Sanin et a. (1994), after examining 400 patients classified according to the IHS criteria, found that, even if the diagnosis of migraine was the most frequent,

in only ¼ of the patients was it the only diagnosis. The majority required at least two, often three or four, diagnoses. This problem relates to that already discussed regarding "chronic daily headache."

In fact, while, as we have seen, some authors consider this headache as an independent headache type, other authors maintain that in this case multiple diagnoses are more correct (Olesen, 1996). This position corresponds to what is suggested by the World Health Organization (1992). Manzoni et al. (1995) maintain an intermediate position and suggest a revised classification of migraine taking account of its evolution and including two more categories, namely, "migraine with interparoxysmal headache" and "chronic migraine." Silberstein et al. (1994) maintain that chronic daily headache is an independent group of headache disorders that includes "chronic tension-type headache" (CTTH), "transformed migraine" (TM), "new daily persistent headache" (NDPH), and "hemicrania continua" (HC).

In childhood and adolescence there may be additional problems. In children the IHS criteria seem to have less sensitivity than those of the Ad Hoc Committee (Mortimer et al., 1992). Seshia et al. (1994) advocate for all pediatric headaches a distinction between "clinically defined" and "clinically probable," while Wober-Bingol et al. (1995) suggest that a modification of the IHS criteria for childhood migraine should consider a reduction of the minimum duration of migraine attacks from two hours to one hour (at least) and the inclusion of severity dimensions – particularly for concomitant symptoms – to improve the sensitivity and the specificity of criteria for tension-type headache. Raieli et al. (1995) and Gallai et al. (1995) made similar propositions.

For cluster headache, Nappi et al. (1992) carefully revised 251 cases seen consecutively, and suggest that the IHS criteria should be revised, in particular to take account of nausea, photophobia, and vomiting, and of the "general" autonomic symptoms, as well as the role instrumental analysis may play in those cases where the signs of autonomic dysfunction are absent or present only at a subclinical level.

Taxonomy of Disorders of the TMJ and the Craniocervicofacial Muscles

The taxonomic assessment of disorders of the temporomandibular joint (TMJ) and the craniocervicofacial muscles has been the subject of considerable controversy. These disorders include numerous pathologies characterized by pain situated at the TMJ or cheek as a consequence of disorders of the TMJ itself and/or of the craniofacial or masticatory muscles. Such disorders have been defined at various times in different ways – "TMJ pain dysfunction syndrome," "myofacial pain dysfunction syndrome," "temporomandibular dysfunction" (TMD), "craniomandibular disorders," and so on.

In the IHS classification, these conditions are considered in two separate groups: "oromandibular dysfunction" and "alteration of the temporomandibular joint." Oromandibular dysfunction is classified within the group of "tension-type headache" as a possible pathogenetic factor and is defined as a condition with "three or more of the following: clicking of the temporomandibular joint on jaw movements, limited or jerky jaw movements, pain on extensive jaw movements, locking of jaw on opening, clenching of teeth, gnashing of teeth (bruxism), other oral parafunction (tongue, lips or cheek biting or pressing)." Diagnostic criteria for "alteration of the TMJ" are as follows: "Pain is mild to moderate and located to the TMJ and/or radiating from there. At least two of the following symptoms are present: tenderness of the TMJ capsule; pain of the jaw precipitated by movement; decreased range of motion; crepitation during joint movements; positive radiographic and/or isotope scintigraphic findings."

It would therefore appear that the state of "oromandibular dysfunction" is considered to be essentially of a "functional" nature, whereas TMJ alterations are of a more "organic" nature. Nevertheless, in a comment following the description of this latter condition, it is stressed that "it cannot be emphasized too strongly that it is rarely due to definable organic disease." Overall, in the descriptions reported above, there is a tendency to group together symptoms typical of muscle parafunction and dysfunction (such as tooth clenching, bruxism, muscular pain, and pain in the temporal or occipital zones) with other symptoms that are more characteristic of intracapsular lesions of the TMJ. This is a consequence of including in a single *nosologic entity* alterations of different types that may often be superimposed in the same patient, and that have some clinical characteristics in common (such as pain in the preauricular area or restriction of jaw movement).

In the IASP classification, the term used is "temporomandibular pain and dysfunction syndrome," but the term "temporomandibular joint disorder" is also given. This is described as a condition characterized by "aching in the muscles of mastication with occasional brief severe pain on chewing, often associated with restricted jaw movement and clicking or popping sounds."

This condition should be distinguished from other pathologies or lesions of the temporomandibular joint and, in particular, from "osteoarthritis of the temporomandibular joint" and "rheumatoid arthritis of the temporomandibular joint."

It seems unjustified and misleading to give one single definition to a group of pathologies characterized by chronic or recurrent craniofacial pain that also extends to the preauricular area. Pathologies currently defined as "craniomandibular disorders" may be very different, even though they may frequently be superimposed on the same patient. To give an example, it is obviously preposterous to define as having a "craniomandibular disorder" a patient with a severe personality disorder, an almost constant headache of tension type, and a joint click. Rather, all pathologies that can be assessed in each patient should be indicated: TMJ intracapsular disorder, myogenic pain due to a neuromuscular factor (with or without an anxiety or depressive disorder), tension-type headache, pain in a somatoform disorder, neuralgic pain, and so on. In the case of superimposition of different pathologies, these should be listed, indicating their time of onset and their relevance. For this a comparative analysis of the data from history and clinical examinations is mandatory (Schiffman et al., 1995, Mongini, 1996).

In this connection, the American Academy of Orofacial Pain (1990), in its guidelines for classification, assessment and management of temporomandibular disorders, suggested additions of the IHS classification to deal with this need. In group 11, "headache or facial pain associated with cranial disorders, disorders of the eyes, ears, nose, sinuses, teeth, mouth or other facial or cranial structures," it suggests adding "masticatory muscles" (11.8) to "temporomandibular joint" (11.7) already present. Table 1.**5** gives the diagnostic criteria recommended for these two subgroups.

Table 1.**5** Integration of the IHS classification proposed by the American Academy of Orofacial Pain

11.7	Temporomandibular joint disorders	
	11.7.1	Change of shape
	11.7.2	Dislocation of meniscus
		11.7.2.1 Dislocation of meniscus with reduction
		11.7.2.2 Dislocation of meniscus without reduction
	11.7.3	Dislocation
	11.7.4	Inflammatory conditions
		11.7.4.1 Synovitis
		11.7.4.2 Capsulitis
	11.7.5	Arthritis
		11.7.5.1 Osteoarthrosis
		11.7.5.2 Osteoarthritis
		11.7.5.3 Polyarthritis
	11.7.6	Ankylosis
		11.7.6.1 Fibrous
		11.7.6.2 Bony
11.8	Masticatory muscle disorders	
	11.8.1	Myofacial pain
	11.8.2	Myositis
	11.8.3	Spasm
	11.8.4	Protective splinting
	11.8.5	Contracture
	11.8.6	Neoplasia

References

Ad Hoc Committee on Classification of Headache: classification of headache, 1962, JAMA, 178 : 717 – 718.

American Academy of Orofacial Pain, *Temporomandibular disorders – Guidelines for classification, assessment, and management*, McNeil C., Quintessence Publishing Co., Chicago, 1990.

American Psychiatric Association, *Diagnostic and statistical manual of mental disorders*, Washington, 4th ed., 1994.

D'Amico D., Leone M., Bussone G., *Side-locked unilaterality and pain localization in longlasting headaches: migraine, tension-type headache, and cervicogenic headache*, Headache, 1994, 34 : 526 – 530.

Fredriksen T., Hovdal H., Sjaastad O., *Cervicogenic headache: Clinical manifestation.* Cephalalgia, 1987, 7 : 147 – 160.

Gallai V., Sarchielli P., Carboni F., Benedetti P., Mastropaolo C., Puca F., *Applicability of the 1988 IHS criteria to headache patients under the age of 18 years attending 21 Italian headache clinics. Juvenile Headache Collaborative Study Group* , Headache, 1995, 35 : 146 – 153.

International Association for the Study of Pain, *Classification of chronic pain: descriptions of chronic pain syndromes and definitions of pain terms*, 2nd ed. IASP Press, Seattle, 1994.

International Headache Society, *Classification and diagnostic criteria for headache disorders, cranial neuralgias and facial pain*, Cephalalgia, 1988, 8 (Suppl. 7):1 – 96.

Iversen H.K., Langemark M., Andersson P.G., Hansen P.E., Olesen J., *Clinical characteristics of migraine and episodic tension-type headache in relation to old and new diagnostic criteria*, Headache, 1990, 30 : 514 – 519.

Leone M., Filippini G., D'Amico D., Farinotti M., Bussone G., *Assessment of International Headache Society diagnostic criteria: a reliability study*, Cephalalgia, 1994, 14 : 280 – 284.

Leone M., D'Amico D., Moschiano F., Farinotti M., Filippini G., Bussone G., *Possible identification of cervicogenic headache among patients with migraine: an analysis of 374 headaches*, Headache, 1995, 35 : 461 – 464.

Manzoni G.C., Granella F., Schianchi C., Zanferrari C., *Nosographic and taxonomic problems about the primary headaches after the IASP and IHS classifications*, Ital. J. Neurol. Sci., 1992, 13 : 17.

Manzoni G.C., Zanferrari C., Sandrini G. et al., *Inability to classify all the chronic daily headache subtypes by IHS criteria*, Cephalalgia, 1993, 13 (Suppl. 13):12.

Manzoni G.C., Granella F., Sandrini G., Cavallini A., Zanferrari C., Nappi G., *Classification of chronic daily headache by International Headache Society criteria: limits and new proposals*, Cephalalgia, 1995, 15 : 37 – 43.

Mathew N.T., Stubits E., Nigam M.P., *Transformation of episodic migraine into daily headache: analysis of factors*, Headache, 1982, 22 : 66 – 68.

Messinger H.B., Spierings E.L.H., Vincent A.J.P., *Overlap of migraine and tension-type headache in the International Headache Society classification*, Cephalalgia, 1991, 11 : 233 – 237.

Michel P., Henry P., Letenneur L., Jogeix M., Corson A., Dartigues J.F., *Diagnostic screen for assessment of the IHS criteria for migraine by general practitioners*, Cephalalgia, 1993, 13 (Suppl. 12):54–59.

Mongini F., *Assessment of craniofacial pain and dysfunction. A multidisciplinary approach*, Cranio, 1990, 8 : 183–200.

Mongini F., *ATM e Muscolatura Cranio-cervico-faciale. Fisiopatologia e Terapia*, Utet, Torino, 1996.

Mongini F., Rocca R., Gioria A., Carpignano V., Ferla E., *Assessment of systemic factors and personality characteristic in tension-type headache and other types of facial pain*, in: Olesen J. (ed.), *Tension-type headache: classification, mechanisms and treatment*, Raven Press, New York, 1993, 231–236.

Mongini F., Defilippi N., Negro C., *Chronic daily headache. A clinical and psychological profile before and after treatment*, Headache, 1997, 37 : 83–87.

Mortimer M.J., Kay J., Jaron A., *Childhood migraine in general practice: clinical features and characteristics*, Cephalalgia, 1992, 12 : 238–243.

Nappi G., Micieli G., Cavallini A., Zanferrari C., Sandrini G., Manzoni G.C., *Accompanying symptoms of cluster attacks: their relevance to the diagnostic criteria*, Cephalalgia, 1992, 12 : 165–168.

Olesen J., *The International Headache Society classification and diagnostic criteria are valid and extremely usefull*, Cephalalgia, 1996, 16 : 293–295.

Pfaffenrath V., Isler H., *Evaluation of the nosology of chronic tension-type headache*, Cephalalgia, 1993, 13 (Suppl. 12):60–62.

Raieli V., Raimondo D., Cammalleri R., Camarda R., *Migraine headaches in adolescents: a student population-based study in Montreale*, Cephalalgia, 1995, 15 : 5–12.

Sanin L.C., Mathew N.T., Bellmeyer L.R., Ali S., *The International Headache Society (IHS) headache classification as applied to a headache clinic population*, Cephalalgia, 1994, 14 : 443–446.

Schiffman E., Haley D., Baker C., Lindgren B., *Diagnostic criteria for screening headache patients for temporomandibular disorders*, Headache, 1995, 35 : 121–124.

Seshia S.S., Wolstein J.R., Adams C., Booth F.A., Reggin J.D., *International headache society criteria and childhood headache*, Dev. Med. Child. Neurol., 1994, 36 : 419–428.

Sjaastad O., Saunte C., Hovdal H., Breivik H., Gronbaeck E., *"Cervicogenic" headache: an hypothesis*, Cephalalgia, 1983, 3 : 249–256.

Sjaastad O., Fredriksen T.A., Sand T., *The localisation of the initial pain attack. A comparison between classic migraine and cervicogenic headache*, Funct. Neurol., 1989, 4 : 73–78.

Sjaastad O., Fredriksen T.A., Plaffenrrath V., *Cervicogenic headache: diagnostic criteria*, Headache, 1990, 30 : 725–726.

Silberstein S.D., *Tension-type and chronic daily headache*, Neurology, 1993, 43 : 1644–1649.

Silberstein S.D., Lipton R.B., Solomon S., Mathew N.T., *Classification of daily and near-daily headaches: proposed revisions to the IHS criteria*, Headache, 1994, 34 : 1–7.

Solomon S., Lipton R.B., Newman L.C., *Evaluation of chronic daily headache comparison to criteria for chronic tension-type headache*, Cephalalgia, 1992 a, 12 : 365–368.

Solomon S., Lipton R.B., Newman L.C., *Clinical features of chronic daily headache*, Headache, 1992 b, 32 : 325–329.

Wilson P.R., *Taxonomy again?*, Clin. J. Pain., 1991, 7 : 171–174.

Wober-Bingol C., Wober C., Karwautz A., Vesely C., Wagner-Ennsgraber C., Amminger G.P., Zebenholzer K., Geldner J., Baischer W., Schuch B., *Diagnosis of headache in childhood and adolescence: a study in 437 patients*, Cephalalgia, 1995, 15 : 13–21.

World Health Organization, *International classification of diseases 10*, Geneva, World Health Organization, 1992.

2 Local Neurological Disorders as Etiological Factors

Anatomy and Physiology

Sensory information from the face, conjunctiva, oral cavity, craniofacial muscles, temporomandibular joint (TMJ), and dura mater is carried, to a great extent, by the trigeminal (V) nerve via its three branches. The "trigeminal-brain stem complex" consists of the primary trigeminal sensory nucleus in the pons and of the mesencephalic and spinal nuclei (Fig. 2.1).

The cell bodies of fibers carrying somatosensory information are located in the Gasserian ganglion. The fibers enter the brain stem through the anterolateral portion of the pons, maintaining a somatotopic distribution inside the nerve root (Leandri et al., 1997) (Fig. 2.2). These fibers end either in the principal sensory nucleus or in the spinal nucleus. Some fibers bifurcate and end in both nuclei. Tactile information is carried by large-diameter axons to the principal sensory nucleus and to the spinal nucleus and is processed differently according to its destination (Bae et al., 1994). In the principal sensory nucleus a complete representation of the ipsilateral half of the face and the oral cavity has been observed (Ro and Capra, 1994). Thermal and painful sensations are conveyed to the

spinal nucleus by thin myelinated and unmyelinated axons; this nucleus is divided into three portions: subnucleus oralis, interpolaris, and caudalis (Fig. 2.1). There is general agreement that the subnucleus caudalis serves as a major relay site for orofacial pain, although the more rostral subnuclei of the V may also contribute to this function (Dubner, 1985; Yokota, 1985; Sessle, 1987, 1990). Opiod agonists inhibit in the substantia gelatinosa of subnucleus oralis action potential evocation by peripheral stimuli (Grudt and Williams, 1994). At the same site, dihydroergotamine inhibits the effects of stimulation of the superior sagittal sinus of the cat (Hoskin et al., 1996).

In addition, nociceptive information to the subnucleus caudalis derives from visceral afferents of the glossopharingeus and vagus nerves (Hu et al., 1981; Sessle et al., 1986), from neck afferents (Sessle et al., 1986), and from dural vessels afferents (Davies and Dostrovsky, 1986; Strassman et al., 1988). Recent studies suggest that such central convergence may contribute to the spread and referral of pain frequently observed in many types of headache and craniofacial pain (Benoist et al., 1985; Sessle, 1987; Wall, 1989; Sessle et al. 1993 a).

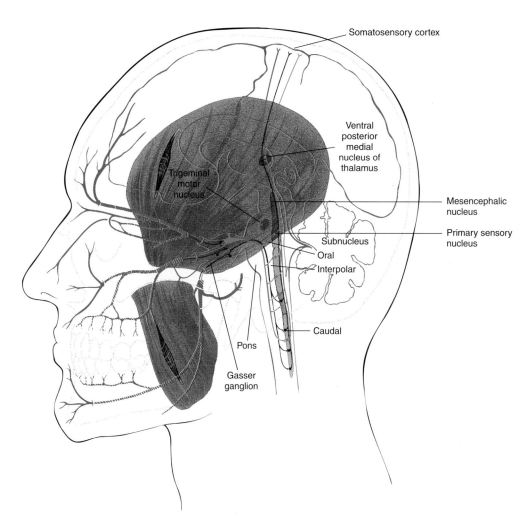

Fig. 2.**1 Afferents and efferents of the trigeminal sensitive complex.** Somatosensory information is shown in blue, thermal and painful information in red, proprioceptive information is in green

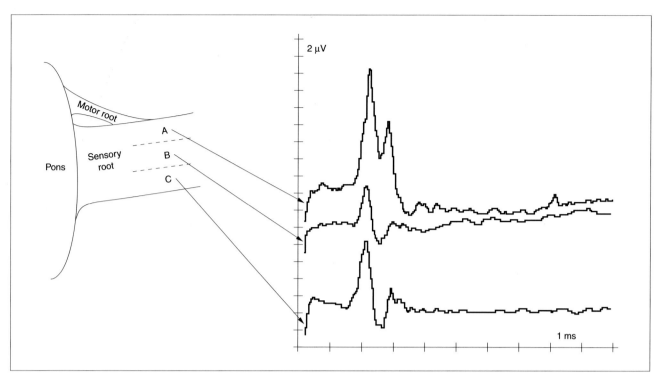

Fig. 2.2 Evoked potentials recorded in the trigeminal root with three pairs of coaxial electrodes after electrical stimulation of the supraorbital nerve. Potentials of higher amplitude were re-corded at the superior portion of the root (A): this demonstrates that the majority of the nerve fibers run in this portion. (From Leandri et al., 1997, with modifications)

Proprioceptive information is also conveyed to the V nucleus. The cell bodies of the proprioceptive sensory afferents are not located in the Gasserian ganglion but in the V mesencephalic nucleus, which is the only site of the central nervous system where primary sensory nervous cell bodies have been found (Dubner et al., 1978; Dubner, 1985).

From the trigeminal brain stem complex the sensory information may be conveyed to the ipsilateral and contralateral thalamus (ventral posterior medial nucleus) (Ro and Capra, 1994), and from the thalamus to the primary somatosensory cortex, where there is a complete representation of the contralateral hemiface and of the perioral region (Fig. 2.1). Some of this information may also be conveyed to brain stem reflex centers involved in autonomic and muscular reflex responses to noxious orofacial stimuli (Sessle, 1987, 1990).

Conduction Disorders

In the afferent fibers the action potential travels from peripheral receptors (in skin, mucosa, joints, muscle, or viscera) to the central nervous system (CNS), where the synaptic terminal is located. The speed of conduction depends on the size of the axon and on the presence and size of a sheath of myelin. The axial resistance to the propagation of the action potential decreases in proportion to the square of the axon diameter. The myelin sheath of the Schwann cells further increases the size and also functions as an insulating material: this greatly increases the speed of action potential (Koester, 1991). The myelin sheath is interrupted every 1 to 2 mm by the "nodes of Ranvier," which contain a large number of sodium channels. Thus the action potential spreads quite rapidly along the internodal areas and slows down at the nodes, hence the definition of "saltatory" conduction (Fig. 2.3).

Alterations of conduction velocity may result from several events, such as stretching, compression, irritation, and infection of nerves. These may lead to segmental demyelination, that is, the loss of portions of the myelin sheath (Beaver et al., 1965; Kerr, 1967; Ludwin, 1981). In the demyelinated axons, sodium channels are dispersed and more numerous (Foster et al., 1980). Hence, the axon membrane may lose its refractory capacity and can become excitable by its own discharges, thus creating "ectopic impulses" traveling in both directions, orthodromically and antidromically (Rasminsky, 1978; Kocsis et al., 1982; Nordin et al., 1984) (Fig. 2.4). Moreover, the loss of insulation of the myelin sheath could lead to "ephaptic transmission," that is to abnormal "cross talk" between neighboring axons (Rasminsky, 1978; Selzer and Devor, 1979; Rasminsky, 1980; Devor and Wall, 1990) (Fig. 2.4) and to an increase in sensitivity to the action of α-adrenergic agonists (Fields and Rowbotham, 1993).

Electrogenic ectopic activity may also occur in the dorsal ganglion roots. In fact, it has been observed that several sensory ganglion cells respond to mechanical and chemical stimulation (Devor et al., 1991; Devor, 1994). Likewise, the existence of a reciprocal cross excitation between ganglion cells has been demonstrated. Repeated excitation of ganglion cells leads to depolarization of neighboring neurons, thus enhancing their probability of responding to subliminal stimulations (Utzschneider et al., 1992). Mechanical sensitivity is usually latent but may be enhanced and become a significant factor for pain in presence of discal herniations or other lesions producing compressive forces on the ganglion (Devor, 1994).

It has been suggested that ectopic impulse generation and ephaptic transmission may be the basis of paresthesias and dysesthesias in the trigeminal nerve system (see review by Sessle, 1987; Cooper and Sessle, 1992; Devor, 1994).

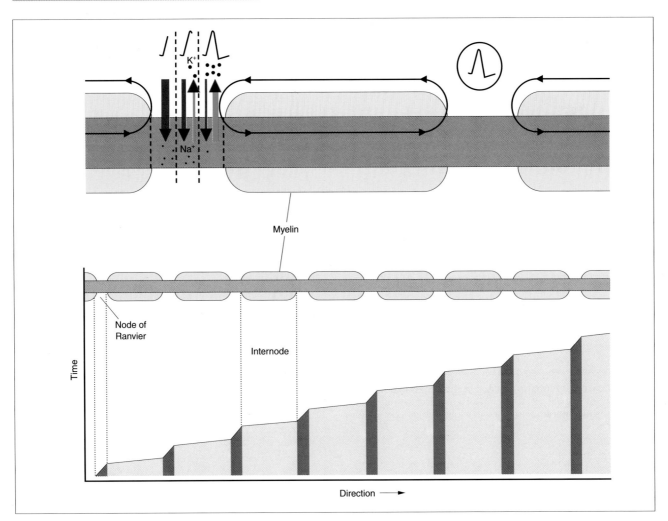

Fig. 2.**3**   The mechanisms of "saltatory conduction" of the action potential along the nerve fiber. Further explanation is given in the text

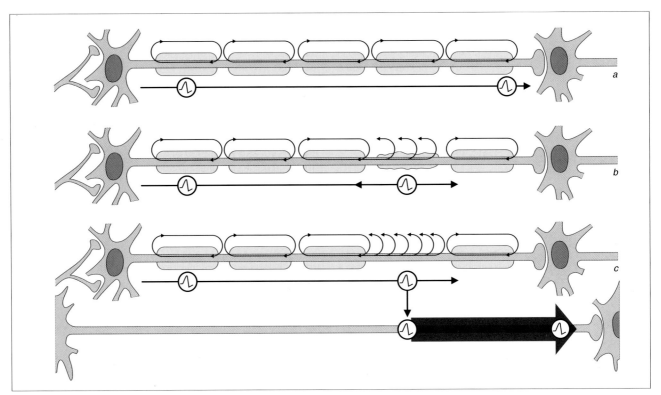

Fig. 2.**4**   **a** Normal conduction of action potential. **b** Delayed conduction and formation of antidromic potentials as a consequence of a segmental demyelination. **c** Ephaptic transmission between a myelinated fiber and an unmyelinated one. (From Cooper and Sessle, 1992, with modifications)

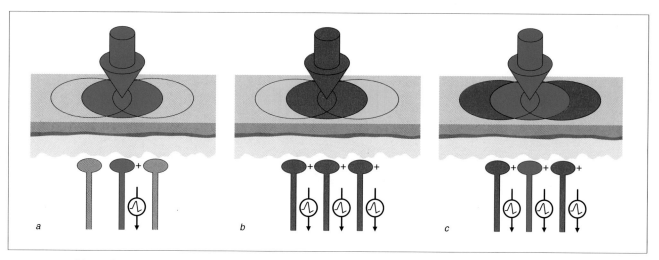

Fig. 2.5 Possible pathogenetic mechanism of trigeminal neuralgia. The diagram shows three wide dynamic range (WDR) neurons with partially superimposed receptive fields. In (**a**), a low threshold stimulus applied at the centre of the receptive field of a neuron causes excitation of this neuron alone and not of the other two. In (**b**), an intense and harmful stimulus applied at the same point causes excitation of all three neurons. In (**c**), as a consequence of the expansion of the low-threshold reception field, a low-threshold stimulus causes excitation of all three neurons, simulating the effect produced in normal conditions by harmful stimuli. (From Dubner et al., 1987, with modifications)

Ephaptic transmission could be one mechanism underlying trigeminal neuralgia (Fromm and Sessle, 1991), a disorder characterized by brief paroxysms of excruciating pain, usually along the second and/or third trigeminal branch. Such fits of pain are most often elicited by light touch stimuli (see Chapter 20). Different mechanisms have been suggested to explain trigeminal pain. According to Dubner (1991) altered nociceptive afferents could be activated by intact mechanoreceptive fields. Moreover, it has been shown that light tough stimuli can activate, as well as low-threshold mechanoceptors, also a population of A-delta and C fiber nociceptors. Normally, such activation is insufficient for the sensation of pain (Van Hees and Gybels, 1981; Adriansen et al., 1983; Cooper, 1993). However, thanks either to a development of ectopic foci or to changes at central termination level, they could acquire the capability of triggering dysesthesic or painful events (Cooper and Sessle, 1992). Also, alterations in the receptive field organization of wide dynamic range (WDR) neurons could be

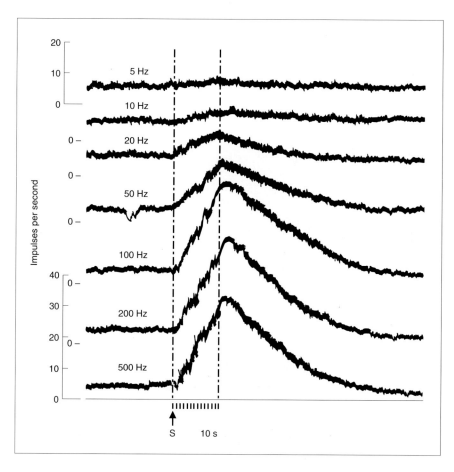

Fig. 2.6 Spontaneous activity recorded from a neuron of a spinal sensory ganglion. Tetanic stimulation (arrow) for ten seconds of axons of neighboring neurons, but not of the recorded neuron itself, triggers an increase in autonomous firing well outlasting the stimulus itself. (From Rappaport and Devor 1994, with modifications)

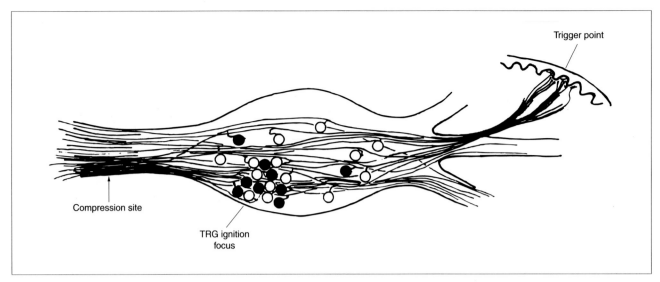

Fig. 2.**7** **The "trigeminal ganglion ignition hypothesis" according to Rappaport and Devor.** A small lesion along the trigeminal root (arrow) promotes ectopic firing in a focal group of trigeminal ganglion neurons (solid circles). When the activity is supplemented by activity of other neighboring neurons (open circles) evoked by tactile stimulation of peripheral trigger points, the spontaneous electrogenic activity may be enhanced (see Fig. 2.**6**)

involved with expansion of their touch receptive field. As a consequence, touch stimuli would produce activity of WDR neurons mimicking the activity normally generated by noxious stimuli (Dubner et al., 1987; Sessle, 1987, 1991) (Fig. 2.**5**).

Recently, Rappaport and Devor (1994) have proposed the hypothesis of the "trigeminal ganglion ignition." This hypothesis is based on the above-mentioned observation of a spontaneous electrogenetic activity of some ganglion neurons. A lesion of the trigeminal root could increase the intrinsic excitability of these neurons and a sequence of discharge would follow that persists after stimulus application ("afterdischarge"). A similar mechanism has been demonstrated experimentally in the dorsal ganglions (Devor and Wall, 1990) (Figs 2.**6**, 2.**7**) and could be also present in the trigeminal ganglion and produce neuralgic pain. Antidromic firing, if it occurs, should produce neurogenic vasodilation (Devor, 1994). Mongini et al. (1990) report a case of a patient with trigeminal

neuralgia in which the neuralgic fit led to local hyperthermia in the pain area, presumably consequent on neurogenic inflammation (Fig. 2.**8**). Other authors, however, are in favor of a central origin of the neuralgic paroxysmal pain that would be produced by an epileptogenetic focus in the brain stem (Fromm et al., 1981; Fromm and Sessle, 1991; Fromm, 1992; Pagni, 1993; Canavero et al., 1995). Indeed, antiepileptic drugs, such as carbamezapine, are also efficacious against trigeminal neuralgia.

A paroxysmal or continuous trigeminal pain has indeed been observed both in patients with brain stem lesions and consequent damage to the trigeminal intraxial pathways, and in those with extraxial pathologies of the nerve, of the ganglion or of the trigeminal root (Coratti et al., 1993, Mongini, unpublished observations) (Figs 2.**9**, 2.**10**).

Paroxysmal or continuous trigeminal pain may be also observed in presence of a "neurovascular conflict" (Janetta, 1967,

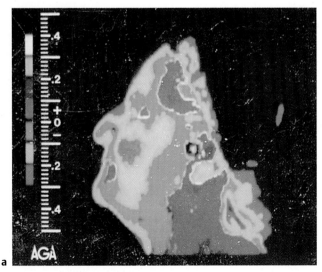

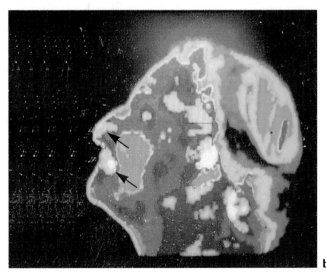

Fig. 2.**8** **Female patient suffering from neuralgia of the second and third branches of the trigeminal nerve.** In basal conditions, thermography findings are normal (**a**). Two marked hyperthermic areas appear at the base of the nose and lip corner (arrows) during the neuralgic fit (**b**). These areas roughtly correspond to trigger points. This phenomenon may be determined by a mechanism of neurogenic vasodilation

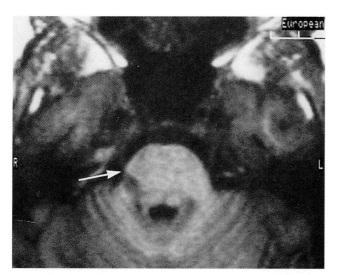

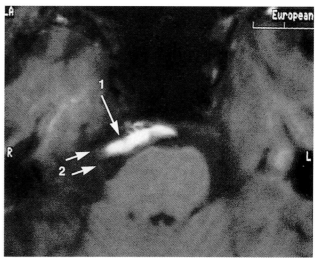

Fig. 2.**9** **Magnetic resonance of a patient with multiple sclerosis and trigeminal neuralgia.** Note a plaque of demyelinization (arrow) in the lateral right portion of the pons in correspondence to the entrance of the trigeminal nerve root. (From Cruccu et al. *Journal of Neurology, Neurosurgery and Psychiatry,* 1990, 53: 1034–1042, with permission)

Fig. 2.**11** **Patient with trigeminal neuralgia.** Magnetic resonance shows a dilated and tortuous basal artery (1) which compresses and dislocates the trigeminal nerve (2) in proximity to its entrance into the pons. (From Cruccu et al., *Journal of Neurology, Neurosurgery and Psychiatry,* 1990, 53: 1034–1042, with permission)

1977; Pagni, 1982). In this situation, the root of the nerve is compressed and irritated by an ectasic or tortuous artery (Fig. 2.**11**).

Neurogenic Inflammation

Neurogenic inflammation, that is, inflammatory response with vasodilatation and plasma extravasation, following on antidromic electrical, chemical or mechanical stimulation of sensory nerves, has long been demonstrated (Bayliss, 1901, 1902; Hinsey and Gasser, 1930; Jancso et al., 1967; Saria et al., 1983; Lundberg et al., 1984; Szolcsànyi, 1988) in different areas of the body. A peripheral injury releases chemical mediators, such as bradikinin, prostaglandin, serotonin and K^+, which, in turn, activate the nociceptors. As a result of antidromic excitation, substance P and other tachykinins, such as calcitonin gene related peptide (CGRP), are released by the peripheral sensory axons with consequent vasodilation (Lembeck and Gamse 1982; Holzer, 1988; Micevych and Kruger, 1992). Moreover, substance P leads to release of histamine from mast cells (Hagermark et al., 1978; Barnes et al., 1986; Ebertz et al., 1987; Eschenfelder et al., 1995; Benrath et al., 1995). Histamine further activates the nociceptors. Thus, substance P is both the main mediator of neurogenic inflammation and a neurotransmitter within primary sensory neurons (Lembeck, 1953) (Fig. 2.**12**).

Indeed, neurogenic inflammation has been demonstrated almost exclusively in tissues containing substance P-releasing nerve fibers innervating blood vessels, and can be attenuated by substance P-releasing nerve fibers innervating blood vessels, and can be attenuated by substance P receptor blockers (Rosell et al., 1981) or drugs inhibiting substance P release (Lembeck et al., 1981, 1982; Lembeck and Donnerer, 1985). Substance P, neurokinin A and CGRP are also released by peripheral trigeminal endings of the pial and dural vessels, with consequent vasodilation and plasma extravasation (Markowitz et al., 1987; Moskowitz et al., 1983, 1989; Uddman and Edvinsson, 1989; Jansen et al., 1991; Beattie et al., 1993; Escott et al., 1995; Williamson et al., 1997) (Fig 2.**13**). Markowitz et al. (1987) caused vasodilation and release of plasma proteins from blood vessels of the dura mater in adult rats subjected to electrical stimulation of the trigeminal ganglion or to intravenous injection of capsaicin (Fig. 2.**14**). These effects were not found in rats lacking C fibers: this suggests that neurogenic inflammation is mediated by these fibers also

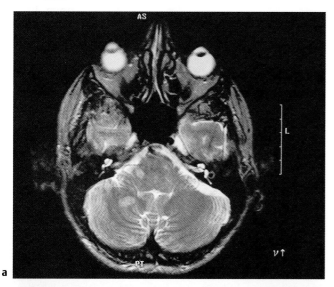

a

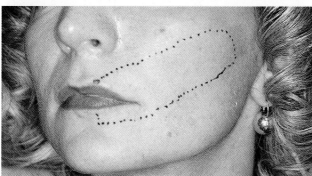

b

Fig. 2.**10** **Another case of multiple sclerosis in a young woman.** **a** Magnetic resonance shows plaques of demyelinization in the pons. **b** The patient had a constant burning pain in the territory of the second and third trigeminal branches

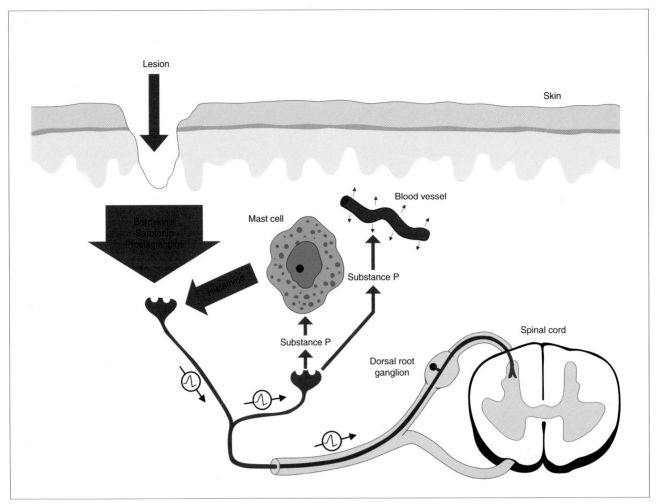

Fig. 2.12   The mechanisms of neurogenic inflammation. Stimulation of the nociceptors due to the release of chemical mediators causes substance P to be released from the peripheral sensitive endings, via antidromic excitation. Substance P in turn causes histamine to be released by the mastocytes and the blood vessels to dilate. (From Lembech and Gamse, 1982, with modifications)

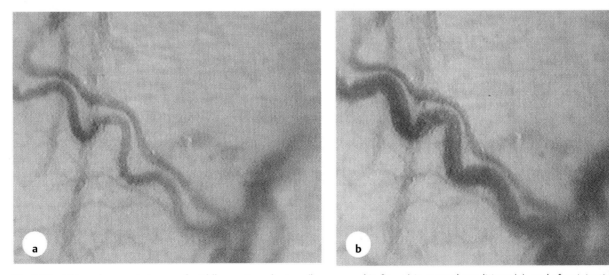

Fig. 2.13   Videomicroscopic image of middle meningeal artery (lower vessel in figure) in normal conditions (**a**), and after injection of substance P (**b**). (From Williamson et al., 1997, with permission)

in the dura mater. The stimulation of the trigeminal ganglion increases the substance P and CGRP in the venous intracranial circulation but not in the peripheral circulation: this confirms that such peptide release is a local phenomenon (Goadsby et al., 1988). Moreover, plasma extravasation consequent on elec-trical stimulation of the trigeminal ganglion can be suppressed by agonists of serotonin receptors 5-HT 1 d, which are active against migraine (Moskowitz, 1992) (see Chapter 5), and by neurokinin 1 receptor antagonists (Shepheard et al., 1993). In man, vasodilation has been observed in the facial area after le-

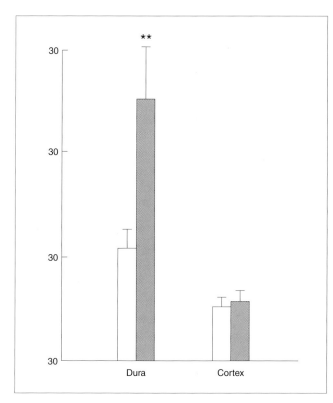

Fig. 2.**14** Unilateral electric stimulation of the trigeminal ganglion in the rat causes extravasation in the dura mater of albumin previously injected to a greater extent (solid bars) than in control animals (open bars). The phenomenon is not observed in the cerebral cortex because of the cerebrovascular barrier. ★★ = P < 0.01. (From Markowitz et al., 1987, with modifications)

sions of the trigeminal ganglion (Sweet and Wepsic, 1974; Drummond et al., 1983) or after thermal or electric stimulation (Goadsby et al., 1988).

Moskowitz (1984, 1991) suggests that a similar mechanism might underlie some types of headache in which a vasomotor component is present. This author advances the hypothesis that some form of "insult" to the blood vessels or to the surrounding cerebral tissue leads to the release of the chemical mediators mentioned above. These would cause orthodromic impulses that would convey the perception of pain to the brain stem and thence to the higher centers, whereas a mechanism of antidromic conduction would, as stated above, determine release of substance P and of other mediators (and, in particular, of CGRP) in the vessel walls, not only at the depolarization site but also in adjacent areas, with consequent vasodilation. Furthermore, substance P provokes the synthesis of thromboxanes by the macrophages and the release of histamine by the mastocytes. Local inflammation would then develop.

Evidence has also been produced that nitric oxide (NO) may actively participate in these peripheral mechanisms of pain modulation (Haley et al., 1992; Kitto et al., 1992; Meller et al., 1992, 1993; Babbedge et al., 1993; Radhakrishnan and Henry, 1993; Sorkin, 1993; Benrath et al., 1995). NO is an unstable molecule that plays an important role as a mediator of molecular and cellular processes in the peripheral tissues and in the CNS. In particular, it was shown that NO plays a protective role against cerebral ischemia, while excessive production of NO in the neurons facilitates or mediates neurotoxicity phenomena (see below) (Dalkara and Moskowitz, 1994; Dal-

kara et al., 1994). Systemic administration of L-arginine analogues (NO-synthetase inhibitors) produces an antinociceptive activity against neuropathic pain (Meller et al., 1922) and chemically induced pain (Dalkara and Moskowitz, 1994; Dalkara et al., 1994).

Several authors (Olesen, 1993; Olesen et al., 1993, 1995; Thomsen et al., 1993; Iversen and Olesen, 1994) suggest that NO also plays an important role in headache of migraine type. These authors have observed that, whereas the venous infusion of nitroglycerin causes, in the short term, in all subjects, a pulsating headache with dilation of intracranial and extracranial arteries, in the long term it produces headache with migraine characteristics only in migraine patients. They hypothesize that this is due to the fact that NO, derived from the nitroglycerin, activates the trigeminal system.

Hyperalgesia, Referred Pain and Neuron Plasticity

Intense mechanical or thermal stimuli produce an area of "primary hyperalgesia." Hyperalgesia is defined as "a leftward shift of the stimulus – response function that relates magnitude of pain to stimulus intensity" (Manning et al., 1991; Meyer et al., 1994; Dalkara and Moskowitz, 1994; Dalkara et al., 1994) (Fig. 2.**15**). Primary hyperalgesia is consequent on "sensitization" of peripheral nociceptors (Meyer and Campbell, 1981 a, b; LaMotte et al., 1982; Simone et al., 1989 a, b; Woolf, 1991). "Sensitization" is described as "a leftward shift of the stimulus – response function that relates magnitude of the neural response to stimulus intensity" (Kahn et al., 1992; Meyer et al., 1994) (Fig. 2.**15**). However, while the peripheral sensitization can explain the "primary hyperalgesia" at the esite of tissue damage, it does not readily explain the "secondary hyperalgesia" of the surrounding undamaged tissues.

According to the majority of the authors, this secondary hyperalgesia implies a lower pain threshold for mechanical stimuli but *not* for thermal stimuli (LaMotte et al., 1983; LaMotte, 1984; Raja et al., 1984; Treede et al., 1992) (Fig. 2.**16**). More recently, a secondary hyperalgesia to heat stimuli after burn injury in man was also described (Pedersen and Kehlet, 1998). At any rate, accumulatory evidence suggests that central neuronal changes involving "unmasking" of convergent afferent inputs and perhaps "excitoxicity" (see below) may contribute to some forms of hyperalgesia (Woolf, 1983, 1991; Sessle, 1991; Dubner, 1991; Kilo et al., 1994; Sang et al., 1996).

Innocuous mechanical stimuli activate large-diameter myelinated fibers that never evoke painful sensations under normal circumstances. Painful sensations are carried by small-diameter, thin myelinated A delta fibers or unmyelinated C fibers. To explain the selective secondary hyperalgesia to normally innocuous mechanical stimulation, it has been suggested that dorsal horn processing could be initiated by the persistent peripheral input and then maintained by the same input or by mechanisms within the spinal horn itself (Raja et al., 1984; Woolf, 1991). A peripheral injury could provoke an alteration to the central nervous system, so that signals from low-threshold mechanoreceptors might ultimately be misinterpreted as coming from nociceptors (Fig. 2.**17**) (Woolf, 1991, 1994). Alternatively, an intense and prolonged stimulation of peripheral nociceptors may lead to a selective modulation of the central nociceptors (central pain-signaling neurons) such that the input from low-threshold receptors is augmented. Such selective sensitization may be due to an increase of the synaptic efficacy of the low-threshold mechanoreceptors onto the central nociceptors. Thus, light tactile

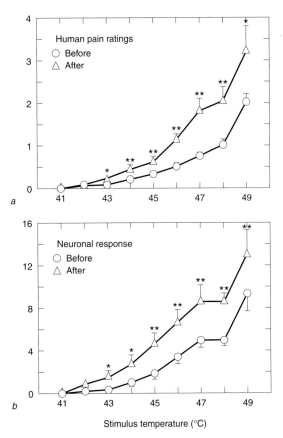

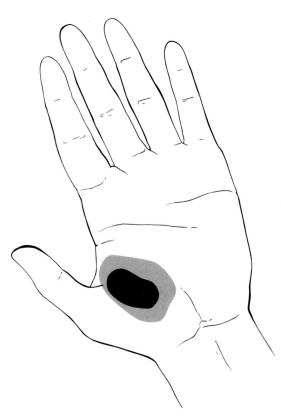

Fig. 2.**15** Intradermal injection of bradikinin produces thermal hyperalgesia in man and sensitization in the experimental animal. **a** After bradikinin injection in man there is an increase of pain ratings to heat stimuli presented to the volar forearm (hyperalgesia). (From Manning et al., 1991, with modifications). **b** In the experimental animal after bradikinin injection an increase of the neuronal response to heat stimuli is observed (sensitization). (From Khan et al., 1992, with modifications). ** = P < 0.01

Fig. 2.**16** Area of primary hyperalgesia (to mechanical and heat stimuli) (red), and of secondary hyperalgesia (to mechanical stimuli only) (pink) on the palm of the hand consequent on painful heat stimulation at the points indicated in black. (From Raja et al., 1984, with modifications)

stimuli that activate low-threshold mechanoreceptors produce action potentials that now gain enhanced access to the central nociceptors with consequent perception of pain (Meyer et al., 1994) (Fig. 2.**18**).

Dubner (1991, 1993), Dubner and Ruda (1992), Torebjörk et al. (1992), and Torebjörk (1993) suggest that the increased peripheral input after a peripheral injury could lead to an increased depolarization of dorsal horn receptors for glutamate and N-methyl-D-aspartate (NMDA), which are the excitatory amino acids (EEA) mediating the more rapid excitatory events in nociceptive neurons. Their depolarizing action is facilitated by the release of neuropeptides (substance P, dynorphin, CGRP). The excitation of the cells and the prolonged depolarization would produce an excessive accumulation of excitatory amino acids, with a consequent neuronal dysfunction due to neurotoxicity (or "excitotoxicity"): this, in turn, could result in neuron hyperexcitability with progressive increase of the firing rate of the dorsal horn neurons, a phenomenon known as "wind-up," and formation of more expanded receptive fields (Fig. 2.**19**). The "wind-up" is blocked by administration of ketamine, and NMDA receptor antagonist (Davies and Lodge, 1987; Dickenson and Sullivan, 1987; Warncke et al., 1997). This would explain the results of a preliminary study that demonstrated that ketamine may induce a reduction of neuropathic peripheral and central pain (Backonja et al., 1994).

Moreover, it has been shown that repetitive peripheral input on the glutamate receptors leads to a cascade of events that stimulates in the nucleus of the dorsal horn neurons the expression of protooncogenes ("early genes") c-*fos* and c-*jun* (Hunt et al., 1987; Menetrey et al., 1989; Bullit, 1990; Wisden et al., 1990; Zimmermann and Herdegen, 1994; Dubner and Basbaum, 1994; Carli and Zimmermann, 1996) (Fig. 2.**20**). Expression of fos-like immunoreactivity consequent on painful stimulations was also detected in the medullary dorsal horn and the first segment of the spinal cord (Iwata et al., 1998), in the trigeminal spinal nucleus, and in the hippocampal section (Wisden et al., 1990; Aloisi et al., 1997) (Fig. 2.**21**). These genes lead to transcription of a RNA messenger that is released in the cytoplasm and induces the production of protein molecules containing sequences of active peptides. This mechanism has long-term effects (hours, days) and may be prevented by systemic or spinal morphine injections (Tölle et al., 1990; Abram and Yaksh, 1993).

Nitrous oxide is also probably involved in these mechanism. Repetitive stimulation of NMDA receptors leads to opening of the calcium channels and to consequent production of NO-synthetase and, eventually, NO. NO would, in turn, potentiate the synaptic transmission in the dorsal horn through protooncogene production, thus leading to neuronal toxicity (Meller et al., 1993). In addition, NO diffuses in the

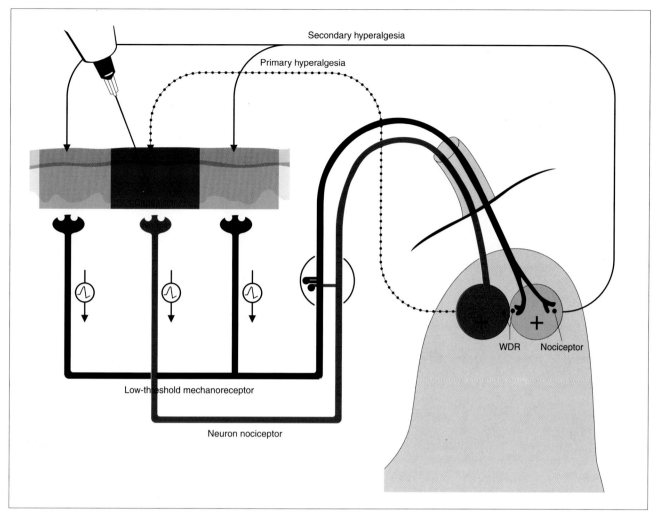

Fig. 2.17 Primary and secondary hyperalgesia mechanisms according to Wolf (1991). A peripheral insult (for example, injection of capsaicin) would cause the increase in excitability of "wide dynamic range" neurons (WDR) and nociceptors at the dorsal norm of the spinal cord. In this way, signals from the nociceptive neurons would cause primary hyperalgesia, whereas those from low threshold mechanoceptive neurons would be falsely interpreted as though they were from nociceptors, and would cause secondary hyperalgesia

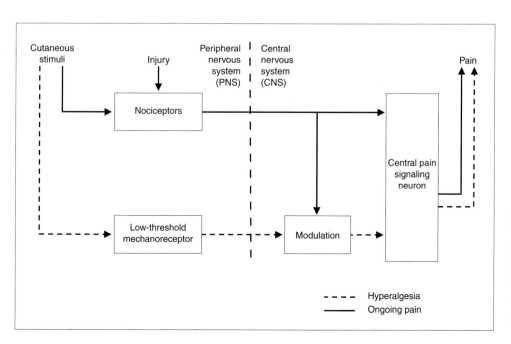

Fig. 2.18 An alternative model of secondary hyperalgesia to mechanical stimuli. A peripheral injury promotes sensitization of the central nociceptors and consequent increase of their response to input from low-threshold mechanoceptors. (From Meyer et al., 1994, with modifications)

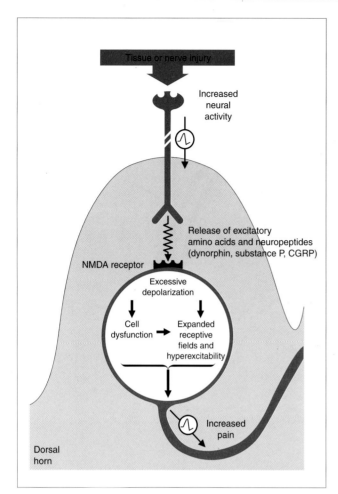

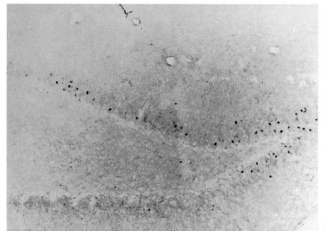

Fig. 2.**19   Possible chain of events in the dorsal horm of the spinal cord consequent on a peripheral tissue and nerve injury.** The increase in neuron activity causes the release of excitatory amino acids and neuropeptides with consequent increased depolarization of NMDA receptors. The excitation and increased depolarization would cause a chain of events with consequent increase in pain. (From Dubner, 1991, with modifications)

Fig. 2.**21**   Expression of Fos-like immunoreactivity in the dorsal hippocampus of the rat (**a**) before and (**b**) after subcutaneous formalin injection. (From Aloisi et al., 1997, with permission)

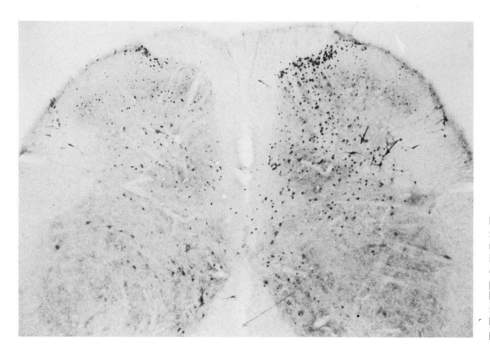

Fig. 2.**20   Photomicrograph showing Fos-protein like immunoreactivity produced by formalin injection into the right hind paw of the rat.** The immunoreactivity is particularly evident in the medial half of the ipsilateral superficial dorsal horn (laminae I and II). (From Dubner and Basbaum, 1994, with permission)

presynaptic neuron, modulating its excitability (thus acting as a "retrograde transmitter") (Baringa, 1991) (Fig. 2.**22**).

Another possibility is that usually inexcitable afferent fibers are modified by injury and become sensitive to low-intensity mechanical stimuli ("unmasking"). Such "silent" afferents have indeed been demonstrated in the skin and joints (Mayer et al., 1984; Schaible and Schmidt, 1988; Schmidt, 1993).

These concepts implicate a centrally based process, so-called "functional plasticity" or "central sensitization," as a main factor leading to the development of prolonged pain, but peripheral mechanisms related to sensitization may be involved, as noted above.

That hyperalgesia and referred pain may not be explained only by convergence mechanisms, but are partly due to CNS changes, is suggested by the fact that it can spread to regions that do not share the same dermatomes with the triggering lesion (Lewis, 1942; Livingston, 1943, quoted by Coderre et al., 1993).

An elegant experimental demonstration of this plasticity and central sensitization was obtained by injecting mustard essence into the masseter (Hu et al., 1992) and lingual muscles (Sessle et al., 1993 b); in the nociceptors of the trigeminal nucleus this caused an expansion of their cutaneous reception area to mechanical stimuli as well as an increase in their spontaneous activity and their response to electrical stimuli. More recently, Torneck et al. (1996) found neuroplastic changes of

low-threshold mechanoreceptors in the trigeminal subnucleus oralis consequent on tooth-pulp inflammation.

Neuroplastic changes were also observed in the trigeminal system after deafferentiation. "Deafferentation" refers to the loss of sensory afferent fibres in a given region of the body. Following deafferentation, anatomic and functional changes have been observed in the spinal cord (Devor and Wall, 1981 a, b; Wall et al., 1982; Woolf, 1985; Wall, 1989; Devor, 1994) that may account for the painful phenomenon known as "phantom limb." In the trigeminal system, anatomic and functional alterations in the V brain stem sensory complex have been reported following tooth-pulp deafferentation in adult cats (Sessle, 1985, 1987; Hu et al., 1986). In particular, alterations in the somatotopic distribution of the sensory cells were observed, with a statistically significant increase of neurons with an extensive mechanoreceptive field (Fig. 2.**23**), together

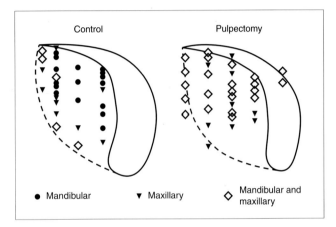

Fig. 2.**23** Neurons of the trigeminal sensitive nucleus in the adult cat with afferents of the second or third branch of the trigeminal nerve, or of both, before and after experimental pulpotomy. After pulpotomy the number of neurons with afferents from two branches increased markedly. (From Sessle, 1985, with modifications)

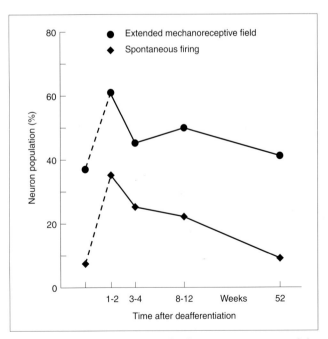

Fig. 2.**24** **Effects of experimental pulpotomy on neurons of the trigeminal oral nucleus in the adult cat.** After pulpotomy there is a marked increase in neurons with extended receptive field and with spontaneous activity. This phenomenon tends to regress progressively over time. (From Sessle, 1987, with modifications)

Fig. 2.**22** **Interactive mechanisms consequent on NMDA receptor activation and nitric oxide (NO) production.** (NOS, NO-syntetase; glu, glutamate; SP, substance P; CGRP, calcitonin gene-related peptide; CaM, calmodulin). (From Meller and Gebart, 1993, with modifications)

with signs of increased neuronal excitability (Fig. 2.**24**). It has been suggested that such alterations might contribute to the development of chronic facial pain (Sessle, 1985), although most of these changes have not yet been documented in nociceptive V brain stem neurons.

Sympathetically Maintained Pain

While nociceptor activation induces an increase of sympathetic discharge, in normal conditions sympathetic activity has no influence on nociceptor activity. However, this may occur in certain pathological conditions in which a painful condition is evoked or sustained by the activity of the sympathetic endings, or by catecholamines circulating in the body region involved. This situation is referred to as "sympathetically maintained pain" (SMP) (Roberts, 1986). SMP can be manifest in pain that arises from acute herpes zoster, soft-tissue trauma, nerve injury, metabolic neuropathies, and other conditions (Meyer et al., 1994).

SMP may be associated with other painful syndromes described as "reflex sympathetic dystrophy" and "causalgia." The term reflex sympathetic dystrophy is controversial, because not all cases defined as such seem to have sympathetically maintained pain, and not all are dystrophic (International Association for the Study of Pain, 1994). Causalgia refers to "a syndrome of sustained burning pain, allodynia and hyperpathia after a traumatic nerve lesion, often combined with vasomotor and sudomotor dysfunction and later trophic changes" (International Association for the Study of Pain, 1994). In any case, according to the International Association for the Study of Pain, reference should be made to the "complex regional pain syndrome."

As mentioned, these syndromes normally follow a skin or nervous lesion consequent on trauma. Typically, both the anaesthetic blocking of the sympathetic ganglion (Hannington-Kiff, 1974; Loh and Nathan, 1978; Bonica et al. 1979; Casale et al., 1991) and the regional administration of guanetidine, which presumably cause of depletion of norepinephrine in the sympathetic nerve endings (Hannington-Kiff, 1974), and the intravenous administration of

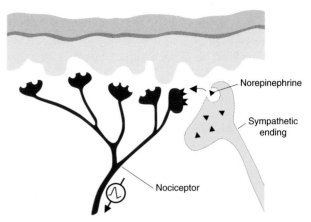

Fig. 2.**25** The activation of the α_1 receptors and peripheral nociceptors by the norepinephrine released by the sympathetic nerve endings might cause or increase painful sensations

phentolamine, an α-adrenergic antagonist (Raja et al., 1991) cause a remission of symptoms.

Numerous observations suggest that the adrenergic receptors participate in the phenomenon of sympathetically maintained pain (Ghostine et al., 1984; Treede et al., 1991; Raja et al., 1991, 1992). In particular, Davis et al. (1991) have shown that the pain is also attenuated by the local application of transdermal-releasing compresses of clonidine. Clonidine is an activator of adrenergic α_2 receptors, which are situated on the end of the efferent sympathetic fibers and which inhibit the release of norepinephrine: the analgesic effect of clonidine must thus be due to this inhibition. This hypothesis is also supported by the fact that the subsequent intradermal injection of phenylephrine (αagonist) causes the pain to reappear.

These observations have given rise to a theory (Raja et al., 1992; Campbell et al., 1992, 1993) according to which the sympathetic nervous system causes pain because norepinephrine would have aquired the ability to activate the nocireceptors (Fig. 2.**25**). Normally, these do not have α_1 receptors but would express them as a consequence of a pheno-

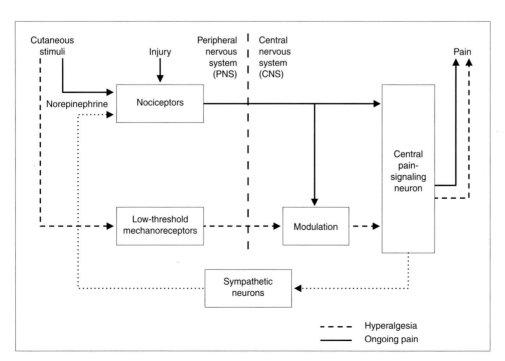

Fig. 2.**26** **Explanatory model of sympathetically mantained pain.** Hyperalgesia (see Figs. 2.**17** and 2.**18**) promotes adrenergic sensitivity of nociceptors and, as a consequence, their spontaneous activity in presence of norepinephrine released by sympathetic neurons. This spontaneous activity maintains the CNS in a sensitized state. (From Meyer et al., 1994, with modifications)

type mutation caused by a skin or nervous lesion. Alternatively, it is possible that these α_1 receptors are already present in the nociceptors but that in normal conditions they are inactive. In any case, in this situation, sympathetic efferent activity leads to a low-grade ongoing activity in the nociceptors. This activity may maintain the central nociceptive neurons in a sensitized state such that input from low-threshold mechanoreceptors produces pain (Meyer et al., 1994) (Fig. 2.**26**).

References

Abram S.E., Yaksh T.L., *Morphine, but not inhalation anesthesia, blocks post-injury facilitation. The role of preemptive suppression of afferent transmission.* Anesthesiology, 1993, 78 : 713 – 721.

Adriansen H., Gybels J., Handwerker H.O., et al., *Response properties of thin myelinated (A-delta) fibers in human skin nerves,* J. Neurophysiol., 1983, 49 : 111 – 112.

Aloisi A.M., Zimmermann T., Herbegent T., *Sex-dependent effects of formalin and restraint ou c-fos expression in the septum and hippocampus of the rat,* Neuroscience, 1997, 81 : 951 – 958.

Babbedge R.C., Wallace P., Gaffen Z.A., Hart S.L., Moore P.K., *LNG-nitro arginine p-nitroanilide (L-NAPNA) is anti-nociceptive in the mouse,* Neuroreport, 1993, 4 : 307 – 310.

Backonja M., Arndt G., Gombar A., Check B., Zimmermann M., *Response of chronic neuropathic pain syndromes to ketamine: a preliminary study,* Pain, 1994, 56 : 51 – 57.

Bae Y.C., Nakagawa S., Yoshida A., Nagase Y., Takemura M., Shigenaga Y., *Morphology and synaptic connections of slowly adapting periodontal afferent terminals in the trigeminal subnuclei principalis and oralis of the cat,* J. Comp. Neurol., 1994, 348 : 121 – 132.

Baringa M., *Is nitric oxide the 'retrograde messenger'?,* Science, 1991, 254 : 1296 – 1297.

Barnes P.J., Brown M.J., Dollery C.T., Fuller R.W., Heavey D.J., Ind P.W., *Histamine is released from skin by substance P but does not act as the final vasodilator in the axon reflex,* Br. J. Pharmacol., 1986, 88 : 741 – 774.

Bayliss W.M., *On the origin from the spinal cord of the vasodilator fibers of the hind limb, and on the nature of these fibers,* J. Physiol., 1901, 28 : 173 – 299.

Bayliss W.M., *Further researches on antidromic nerve-impulses,* J. Physiol., 1902, 28 : 276 – 299.

Beattie D.T., Stubbs C.M., Connor H.E., Feniuk W., *Neurokininduced changes in pial artery diameter in the anaesthetized guinea-pig.,* Br. J. Pharmacol., 1993, 108 : 146 – 149.

Beaver D.L., Moses H.L., Ganote C.E., *Electron microscopy of the trigeminal ganglion,* Arch. Pathol., 1965, 79 : 571 – 582.

Benoist J.M., Kayser V., Gautron M., Guilbaud G., *Changes in responses at ventrobasal thalamic neurons during carrageenin-induced inflammation in the rat,* in: Fields H.L., Dubner R., Cervero F. (eds.), *Advances in pain research and therapy,* Raven press, New York, 1985, 9 : 295 – 303.

Benrath J., Eschenfelder C., Zimmerman M., Gillardon F., *Calcitonin gene-related peptide, substance P and nitric oxide are involved in cutaneous inflammation following ultraviolet irradiation,* Eur. J. Pharmacol., 1995, 26, 293 : 87 – 96.

Bonica J.J., *Causalgia and other reflex sympathetic dystrophies,* in: Bonica J.J., Liebeskind J.C., Albe-Fessard D.G. (eds.), *Advances in Pain Research and Theraphy,* Raven press, New York, 1979, 3 : 141 – 166.

Bullitt E., *Expression of c-fos-like protein as a marker for neuronal activity following noxious stimulation in the rat,* J. Comp. Neurol., 1990, 296 : 517 – 530.

Campbell J.N., Meyer R.A., Davis K.D., Raja S.N., *Sympathetically maintained pain: a unifying hypothesis,* in: Willis W.D. (ed.), *Hyperalgesia,* Raven Press, New York, 1992, 141 – 149.

Campbell J.N., Raja S.N., Meyer R.A., *Pain and the sympathetic nervous system: connecting the loop,* in: Vecchiet L., Albe-Fessard, Lindblom U., Giamberardino M.A. (eds), *New trends in referred pain and hyperalgesia,* Elsevier, Amsterdam, 1993.

Canavero S., Bonicalzi V., Pagni C.A. (1995), Pain, 60 : 230 (letter).

Carli G., *Neurofisiologia del dolore,* in: Tiengo M., Benedetti C., (eds.), *Fisiopatologia e Terapia del Dolore,* Masson, Milano, 1996.

Carli G., Zimmermann M., (eds.), *Towards the Neurobiology of Chronic Pain. Progress in Brain Research,* Vol. 110, Elsevier, Amsterdam, 1996, 278.

Casale R., Glynn C.J., Scarzella G., *The role of the sympathetic skin response (SSR) in the investigation of the patient with sympathetically maintained pain,* in: Bond M.R., Charlton J.E., Woolf C.J. (eds.), *Proceedings of the VIth World Congress on Pain,* Elsevier, Amsterdam, 1991, 395 – 398.

Coderre T.J., Katz J., Vaccarino A.L., Melzack R., *Contribution of central neuroplasticity to pathological pain: review of clinical and experimental evidence,* Pain, 1993, 52 : 259 – 285.

Cooper B.Y., *Contributions of edema to the sensitization of high threshold mechanoreceptors of the goat palatal mucosa,* J. Neurophysiol., 1993.

Cooper B.Y., Sessle B.J., *Anatomy, physiology and pathophysiology of trigeminal system paresthesias and dysesthesias,* Oral Maxillof. Surg. Clin. North Am., 1992, 4 : 297 – 322.

Coratti P., Leardi M.G., Cruccu G., Ferracuti S., Manfredi M., *Neurogenic pain in the craniofacial region is provoked by primary afferent lesions (abs.),* 7 th World Congress on Pain, IASP, Seattle, 1993.

Cruccu G., Leandri M., Feliciani M., Manfredi M., *Idiopathic and symptomatic trigeminal pain,* Journal of Neurology, Neurosurgery and Psychiatry, 1990, 53 : 1034 – 1042.

Dalkara T., Moskowitz M.A., *The complex role of nitric oxide in the pathophysiology of focal cerebral ischemia,* Brain Pathol., 1994, 4 : 49 – 57.

Dalkara T., Yoshida T., Irikura K., Moskowitz M.A., *Dual role of nitric oxide in focal cerebral ischemia,* Neuropharmacology, 1994, 33 : 1447 – 1452.

Davies S.N., Lodge D., *Evidence for involvement of N-methyl-D-aspartate receptors in "wind-up" of class 2 neurones in the dorsal horn of the rat,* Brain Research, 1987, 424 : 402 – 406.

Davis K.D., Dostrovsky J.O., *Activation of trigeminal branstem nociceptive neurons by dural artery stimulation,* Pain, 1986, 25 : 395 – 401.

Davis K.D., Treede R.D., Raja S.N., Meyer R.A., Campbell J.N., *Topical application of clonidine relieves hyperalgesia in patients with sympathetically maintained pain,* Pain, 1991, 47 : 309 – 317.

Devor M., *The pathophysiology of damaged peripheral nerves,* in: Wall D., Melzack R. (eds.), *Textbook of pain,* 3 rd ed., Churchill Livingstone, 1994, 79 – 100.

Devor M., Wall P.D., *The effect of peripheral nerve injury on receptive fields of cells in the cat spinal cord,* J. Comp. Neurol., 1981 a, 199 : 679 – 684.

Devor M., Wall P.D., *Plasticity in the spinal cord sensory map following peripheral nerve injury in rats,* J. Neurosci., 1981 b, 148 : 679 – 684.

Devor M., Wall P.D., *Cross excitation among dorsal root ganglion neurons in nerve injured and intact rats,* J. Neurophysiol., 1990, 64 : 1733 – 1746.

Devor M., Basbaum A.I., Bennet G.J. et al., Group Report: *Mechanisms of neuropathic pain following peripheral injury,* in: Basbaum A.I., Besson J.M. (eds.), *Towards a new pharmacotherapy of pain,* Dahlem Konferenzen, Wiley, Chichester, 1991, 417 – 440.

Dickenson A.H., Sullivan A.F., *Evidence for a role of the NMDA receptor in the frequency dependent potentiation of deep rat dorsal horn nociceptive neurone following C-fibre stimulation,* Neuropharmacology, 1987, 26 : 1235 – 1238.

Drummond P.D., Gonski A., Lance J.W., *Facial flushing after thermocoagulation of the gasserian ganglion,* J. Neurol. Neurosurg. Psychiatry, 1983, 46 : 611 – 616.

Dubner R., *Recent advances in our undestanding of pain,* in Klineberg I., Sessle B. (eds.), *Oro-facial pain and neuromuscular dysfunction. Mechanisms and clinical correlates,* Pergamon press, Oxford, New York, 1985, 3 – 19.

Dubner R., *Neuronal plasticity and pain following peripheral tissue inflammation or nerve injury,* in Bond M.R., Charlton J.E., Woolf C.J. (eds.), *Proceedings of the 6 th World Congress on Pain,* Elsevier, Amsterdam, 1991, 263 – 276.

Dubner R., *Spinal cord neuronal plasticity: mechanisms of persistent pain following tissue damage and nerve injury,* in: Vecchiet L., Albe-Fessard D., Lindblom U., Giamberardino M.A. (eds.), *New trends in referred pain and hyperalgesia,* Elsevier, Amsterdam, 1993, 109 – 177.

Dubner R., Sessle B.J., Storey A.T., *Neural basis of oral and facial function,* Plenum, New York, 1978.

Dubner R., Sharav Y., Gracely R.H., Price D.D., *Idiopathic trigeminal neuralgia: sensory features and pain mechanisms,* Pain, 1987, 31 : 23 – 33.

Dubner R., Ruda M.A., *Activity-dependent neuronal plasticity following tissue injury and inflammation,* TINS, 1992, 15 : 96 – 103.

Dubner R., Basbaum A.I., *Spinal dorsal horn plasticity following tissue or nerve injury,* in: Wall P.D., Melzack R. (eds.), *Textbook of Pain,* Churchill Livingstone, 1994, 225 – 241.

Ebertz J.M., Hirshman C.A., Kettelkamp N.S., Uno H, Hanifin J.M., *Substance P-induced histamine release in human cutaneous mast cells,* J. Invest. Dermat., 1987, 88 : 682 – 685.

Eschenfelder C.C., Benrath J., Zimmermann M., Gillardon F., *Involvement of substance P in ultraviolet irradiation-induced inflammation in rat skin,* Eur. Neurosci., 1995, 1, 7 : 1520 – 6.

Escott K.J., Connor H.E., Brain S.D., Beattie D.T., *The involvement of calcitonin gene-related peptide (CGRP) and substance in feline pial artery diameter responses evoked by capsaicin*, Neuropeptides, 1995, 29 : 129 – 135.

Fields H.L., Rowbotham M.W., *Neurophatic pain: mechanisms and medical management*, 7 th World Congress on Pain, IASP Publications, Seattle, 1993, 369 (abs.).

Foster R.E., Whalen C.C., Waxman S.G., *Reorganization of the axon membrane in demyelinated peripheral nerve fibers: Morphological evidence*, Science, 1980, 210 : 661 – 663.

Fromm G.H., *Physiological rationale for the treatment of neuropathic pain*, Am. J. Pain, 1992.

Fromm G.H., Chattha A.S., Terrence C.F., Glass J.D., *Role of inhibitory mechanisms in trigeminal neuralgia*, Neurology, 1981, 31 : 683 – 687.

Fromm G.H., Sessle B.J. (eds.), *Trigeminal neuralgia: current concepts regarding pathogenesis and treatment*, Butterworth-Heinemann, Boston, MA, 1991, 1 – 230.

Ghostine S.Y., Comair Y.G., Turner D.M., Kassell N.F., Azar C.G., *Phenoxybenzamine in the treatment of causalgia*, J. Neurosurg., 1984, 60 : 1263 – 1268.

Gillardon F., Eschenfelder C., Rush-R.A., Zimmerman M., *Increase in neuronal Jun immunoreactivity and epidermal NGF levels following UV exposure of rat skin*, Neuroreport, 1995, 19, 6 : 1322 – 4.

Goadsby P.J., Edvinsson L., Ekman R., *Release of vasoactive peptides in the extracerebral circulation of humans and the cat during activation of the trigeminovascular system*, Ann. Neurol., 1988, 23 : 193 – 196.

Grudt T.J., Williams J.T., *Mu-Opioid agonists inhibit spinal trigeminal substantia gelatinosa neurons in guinea pig and rat*, J. Neurosci., 1994, 14 : 1646 – 1654.

Hagermark O., Hökfelt T., Pernow B., *Flare and itch induced by substance P in human skin*, Journal of Investigative Dermatology, 1978, 71 : 233 – 235.

Haley J.E., Dickenson A.H., Schachter M., *Electrophysiological evidence for a role of nitric oxide in prolonged chemical nociception in the rat*, Neuropharmacology, 1992, 31 : 251 – 258.

Hannington-Kiff J.G., *Pain relief*, Lippincott, Philadelphia, 1974, 68 – 79

Hinsey J.C., Gasser H.S., *The component of the dorsal root mediating vasodilation and the Sherrington contracture*, Am. J. Physiol., 1930, 92 : 679 – 689.

Holzer P., *Local effector functions of capsaicin-sensitive sensory nerve endings: Involvement of tachykinins, calcitonin gene-related peptide and other neuropeptides*, Neuroscience, 1988, 24 : 739 – 768.

Hoskin K.L., Kaube H., Goadsby P.J., *Central activation of the trigeminovascular pathway in the cat is inhibited by dihydroergotamine. A c-Fos and electrophysiological study*, Brain, 1996, 119 : 249 – 256.

Hu J.W., Dostrovsky J.O., Sessle B.J., *Functional properties of neurons in subnucleus caudalis of the cat. I. Responses to oral-facial noxious and non-noxious stimuli and projections to thalamus and subnucleus oralis*, J. Neurophysiol., 1981, 45 : 173 – 192.

Hu J.W., Dostrovsky J.O., Lenz Y., Ball G., Sessle B.J., *Tooth pulp deafferentation in associated with functional alterations in the properties of neurons in the trigeminal spinal tract nucleus*, J. Neurophysiol., 1986, 56 : 1650 – 1668.

Hu J.W., Sessle B.J., Raboisson P., Dallel R., Woda A., *Stimulation of craniofacial muscle afferents induces prolonged facilitatory effects in trigeminal nociceptive brain-stem neurones*, Pain, 1992, 48 : 53 – 60.

Hunt S.P., Pini A., Evan G, *Induction of c-fos-like protein in spinal cord neurons following sensory stimulation*, Nature, 1987, 328 : 632 – 634.

International Association for the Study of Pain, *Classification of chronic pain: descriptions of chronic pain syndromes and definitions of pain terms*, 2 nd ed. IASP Press, Seattle, 1994.

Iversen H.K., Olesen J. *Nitroglycerin-induced headache is not dependent on histamine release. Support for a direct nociceptive action of nitric oxide*, Cephalalgia, 1994, 14 : 437 – 42.

Iwata K., Takahashi O., Tsubori Y., et al., *Fos protein induction in the medullary dorsal horn and first segment of the spinal cord by tooth-pulp stimulation in cats*, Pain, 1998, 75 : 27 – 36.

Jancso N., Jancso-Gabor A., Szolcsanyl J., *Direct evidence for neurogenic inflammation and its prevention by denervation and by pretreatment with capsaicin*, Br. J. Pharmacol. Chemother., 1967, 31 : 138 – 151.

Jannetta P.J., *Arterial compression of the trigeminal nerve in patients with trigeminal neuralgia*, J. Neurosurg., 1967, 26 : 159 – 162.

Jannetta P.J., *Observation on the etiology of trigeminal neuralgia, hemifacial spasm, acoustic nerve dysfunction and glossopharingeal neuralgia. Definite microsurgical treatment and results in 117 patients*, Neurochirurgia, 1977, 20 : 145 – 154.

Jansen I., Alafaci C., McCulloch J., Uddman R., Edvinsson L., *Tachykinins (substance P, neurokinin A, Neuropeptide K and Neurokinin B) in the cerebral circulation, vasomotor responses in vitro and in situ*. J. Cereb. Blood Flow Metab., 1991, 11 : 567 – 575.

Kerr F.W.L., *Pathology of trigeminal neuralgia: light and electron microscopic observations*, J. Neurosurg., 1967, 26 : 151 – 156.

Khan A.A., Raja S.N., Manning D.C., Campbell J.N., Meyer R.A., *The effects of bradykinin and sequence-related analogs on the response properties of cutaneous nociceptors in monkeys*, Somatos. Mot. Res., 1992, 9 : 97 – 106.

Kilo S., Schmeltz M., Koltzenburg M., Handwerker H.O., *Different patterns of hyperalgesia induced by experimental inflammation in human skin*, Brain, 1994, 117 : 385 – 396.

Kitto K.F., Haley J.E., Wilcox G.L., *Involvement of nitric oxide in spinally mediated hyperalgesia in the mouse*, Neurosci. Lett., 1992, 148 : 1 – 5.

Kocsis J.D., Waxman S.G., Hildebrand C. et al., *Regenerating mammalian nerve fibres: changes in action potential waveform and firing characteristics following blockage of potassium conductance*, Proc. R. Soc. Lond. (Biol.), 1982, 217 : 277 – 287.

Koester J., *Passive membrane properties of the neuron*, in: Kandel E.R., Schwartz J.H., Jessel T.M. (eds.), *Principles of neural sciences*, Elsevier, Amsterdam, 1991, 95 – 103.

La Motte R.H., *Can the sensitization of nociceptors account for hyperalgesia after skin injury?* Hum. Neurobiol., 1984, 3 : 47 – 52.

LaMotte R.H., Thalhammer J.G., Torebjörk H.E., Robinson C.J., *Peripheral neural mechanisms of cutaneous hyperalgesia following mild injury by heat*, J. Neurosci., 1982, 2 : 765 – 781.

La Motte R.H., Thalhammer J.G., Robinson C.J., *Peripheral neural correlates of magnitude of cutaneous pain and hyperalgesia: a comparison of neural events in monkey with sensory judgements in human*, J. Neurophysiol., 1983, 50 : 1 – 26.

Leandri M., Eldridge P.R., Milza J.B., Haggett C., Mackenzie I., *Electrophysiological assessment of fibre distribution within the retrogasserian trigeminal root*, Ital. J. Neurol. Sci., 1997, 18 : 227.

Lembeck F., *Zur fragen der zentralen ubertragung afferenter impulse*, III Mitteilung. *Das vorkommen und die bebeutung der substanz P in dorsalen wurzeln des ruckenmarks*, Naunyn-Schmiedeberg's, Arch. Exp. Pathol. Pharmakol., 1953, 219 : 197 – 213.

Lembeck F., Holzer P., *Substance P as neurogenic mediator of antidromic vasodilation and neurogenic plasma extravasation*. Naunyn-Schmiedebergs Archives of Pharmacology, 1979, 310 : 175 – 183

Lembeck F., Folkers K., Donnerer J., *Analgesic effect of antagonists of substance P*, Biochem. Biophys. Res. Commun., 1981, 103 : 1318 – 1321.

Lembeck F., Gamse R., *Substance P in peripheral sensory processes*, Ciba Foundation Symposium, 1982, 91 : 35 – 54.

Lembeck F., Donnerer J., Bartho L., *Inhibition of neurogenic vasodilation and plasma extravasation by substance P antagonists, somatostatin and [D-Met 2, Pro 3] enkephanilamide*, Eur. J. Pharmacol., 1982, 85 : 171 – 176.

Lembeck F., Donnerer J., *Opioid control of the function of primary afferent substance P fibers*, Eur. J. Pharmacol., 1985, 114 : 241 – 246.

Lewis T., *Pain*, MacMillan, New York, 1942.

Livingston W.K., *Pain mechanisms*, MacMillan, New York, 1943.

Loh L., Nathan P.W., *Painful peripheral states and sympathetic blocks*, J. Neurol., Neurosurg. Psychiatry, 1978, 41 : 664 – 671.

Ludwin S.K., *Pathology of demeyelination and remyelination*, in Waxman S.G., Ritchie J.M. (eds.), *Demyelination diseases: basic and clinical electrophysiology*, Advances in neurology, vol. 31, Raven Press, New York, 1981, 123.

Lundberg J.M., Brodin E., Hua H.Y., Saria A., *Vascular permeability changes and smooth muscle contraction in relation to capsaicin-sensitive substance P afferents in guinea pig*, Acta Physiol. Scand., 1984, 120 : 217 – 227.

Manning D.C., Raja S.N., Meyer R.A., Campbell J.N., *Pain and hyperalgesia after intradermal injection of bradykinin in humans*, Clin. Pharmacol. Ther., 1991, 50 : 721 – 729.

Markowitz S., Saito K., Moskowitz M.A., *Neurogenically mediated leakage of plasma protein occurs from blood vessels in dura mater but not brain*, J. Neurosci., 1987, 7 : 4129 – 4136.

Mayer M.L., Westbrook G., Guthrie P.B., *Voltage-dependent block by Mg 2 of NMDA responses in spinal cord neurones*, Nature, 1984, 309 : 261 – 263.

Meller S.T., Pechman P.S., Gebhart G.F., Maves T.J., *Nitric oxide mediates the thermal hyperalgesia produced in a model of neuropathic pain in the rat*, Neuroscience, 1992, 50 : 7 – 10.

Meller S.T., Gebhart G.F., Nitric Oxide (NO) and nociceptive processing in the spinal cord. Pain, 1993, 52 : 127 – 136.

Meller S.T., Takagi H., Valtschanoff, Wilcox G., *Nitric oxide and pain*, 7 th World Congress on Pain, IASP Publications, Seattle, 1993, 122, *(abs.)*.

Menetrey D., Gannon A., Levine J.D. and Basbaum A.I., *The expression of c-fos protein in presumed-nociceptive interneurons and projection aeurons of the rat spinal cord: anatomical mapping of the central effects of noxious somatic, articular and visceral stimulation*, J. Comp. Neurol., 1989, 258 : 177 – 195.

Meyer R.A., Campbell J.N., *Myelinated nociceptive afferents account for the hyperalgesia that follows a burn to the hand*, Science, 1981 a, 213 : 1527 – 1529.

Meyer R.A., Campbell J.N., *Peripheral neural coding of pain sensation*, Johns Hopkins Applied Physic Laboratory Technical Digest, 1981 b, 2 : 164 – 171.

Meyer R.A., Campbell J.N., Raja S.N., *Peripheral neural mechanisms of nociception*. In: Wall P.D., Melzac R. (eds.), *Textbook of Pain*. Churchill Livingstone, Edinburgh, 1994, 13 – 44.

Micevych P.E., Kruger L., *The status of calcitonin gene-related peptide as an effector peptide*, Ann. NY Acad. Sci., 1992, 657 : 379 – 396.

Mongini F., Caselli C., Macrí V., Tetti C., *Thermographic findings in craniofacial pain*, Headache, 1990, 30 : 497 – 504.

Moskowitz M.A., *The neurobiology of vascular head pain*, Ann. Neurol., 1984, 16 : 157 – 168.

Moskowitz M.A., *The visceral organ brain: implications for the pathophysiology of vascular head pain*, Neurology, 1991, 41 : 182 – 186.

Moskowitz M.A., *Neurogenic versus vascular mechanisms of sumatriptan and ergot alkaloids in migraine*, Trends Pharmacol. Sci., 1992, 13 : 307 – 11.

Moskowitz M.A., Brody M., Liu-Chen L.Y., *In vitro release of immuno-reactive substance P from putative afferent nerve endings in bovine pia-arachnoid*, Neuroscience, 1983, 9 : 809 – 814.

Moskowitz M.A., Buzzi M.G., Sakas D.E., Linnik M.D., *Pain mechanisms underlying vascular headaches*, Rev. Neurol., 1989, 145 : 181 – 193.

Nordin M., Nystrom B., Wallin U. et al., *Ectopic sensory discharges and paresthesia in patients with disorders of peripheral nerves dorsal roots and dorsal columns*, Pain, 1984, 20 : 231 – 245.

Olesen J., *Pathophysiology of human vascular headache*, 7 th World Congress of Pain, IASP Publications, Seattle, 1993, 252 (abs.).

Olesen J., Iversen H.K., Thomsen L.L., *Nitric oxide supersensitivity. A possibile molecular mechanism of migrain pain*, Neuroreport, 1993.

Olesen J., Thomsen L.L., Lassen L.H., Olesen J.J., *The nitric oxide hypothesis of migraine and other vascular headaches*, Cephalalgia, 1995, 15 : 94 – 100.

Pagni C.A., *Trigeminal neuralgia*, Panminerva. Med., 1982, 24 : 113 – 136.

Pagni C.A., *The origin of tic douloureux: a unified view*, J. Neurosurg. Sci., 1993, 37 : 185 – 194.

Pedersen J.L., Kehlet H., *Secondary hyperalgesia to heat stimuli after burn injury in man*, Pain, 1998, 76 : 377 – 384.

Radhakrishnan V., Henry J.L., *L-NAME blocks responses to NMDA, substance P and noxious cutaneous stimuli in cat dorsal horn*, Neuroreport, 1993, 4 : 323 – 326.

Raja S., Campbell J.N., Meyer R.A., *Evidence for different mechanisms of primary and secondary hyperalgesia following heat injury to the glabrous skin*, Brain, 1984, 107 : 1179 – 1188.

Raja S.N., Treede R.D., Davis K.D., Campbell J.N., *Systemic alpha-adrenergic blockade with phentolamine: a diagnostic test for sympathetically maintained pain*, Anesthesiology, 1991, 74 : 691 – 698.

Raja S.N., Davis K.D., Campbell J.N., *The adrenergic pharmacology of sympathetically maintained pain*, J. Reconstr. Microsurg., 1992, 8 : 63 – 69.

Rappaport Z.H., Devor M., *Trigeminal neuralgia: the role of self-sustaining discharge in the trigeminal ganglion*, Pain, 1994, 56 : 127 – 138.

Rasminsky M., *Ectopic generation of impulses and cross-talk in spinal nerve roots of dystrophic mice*, Ann. Neurol., 1978, 3 : 351 – 357.

Rasminsky M., *Ephaptic transmission between single nerve fibres in the spinal nerve roots of dystrophic mice*, J. Physiol., 1980, 305 : 151 – 169.

Ro J.Y., Capra N.F., *Receptive field properties of trigeminothalamic neurons in the rostral trigeminal sensory nuclei of cats*, Somatosens. Mot. Res., 1994, 11 : 119 – 130.

Roberts W.J., *A hypothesis on the physiological basis for causalgia and related pains*, Pain, 1986, 24 : 297 – 311.

Rosell S., Olgart L., Gazelius B., Panopoulos P., Folkers K., Horing J., *Inhibition of antidromic and substance P induced vasodilatation by a substance P antagonist*, Acta Physiol. Scand., 1981, 111 : 381 – 382.

Sang C.N., Gracely R.H., Max M.B., Bennet G.J., *Capsaicin-evoked mechanical allodynia and hyperalgesia cross nerve territories. Evidence for a central mechanism*, Anesthesiology, 1996, 85 : 491 – 496.

Saria A., Lundberg J.M., Skofttsch G., Lembeck F., *Vascular leakage in various tissues induced by substance P, capsaicin, bradykinin, serotonin, histamine and by antigen challenge*, Naunyn Schmedeberg's Arch. Pharmacol., 1983, 324 : 212 – 218.

Schaible H.G., Schmidt R.F, *Direct observation of the sensitization of articular afferents during an experimental arthritis*, in: Dubner R., Gebhart G.F., Bond M.R. (eds.), *Proceedings of the Vth World Congress on Pain*, Pain Research and Clinical Management, Elsevier, Amsterdam, 1988, 3 : 44 – 50.

Schmidt R.F., *The nociceptor as a dynamic entity*, 7 th World Congress on Pain, IASP Publications, Seattle, 1993, 128 (abs.).

Selzer Z., Devor M., *Ephaptic transmission in chronically damaged peripheral nerves*, Neurology, 1979, 29 : 1061 – 1064.

Sessle B.J., *Dental deafferentation can lead to the development of chronic pain*, in: Klineberg I., Sessle B. (eds.),*Orofacial pain and neuromuscular dysfuction: mechanisms and clinical correlates*, Pergamon, Oxford, 1985, 115 – 129.

Sessle B.J., *The neurobiology of facial and dental pain: present knowledge, future directions*, J. Dent. Res., 1987, 66 : 962 – 981.

Sessle B.J., *Anatomy, physiology and pathophysiology of orofacial pain*, in: Jacobson A.L., Donlon W.C. (eds.), *Headache and facial pain*, Raven Press, New York, 1990, 1 – 24.

Sessle B.J., *Physiology of the trigeminal system*, in: Fromm G.H., Sessle B.J. (eds.), *Trigeminal neuralgia: current concepts regarding pathogenesis and treatment*, Butterworth-Heinemann, London, 1991, 72 – 104.

Sessle B.J., Hu J.W., Amano N. et al., *Convergence of cutaneous, tooth pulp, visceral, neck and muscle afferents onto nociceptive and non-nociceptive neurones in trigeminal subnucleus caudalis (medullary dorsal horn) and its implications for referred pain*, Pain, 1986, 27 : 219 – 235.

Sessle B.J., Hu J.W., Yu X.M., *Brainstem mechanisms of referred pain and hyperalgesia in the orofacial and temporomandibular region*, in: Vecchiet L., Albe-Fessard D., Lindblom U., Giamberardino M.A. (eds.), *New trends in referred pain and hyperalgesia*, Elsevier, Amsterdam, 1993 a, 59 – 71.

Sessle B.J., Yu X.M., Hu J.W., *Trigeminal (V) brainstem neuronal plasticity induced by application of inflammatory irritant to cutaneous and deep tissues*, 7 th World Congress on Pain, IASP Publications, Seattle, 1993 b, 28 (abs.).

Shepheard S.L., Williamson D.J., Hill R.G., Hargreaves R.J., *The non-peptide neurokinin, receptor antagonist RP67580 blocks neurogenic plasma extravasation in the dura mater of rats*, Br. J. Pharmacol., 1993, 108 : 11 – 12.

Simone D.A., Baumann T.K., Collins J.G., La Motte R.H., *Sensitization of cat dorsal horn neurons to innocuous mechanical stimulation after intradermal injection of capsaicin*, Brain Res., 1989 a, 486 : 185 – 189.

Simone D.A., Baumann T.K., La Motte R.H., *Dose-dependent pain and mechanical hyperalgesia in humans after intradermal injection of capsaicin*, Pain, 1989 b, 39 : 99 – 107.

Sorkin L.S., *NMDA evoked an L-NAME sensitive spinal release of glutamate and citrulline*, Neuroreport, 1993, 4 : 479 – 482.

Strassman A., Potrebic S., Moskowitz M., Maciewicz R., *Morphology and projections of intracellularly labelled brainstem trigeminal vascular convergence neurons*, Soc. Neurosci., 1988, 18 : 1163.

Sweet W.H., Wepsic J.G., *Controlled thermocoagulation of trigeminal ganglion and rootlets for differential destruction of pain fibers, part I: Trigeminal neuralgia*, J. Neurosurg., 1974, 40 : 143 – 156.

Szolcsànyi J., *Antidromic vasodilation and neurogenic inflammation*, Agents Actions, 1988, 23 : 4 – 1.

Thomsen L.L., Iversen H.K., Brinck T.A., Olesen J., *Nitroglycerin (NTG) induced headache (NTGH) in migraineurs and controls*, 7 th World Congress on Pain, IASP Publications, Seattle, 1993, 12.

Tölle T.R., Castro L.J., Coimbra A., Zieglgänsberger W, *Opiates modify induction of c-fos proto-oncogene in the spinal cord of the rat following noxious stimulation*, Neurosci. Lett., 1990, 111 : 46 – 51.

Torebjörk H.E., *Nociceptor dynamics in humans*, 7 th World Congress on Pain, IASP Publications, Seattle, 1993, 130 (abs.).

Torebjörk H.E., Lundberg L.E., La Motte R.H., *Central changes in processing of mechano receptive input in capsicum-induced secondary hyperalgesia in man*, J. Physiol., 1992, 448 : 765 – 780.

Torneck C.D., Kwan C.L., Hu J.W., J. Dent. Res, 1996, 75 : 553 – 561.

Treede R.D., Raja S.N., Davis K.D., Meyer R.A., Campbell J.N., *Evidence that peripheral alfa-adrenergic receptors mediate sympathetically maintained pain*, in: Bond M.R., Charlton J.E., Woolf C.J. (eds.), *Proceedings of the VIth World Congress on Pain*, Elsevier, Amsterdam, 1991, 377 – 382.

Treede R.D., Meyer R.A., Raja S.N., Campbell J.N., *Peripheral and central mechanisms of cutaneous hyperalgesia*, Prog. Neurobiol., 1992, 38 : 397 – 421.

Uddman R., Edvinsson L., *Neuropeptides in the cerebral circulation*, Cerebrovasc. Brain Metab. Rev., 1989, 1 : 230 – 252.

Utzchneider D. Kocsis J., Devor M., *Mutual excitation among dorsal root ganglion neurous in the rat*, Neurosci. Lett., 1992, 146 : 53 – 56.

Van Hees J., Gybels J., *C nociceptor activity in human nerve during painful and non painful skin stimulation*, J. Neurol. Neurosurg. Psychiatry, 1981, 44 : 600 – 607.

Vighetti S., Asteggiano G., Mongini F., Bergamasco L., Mattiuzzi M., *EPS-ERPS Mapping in migraine patients*, It. J. Neurol. Sc., 1997, 18, 229 – 230.

Wall P.D., *The dorsal horn*, in: Wall P.D., Melzack R. (eds.), *Textbook of pain*, Churchill Livingstone, Edinburgh,1989.

Wall P.D., Fitzgerald M., Nussbaumer J.C., Van Der Loos H., Devor M., *Somatotopic maps are disorganized in adult rodents treated neonatally with Capsaicin*, Nature, 1982, 295 : 691 – 693.

Warncke T., Stubhaug A., Jørum E., *Ketamine, an NMDA receptor antagonist, suppresses spatial and temporal properties of burn-induced secondary hyperalgesia in man: a double-blind, cross-over comparison with morphine and placebo*, Pain, 1997, 72 : 99 – 106.

Wilcox G.L., *Excitatory neurotransmitters and pain*. In: Bond M.R., Charlton J.E., Woolf C.J. (eds.) *Proceedings of the VIth World Congress on Pain*, Elsevier, Amsterdam, B.V., 1991, 97 – 117.

Williamson D.J., Hargreaves R.J., Hill R.G., Shepheard S.L., *Intravital microscope studies on the effects of neurokinin agonists and calcitonin gene-related peptide on dural vessel diameter in the anaesthetized rat*, Cephalalgia, 1997, 17 : 518 – 524.

Wisden W., Errington M.L., Williams S., Dunnett S.B., Waters C., Hitchcock D., Evan G., Bliss T.V. and Hunt S.P., *Differential expression of immediate early genes in the hippocampus and spinal cord.*, Neuron., 1990, 4 : 603 – 614.

Woolf C.J., *Evidence for a central component of postinjury pain hypersensitivity*, Nature, 1983, 308 : 686 – 688.

Woolf C.J., *Functional plasticity of the flexor vithdrawal reflex in the rat following peripheral tissue injury*, in: Fields H.L., Dubner R., Cervero F. (eds.), *Advances in pain research and therapy*, Raven Press, New York, 1985, 9 : 193 – 201.

Woolf C.J., *Central mechanisms of acute pain*, in: Bond M.R., Charlton J.E., Woolf C.J. (eds.), *Proceedings of the VIth World Congress on Pain*, Elsevier, Amsterdam., 1991, 25 – 34.

Woolf C.J., *The dorsal horn: state - dependent sensory processing and the generation of pain*, in: Wall P.D., Melzack R. (eds.), *Texbook of pain*, Churchill Livingstone, Edinburgh, 1994, 101 – 112.

Woolf C.J., Thompson S.W.N. et al., *Prolonged primary afferent induced alterations in dorsal horn neurones, an intracellular analysis in vivo and invitro*. J. Physiol., 1989, 83 : 255 – 266.

Yokota T., *Neural mechanisms of tigeminal pain*, in Fields H.L., Dubner R. and Cervero F. (eds.), *Advances in pain research and therapy*, Raven Press, New York, 1985, 9, 221 – 232.

Zimmermann M., Herdegen T., *Control of gene transcription by Jun and Fos proteins in the nervous system*, Am. Pain Soc. J., 1994, 3 : 33 – 48.

3 Muscle Disorders

The Neuromuscular Junction and Principles of Muscle Physiology

The muscle fibers are made of longitudinal bundles of *myofibrils* associated with the *sarcoplasmatic reticulum*, and a number of mitochondria. Each motor fiber before ending splits into several branches: each of these branches innervates only a single muscle cell. The complex represented by one motor fiber, its branches, and the relevant muscle cells is a defined "motor unit" (of Sherrington). Motor fibers connect to a special region of the muscle membrane, the *muscle end-plate*. In this region, the muscle membrane forms folds, the *junctional folds,* where many acetylcholine (ACh) receptors are located. Directly opposed to the muscle end-plate are the *synaptic boutons,* small varicosities located at the extremity of the thin branches into which each motor neuron splits near its end (Fig. 3.**1**).

When an action potential arrives at a synaptic bouton, ACh is released from the boutons into the synaptic cleft. The interaction of ACh with the receptors in the junctional folds produces an *end-plate potential,* which conversely opens the voltage-gated sodium channels of the muscle end-plate: thus, an *action potential* is produced inside the muscle fiber. The action potential drives along the muscle fiber membrane (that is, the *sarcolemma*) to its minute invaginations, called *transverse tubules* (Fig. 3.**2**).

Each muscle fiber contains longitudinal bundles of *myofibrils* associated with the *sarcoplasmatic reticulum,* and a number of mitochondria (Fig. 3.**2**). The depolarization along the transverse tubules produces the opening of voltage-gated

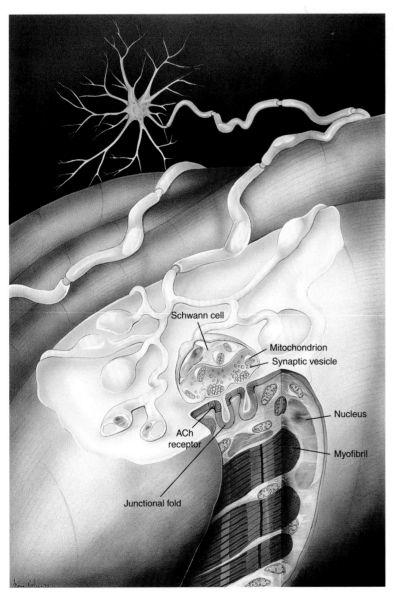

Fig. 3.**1** The neuromuscular junction

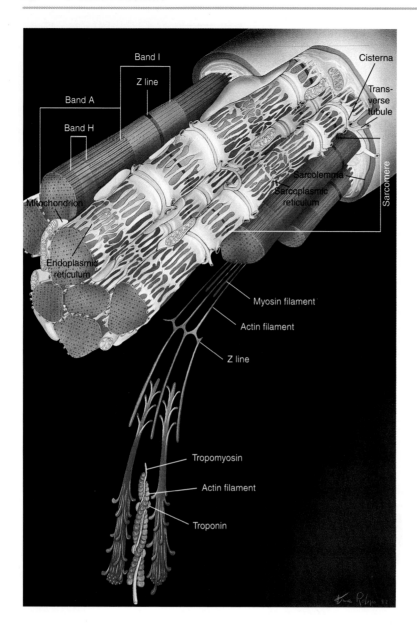

Band I
Z line
Band A
Band H
Cisterna
Trans-verse tubule
Mitochondrion
Sarcolemma
Sarcoplasmic reticulum
Sarcomere
Endoplasmic reticulum
Myosin filament
Actin filament
Z line
Tropomyosin
Actin filament
Troponin

Fig. 3.**2**   The muscle fiber

calcium channels of the sarcoplasmatic reticulum. This process, together with the presence of adenosine triphosphate (ATP), is essential for muscle contraction. With phase-contrast microscopy, two regions can be recognized in the myofibrils; dark bands, *A* (anisotropic) bands, and light *I* (isotropic) bands. The I bands are bisected by a protein structure, the *Z line.*

The smallest contractile unit of a muscle fiber is the *sarcomere,* which extends from one Z line to the next. Each sarcomere is composed of two fibrillar proteins, the thick and the thin filaments. The thick filaments contain myosin, a rod-shaped molecule, while the thin filaments contain pairs of monomers of actin, arranged as helixes, and two other proteins, tropomyosin and troponine (Fig. 3.**2**). Muscle contraction occurs by the interaction between actin and myosin. This is made possible because the calcium binds to troponin, thus producing a conformational change in the actin, which exposes a receptor for the myosin head. The myosin heads attach to the actin filaments, which are drawn toward the center of the sarcomere, which in consequence shortens. When the myosin is attached to the actin to form actomyosin, it has an ATPase activity that catalyses the breakdown of ATP into adenosine diphosphate (ADP) and inorganic phosphate (P). When the depolarization ends, calcium ions are pumped back into

the sarcoplasmic reticulum, and the cross-bridges between myosin and actin detach. The presence of ATP is essential for such detachment, that is, for muscle relaxation. If ATP is lacking, the muscle becomes rigid and *contracture* occurs: in this situation no EMG muscle activity (see below) is present (Layzer, 1994; Simons and Mense, 1998). Thus muscle tissue, like other tissues, requires a constant supply of ATP. However, unlike other tissues, the muscle under contraction may require as much as 200 times the quantity of ATP it does when at rest (Smith et al., 1985). During muscle exercise, such an enormous need for metabolic energy is satisfied by glycolysis of the glycogen stored in the muscle, as well as of the blood glucose. By a sequence of reactions, the glucose is transformed into lactate and ATP is formed. This pathway is unique in that it occurs in the absence of oxygen, which, as we shall see, is at very low concentrations in the muscle under contraction. Sustained muscle activity promotes the release of lactate and K^+ from the muscle fibers: these ions diffuse into the interstitial fluid and the venous blood, and thence into noncontractile tissues: this, in turn, ensures that favorable concentration gradients are maintained so that the ions may further circulate from the muscle interstitial fluid to the venous blood (Lindinger et al., 1995). Nevertheless, prolonged muscle activity leads to an "oxygen debt," that is, to the need, which continues after the activity has stopped, for oxygen consumption well above the base rate, in order to oxidize the lactic acid.

Muscle Contraction

Muscle contraction is most effective and economical when the muscle is at its optimal length (Astrand and Rodahl, 1986; Jones and Round, 1990).

Basically, three patterns of muscle contraction can be distinguished: isotonic, isometric, and eccentric contraction. During isotonic contraction, the muscle shortens progressively; during isometric contraction, it stays the same length; while during eccentric contraction it is elongated by forces directed against its direction of contraction.

Repeated eccentric contraction provokes muscle soreness (Friden et al., 1981; Friden, 1984; Jones et al., 1986; Vecchiet et al., 1987; Newham, 1988; Kroon and Naeije, 1988; Stauber, 1989); it has also been shown to evoke longer-lasting changes in EMG signals, with comparatively fewer motor units being active than during concentric contraction (Bigland-Ritchie, 1981). As a consequence, the tension per active motor unit increases, and muscle fiber damage may result (Friden et al., 1981).

The axons descending from the motor cortex to innervate the spinal motor neuron also send collaterals to interneurons, which inhibit the motor neurons innervating the antagonist muscles (Jankowska et al., 1976) (Fig. 3.**3**). This reciprocal innervation provides for a very efficient energy consumption, but requires the load to be acurately known. Sometimes it may be necessary to contract agonist and antagonist muscles simultaneously to perform precise movementes and to stabilize the joint (Gordon, 1991) (Fig. 3.**4**). This co-contraction uses more energy, but does not require the load to be known

as precisely as during reciprocal innervation: since the joint is stiffer during co-contraction, a difference between the actual and the expected load will have little effect on the limb position. During co-contraction, the antagonist muscles undergo eccentric contraction, with the possible consequences mentioned above. The process of learning a movement sequence implies that the systems switches from co-contraction to reciprocal innervation (Gordon, 1991).

Muscles contain two kinds of receptors: the Golgi tendon organs and the muscle spindles. The Golgi tendon organs are located between the muscles and the tendons and sense changes in muscles tension (Fig. 3.**5**). The muscle spindles are encapsulated structures running parallel to the muscle fibers, which have specialized muscle fibers, the *intrafusal fibers* (Fig. 3.**6**). They are sensitive to muscle elongation: in fact, the stretching of the intrafusal fibers brought about by muscle elongation leads to firing of the afferent nerve fibers by the spindles. Spindles are also innervated by efferent fibers of the gamma motor neurons. It has been shown (Granit, 1970) that stimulation of the cortex and other higher centers leads to stimulation of both the alpha and the gamma motoneurons. This *alpha gamma coactivation* is essential to keep the intrafusal fibers active while the muscle shortens during contraction (Hunt and Kuffler, 1951; Granit, 1970; Vallbo, 1981; Gordon and Ghez, 1991). The performance of difficult tasks or experience of unpredictable situations increases gamma system activity. The afferent spindle fibers make monosynaptic connection with the alpha motoneurons. Thus, muscle elongation produces excitatory potentials in the motoneurons, which, in turn, lead to the contraction of the muscle. This "stretch reflex" is essential in maintaining posture. The mandibular elevator muscles are rich in muscle spindles (Freimann, 1954; Cooper, 1960; Hosokawa, 1961). Their stimulation as a consequence of mandibular drop leads to reflex contraction of the muscle. Here, the *stretch* or *jaw-closing reflex* is mediated

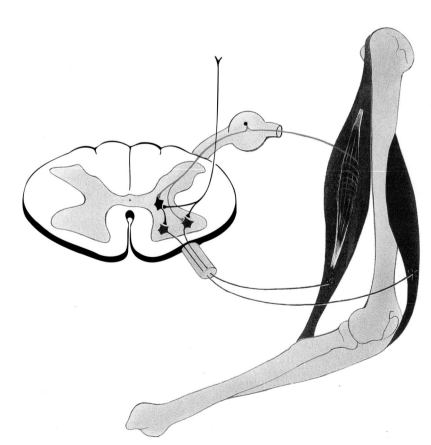

Fig. 3.**3 Reciprocal innervation.** Black: axon from the motor cortex and inhibitory interneuron. Red: alpha motoneurons of agonist and antagonist muscles. Green: proprioceptive afferences from neuromuscular spindles

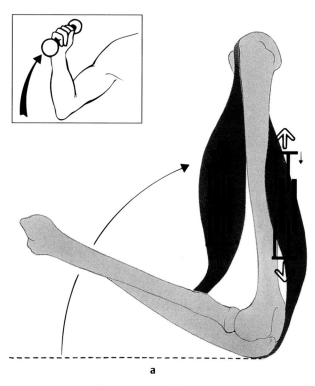
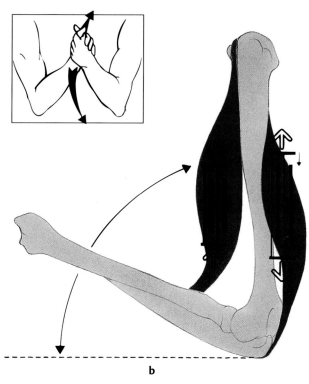

Fig. 3.**4 a** Reciprocal innervation with contraction and shortening of agonist muscle and decontraction and lengthening of antagonist muscle. **b** Co-contraction of the agonist muscle (with consequent shortening) and of the antagonist muscle (with lengthening) and consequent eccentric contraction of the latter

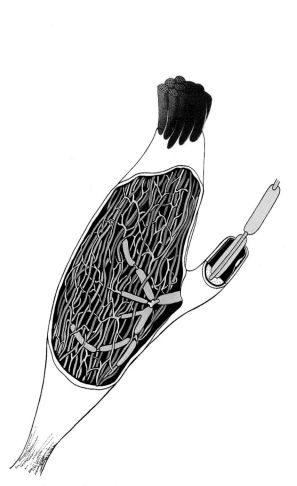

Fig. 3.**5 Golgi muscle tendon organ.** Note the close relation between nerve fibers (in gray) and the bands of the muscle tendon organ (in light blue)

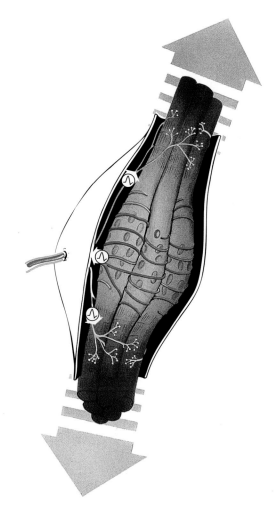

Fig. 3.**6 Neuromuscular spindle.** Green, the proprioceptive afferents from the spindle; pink, the efferent fibers of the gamma motoneurons

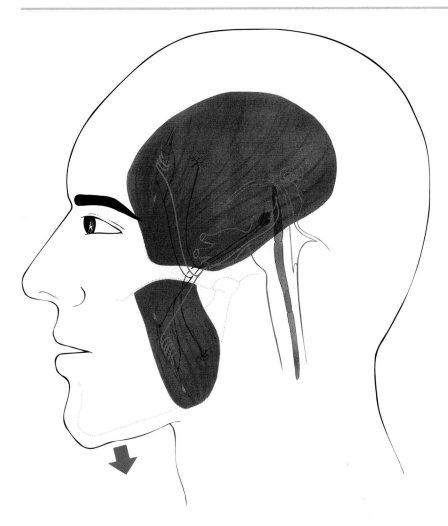

Fig. 3.**7** **Paths of the mandible closing reflex.** As the mandible drops, the neuro-muscular spindles are stretched and in consequence the afferent fibers to the mesencephalic nucleus of the trigeminal nerve are excited (green); this causes excitation of the alpha motoneurons of the trigeminal motor nucleus (red) and reflex muscle contraction. An increased activity of the gamma motoneurons (pink) due to input from the reticular substance or higher centers (grey) enhances the closing reflex

through the mesencephalic component of the trigeminal sensory complex and the motor nucleus of the same nerve. The jaw-closing reflex is considered one of the main factors responsible for the postural position of the mandible (Dubner et al., 1978) (Fig. 3.**7**). An increase in the gamma activity in this area increases the reaction to stretch, and may change the postural position of the mandible.

Muscle Blood Flow. Muscle Fatigue

The amount of muscle blood flow varies with the type of muscle: muscles with white, fast-twitch fibers have less blood flow than those with an abundance of red, slow-contracting fibers. During rest, blood flow maintains the homeostasis and the oxygen tension necessary to restore the energy substrate (Sjögaard et al., 1988). During contraction, the muscle blood flow (MBF) depends on the local vasodilatation and on the systemic cardiovascular response, which tends to increase the flow (Forbes et al., 1979), and also on the increase of intramuscular pressure and tissue displacement, which tend to decrease it (Hill, 1948; Edwards et al., 1972; Möller et al., 1979). The increase in intramuscular pressure is proportional to the mean velocity of contraction. The level of isometric contraction that can arrest MBF varies in the different muscles (Barcroft and Millen, 1939; Edwards et al., 1972; Bonde-Petersen and Christensen, 1973); differing values are reported in the masseter muscles. According to Möller (1981), tooth-clenching at 25% of full effort may lead to significant impairment of blood flow to the temporal and masseter

muscles. This author maintains that, in these muscles, even a sustained contraction as low as 10% of maximum voluntary contraction may result in blood flow alterations in some subjects. However, Monteiro and Kopp (1988) found that, during sustained contraction, there may be an increase in blood flow compared to rest values, but that this may be insufficient to meet the demand due to the much higher increase in muscle activity. As a consequence, after contraction, a pronounced hyperemia occurs (Monteiro and Kopp, 1989).

During sustained contraction, muscle fatigue develops. Muscle fatigue has been defined in different ways by different authors. However, there is substantial agreement that muscle fatigue is characterized by a decrease of the capability of the neuromuscular system to produce force to accomplish a given task (Edwards, 1978; Bigland-Richtie, 1981; Hainaut and Duchateau, 1989). Such a decrease may be a consequence of reduced activity of the central nervous system on the muscle (neurological central fatigue), on an alteration of the signal transmission at neuromuscular level (neuromuscular central fatigue), or on an alteration of the contraction capability of the muscle cell (neuromuscular peripheral fatigue) (Asmussen, 1979; Junge and Clark, 1993). A further distinction may be drawn between "lactacid" and "non-lactacid" muscle fatigue. During prolonged isometric contraction, glycolysis leads to the accumulation of lactic acid and consequent oxygen deficit and intracellular acidosis. As a result, ATP production is lower, and the force due to actin–myosin interaction is reduced (lactacid fatigue). However, this mechanism requires some time to develop: it therefore does not fully explain some typical changes in the electromyographic activity that, as we shall see, occur over a short time and must therefore be, at least in part, the consequence of other mechanisms (non-lactacid fatigue). Moreover, one should consider that during sustained isometric contraction of the masseter muscles the force exerted decreases gradually as the pain produced by the exercise increases (Clark and Carter, 1985). This is not a true muscle fatigue but a reflex central mechanism.

Muscle fatigue is characterized by a shift of the EMG power spectrum toward lower frequencies (Viitasolo and Komi, 1977, 1980; Palla and Ash, 1981; Naeije and Zorn, 1981, 1982; Basmajian and De Luca, 1985; Kroon et al., 1986; Merletti et al., 1990; Hori et al., 1995). This phenomenon was attributed to the decreased speed of conduction in the muscle fiber (Lindstrom et al., 1970; Sadoyama and Miyano, 1981; Naeije and Zorn, 1982; Kranz et al., 1983; Zwarts, 1989) and to the synchronization of the motor units (Person and Mishin, 1964; O'Donnell et al., 1973; Weyjens and van Steenberghe, 1984).

To study masseter muscle fatigue, Mongini et al. (1995) employed a device previously developed and employed on the long muscles (Knaflit et al., 1990). This device is linked to a gnathodymometer, developed to be located between the dental arches during the tests (Fig. 3.**8**). The myoelectric signal is detected by a four-bar surface electrode (Fig. 3.**9**). The single differential output is obtained from the two central bars and used to analyze the spectral parameters. This allows a more precise signal analysis than with electromyographs with conventional surface electrodes. Using this system, healthy subjects were asked to clench their teeth at 30% and at 60% of the maximal voluntary contraction (MVC). In both cases there was a decrease of the mean frequency of the signal during the test. However, the mean reduction of EMG frequency at 60% of the MVC was significantly higher than that at 30% of the MVC (Fig. 3.**10**). In other words, as expected, the degree of masseter fatigue at 60% of the MVC was higher than at 30%. Frequency values at the beginning of each test were, in the majority of cases, higher at 30% that at 60% of the MVC (Fig. 3.**11**). This finding is in agreement with those of other authors (Duxbury et al., 1976; Palla and Ash, 1981; Hagberg and Hagberg, 1988;

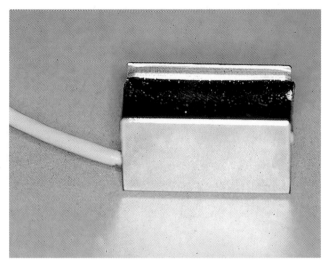

Fig. 3.**8**   Gnathodynamometer to be inserted between the dental arches in order to measure the force exerted during tooth clenching

Clark et al., 1988) and is contrary to what has been observed in the long muscles, such as the tibialis anterior, in which higher forces are associated with higher EMG frequencies at the beginning of the test (Merletti et al., 1990). This difference is probably due to the difference in structure of the muscles. Histochemical studies have shown that craniomandibular muscles, in contrast to the long muscles, have more fatigue-resistant slow fibers (type I fibers) than nonresistant fast fibers (type IIB fibers) (Eriksson and Thornell, 1983; Clark et al., 1991). It has been speculated that in the masseter the amount of activated type I fibers (slow fibers) may increase as the intensity of contraction increases (Westbury and Shaughnessy, 1987).

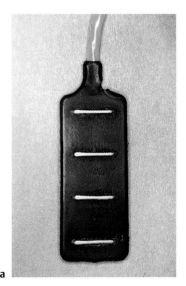
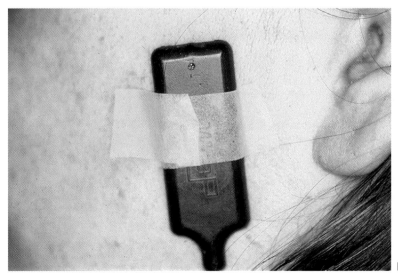

a   **b**

Fig. 3.**9**   Surface electrode with four bars (**a**) applied on the masseter region (**b**) to assess the myoelectric signal

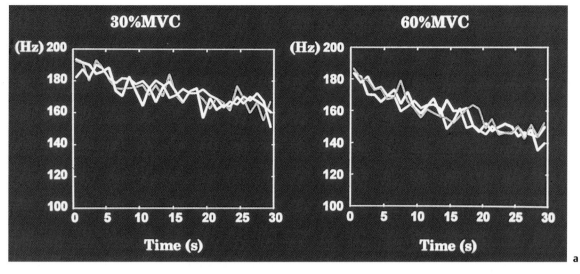

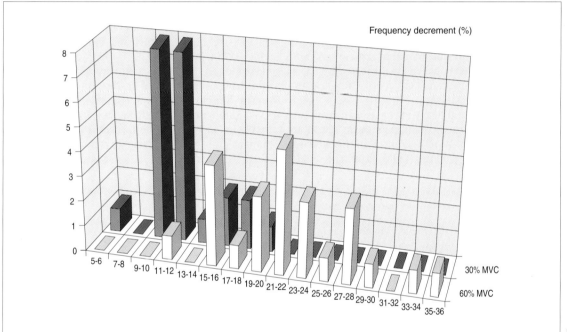

Fig. 3.**10** **a** Data from three clenching tests at 30% and 60% of the maximal voluntary contraction. Values of the frequency of the myo-electric signal are given in hertz (Hz). There is a gradual shift toward lower frequencies over time. This shift is more pronounced at the 60% of the maximal voluntary contraction. **b** At 30% of contraction force the decrement in frequency of the signal ranges between 9% and 12%, at 60% of contraction force the decrement ranges between 15% and 28%

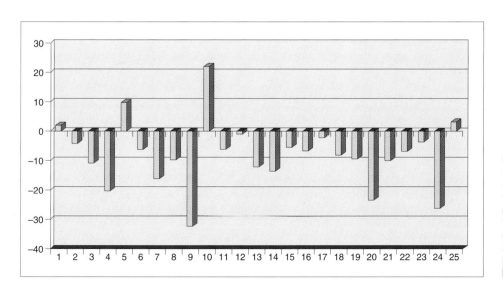

Fig. 3.**11** Difference between the frequency values of the myo-electric signal at the beginning of the test at 60% and 30% of the maximal voluntary contraction. In the majority of cases the difference values are negative because at 30% of contraction force the initial frequency of the signal is higher than at 60%

Muscle Pain

Muscle fatigue is accompanied by muscle pain in a relatively short time (Jones et al., 1987; Vecchiet et al., 1987), although the two factors are not necessarily concomitant: in fact, the EMG signs of muscle fatigue previously described may be present in the absence of pain and, conversely, painful sensations may be present before the EMG alterations are evident. Several causes may produce muscle pain. As we have seen, one reason is local acidosis, which stimulates pain receptors (Edwards, 1985, 1986). In fact, nociceptors, mainly with free endings, have been shown to be present in muscle tissue; these are activated only by intense stimulation (Paintal, 1960; Bessou and Laporte, 1961; Mense and Meyer, 1985) and show an increased excitability in conditions of ischemia (Mense and Stahnke, 1983; Kaufman et al., 1984) (Fig. 3.**12**). This mechanism, however, requires a certain time to develop and may therefore not account for the pain in the very short term. Indeed, Clark et al. (1989) have shown that healthy subjects very quickly display a sharp pain in the masseter during maximal clench. This pain disappears rapidly after cessation of the task. These authors therefore expressed doubt that prolonged isometric contraction is a valuable model to explain subacute or chronic pain in this area, as has been advocated by other authors (Direnfeld, 1967; Scott and Lundeen, 1980; Christensen, 1981; Bowley and Gale, 1987).

Finally, unaccustomed and heavy exercise of the muscles may provoke long-lasting muscle pain; pain arises after 8 to 24 hours and reaches its peak 24 to 72 hours after the exercise. This *delayed onset of muscle soreness* (DOMS) could be due to

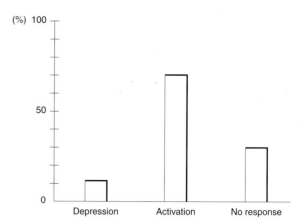

Fig. 3.**12** **Effect of hypoxia on nociceptors of the diaphragmatic muscle.** The percentage of nociceptors that are activated is much higher than that of those that are depressed. (From Mense, 1993, with modifications)

local tissue damage with alterations of the microstructure of the muscle fibers (Armstrong et al., 1983; Sjöström and Friden, 1984; Jones et al., 1987, 1990; Larsson et al., 1990; Henriksson et al., 1993). Degenerative and inflammatory alterations have been observed in the induction of DOMS after eccentric muscle contraction (Newham et al., 1983; Newham, 1984; Stauber et al., 1990; Faulkner et al., 1990) (Fig. 3.**13**). A significant increase of plasma creatine kinase was observed in humans after repetitive eccentric muscle contractions in the lower (Newham et al., 1983) and upper (Clarkson and Trem-

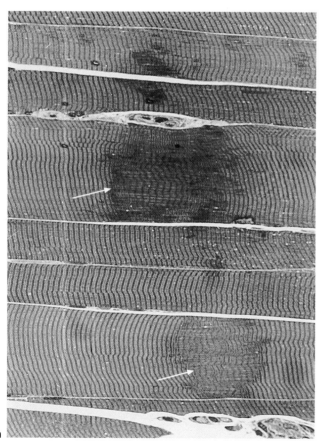

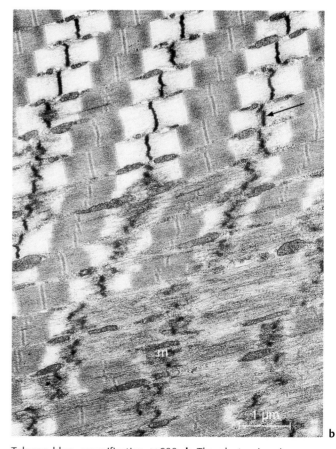

a

b

Fig. 3.**13** **Biopsy of soleus muscle of a young man after prolonged intense eccentric contraction followed by delayed muscular pain. a** The optical microscope shows numerous focal alterations of the striated fibers, particularly extensive in some of them (arrows).

Toluene blue, magnification ×600. **b** The electronic microscope shows that these alterations originate from the Z bands, which appear dilated (arrow), deformed and interrupted in places. m, mytochondria. (From Sjöström and Friden, 1984, with permission)

blay, 1988) limbs. Similarly, Hutchings et al. (1995) reported a significant increase of plasma creatine kinase of mice after repetitive masseter eccentric contractions.

In conclusion, different mechanisms may determine craniofacial pain of myogenic origin. Pain in the short term during a prolonged isometric contraction may be a protective mechanism related to the fact that in the mandible elevator muscles the fast contracting fatigue-resistant (type IIA) fibers are few (Mao et al., 1992; Mao, 1993). This mechanism may be both central and peripheral (with stimulation of the usually *silent* nociceptors (Mense, 1991, 1993). Subacute pain is probably a consequense of local acidosis due to the oxygen debt; this, as we have seen, may be accompanied by muscle contraction. Finally, the delayed pain is probably explained by the mechanisms of DOMS described above: this applies in particular, as we will see, to the *trigger points* that are frequently found in the craniocervical muscles.

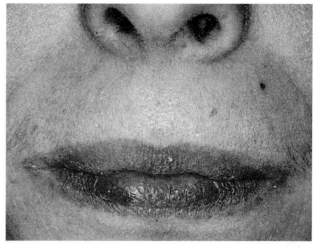

Fig. 3.**14**   Labial seal with excessive perioral muscle contraction

Muscle Hyperactivity and Parafunction

Within the craniofacial, neck and shoulder muscles, hyperfunction and/or parafunction are common. In some situations, hyperactivity may be of some functional significance. For instance, individuals with morphological characteristics deviating from normal may increase muscle activity to decrease the effects of the malformation. Thus, some subjects with tooth malposition maintain lip seal by continuous acti-

vation of the circumoral muscles for much of the day (Fig. 3.**14**); others with mandibular micrognathism keep the mandible in a protracted position by activating the lateral pterygoid muscles (Fig. 3.**15**) (Yemm et al., 1978; Yemm, 1979). Similarly, postural problems, which will be discussed later, often lead to hyperfunction of the neck musculature.

However, parafunctional muscle activities without functional significance are frequent. Teeth clenching during

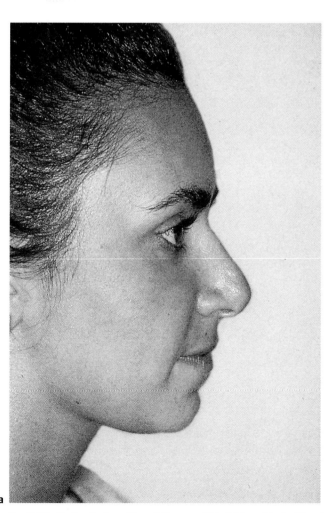

a

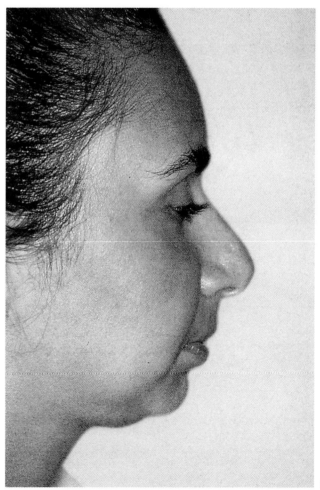

b

Fig. 3.**15**   Protracted position of the mandible (**a**) in subject with micromandibolism (**b**). (From Mongini, 1984)

day and/or night results in excessive and prolonged isometric contraction of the masseter and temporal muscles. Hyperactivity of these muscles, together with that of the lateral pterygoid muscles, is also present in bruxism, a very common problem among subjects of all ages with or without craniofacial pain (Reding, 1966; Dubner et al., 1978; Rugh and Solberg, 1979; Solberg et al., 1979; Glaros, 1981; Clarke and Townsend, 1984; Rugh and Harlan, 1988; Okeson et al., 1990, 1991; Widmalm et al., 1955).

Other parafunctional habits include tongue thrust (Fig. 3.**16**), nail biting (Fig. 3.**17**) or lip biting (Fig. 3.**18**), and sustained contraction of the frontal muscles (Fig. 3.**19**). Hyperfunction of the neck muscles is frequently observed in subjects under stress, with consequent decrease or loss of the cervical curvature.

On inspection, a sign of muscle parafunction may be hypertrophy of the masseter or the temporal or both muscles (Figs 3.**20**–3.**22**). Muscle palpation may elicit pain and reveal sites of muscle contraction and trigger points (see below).

When the mandible is in a position of posture, the activity of the elevator muscles (masseter, temporal, medial pterygoid) may vary (Fig. 3.**23**). Some researchers state that the activity of such muscles in the postural position of the mandible is normally minimal (Shpuntoff and Shpuntoff, 1956; Hickey et al. 1961). On the other hand, spontaneous muscular activity has been reported by several authors (Kawamura and Fujimoto, 1957; Rugh and Drago, 1981; Manns et al., 1981) and it has been shown that in this position, activity is indeed higher than the minimum muscle activity (Rugh and Drago, 1981; Manns et al., 1981) (Fig. 3.**24**).

As previously stated, the postural portion of the mandible is conditioned by the jaw-closing or stretch reflex, among other factors: stimulation of the neuromuscular spindles of the elevator muscles as a consequence of mandibular drop leads to reflex contraction of these muscles (Fig. 3.**7**). During situations of stress, an increase of the gamma activity may in-

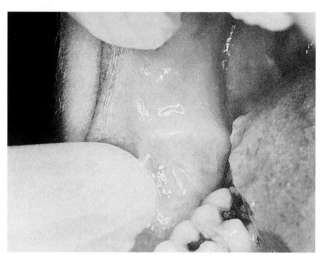

Fig. 3.**16**   Typical festooning of the lingual border due to prolonged lingual pressure against the tooth arches

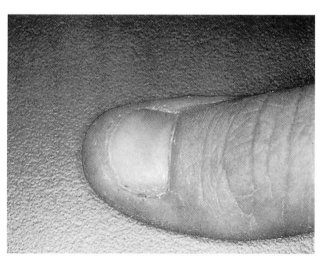

Fig. 3.**17**   Thumb of nail-biting patient

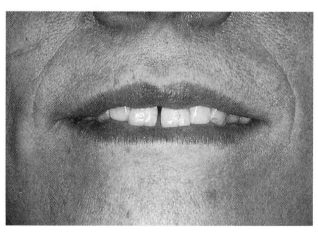

Fig. 3.**18**   Biting of lower lip

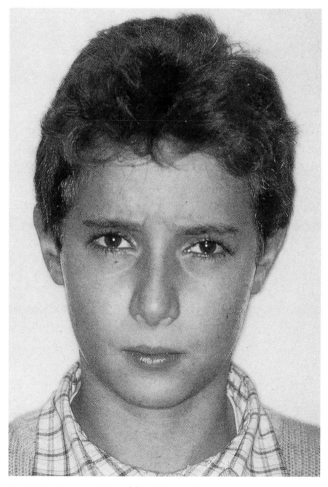

Fig. 3.**19**   Hyperactivity of frontal muscles

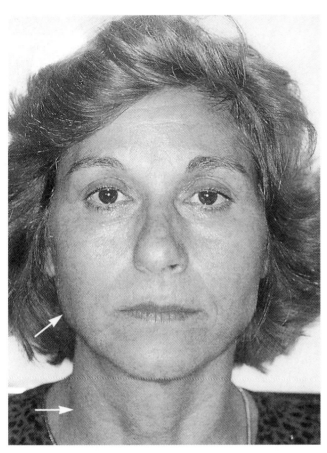

Fig. 3.**20 Hyperactivity of cervical and craniomandibular muscles.** The arrows indicate the hypertrophic sternocleidomastoid and masseter muscles

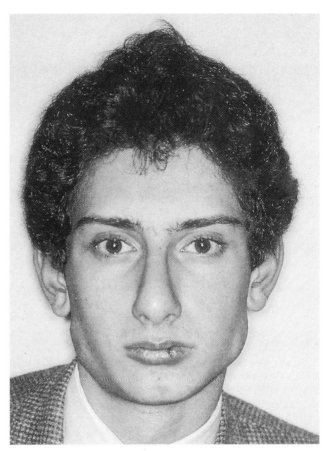

Fig. 3.**21** Marked hypertrophy of the masseters in patient with pronounced muscular hyperparafunction

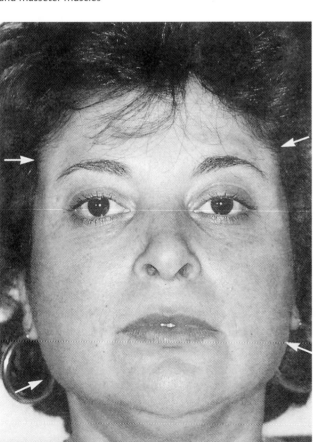

Fig. 3.**22** Hypertrophy of the masseter and temporal muscles (arrows) due to parafunction

crease the reaction to stretch, leading to an increase of elevator muscle activity, independent of the above-mentioned parafunctions, and consequently to a change in the postural position of the mandible. However, EMG studies on the resting level activity of craniomandibular muscle in patients with muscle pain led to controversial results (see Lund and Widmer, 1989, for a review). Several authors state that in these patients a postural hyperactivity is present (Copeland, 1954; Perry, 1957; Franks, 1965; De Vries, 1966; Lous et al., 1970; Griffin and Munro, 1971; Möller et al., 1971; Chaco, 1973; Cobb et al., 1975; Möller, 1985; Sheikholeslam, 1985; Gervais et al., 1989) or, at least, can be more easily induced than in normal subjects by stressful conditions (Perry et al., 1960; Yemm, 1969a, b, 1971; Mercuri et al., 1979; Dahlstrom et al., 1985; Rugh and Montgomery, 1987; Kapel et al., 1989; Flor et al., 1991); other authors (Majewski and Gale, 1984; Carlson et al., 1993) reject this hypothesis.

During a test performance, postural muscle activity may be normal, but it might increase if the test becomes particularly hard (Yemm, 1969b). This activity may also increase at certain times of the day or week, as has been shown by experiments using portable EMG devices (Rugh and Solberg, 1979). Muscle fatigue and contraction could follow: this is, as we have seen, a situation in which the muscle is electrically silent but cannot decontract because of lack of ATP. This would explain observations made in other studies that the ability of painful muscle to contract forcefully is reduced (Molin, 1972; Sheikholeslam et al., 1980).

The relation between parafunction, fatigue of the craniofacial muscles and tension-type headache is still debated. As we have seen (see Chapter 1), the classification of the International Headache Society (1991) makes a distinction be-

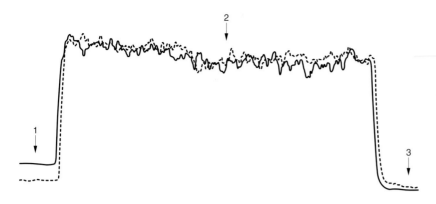

Fig. 3.**23**   Mean electromyographic activity of the right (broken line) and left masseter (solid line) before (1), during (2) and after (3) prolonged isometric contraction. Note that after isometric contraction, postural activity of the two masseters is much reduced. (From Mongini, 1984, with modifications)

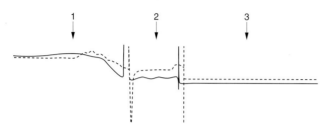

Fig. 3.**24**   Mean EMG activity of masseter muscles during posture (1), after a biofeedback session (2) and after a training autogenous session (3). Note that in posture activity is much higher than in the other conditions. (From Mongini, 1984, with modifications)

tween "tension-type headache *with and without* disorders of the pericranial muscles." This is because a relationship between muscle tenderness and headache severity is not always found. On the other hand, an increase of tenderness of the pericranial muscles in patients with tension-type headache compared with asymptomatic subjects was demonstrated by accurate double blind studies (Langemark and Olesen 1987; Hatch et al., 1992; Jensen et al., 1993; Lipchik et al., 1997). Moreover, muscle tenderness increases during the cephalalgic attacks (Jensen, 1990, 1996). It has also been demonstrated that the EMG activity of the temporal muscle of patients with tension-type headache, as examined in the intercritical periods, is higher than the activity of headache-free subjects (Jensen et al., 1994; Jensen, 1996). Mongini et al. (1997) have observed in patients with tension-type headache a higher prevalence of muscle elevator hypertrophy with respect to patients with other headache types (Fig. 3.**25**). Attacks of tension-type headache may be induced by prolonged tooth clench (Jensen and Olesen, 1996). Gay et al. (1994) have observed that the masseter and temporal muscles of patients with myogenic facial pain show a lower endurance and a higher decrease of signal frequency.

Similarly, there is a great variety of opinions whether hyperfunctional and parafunctional activities may produce TMJ intracapsular alterations. Several authors maintain that bruxism and the consequent dental attrition are etiological factors of dysfunction (Laskin, 1969; Christiansen, 1970; Randow et al., 1976; Keith, 1983; Moss and Garret, 1984; Allen et al., 1990; Lieberman et al., 1985; Ash, 1986; De Laat, 1986; Lundh et al., 1987; Runge, 1989; Parker, 1990), while others doubt about the existence of a strict cause – effect relationship between the two factors (Lederman and Clayton, 1982; Droukas et al., 1984; Seligman and Pullinger, 1989; Meng et al., 1987; Roberts et al., 1987; Seligman et al., 1988 a, b; De Kanter et al., 1989).

Different mechanisms may be hypothesized as to how muscle hyperfunction and parafunction may induce TMJ dys-

function. Prolonged daily and nightly tooth grinding, with excessive anteroposterior and/or lateral mandibular and condylar movement, may lead to stretching and tearing of the joint capsule and ligaments and, eventually, to consequent disk displacement. Moreover, bruxing habits over the years may lead to severe tooth wear and consequent alterations of the jaw relationship, and thus a "structural factor" (see Chapter 4) (Fig. 3.**26**).

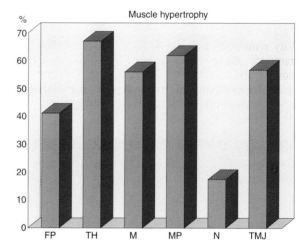

Fig. 3.**25**   Prevalence of hypertrophy of the mandible elevator muscles in patients with tension-type headache (TH), migraine (M), facial pain disorder (FP), myogenic pain (MP), trigeminal neuralgia (N) and TMJ dysfunction (TMJ). (From Mongini et al., 1997)

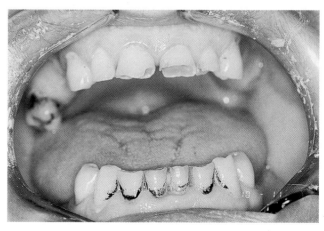

Fig. 3.**26   Severe dental attrition consequent on chronic tooth grinding in an elderly woman with depressive disorder and chronic daily headache.** Parafunction has, in turn, produced an aggravation of the alteration of the jaw structure

Muscle Dysfunction and TMJ Disorders

Animal experiments have given evidence that TMJ intracapsular lesions may provoke direct muscle function alterations with increased contraction activity in the jaw elevators. An increase of EMG activity at the ipsilateral anterior digastric temporals and genioglossus muscles was observed by Broton and Sessle (1988) after injection of algesic chemicals (7 % NaCl, KCl and histamine) into the joint of an anesthetized cat. Such findings were confirmed by Yu et al. (1992) after mustard oil injection in the TMJ of a rat. The authors concluded that "increased activity of jaw muscles may be associated with TM inflammatory condition and may serve to protect the masticatory system from potentially damaging movements and stimuli." This EMG response is probably mediated by central and peripheral NMDA receptors (Yu et al., 1996) and NK-1 and NK-2 tachykinin receptors (Bakke et al., 1998).

A number of authors have described patterns of EMG activity alterations as a consequence of TMJ disorders in man (Möller, 1970; Bessette et al., 1971; Bessette and Shatkin, 1979; De Laat et al., 1985).

Mongini et al. (1986, 1989) studied the different parameters of masticatory function in normal individuals and patients with TMJ dysfunction, using a system which allowed simultaneous assessment of mandibular movements and velocity and EMG activity of the elevator muscles.

In a healthy individual, habitual mastication is a rhythmic activity with different envelopes of motion that alternate characteristically in each subject (Fig. 3.**27**). When mean data of movements and EMG activity of the mandibular elevators are examined, a typical pattern can be observed. During mouth opening, activity of these muscles is minimal, with a slight increase in the last phase of opening. During closing, two phases may be distinguished: during the first half of closing there is a parallel increase in velocity of movements and EMG activity, indicating that the muscle contraction pattern is prevalently isotonic in this phase. In the second half of closing, however, muscle contraction increases further, while velocity decreases (Fig. 3.**28**). In this phase, the muscle contraction is predominantly isometric, and pressure is applied to the bolus and the TMJ.

Where TMJ lesions are present, several alterations of the masticatory parameters are observed. In particular, movements tend to be repetitive and deviated toward the lesion side (Fig. 3.**29**). In addition, a general restriction of movements is observed, and the isometric phase of muscle contrac-

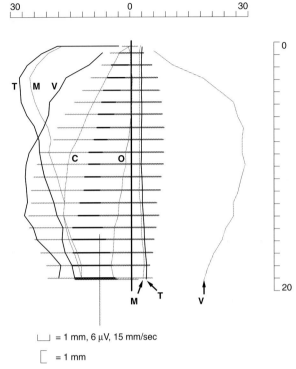

$$\llcorner\lrcorner = 1 \text{ mm, } 6 \text{ μV, } 15 \text{ mm/sec}$$

$$\ulcorner = 1 \text{ mm}$$

Fig. 3.**28 Mean masticatory movements, velocity and EMG activity in a group of healthy subjects.** O, opening movement; C, closing movement; V, velocity; M, EMG activity of the masseter; T, EMG activity of the temporal. The movements are reported on the frontal plane. V, M and T on the right refer to values during opening; on the left to values during closing. Note how the EMG activity and velocity are roughly parallel in the first half of the closing movement whereas they diverge in the second half. Further explanation is given in the text. (From Mongini et al., 1986)

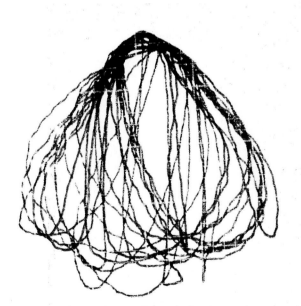

Fig. 3.**27 Movements of the mandible viewed in the frontal plane in a normal subject.** Note how, despite the variability of movements, these are distributed in a relatively symmetrical manner. (From Monigini et al., 1986)

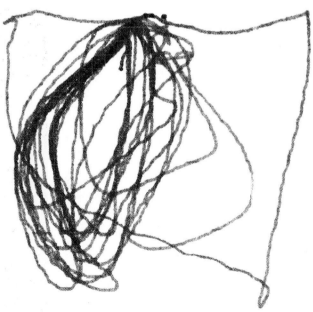

Fig. 3.**29 Subject with intracapsular lesion of the right TMJ.** The masticatory movements appear limited, deviated to the side of the lesion and more repetitive

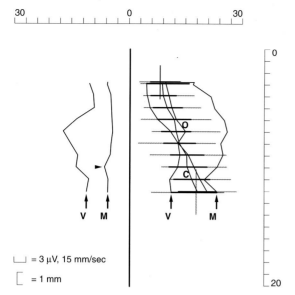

```
30            0           30
```

= 3 µV, 15 mm/sec

= 1 mm

Fig. 3.**30** **Movements, velocity and EMG activity during mastication in a subject with disk displacement without reduction of the right TMJ.** Symbols used are as in Fig. 3.**28**. Note how the opening (O) and closing (C) movements deviate to the lesion side and are very limited. Also note that the EMG activity of the masseter on closing is parallel to the velocity during the entire closing movement. This indicates that the phase normally present of predominantly isometric muscle contraction (see Fig. 3.**28**) is here suppressed. During opening, the same muscle shows above-normal activity (arrow). (From Mongini et al., 1989)

tion tends to be reduced or suppressed (Fig. 3.**30**). This can be due to a protective mechanism aimed at suppressing load on the impaired joint. Finally, a definitive increase of EMG activity of the muscle elevators *during opening* is observed (Fig. 3.**30**). In other words, there seems to be a shift from a mechanism of *reciprocal innervation* to a *co-contraction,* during which the elevator muscles undergo eccentric con-

traction (this is contraction and elongation at the same time because the action of the jaw-depressing muscles prevails). This functional situation makes it easier to perform sudden movement, stops or deviations, which might be required by the impaired joint. But, as mentioned, this could induce mechanical damage to the muscle and *delayed onset muscle soreness* as a consequence.

Tender and Trigger Points

Localized spots tender on palpation are frequent in the muscles. These *tender points* should be kept separate from the *trigger points* (TPs), which are muscle sites of fairly constant location, exquisitely more tender on palpation than adjacent areas. Objectively, one may feel a nodule or a "taut fiber band." Typically, palpation may elicit a twitch response and produces a referred pain in characteristic sites (Simons, 1988). The pressure tolerance threshold is markedly reduced (Fischer, 1986; Reeves et al., 1986; Fischer, 1988). Irritability of trigger points may be intense or average, or they may be *latent* (Simons, 1988; Vecchiet et al., 1990). In patients with intense painful symptomatology and with very irritable trigger points, the pain in the target area is present in the skin, in the subcutaneous area and in the muscle layer, whereas in patients with more limited symptomatogy, the pain may be confined to the muscle layer (Vecchiet et al., 1991, 1993). Limited hyperthermic zones are frequently observed in relation to trigger points (Fischer and Chang, 1986; Mongini et al., 1990). These areas may be surrounded by hypothermic bands (Mongini et al., 1990) (Figs 3.**31**, 3.**32**).

TPs are a frequent finding in head and neck muscles and, hence, they represent a fairly common source of craniofacial pain. Detailed descriptions have been provided which are actual maps of the sites of pain localization of the referred pain (Travell and Simons, 1983; Simons, 1988). Thus the trigger points in the masseter muscle may reflect pain in the cheeks, teeth, or ear (Fig. 3.**33**); in the temporal muscle, they may pro-

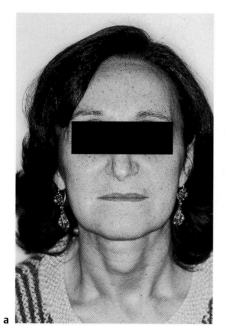

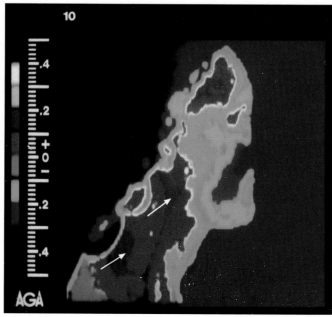

Fig. 3.**31**   **Patient with cervical and craniofacial pain. a** Note the contraction of the sternocleidomastoid muscles. **b** On thermography, highly hyperthermic sites (in red) are observed on the sternocleidomastoid and trapezius muscles (arrows). These sites correspond to trigger points that on palpation produce pain locally and in different craniofacial areas

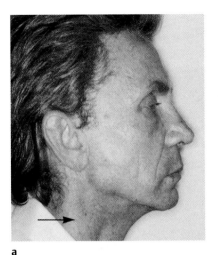

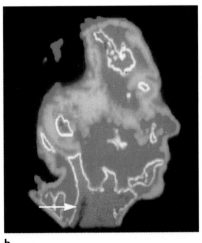

Fig. 3.32 Patient with postural defects and cervicofacial pain. a Hypertrophy of sterno-cleidomastoid muscle (arrow). **b** Thermography shows hyperthermic areas at neck (arrow) related to trigger points of the sternocleido-mastoid muscle

a **b**

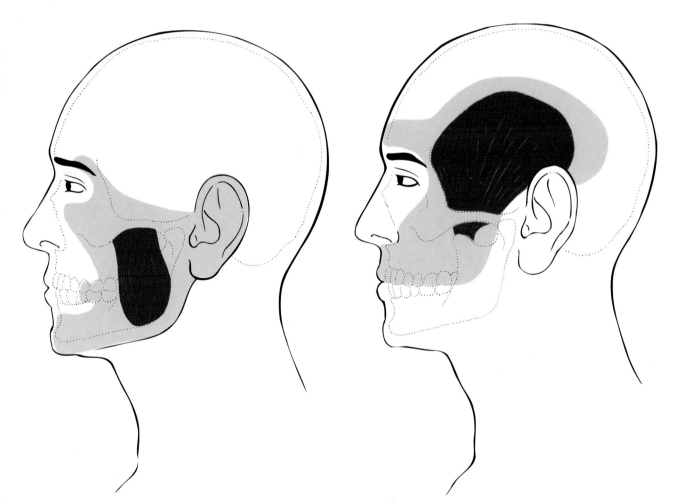

Fig. 3.**33** Areas of possible referred pain from the masseter muscle

Fig. 3.**34** Areas of possible referred pain from the temporal muscle

voke referred pain to the upper jaw or the orbit, and may cause a periorbital or temporal headache (Fig. 3.**34**). Referred pain of TPs in the lateral pterygoid muscle may be in the anteroauricular region, thus simulating pain due to dysfunction of the temporomandibular joint (Fig. 3.**35**). In the neck, TPs are frequent in the sternocleidomastoid muscle, where taut bands may easily be palpated under the skin. Referred pain may be periorbital, or located in the vertex or the front (Fig. 3.**36**). TPs are also often found in the trapezoid muscle,

and may project pain to the temporal area and/or the corner of the mandible. These indications must nevertheless be considered with some care, in the light of the marked variations which may be found among patients and the possible diversity of evaluation among clinicians (McCain, 1993 a). In fact, in blind studies trigger points have shown a low interrater reproducibility and the presence of false positives in healthy subjects (Wolfe et al., 1992; Nice et al., 1992; Bohr, 1995). Interrater reproducibility improves when the examiners have

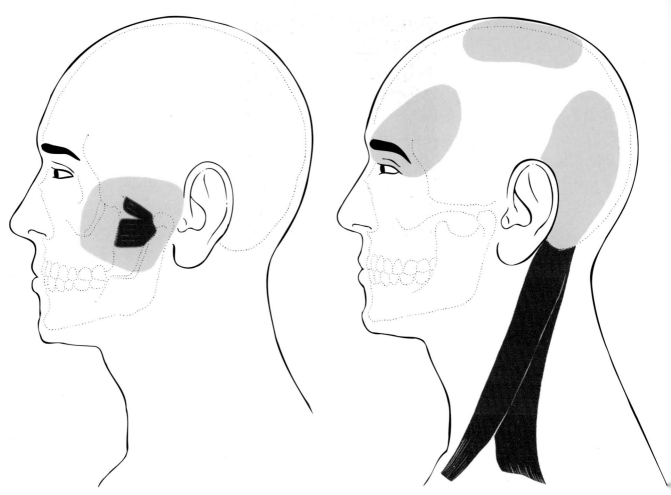

Fig. 3.**35** Areas of referred pain from the lateral pterygoid muscle

Fig. 3.**36** Areas of referred pain from the sternocleidomastoid muscle

previously attended theoretical and practical training sessions (Gerwin et al., 1997). Furthermore, an almost identical situation may be found in cases of pain originating from a zygoapophyseal joint among the cervical vertebrae (Aprill et al., 1990; Dwyer et al., 1990; Bogduk and Aprill, 1993). Some 80% of posttraumatic cervical pain (in particular after whiplash) is due to the injury of such joints (Aprill and Bogduk, 1992).

Tender points and trigger points can be caused by muscle overloading, either acute or chronic (Simons, 1988). As we have seen, this overloading, especially if due to eccentric contractions, may lead to lesions of the muscle fibers (Stauber et al., 1990; Larsson et al., 1990; Henriksson et al., 1993). Mense (1987, 1991, 1993) hypothesizes that the consequent liberation of vasoactive substances (prostaglandin, bradykinin, histamine, etc.) provokes local edema and, in consequence, a disorder of the microcirculation and ischemia. A reduction of ATP, with localized and persistent contraction, would follow. Stimulation of the nociceptive endings (made more excitable by the ischemia) would cause local pain (Fig. 3.**37**).

Muscle overloading is frequently found in the craniocervicofacial muscles. As we will see (Chapter 4), these muscles play an important role in the posture of the head respect to the neck and the shoulders. They are therefore involved in all posture alterations of these structures.

Furthermore, functional overload may result from the hyperfunctional and parafunctional activities previously described. This is true for the craniomandibular muscles (as in

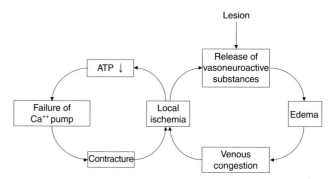

Fig. 3.**37** Possible formation mechanism of muscular trigger points. (From Mense, 1993, with modifications)

bruxism and tooth clenching) and for the craniocervical muscles, which may become contracted, thus leading to decrease or loss of the cervical curvature. Moreover, bruxing movements lead to lengthening of the mandibular elevator muscles while they are contracted. In these situations one may assume that, besides pain consequent on muscle fatigue, sudden additional effort may provoke microlesions and tender and trigger points (Christensen and Hutchings, 1992).

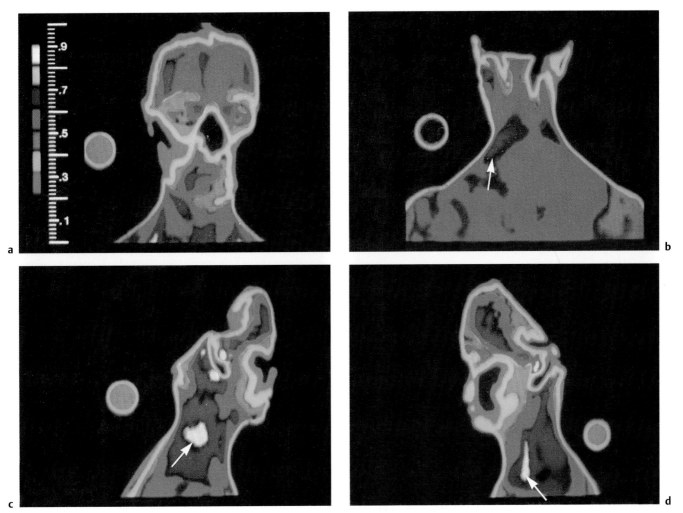

Fig. 3.38 Patient suffering from primary fibromyalgia. Thermography shows hyperthermic zones (arrows) corresponding to trigger points

Primary Fibromyalgia and Myofascial Pain Syndrome

Primary fibromyalgia is a systemic disorder of the skin and muscles whose classification is still uncertain, and which has gained particular importance in recent years (Yunus et al., 1981; Campbell et al., 1983; Wolfe et al. 1985, 1992; Goldenberg, 1987; Merskey, 1993; Wall, 1993; Wolfe, 1993). This condition, which mainly affects women, is characterized by a generalized muscle pain and by many muscle points painful to palpation (Fig. 3.38). In the muscles of these patients, alterations have been found that suggest a peripheral origin of the pain. These alterations are abnormal tissue oxygenation, changes in collagen, and alterations of muscle morphology (Bengtsson et al., 1986 a, b, c; Henriksson, 1988; Henriksson and Bengtsson, 1991; Henriksson et al., 1993). Among the latter, the presence of "ragged fibers" has been described in particular (Fig. 3.39), although, as we have seen, these may also be observed in other patients. They are due to mitochondrial proliferations and accumulation at the periphery of the myocells: this phenomenon might compensate for an alteration of the oxidative metabolism or for a state of hypoxia of the muscle tissue (Bengtsson et al., 1986b, Henriksson et al., 1993). Other authors reject the hypothesis that fibromyalgia is a distinctive entity. They speculate that, for instance, numerous painful sites in these patients are not specific but correspond to those of rheumatoid arthritis (McCain, 1993a, b),

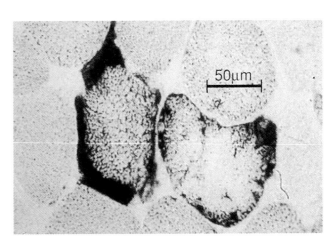

Fig. 3.39 Muscle fiber alteration that may be found in primary fibromyalgia. The excessive accumulation of mitochondria (dark areas on the edges of the myofibrils) causes a characteristic "ragged fiber" appearance. Stained with succinate dehydrogenase. (From Henriksson et al., 1993, with permission)

and that even sites that are not considered to be standard for tender points may elicit more pain at palpation than in normal subjects (Bohr, 1996). It has also been underlined that tenderness is frequently accompanied by shortening of the axial and limb muscles and consequent myogenous pain and

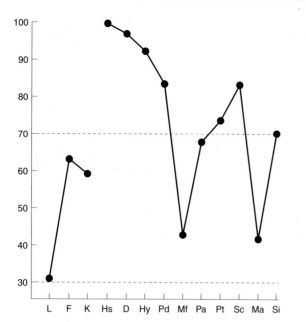

Fig. 3.**40**   **The same patient as in Fig. 3.28.** The MMPI psychological profile shows elevation of the neurotic scales and of several psychotic scales (see Chapters 8 and 10)

pain consequent on pulling upon tendons and ligaments (Gunn, 1990). Shortening of paraspinal muscles may, in turn, compress the intervertebral disk and irritate the nerve root (Gunn, 1995). Finally, some EEG sleep alterations described in these patients (with alpha waves superimposed over delta waves) (Moldofsky, 1986, 1989a, b, c) are found in other conditions, such as nocturnal myoclonus, periodic prolonged apnea and rheumatoid arthritis (McCain, 1993a).

Many authors stress the importance of psychogenic and psychosocial factors in the etiopathogenesis of this disorder (Payne et al., 1982; Ahles et al., 1984; Wolfe et al., 1984; Ellersten et al., 1991, 1993; Wolfe, 1998) (Fig. 3.**40**). Frequently these are patients suffering from simple phobia, social phobia, generalized anxiety disorders, somatization, etc., disorders that were present before the onset of pain (Hudson and Pope, 1989; Hudson et al., 1992; Bradley, 1993).

Fibromyalgia must be distinguished from the *myofascial pain syndrome*. The most important distinctive criterion is the presence of tender points and of aspecific and generalized pain accounting for a generalized disturbance of pain modulation in fibromyalgia (Wolfe, 1998; Morris et al., 1998; Weigent et al., 1998) with respect to regional trigger points, and taut bands and local and stereotypical referred pain in the myofascial pain syndrome. This pathology is strictly regional, trigger points are an element that further characterizes it, and the prognosis is definitely better (McCain, 1993a, b; Vecchiet et al., 1994). When this syndrome is located in the craniocervical area it is often ascribed to the group of pathologies generically referred to as *craniomandibular dysfunctions*. This, as we have seen in Chapter 1, does note seem justified by rational criteria.

References

Ahles T.A., Yunus M.B., Riley S.D., Bradley J.M., Masi A.T., *Psychological factors associated with primary fibromyalgia syndrome*, Arthritis Rheum., 1984, 27 : 1101 – 1106.

Allen J.D., Rivera-Morales W.C., Zwemer J.D., *The occurence of temporomandibular disorder symptoms in healthy young adults with and without evidence of bruxism*, Cranio, 1990, 8 : 312 – 318.

Aprill C., Bogduk N., *The prevalence of cervical zygapophysial joint pain: a first approximation*, Spine, 1992, 17 : 744 – 747.

Aprill C., Dwyer A., Bogduk N., *Cervical zygapophyseal joint pain patterns*, II., A clinical evaluation, Spine, 1990, 15 : 458 – 461.

Armstrong R., Ogilvie R., Schwane J., *Eccentric exercise-induced injury to rat skeletal muscle*, Appl. Physiol., 1983, 54 : 80 – 93.

Ash M.M., *Current concepts in the aetiology, diagnosis and treatment of TMJ and muscle dysfunction*, J. Oral Rehabil., 1986, 13 : 1 – 20.

Asmussen E., *Muscle fatigue*, Med. Sci. Sports, 1979, 11 : 313 – 321.

Astrand P.O., Rodahl K., *Textbook of work physiology, Physiological bases of exercise*, McGraw-Hill, 1986.

Bakke M., Hu J.W., Sessle B.J., *Involvement of NK-1 and NK-2 tachykinin receptor mechanisms in jaw muscle activity reflexly evoked by inflammatory irritant application to the rat in the temporomandibular joint*, Pain, 1998, 75(2 – 3):219 – 227.

Barcroft J., Millen J.L.E., *Blood flow through muscle during sustained contraction*, J. Physiol., 1939, 97 : 17 – 31.

Basmajian J.V., De Luca C.J., *Muscles alive: Their functions as revealed by electromyography*, (5 th ed.), Williams Wilkins, Baltimore, 1985.

Bengtsson A., Henriksson K.G., Jorfeldt L., Kagedal B., Lennmarken C., Lindstrom F., *Primary fibromyalgia. A clinical and laboratory study of 55 patients*, Scand. J. Rheumatol., 1986a, 15 : 340 – 347.

Bengtsson A., Henriksson K.G., Larsson J., *Reduced high-energy phosphate levels in the painful muscles of patients with primary fibromyalgia*, Arthritis Rheum., 1986b, 29 : 817 – 821.

Bengtsson A., Henriksson K.G., Larsson J., *Muscle biopsy in primary fibromyalgia. Light-microscopical and histochemical findings*, Scand. J. Rheumatol., 1986c, 15 : 1 – 6.

Bessette R., Bishop B., Mohl N., *Duration of masseter silent period in patients with TMJ-syndrome*, J. Appl. Physiol., 1971, 216 : 16 – 21.

Bessette R.W., Shatkin S.S., *Predicting by electromyography the results of nonsurgical treatment of temporomandibular joint syndrome*, Plast. Reconstr. Surg., 1979, 64 : 232 – 238.

Bessou P., Laporte Y., *Étude des récepteurs musculaires innervés par les fibres afférentes du groupe III (fibres myélinisées fines) chez le chat*, Arch. Ital. Biol., 1961, 99 : 293 – 321.

Bigland-Ritchie B., *EMG/Force relations and fatigue of human voluntary contractions*, Exerc. Sport Sci. Rev., 1981, 9 : 75 – 117.

Bogduk N., Aprill C., *On the nature of neck pain, discography and cervical zygapophysial joint blocks*, Pain, 1993, 54 : 213 – 217.

Bohr T.W., *Fibromyalgia and myofascial pain syndrome: do they exist?*, Neurol. Clin. North Am., 1995, 13 : 365 – 381.

Bohr T.W., *Problems with myofascial pain syndrome and fibromyalgia syndrome*, Neurology, 1996, 46 : 593 – 597.

Bonde-Petersen F., Christensen L.V., *Blood flow in human temporal muscle during tooth grinding and clenching as measured by 133 xenon clearance*, Scand. J. Dent. Res., 1973, 81 : 272 – 275.

Bowley J.F., Gale E.N., *Experimental masticatory muscle pain*, J. Dent. Res., 1987, 66 : 1765 – 1769.

Bradley L., in: Wolfe F., *Fibromyalgia program*, 7 th World Congress on Pain, IASP Publications, Seattle, 1993, 607, (abs.).

Brazeau G., Watts S., Mathews L., *Role of calcium and arachidonic acid metabolites in creatine kinase from isolated rat skeletal muscles damaged by organic cosolvents*, J. Parenter. Sci. Technol., 1992, 46 : 25 – 30.

Broton J.G. and Sessle B.J., *Reflex excitation of masticatory muscles induced by algesic chemicals applied to the temporomandibular joint of the cat*, Arch. Oral. Biol., 1988, 33 : 741 – 747.

Campbell S.M., Clark S., Tindall E.A., Forehand M.E., Bennett R.M., *Clinical characteristics of fibrositis*, I: A controlled study of symptoms and tender points, Arthritis Rheum., 1983, 26 : 817 – 824.

Carlson C.R. Okeson J.P., Falace D.A., Nitz A.J., Currans S.L., Anderson D., *Comparison of psychologic and physiologic functioning between patients with masticatory muscle pain and matched controls*, J. Orofac. Pain, 1993, 7 : 15 – 22.

Chaco J., *Electromyography of the masseter muscles in Costen's syndrome*, J. Oral Med., 1973, 28 : 45 – 46.

Christensen L.V., *Jaw muscle fatigue and pains induced by experimental tooth clenching: a review*, J. Oral Rehabil., 1981, 8 : 27 – 36.

Christensen L.V., Hutchings M.O., *Methodological observations on positive and negative work (teeth grinding) by human jaw muscles*, J. Oral Rehabil., 1992, 19 : 399 – 411.

Christiansen J., *Effect of occlusion-raising procedure on the chewing system*, Dent. Pract., 1970, 20:233–238.

Clark G.T., Carter M.C., *Electromyographic study of human jaw-closing muscle endurance, fatigue and recovery at variousisometric force levels*, Arch. Oral Biol., 1985, 30:563–569.

Clark G.T., Carter M.C., Beemsterboer P.L., *Analysis of electromyographic signals in human jaw closing muscles at various isometric force levels*, Arch. Oral Biol., 1988, 33:833–837.

Clark G.T., Jow R.W., Lee J.J., *Pain and stiffness levels after repeated maximum voluntary clencing*, J. Dent. Res., 1989, 69–71.

Clark G.T., Adler R.C., Lee J.J., *Jaw pain and tenderness levels after repeated sustained maximum voluntary protrusion*, Pain, 1991, 45:17–22.

Clarke N.G., Townsend G.C., *Distribution of nocturnal bruxing patterns in man*, J. Oral. Rehabil., 1984, 11:529–534.

Clarkson P., Tremblay I., *Exercise-induced muscle damage, repair, and adaptation in humans*, J. Appl. Physiol., 1988, 65:1–6.

Cobb C.R., De Vries H.A., Urban R.T., Luekens C.A., Bagg R.J., *Electrical activity in muscle pain*, Am. J. Phys. Med., 1975, 54:80–87.

Cooper S., *Muscle spindle and other muscle receptors*, in: Bourne G.H. (ed.), *The structure and function of muscle*, Academic Press, New York, 1960, 381–420.

Copeland J., *Abnormal muscle tension and the mandibular joint*, Dent. Rec., 1954, 74:331–335.

Dahlstrom L., Carlsson S.G., Gale E.N., Jansson T.G., *Stress-induced muscular activity in mandibular dysfunction: Effects of biofeedback training*, J. Behav. Med., 1985, 8:191–200.

De Kanter R.J.A.M., Van Bladel A.J.W.P., Partman S.R.K., Van 'T Hof M.A., *Mandibular dysfunction and attrition, age and sex influences*, J. Dent. Res., 1989, 68, 4:(Spec. Issue) 635.

De Laat A., Van der Glas H.W., Weytjens J.L.F., Van Steenberghe D., *The masseteric post-stimulus electromyographic-complex in people with dysfunction of the mandibular joint*, Arch. Oral Biol., 1985, 30:177–180.

De Laat A., Van Steenberghe D., Lesaffre E., *Occlusal relationships and temporomandibular joint dysfunction. II: Correlations between occlusal and articular parameters and symptoms of TMJ dysfunction by means of stepwise logistic regression*, J. Prosthet. Dent., 1986, 55:116–121.

De Vries H.A., *Quantitative electromyographic investigation of the spasm theory of muscle pain*, Am. J. Phys. Med., 1966, 45:119–134.

Direnfeld V., *Muscle endurance test in patients with temporomandibular joint dysfunction*, MS Thesis, University of Illinois Medical Center, 1967.

Droukas B., Lindee C., Carlsson G.E., *Relationship between occlusal factors and signs and symptoms of mandibular dysfunction*, Acta Odontol. Scand., 1984, 42:277–283.

Dubner R., Sessle B.J., Storey A.T., *The neural basis of oral and facial function*, Plenum Press, New York, 1978.

Duxbury A.J., Hughes D.F., Clark D.E., *Power spectral distribution of the masseter electromyogram from surface electrodes*, J. Oral Rehabil., 1976, 3:333–339.

Dwyer A., Aprill C., Bogduk N., *Cervical zygapophyseal joint pain patterns, I. A study in normal volunteers*, Spine, 1990, 15:453–457.

Edwards R.H.T., Hill D.K., McDonnell M., *Myothermal and intramuscular pressure measurements during isometric contraction of the human quadriceps muscle*, J. Physiol., 1972, 224:58–59.

Edwards R.H.T., *Physiological analysis of skeletal muscle weakness and fatigue*, Clin. Sci. Mol. Med., 1978, 54:463–470.

Edwards R.H.T., *Muscle fatigue and pain*, Acta Med. Scand. Suppl., 1985, 711:179–188.

Edwards R.H.T., *Interaction of chemical with electromechanical factors in human skeletal muscle fatigue*, Acta Physiol. Scand., 1986, 128:149–155.

Ellertsen B., Vaeröy H., Endresen I., Förre O., *MMPI in fibromyalgia and local nonspecific myalgia*, New Trends Exp. Clin. Psychiatry, 1991, 7:53–62.

Ellertsen B., Troland K., Vaeröy H., *Psychological assessment of patients with musculoskeletal pain*, in: Vaeröy H., Merskey H. (eds.), *Progress in fibromyalgia and myofascial pain*, Elsevier Amsterdam, 1993, 93–99.

Eriksson P.O., Thornell L.E., *Histochemical and morphological muscle-fiber characteristics of human masseter, the medical pterygoid and the temporal muscles*, Arch. Oral Biol., 1983, 28:781.

Faulkner J.A., Zerba E., Brooks S.V., *Contraction-induced injury to skeletal muscle tibers*, in: Sutton J.R., Coates G., Remmers J.E. (eds.), *Hypoxia: The adaptations*, B.C. Decker Inc., Philadelphia, 1990, 225–230.

Fischer A.A., *Pressure threshold meter: its use for quantification of tender spots*, Arch. Phys. Med. Rehabil., 1986, 67:836–838.

Fischer A.A., *Documentation of myofascial trigger points*, Arch. Phys. Med. Rehabil., 1988, 69:286–291.

Fischer A.A., Chang C., *Temperature and pressure threshold measurements in trigger points*, Thermology, 1986, 1:212–215.

Flor H., Birbaumer N., Schulte W., Roos R., *Stress-related electromyographic responses in patients with chronic temporomandibular pain*, Pain, 1991, 46:145–152.

Forbes J., Abbey L.M., Burch J.G., Secreti A.C., *Cardiovascularresponses to isometric and dynamic jaw-muscle exercise in man*, Arch. Oral Biol., 1979, 24:205–210.

Franks A.S.T., *Masticatory muscle hyperactivity and temporomandibular joint dysfunction*, J. Prosthet. Dent., 1965, 15:1122–1131.

Freimann V.R., *Untersuchungen über Zahl und Anordnung der Muskelspindeln in den Kaumuskeln des Menschen*, Anat. Anz., 1954, 100:258.

Friden J., *Changes in the human skeletal muscle induced by long-term eccentric exercise*, Cell. Tissue Res., 1984, 236:365–372.

Friden J., Sjostrom M., Ekblom B., *A morphological study of delayed muscle soreness*, Experientia, 1981, 37:506–507.

Gay T., Maton B., Rendell J., Majourau A., *Characteristics of muscle fatigue in patients with myofascial pain-dysfunction syndrome*, Arch. Oral Biol., 1994, 39:847–852.

Gervais R.O., Fitzsimmons G.W., Thomas N.R., *Masseter and temporalis electromyographic activity in asymptomatic, subclinical and temporomandibular joint dysfunction patients*, The Journal of Craniomandibular Practice, 1989, 7:52–57.

Gerwin R.D., Shannon S., Hong C.Z., Hubbard D., Gevirtz R., *Interrater reliability in myofascial trigger point examination*, Pain, 1997, 69:65–73.

Glaros A., *Incidence of diurnal and nocturnal bruxism*, J. Prosthet. Dent., 1981, 45:545–549.

Goldenberg D.L., *Fibromyalgia syndrome: an emerging but controversial condition*, JAMA, 1987, 25:2782–2787.

Gordon J., *Spinal mechanisms of motor coordination*, in: Kandel E.R., Schwartz J.H., Jessel T.M. (eds.), *Principles of neural science*, Elsevier, Amsterdam, 1991, 581–595.

Gordon J., Ghez C., *Muscles receptors and spinal reflexes: the stretch reflex*, in: Kandel E.R., Schwartz J.H., Jessel T.M. (eds.), *Principles of neural science*, Elsevier, Amsterdam, 1991, 564–580.

Granit R., *The basis of motor control*, Academic Press, London, 1970.

Griffin C.J., Munro R.R., *Electromyography of the masseter and anterior temporalis muscles in patients with temporomandibular dysfunction*, Arch. Oral Biol., 1971, 16:929–949.

Gunn C.C., *The mechanical manifestations of neuropathic pain*, Ann. Sports Med., 1990, 5:138–141.

Gunn C.C., *Fibromyalgia-what have we created? (Wolfe 1993) [letter]*, Pain, 1995, 60:349–350.

Hagberg C., Hagberg M., *Surface EMG frequency dependence on force in the masseter and the anterior temporal muscles*, Scand. J. Dent. Res., 1988, 96:451.

Hainaut K., Duchateau J., *Muscle fatigue, effects of training and disuse*, Muscle Nerve, 1989, 12:660.

Hatch J., Moore P., Cyr-Provost M., Boutros N., Seleshi E., Borcherding S., *The use of electromyography and muscle palpation in the diagnosis of tension-type headache with and without pericranial muscle involvement*, Pain, 1992, 49:175–178.

Henriksson K.G., *Muscle pain in neuromuscular disorders and primary fibromyalgia*, Eur. J. Appl. Physiol., 1988, 57:348–352.

Henriksson K.G., Bengtsson A., *Fibromyalgia and clinical entity?*, Can. J. Physiol. Pharmacol., 1991, 69:672–677.

Henriksson K.G., Bengtsson A., Lindman R., Thornell L.E., *Morphological changes in muscle in fibromyalgia and chronic shoulder myalgia*, in: Vaeröy H., Merskey H. (eds.), *Progress in fibromyalgia and myofascial pain*, Elsevier, Amsterdam, 1993, 61–73.

Hickey C., Williams B.H., Woelfel J.B., *Stability of mandibular rest position*, J. Prosthet. Dent., 1961, 11:566.

Hill A.V., *The pressure developed in muscle during contraction*, J. Physiol., 1948, 107:518–526.

Hori H., Kobayashi H., Hayashi T., Kohno S., *Mean power frequency shift during fatigue and recovery in patients with craniomandibular disorders*, J. Oral Rehabil., 1995, 22:159–165.

Hosokawa H., *Proprioceptive innervation of striated muscles in the territory of the cranial nerves*, Tex. Rep. Biol. Med., 1961, 19:405.

Hudson J., Pope H., *Fibromyalgia and psychopathology: is fibromyalgia a form of "affective spectrum disorder?"*, J. Rheumatol., 1989, 16 (Suppl. 19):15–22.

Hudson J., Goldenberg D., Pope H., *Comorbidity of fibromyalgia with medical and psychiatric disorders*, Am. J. Med., 1992, 92:363–367.

Hunt C.C., Kuffler S.W., *Stretch receptor discharges during muscle contraction*, J. Physiol., 1951, 113:298–315.

Hutchings M.O., Skjonsby H.S., Brazeau G.A., Parikh U.K., Jenkins R.M., *Weakness in mouse masticatory muscles by repetitive contractions with forced lengthening*, J. Dent. Res., 1995, 74:642–648.

International Headache Society, *Classification and diagnostic criteria for headache disorders, cranial neuralgias and facial pain*, Cephalalgia, 1988, 8 (Suppl. 7):1–96.

Jankowska E., Padel Y., Tanaka R., *Synaptic inhibition of spinal motoneurons from the motor complex in the monkey*, J. Physiol., 1976, 258:467–487.

Jensen R., *Quantification of tenderness by palpation and use of pressure algometer*, Adv. Pain Res. Ther., 1990, 17:165–181.

Jensen R., *Mechanisms of spontaneous tension-type headaches: an analysis of tenderness, pain thresholds and EMG*, Pain, 1996, 64:251–256.

Jensen R., Rasmussen B.K., Olesen J., *Muscle tenderness and pressure pain threshold in tensiontype headache and migraine*, Pain, 1993, 52:193–199.

Jensen R., Fuglsang-Frederiksen A., Olesen J., *Quantitative surface EMG of pericranial muscles in headache. A population study*, Electroencephalogr. Clin. Neurophysiol., 1994, 93:335–44.

Jensen R., Olesen J., *Initiating mechanisms of experimentally induced tension-type headache*, Cephalalgia, 1996, 16:175–182.

Jones D.A., Newham D.J., Round J.M., Tolfree S.E.J., *Experimental human muscle damage: morphological changes in relation to other indices of damage*, J. Physiol., 1986, 375:435–448.

Jones D.A., Newham D.J., Obletter G., Giamberardino M.A., *Nature of exercise induced muscle pain*, in: Tiengo M., Eccles. J., Cuello A.C., Ottoson D. (eds.), *Advances in pain research and therapy*, vol. 10, Raven Press, New York, 1987, 207–218.

Jones D., Round J. (eds.), *Skeletal muscle in health and disease: A textbook of muscle physiology*, Manchester University Press, Manchester, 1990, 134–157.

Junge D., Clark G.T., *Electromyographic turns analysis of sustained contraction in human masseter muscles at various isometric force levels*, Arch. Oral Biol., 1993, 38, 583–588.

Kapel L., Glaros A.G., McGlynn F.D., *Psychophysiological responses to stress in patients with myofascial pain-dysfunction syndrome*, J. Behav. Med., 1989, 12:397–406.

Kaufman M.P., Rybichi K.J., Waldrop T.G., Ordway G.A., *Effect of ischemia on responses of groups III and IV afferents to contraction*, J. Appl. Physiol., 1984, 57:644–650.

Kawamura Y., Fujimoto J., *Some physiologic considerations on measuring rest position of the mandible*, Med. J. Osaka Univ., 1957, 247–255.

Keith D.A., *Etiology and diagnosis of temporomandibular pain dysfunction: Organic pathology (other than arthritis)*, in: Laskin D.M., Greenfield W., Gale E., Rugh J., Neff P., Alling C., Ayer W.A. (eds.), *The President's conference on the examination, diagnosis, and management of temporomandibular disorders*, Am. Dent. Assoc., 1983, 118–122.

Knaflitz M., Merletti R., De Luca J., *Inference of motor unit recruitment order in voluntary and electrically elicited contractions*, J. Appl. Physiol., 1990, 68:1657–1667.

Kranz H., Williams A.M., Cassell J., Caddy D.J., Silberstein R.B., *Factors determining the frequency content of the electromyogram*, J. Appl. Physiol.: Respir. Environ. Exerc. Physiol., 1983, 55:392–399.

Kroon G.W., Naeije M., Hansson T.L., *Electromyographic power-spectrum changes during repeated fatiguing contractions of the human masseter muscles*, Arch. Oral Biol., 1986, 31:603–608.

Kroon G.W., Naeije M., *Recovery following exhaustive dynamic exercise in the human biceps muscle*, Eur. J. Appl. Physiol., 1988, 58:228–232.

Langemark M., Olesen J., *Pericranial tenderness in tension headache*, Cephalalgia, 1987, 7:249–55.

Larsson S.E., Bodegård L., Henriksson K.G., Öberg P.Å., *Chronic trapezius myalgia. Morphology and blood flow studied in 17 patients*, Acta Orthop. Scand., 1990, 61:394–398.

Laskin D.M., *Etiology of the pain-dysfunction syndrome*, J. Am. Dent. Assoc., 1969, 79:147–153.

Layzer R.B., *Muscle pain, cramps, and fatigue*, in: Engel A.G., Franzini-Armstrong C., (eds.), *Myology*, vol. 2, 2d ed., McGraw-Hill, New York, 1994, 1754–1768.

Lederman K.H., Clayton J.A., *Restored occlusions. II: The relationship of clinical and subject symptoms to varying degrees of TMJ dysfunction*, J. Prosthet. Dent., 1982, 47:303–309.

Lieberman M.A., Gazit E., Fuchs C., Lilos P., *Mandibular dysfunction in 10–18 year old schoolchildren as related to morphological malocclusion*, J. Oral Rehabil., 1985, 12:209–214.

Lindinger M.I., McKelvie R.S., Heigenhauser G.J., *K+ and Lac- distribution in humans during and after high-intensity exercise: role in muscle fatigue attenuation?*, J. Appl. Physiol., 1995, 78:765–777.

Lindstrom L., Magnusson R., Peterseon I., *Muscular fatigue and action potential conduction velocity changes studied with frequency analysis of EMG signals*, Electromyography, 1970, 4:341–356.

Lipchik G.L., Holroyd K.A., Talbot F., Greer M., *Pericranial muscle tenderness and exteroceptive suppression of temporalis muscle activity: a blind study of chronic tension-type headache*. Headache, 1997, 37:368–376.

Lous I., Sheikoleslam A., Möller E., *Postural activity in subjects with functional disorders of the chewing apparatus*, Scand. J. Dent. Res., 1970, 78:404–410.

Lund J.P., Widmer C.G., *An evaluation of the use of surface electromyography in the diagnosis, documentation, and treatment of dental patients*, J. Craniomandib. Disord. Facial Oral Pain, 1989, 3:125–137.

Lundh H., Westesson P.L., Kopp S., *A three-year follow-up of patients with reciprocal temporomandibular joint clicking*, Oral Surg. Oral Med. Oral Pathol., 1987, 65:530–533.

Majewski R.F., Gale E.N., *Electromyographic activity of anterior temporal area pain patients and non-pain subjects*, J. Dent. Res., 1984, 63:1228–1231.

Manns A., Miralles R., Guerrero F., *The changes in electrical activity of the postural muscles of the mandible upon varying the vertical dimension*, J. Dent. Res., 1981, 45:438.

Mao J., *Fatigue in human jaw muscles: a review*, J. Orofacial, Pain, 1993, 7:135–142.

Mao J., Osborn J.W., Stein R.B., *The fiber type and composition of mammalian jaw muscles: A review*, J. Craniomandib. Disord. Facial Oral Pain, 1992, 6:192–201.

McCain G.A., *Chronic musculoskeletal pain syndromes – Overlapping features of myofascial pain and fibromyalgia*, 7th World Congress on Pain, IASP Publications, Seattle, 1993a, 495, (abs.).

McCain G.A., *The clinical features of the fibromyalgia syndrome*, in: Vaeröy H., Merskey H. (eds.), *Progress in fibromyalgia and myofascial pain*, Elsevier, Amsterdam, 1993b, 195–215.

McCain G.A., *Fibromyalgia and myofascial pain syndromes*, in: Wall P.D., Melzack R. (eds.), *Textbook of Pain*, 3rd ed. Churchill Livingstone, Edinburgh, 1994, 475–493.

Mense S., *Anatomical and neurophysiological basis of muscle pain*, Pain, 1987, (Suppl. 4):209.

Mense S., *Considerations concerning the neurobiological basis of muscle pain*, Can J. Physiol. Pharmacol., 1991, 69:610–616.

Mense S., *Neurophysiology of muscle in relation to pain*, in: Vaeröy H., Merskey H., *Progress in fibromyalgia and myofascial pain*, Elsevier, Amsterdam, 1993, 23–39.

Mense S., Stahnke M., *Responses in muscle afferent fibres of slow conduction velocity to contractions and ischaemia in the cat*, J. Physiol., 1983, 342:383–397.

Mense S., Meyer H., *Different types of slowly conducting afferent units in cat skeletal muscle and tendon*, J. Physiol., 1985, 363:403–417.

Mercuri L.G., Olsen R.E., Laskin D.M., *The specificity of response to experimental stress in patients with myofascial pain dysfunction syndrome*, J. Dent. Res., 1979, 58:1866–1871.

Merletti R., Knaflitz M., De Luca C.J., *Myoelectric manifestations of fatigue in voluntary and electrically elicited contractions*, J. Appl. Physiol., 1990, 69:1810–1820.

Merskey H., *The classification of fibromyalgia and myofascial pain*, in: Vaeröy H., Merskey H. (eds.), *Progress in fibromyalgia and myofascial pain*, Elsevier, Amsterdam, 1993, 191–194.

Moldofsky H., *Sleep and musculoskeletal pain*, Am. J. Med., 1986, 81 (Suppl. 3A):85–89.

Moldofsky H., *Sleep-wake mechanism in fibrositis*, J. Rheumatol., 1989a, 16 (Suppl. 19):4748.

Moldofsky H., *Non-restorative sleep and symptoms after a febrile illness in patients with fibrositis and chronic fatigue syndrome*, J. Rheumatol., 1989b, 16 (Suppl. 19):150–153.

Moldofsky H., *Sleep and fibrositis syndrome*, Rheum. Dis. Clin. N. Am., 1989c, 15:91–103.

Molin C., *Vertical isometric muscle forces of the mandible*, Acta Odontol. Scand., 1972, 30:485–499.

Möller E., *Computer analysis of electromyographic data in clinical studies of oral function*, Scand. J. Dent. Res., 1970, 78:411–416.

Möller E., *The Myogenic factor in headache and facial pain*, in: Kawamura Y., Dubner R. (eds.), *Oral-facial sensory and motor function*, Quintessence, Tokyo, 1981, 225–239.

Möller E., *Muscle hyperactivity leads to pain and dysfunction: Position paper*, in: Klineberg I, Sessle B. (eds.), *Oro-facial pain and neuromuscular dysfunction*, Pergamon Press, Oxford, 1985, 69–92.

Möller E., Sheikoleslam A., Lous I., *Deliberate relaxation of the temporal and masseter muscles in subjects with functional disorders of the chewing apparatus*, Scand. J. Dent. Res., 1971, 79:478–482.

Möller E., Rasmussen O.C., Bonde-Petersen F., *Mechanism of ischemic pain in human muscles of mastication: intramuscular pressure. EMG, force and blood flow of the temporal and masseter muscles during biting*, in: Bonica J.J., Liebeskind C.J., Albe-Fessard D.G. (eds.), *Advances in pain research therapy*, vol. 3, Raven Press, New York, 1979, 271–281.

Mongini F., *The stomatognathic system*. Quintessence, Chicago-Berlin, 1984.

Mongini F., Tempia-Valenta G., Benvegnù G., *Computer based assessment of habitual mastication*, J. Prosthet. Dent., 1986, 55:638–649.

Mongini F., Tempia-Valenta G., Conserva E., *Habitual mastication in dysfunction: a computer-based analysis*, J. Prosthet. Dent., 1989, 61 : 484–94.

Mongini F., Caselli C., Macry V., Tetti C., *Thermographic findings in craniofacial pain*, Headache, 1990, 30 : 497–504.

Mongini F., Knaflitz M., Ecclesia P., Balestra G., Bezzan M., *A new methodology to study muscle fatigue in normal and headache patients*, in: Olesen J. (ed.), *Experimental headache models in animal and man*, Raven Press, New York, 1995, 319–323.

Mongini F., Poma M., Bava M., Fabbri G., *Phychosomatic symptoms in different types of headache and facial pain*, Cephalalgia, 1997, 17 : 274, 1997, (abs.).

Monteiro A.A., Kopp S., *Estimation of blood flow by 133 Xe clearance in human masseter muscle during rest, endurance of isometric contraction, and recovery*, Arch. Oral Biol., 33, 1988, 8 : 561–565.

Monteiro A.A., Kopp S., *The sufficiency of blood flow in human masseter muscle during endurance of biting in the intercuspal position and on a force transducer*, Proc. Finn. Dent. Soc., 1989, 85 : 261–272.

Morris V., Cruwys S., Kidd B., *Increased capsaicin-induced secondary hyperalgesia as a marker of abnormal sensory activity in patients with fibromyalgia*, Neurosci. Lett., 1998, 250(3): 205–207.

Moss R.A., Garret J.C., *Temporomandibular joint dysfunction syndrome and myofascial pain dysfunction syndrome: A critical review*, J. Oral. Rehabil., 1984, 11 : 3–28.

Naeije M., Zorn H., *Changes in the power spectrum of the surface electromyogram of the masseter muscle due to local muscular fatigue*, Arch. Oral Biol., 1981, 26 : 409–412.

Naeije M., Zorn H., *Relation between EMG power spectrum shifts and muscle fibre action potential conduction velocity changes during local muscular fatigue in man*, Eur. J. Appl. Physiol., 1982, 50 : 23–33.

Newham D.J., Jones D.A., Edwards R.H.T., *Large delayed plasma creatine kinase changes after stepping exercise*, Muscle Nerve, 1983, 6 : 380–385.

Newham D.J., *Exercise induced pain and damage in human skeletal muscle*, Thesis Polytechnic of North London and Department of Medicine, London University, 1984.

Newham D.J., *The consequences of eccentric contractions and their relationship to delayed onset muscle pain*, Eur. J. Appl. Physiol., 1988, 57 : 353–359.

Nice D., Riddle D., Lamb R. et al., *Inter-tester reliability of judgements of the presence of trigger points in patients with low back pain*, Arch. Phys. Med. Rehabil., 1992, 73 : 893–898.

O'Donnell R.D., Rapp J., Berkhout J., Adey W.R., *Autospectral and coherence patterns from two locations in the contracting biceps*, Electromyogr. Clin. Neurophysiol., 1973, 13 : 259–269.

Okeson J.P., Phillips B.A., Berry D.T.R., Cook Y., Paisani D., Galante J., *Nocturnal bruxing events in healthy geriatric subjects*, J. Oral Rehabil., 1990, 17 : 411–418.

Okeson J.P., Philips B.A., Berry D.T., Cook Y., Cabelka J.F., *Nocturnal bruxing events in subjects with sleep-disordered breathing and control subjects*, J. Craniomandib. Disord. Facial Oral Pain, 1991, 5 : 258 : 264.

Paintal A.S., *Functional analysis of group III afferent fibres of mammalian muscles*, J. Physiol., 1960, 152 : 250–270.

Palla S., Ash M.M. jr., *Power spectral analysis of the surface electromyogram of the human jaw muscles during fatigue*, Arch. Oral Biol., 1981, 26 : 547 : 553.

Parker M.W., *A dynamic model of etiology in temporomandibular disorders*, J. Am. Dent. Assoc., 1990, 120 : 283–290.

Payne T.C., Leavitt F., Garron D.C.,et al. *Fibrositis and psychological disturbance*, Arthritis Rheum., 1982, 25 : 213–217.

Perry H.T., *Muscular changes associated with temporomandibular joint dysfunction*, J. Am. Dent. Assoc., 1957, 54 : 644–653.

Perry H.T., Lammie G.A., Main J., Teuscher G.W., *Occlusion in a stress situation*, J. Am. Dent. Assoc., 60 : 626–633, 1960.

Person R.S., Mishin L.N., *Auto- and cross-correlation analysis of the electrical activity of muscles*, Med. Electron. Biol. Eng., 1964, 2 : 155–159.

Randow K., Carlsson K., Edlund J., Öberg T., *The effect of an occlusal interference on the masticatory system*, Odontol. Rev., 1976, 27 : 245–256.

Reding G.R., *Incidence of bruxism*, J. Dent. Res., 1966, 45 : 1198.

Reeves J.L., Jaeger B., Graff-Radford S.B., *Reliability of pressure algometer as a measure of myofascial trigger point sensitivity*, Pain, 1986, 24 : 313–321.

Roberts C.A., Tallents R.H., Katzberg R.W., Sanchez-Woodworth R.E. Espeland M.A., Handelman S.L., *Comparison of internal derangements of the TMJ with occlusal findings*, Oral Surg. Oral Med. Oral Pathol., 1987, 63 : 645–650.

Rugh J.D., Solberg W.K., *Psychological implications in temporomandibular pain and dysfunction*, in: Zarb G.A., Carlsson G.E. (eds.), *Temporomandibular joint, function and dysfunction*, C.V. Mosby Co., St. Louis, 1979.

Rugh J.D., Drago C.J., *Vertical dimension: a study of clinical rest position and jaw muscle activity*, J. Prosthet. Dent., 1981, 45 : 670.

Rugh J.D., Montgomery G.T., *Physiological reactions of patients with TM disorders vs. symptom-free controls on a physical stress task*, J. Craniomandib. Disord. Facial Oral Pain, 1987, 1 : 243–250.

Rugh J.D., Harlan J., *Nocturnal bruxism and temporomandibular disorders*, in: Jankovic J., Tolosa E. (eds.), *Advances in neurology*, Raven Press, New York, 1988, 329–341.

Runge M.E., Sadowsky C., Sakols E., Begole E.A., *The relationship between temporomandibular joint sounds and malocclusion*, Am. J. Orthodont., 1989, 96 : 36–42.

Sadoyama T., Miyano H., *Frequency analysis of surface EMG to evaluation of muscle fatigue*, Eur. J. Appl. Physiol., 1981, 47 : 239–246.

Scott D.S., Lundeen T.F., *Myofascial pain involving the masticatory muscles: an experimental model*, Pain, 1980, 8 : 207–215.

Seligman D.A., Pullinger A.G., Solberg W.K., *The prevalence of dental attrition and its association with factors of age, gender, occlusion, and TMJ symptomatoloy*, J. Dent. Res., 1988 a, 67 : 1323–1333.

Seligman D.A., Pullinger A.G., Solberg W.K., *Temporomandibular disorders. III: Occlusal and articular factors associated with muscle tenderness*, J. Prosthet. Dent., 1988 b, 59 : 483–489.

Seligman D.A., Pullinger A.G., *Association of occlusal variables among refined TM patient diagnostic groups*, J. Craniomandib. Disord. Facial Oral Pain, 1989, 3 : 227–236.

Sheikoleslam A., *Clinical and electromyographic studies on function and dysfunction of the temporal and masseter muscles*, Thesis Karolinska Institutet, Stockholm, 1985.

Sheikoleslam A., Möller E., Lous I., *Pain, tenderness and strength of human mandibular elevators*, Scand. J. Dent. Res., 1980, 88 : 60–66.

Shpuntoff H., Shpuntoff W., *A study of physiological rest position and centric position by electromyography*, J. Prosthet. Dent., 1956, 6 : 621.

Simons D.G., *Myofascial pain syndromes of head, neck and low back*, in: Dubner R., Gebhart G.F., Bond M.R. (eds.), *Procedings of the Vth World Congress on Pain*, Elsevier, Amsterdam, 1988, 186–200.

Simons D.G., Mense S., *Understanding and measurement of muscle tone as related to clinical muscle pain*, Pain, 1998, 75 : 1–17.

Sjögaard G., Savard G., Juel C., *Muscle blood flow during isometric activity and its relation to muscle fatigue*, Eur. J. Appl. Physiol., 1988, 57 : 327–335.

Sjöstrom M., Friden J., *Muscle soreness and muscle structure*, Med. Sport Sci., 1984, 17 : 1109–1186.

Smith E.L., Hill R.L., Lehman I.R., Lefkowitz R.J., Handler P., White A., *Muscle*, in: *Principles of biochemistry: mammalian biochemistry*, McGraw-Hill, 1985, 273–295.

Solberg W.K., Woo M.W., Houston J.B., *Prevalence of mandibular dysfunction in young adults*, J. Am. Dent. Assoc., 1979, 98 : 25–34.

Stauber W.T., *Eccentric action of muscles: physiology, injury, and adaptation*, Exerc. Sports Sci. Rev., 1989, 17 : 157–185.

Stauber W.T., Clarkson P.M., Fritz V.K., Evans W.J., *Extracellular matrix disruption and pain after eccentric muscle action*, J. Appl. Physiol., 1990, 69 : 868–874.

Travell J.G., Simons D.G., *Myofascial pain and dysfunction: trigger point manual*, Williams & Wilkins, Baltimore, 1983.

Vallbo A.B., *Basic patterns of muscle spindle discharge in man*, in: Taylor A., Prochazka A. (eds.), *Muscle receptors and movement*, Macmillan, London, 1981, 219–228, 263–275.

Vecchiet L., Giamberardino M.A., Marini I., *Immediate muscular pain from physical activity*, in: Tiengo M., Eccles J., Cuello A.C., Ottoson D. (eds), *Advances in pain research and therapy*, vol. 10, Raven Press, New York, 1987, 193–206.

Vecchiet L., Giamberardino M.A., Saggini R., *Myofascial pain syndromes: clinical and pathophysiological aspects*, Clin. J. Pain, 1991, 7 (Suppl.): 16–22.

Vecchiet L., Dragani L., De Bigontina P., Obletter G., Giamberardino M.A., *Experimental referred pain and hyperalgesia from muscles in humans*, in: Vecchiet L., Albe-Fessard D., Lindblom U., Giamberardino M.A., *New trends in referred pain and hyperalgesia*, Elsevier, Amsterdam, 1993, 239–249.

Vecchiet L., Giamberardino M.A., De Bigontina P., Dragani L., *Comparative sensory evaluation of parietal tissues in painful and nonpainful areas in fibromyalgia and myofascial pain syndrome*, in: Gebhart G.F., Hammond D.L., Jensen T.S. (eds.), *Progress in Pain Research and Management*, IASP Press, Seattle, 1994, 177–185.

Viitasalo J.H.T., Komi P.V., *Signal characteristics of EMG during fatigue*, Eur. J. Appl. Physiol., 1977, 37 : 111–121.

Viitasalo J.H.T., Komi P.V., *Isometric endurance, EMG power spectrum, and fibre composition in human quadriceps muscle*, Biomechanics, 1980, VI-A, 244–250.

Wall P.D., *The mechanism of fibromyalgia: a critical essay*, in: Vaeröy H., Merskey H. (eds.), *Progress in fibromyalgia and myofascial pain*, Elsevier, Amsterdam, 1993, 53–59.

Weigent D.A., Bradley L.A., Blalock J.E., Alarcon G.S., *Currrent concepts in the pathophysiology of abnormal pain perception in fibromyalgia*, Am. J. Med. Sci., 1998, 315(6):405–412.

Westbury J.R., Shaughnessy T.G., *Associations between spectral representation of the surface electromyogram and fiber type distribution and size in human masseter muscle*, Electromyogr. Clin. Neurophysiol., 1987, 27:427–435.

Weytjens J.L.F., Van Steenberghe D., *The effects of motor unit synchronization on the power spectrum of the electromyogram*, Biol. Cybern., 1984, 51:71–77.

Widmalm S.E., Christiansen R.L., Gunn S.M., *Oral parafunctions as temporomandibular disorder factors in children*, Cranio, 1995, 13, 242–246.

Wolfe F., *Fibromyalgia and problems in classification of musculoskeletal disorders*, in: Vaeröy H., Merskey H. (eds.), *Progress in fibromyalgia and myofascial pain*, Elsevier, Amsterdam, 1993, 217–235.

Wolfe F., *What use are fibromyalgia control points?* J. Rheumatol., 1998, 25(3):546–550.

Wolfe F., Cathey M.A., Kleinheksel S.M., et al., *Psychological status in primary fibrositis and fibrositis associated with rheumatoid arthritis*, J. Rheumatol., 1984, 11:500–506.

Wolfe F., Hawley D.J., Cathey M.A., Caro X., Russell I.J., *Fibrositis, symptom frequency and criteria for diagnosis*, J. Rheumatol., 1985, 12:1159–1163.

Wolfe F., Simons D., Fricton J. et al., *The fibromyalgia and myofascial pain syndromes: a preliminary study of tender points and trigger points in persons with fibromyalgia, myofascial pain syndrome and no disease*, J. Rheumatol., 1992, 19:944–951.

Yemm R., *Masseter muscle activity in stress: adaptation of response to a repeated stimulus in man*, Arch. Oral Biol., 1969a, 14:1437–1439.

Yemm R., *Varieties in the electrical activity of the human masseter muscle occuring in association with emotional stress*, Arch. Oral Biol., 1969b, 14:873–878.

Yemm R., *A comparison of the electrical activity of masseter and temporal muscles of human subjects during experimental stress*, Arch. Oral Biol., 1971, 16:269:273.

Yemm R., *Causes and effects of hyperactivity of jaw muscles*, in: Bryant P.S., Gale E., Ruth J.D. (eds.), *Oral motor behavior*, NIH Publication, 79–1845, 1979, 138–156.

Yemm R., El-Sharkawy M., Stephens C.D., *Measurement of lip posture and interaction between lip posture and resting facial height*, J. Oral Rehabil., 1978, 391–402.

Yu X.M., Hu J.W., Vernon H., Sessle B.J., *Temporomandibular inflammatory irritant induces increased activity of jaw muscles*, J. Dent. Res., 1992, 71:603 (abs.).

Yu X.M., Sessle B.J., Haas D.A., Izzo A., Vernon H., Hu J.W., *Involvement of NMDA receptor mechanisms in jaw electromyographic activity and plasma extravasation induced by inflammatory irritant application to temporomandibular joint region of rats*, Pain, 1996, 68:169–178.

Yunus M.B., Masi A.T., Calabro J.J., Miller K.A., Feigenbaum S.L., *Primary fibromyalgia (fibrositis): clinical study of 50 patients with matched normal controls*, Semin. Arthritis Rheum., 1981, 11:151–171.

Zwarts M.J., *Applications of muscle fibre conduction velocity. A surface EMG study*, Thesis, University of Groningen, 1989.

4 Posture and Structure Alterations

Head, Neck, and Shoulder Posture Disorders

In normal conditions the cervical column is vertically oriented on the frontal plane and shows a slight anterior convexity (cervical lordosis) (Fig. 4.1). The skull is connected to the column through the articulating surfaces of the occipital condyles of the skull and the superior articular surfaces of the atlas. The position of the head is secured by a number of muscles located anteriorly and posteriorly with respect to the cervical column. Of the anterior muscles, some connect the mandible indirectly to the sternum and the clavicula by inserting to the hyoid bone (Figs. 4.2, 4.3).

The baricenter of the skull is approximately located at the sella turcica and is, therefore, ahead of the craniovertebral fulcrum, that is, of the occipital condyles (Rocabado, 1983) (Fig. 4.4). Therefore, the force of gravity must be counterbalanced by the action of the posterior neck muscles, which are stronger than the anterior ones (Fig. 4.3).

A frequent cause of alteration of head and neck posture is the failure of the posterior neck muscles to counteract the skull weight. This results in an anterior displacement of head, neck and shoulders (Fig. 4.5). As a consequence, the cervical curvature is lost or inverted (Figs. 4.6, 4.7). With time, this may lead to arthrotic degeneration of the cervical vertebrae (Rocabado, 1982, 1983) (Fig. 4.8). Partial or total loss of curvature may also be functional, due to neck muscles contracting in a stressed patient. Such alterations result in a relative displacement of the hyoid bone (Figs. 4.6, 4.7) and, as a consequence, may result in alterations of the mandibular postural position.

Another frequent condition is a misalignment of the shoulders, that is, one shoulder being higher than the other. This can be observed on inspecting the patient while standing (Fig. 4.9). This situation may be due to different lengths of the two legs, with consequent misalignment of the hips, and/or to column alterations (Figs. 4.10, 4.11). In other cases, the disorder is, at least at first, only functional, due to the patients habits. As a consequence, in order to keep the bipupillar line horizontal, the neck is deviated towards the higher shoulder, which thus appears shorter (Figs. 4.9, 4.10). Radiographically, one may observe the deviation of the cranial column and an asymmetry in the position of the skull with respect to the column (Fig. 4.12). Such a situation requires extra work from the neck muscles, in particular from the sternocleidomastoid and trapezius muscles ipsilateral to the lower shoulder.

Alterations of the normal cervical curvature are frequently superimposed on the shoulder posture disorders. Severe alterations of muscle function of head, neck, and shoulder girdle muscles may result from the situations mentioned above. The constant change of muscle activity, orientation and length results in muscle functional overload and may lead to formation of points that are tender on palpation, taut bands, and, possibly, trigger points.

The relationship between posture disorders and headache and facial pain is still disputed. One reason for this lack of consensus again relates to the imprecise categorization of the different pain syndromes involved. Thus, a number of authors examined this problem in patient populations suffering from so-called *craniomandibular disorders* or *temporomandibular disorders*. Some authors (Fricton et al., 1985; Huggare and Raustia, 1992; Watson and Trott, 1993) found a relation between pathologies so defined and posture disorders of head and neck, while others found no relation between the two factors (Darlow et al., 1987; Hackey et al., 1993) or found a very limited one (Lee et al., 1995). The reasons why the above terminology should be avoided when defining patients with craniofacial pain of different types localized in the cheek of the preauricular area have been discussed (see Chapter 1). While a significant relation between true intracapsular TMJ lesions and posture disorders has not been demonstrated the clinical observation of concomitant facial myogenous pain, tension-type headache, neck pain, and posture disorders is frequent. However, the presence of numerous variables makes it difficult to establish the presence of a cause–effect relationship. As we have seen (Chapter 3), trigger points in the cervical muscles may produce referred pain in different sites of the head (Travell and Simons, 1983): it has been asserted that tension-type headache might be caused by overlapping referral patterns of pain from the temporalis and some of the neck muscles (Simons and Mense, 1998). Moreover, individuals under stress with the parafunctional behaviors described in Chapter 3 may also increase the activity of the long muscles of the neck. When this occurs in a situation in which function

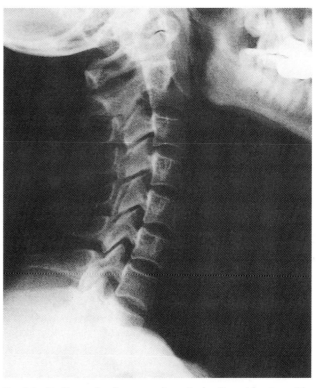

Fig. 4.**1 Radiograph of a normal cervical spine, side view.** Observe the normal anterior convexity (cervical lordosis)

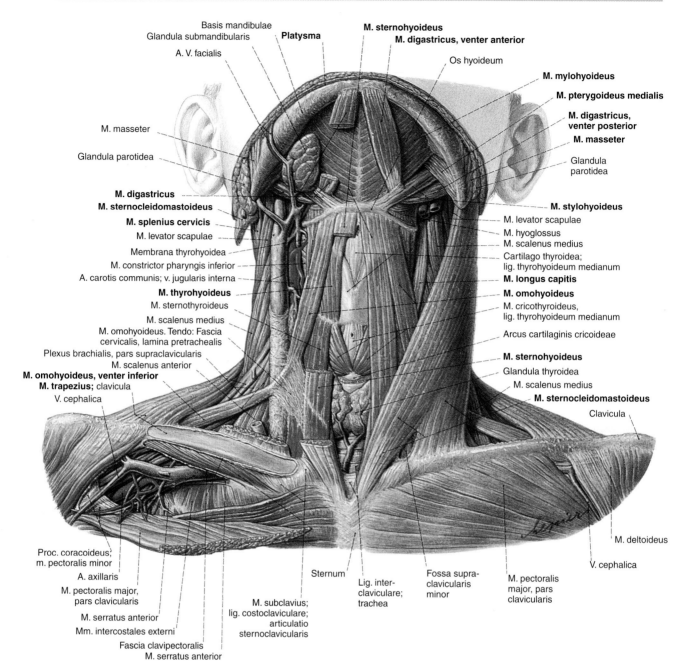

Fig. 4.**2**   Ventral view of the muscles of the neck and of the floor of the mouth. (From Sobotta, Atlas der Anatomie des Menschen, 20th ed., Urban und Schwarzenberg, München, 1993, with permission)

is already impaired by posture disorders, it is more likely that cervical pain will occur, together with facial pain and, possibly, tension-type headache (Fig. 4.**13**).

In a study performed on a consistent number of patients with headache and facial pain of different types it was found that the tension-type headache group showed a higher prevalence of posture disorders (Mongini et al., 1997) (Fig. 4.**14**).

Posture disorders and cervical column alterations may be relevant in *cervicogenic headache,* according to some authors (see Pöllmann et al., 1997, for a review). As we have seen in Chapter 1, in this type of headache pain initiates in the occipi-

tal area and then spreads to the frontal and temporal areas. The anatomical basis for the frontal spreading is the connections between the trigeminal spinal nucleus and the first three cervical nerve roots (Kerr, 1972; Bogduk, 1984, 1989). In fact, a pressure applied corresponding to the C2 root may produce pain in the corresponding dermatome and along the distribution territory of the trigeminal branches (Travell and Simons, 1983).

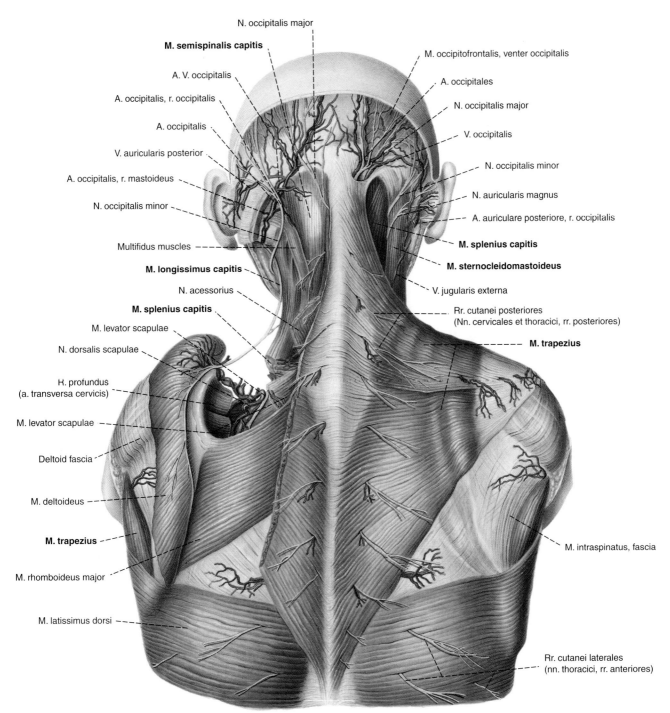

Fig. 4.**3** Superficial and middle layers of muscles, vessels, and nerves of the posterior region of the neck and of the back. On the left side the trapezius, sternocleidomastoid and splenius muscles are sectioned. (From Sobotta, Atlas der Anatomie des Menschen, 20th ed. Urban und Schwarzenberg, München, 1993, with permission)

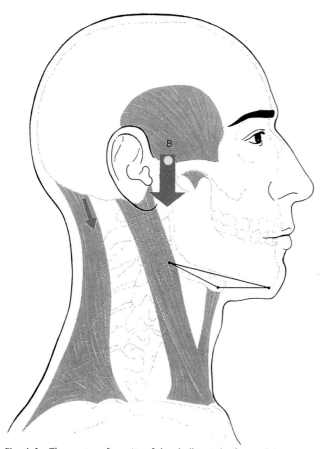

Fig. 4.**4** The center of gravity of the skull is at the front of the vertebral fulcrum

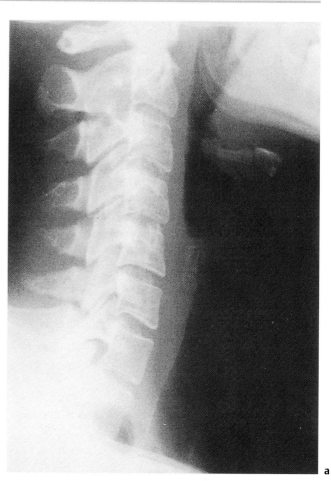

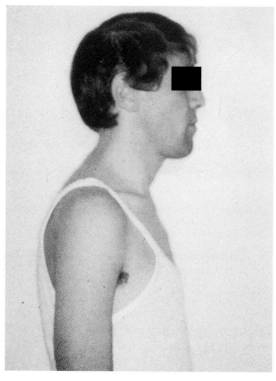

Fig. 4.**5** Patient with head, neck, and shoulders dislocated forwards

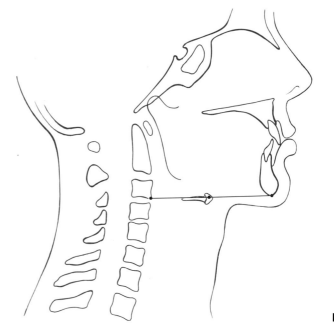

Fig. 4.**6** Radiograph (**a**) and drawing (**b**) showing loss of cervical lordosis

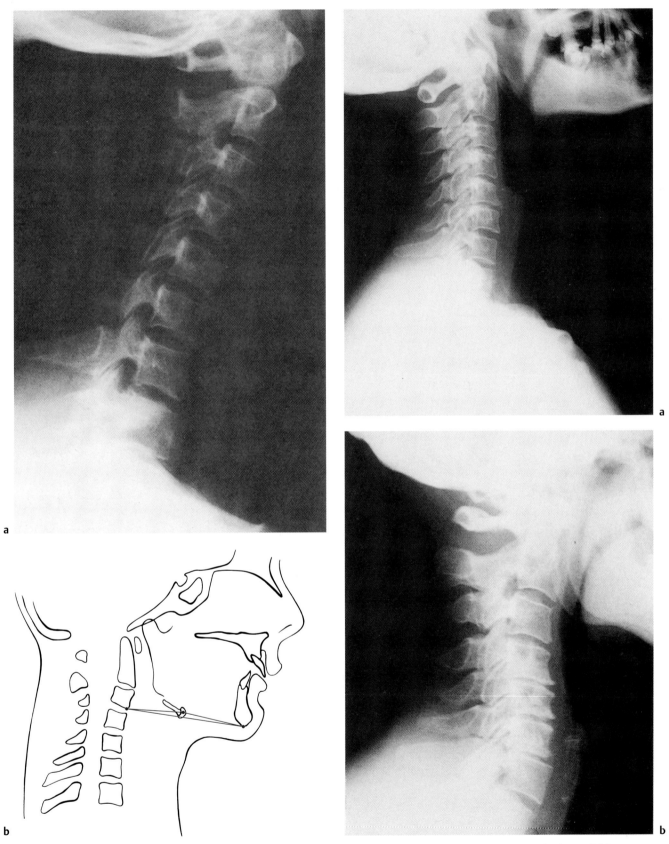

Fig. 4.**7** Radiograph (**a**) and drawing (**b**) showing inversion of spine curvature. In these cases the hyoid bone undergoes a relative dislocation

Fig. 4.**8** Arthrotic lesion of average (**a**) and advanced (**b**) extent in patients with loss and inversion of curvature of spine, respectively

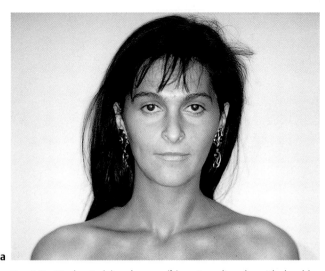
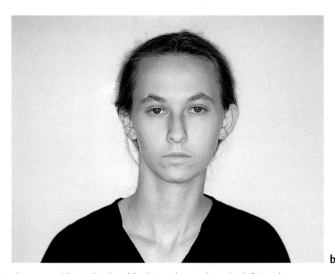

a   b

Fig. 4.**9**   Moderate (**a**) and severe (**b**) posture disorder with shoulder misalignment (the right shoulder being lower than the left) and compensatory cervical scoliosis

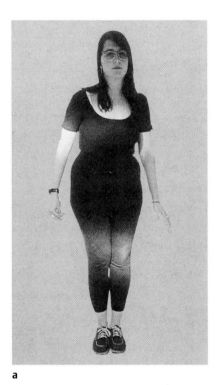
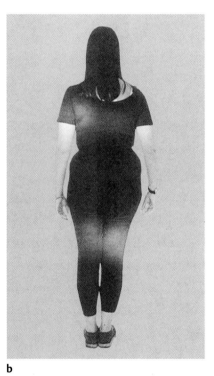
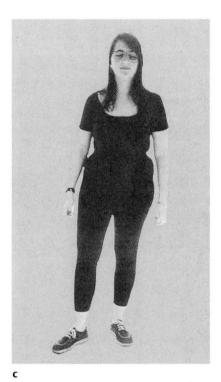

a   b   c

Fig. 4.**10**   Patient with serious posture disorder with shoulders and hips at different levels in standing position (**a, b**) and consequent compensatory posture (**c**)

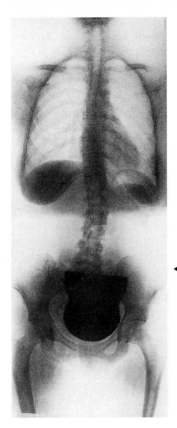

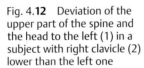

◄Fig. 4.**11**　**Same patient as in Fig. 4.10.** The radiograph of the spine shows a serious thoracolumbar scoliosis

Fig. 4.**12**　Deviation of the upper part of the spine and the head to the left (1) in a subject with right clavicle (2) lower than the left one　►

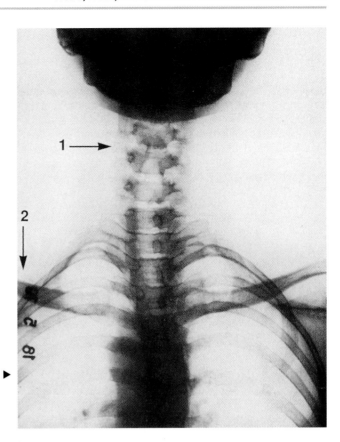

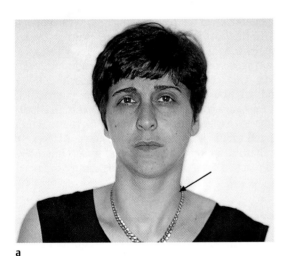

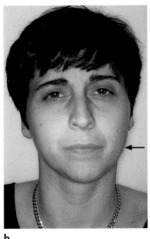

Fig. 4.**13**　**Patient with tension-type headache postural defects and cervico-facial pain. a** A posture disorder is observed, with loss of normal cervical curve, lower left shoulder, a compensative deviation of the head to the right and consequent increase of the activity of the cervical muscles (arrow). **b** The situation is aggravated by parafunctional behaviors, also shown by the hypertrophy of the left masseter muscle (arrow)

a

b

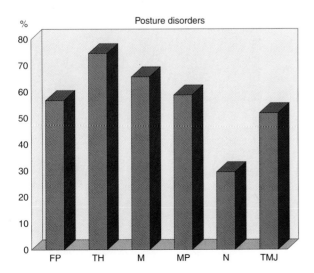

Fig. 4.**14**　Prevalence of posture disorders in patients with tension-type headache (TH), migraine (M), facial pain disorder (FP), myogenic pain (MP), trigeminal neuralgia (N), and TMJ dysfunction (TMJ). (From Mongini et al., 1997)

Anatomy and Function of Jaw and TMJ

The stomatognathic system consists of: (1) the temporomandibular joint (TMJ); (2) the masticatory and paramasticatory muscles; (3) the jaws and associated dental and periodontal structures; and (4) the pertinent part of the central and peripheral nervous system. The TMJ is made up of the mandibular condyle, the glenoid cavity, the articular tuberosity, the articular disk and the capsule with ist reinforcing ligaments (Fig. 4.15). The articular disk lies between the articular surfaces of the condyle and the temporal bone. It is a complex fibrocartilaginous structure, whose posterior portion is thick and concave downward; the middle portion is thin, and the anterior is thicker than the middle portion and is concave upward (Fig. 4.16). The disk is connected to the articular capsule by lateral and posterior attachments, thus dividing the articular space into upper and lower compartment. The posterior attachment has two layers of fibers, with an extended zone of loose connective tissue, rich in vessels and nervous fibers, interposed (Rees, 1954; Choukas and Sicher, 1960; Dixon, 1962; Wilkes, 1978 a, b; Mahan, 1980). The superior layer attaches to the petrotympanic fissure (Fig. 4.17) and has abundant elastic fibers (Griffin and Sharpe, 1960; Ridall et al., 1982). Inferiorly the disk is tightly attached to the lateral and medial poles of the mandibular condyle (Choukas and Sicher, 1960; Mahan, 1980). Anteriorly, the disk is connected to some fibers of the superior head of the pterygoid muscle through the anterior capsular wall, whose medial half is not well defined.

The lateral pterygoid muscle extends anteriorly and medially to the lateral surface of the pterygoid process of the sphenoid bone. The inferior head of the muscle joins the external surface of this process at the pterygoid fovea of the condyle. Recent studies (Wilkinson, 1988; Tanaka, 1991; Bittar et al., 1994; Heylings et al., 1995) have demonstrated that most of the fibers of the superior head also insert to the condyle.

With mouth closed, in the situation of maximum upper and lower jaw approach, the mandibular and condylar position is conditioned by the *occlusion* that is, by the pattern in which the upper and lower teeth intercuspate. Such a situation is also known as *maximum intercuspation.* In normal conditions, at rest, the mandible lies in a position of *posture,* so that the upper and lower teeth do not touch. As we have seen (Chapter 3), in this *postural position,* the elevator muscle activity is usually low, but not minimal as it is, for instance, during certain stages of sleep (Kawamura and Fujimoto, 1957; Möller, 1970). One conditioning factor of muscle activity during mandibular posture is the activity of the gamma system, which may vary considerably and, under certain conditions, may be excessive and lead to muscle hyperfunction with prolonged tooth clench in some cases (see Chapter 3). Apart from these situations, the position of maximum intercuspation is reached for a few milliseconds during the mas-

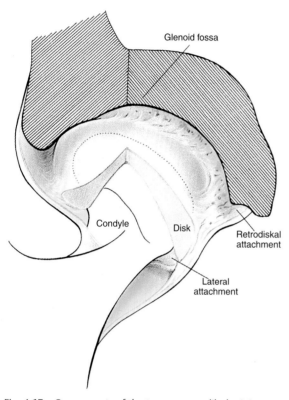

Fig. 4.**15**   Components of the temporomandibular joint

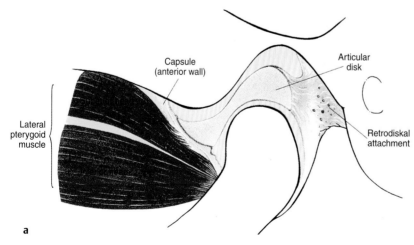

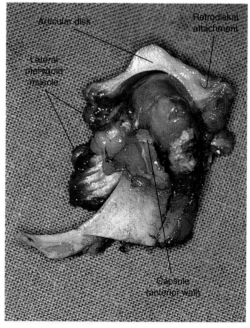

Fig. 4.**16**   **The disk and the other TMJ components. a** Schematic drawing. **b** An autopsy specimen: here the disk was sectioned sagitally to show the underlying condyle. (Courtesy of Professor F. Mela, University of Turin)

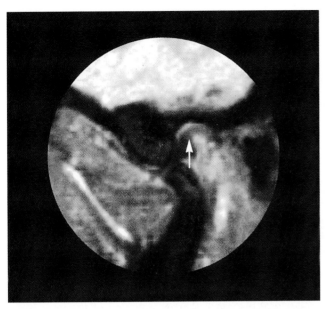

Fig. 4.**17** **Magnetic resonance image at open mouth of a healthy TMJ.** The superior posterior attachment is seen as a low-signal area (arrow)

ticatory cycle and, sometimes for a longer period, during swallowing (Gibbs et al., 1971; Gibbs and Lundeen, 1982; Mongini et al., 1986). In normal conditions, the transition from the postural position of the mandible to maximum intercuspation implies that the mandible performs a small upward vertical movement with an almost barely rotatory movement of the condyle. In the postural position and with mouth closed, the condyle sits on the posterior portion of the disk (which, as we have said, is the thicker part) (Fig. 4.**16**). During mouth opening, the condyle translates forward, by the contraction of the inferior head of the lateral pterygoid muscle, and the disk is pulled forward by the tension of its attachment to the lateral and medial condyle poles. During this movement, the superior head of the muscle is not activated. This movement of the disk is counteracted by the tension of the elastic fibers of the posterior disk attachment. Therefore, the

forward translating condyle is related to progressively more anterior sectors of the disk.

During mouth closure the condyle is brought backward by the elevator muscles and, in particular, by the temporal muscle. In this phase the superior head of the lateral pterygoid muscle is activated, while the inferior head remains silent. During this movement the disk is no longer kept forward by the disk–condyle attachments, which are no longer in tension: however, a smooth and progressive reestablishment of the initial disk position at closed mouth is assured by the balanced action of the elastic fibers of the posterior attachment, which being in tension, tend to draw the disk backward, and that of the fibers of the lateral pterygoid muscle inserting on the disk. Thus, a too abrupt posterior disk movement is be avoided (Mahan, 1980; Bell, 1982). However, it has been suggested that the decreased tension of the elastic fibers could facilitate the expulsion of blood consequent upon the movement of the condyle back inside the glenoid cavity. This would allow the "puffer" function of the posterior attachment to counteract the "pistonlike" movements of the condyle (Scapino, 1991).

Jaw Alterations and TMJ Dysfunction

Jaw structure alteration may be genetic or acquired. In the congenital or genetic type, the deformity is usually severe, entailing marked functional disorders (Cherrik, 1979; Sarnat, 1979) (Fig. 4.**18**). In other cases, alterations may be induced by trauma, infection, or radiation (Sarnat, 1979; Tanaka, 1986). Trauma may be directly to the joint, or indirect, such as a blow to the chin, with or without condylar fracture.

Infection of the TMJ is usually the consequence of an infection spreading from adjacent structures such as the teeth, the parotid gland, or the mandibular body, or, more rarely, of hematogeneous spread from distant regions. Other inflammatory joint diseases that may involve the TMJ are rheumatoid arthritis and ankylosing spondylitis. Rheumatoid arthritis is a general disease that involves dfferent joints progressively with typically intermittent periods of activity (Fig. 4.**19**) (Blackwood, 1963, 1969; Marbach and Spiera, 1967; Kreutziger and Mahan, 1975; Mahan, 1980; Wenneberg,

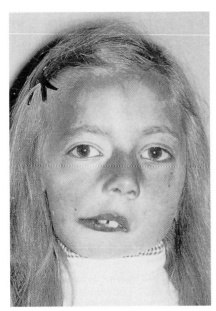

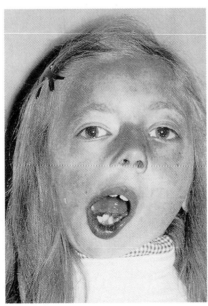

Fig. 4.**18** Very serious structural alteration in a young girl with hemifacial microsomy. (From Mongini and Schmid, 1989)

a   b

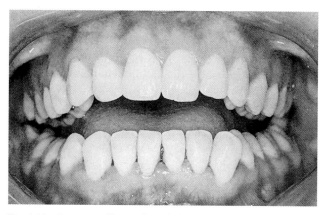 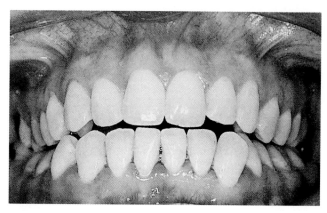

Fig. 4.**19**   **Patient suffering from bilateral rheumatoid arthritis of the TMJ.** In the acute phase (**a**) the patient presents a marked anterior open bite which disappears almost entirely during remission periods (**b**). (From Mongini and Schmid, 1989)

1983; Stabrun et al., 1984; Stabrun, 1985). Ankylosing spondylitis is a chronic disease in which the inflammatory changes of the joint ligaments are gradually followed by ossification and consequent severe restriction of movement (Wenneberg et al., 1983). This disease typically affects the spine and the sacroiliac joints, but may also affect the TMJ, with a frequency reported variously as being between 4% and 32% (Wenneberg and Kopp, 1982). The TMJ may also be involved in gout, Reiter syndrome (Wright, 1963) and psoriasis (Könönen, 1966; Rasmussen and Bakke, 1982).

Radiation therapy for tumors in adjacent regions can also result in permanent damage of the condylar growth center during growth and, consequently, in permanent jaw structure alteration.

Occlusal disorders, that is, alteration of the intercuspation, either genetic and/or acquired, are a relatively frequent finding in both growing and adult populations. These disorders may lead to mandibular deviation and displacement when the position of maximum intercuspation is reached (Fig. 4.**20**). Mandibular displacement involves condyle displacement and, as a consequence, an alteration of the reciprocal disk–condyle position; condyle displacement is three-dimensional. A frequent condition involves posterior and lateral condyle displacement, which may lead to intracapsu-

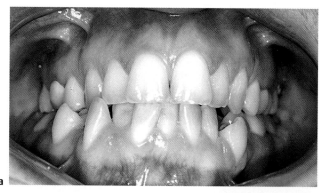 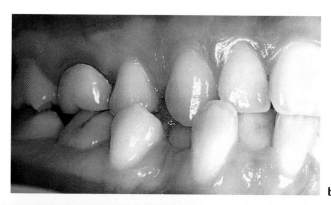

a   b

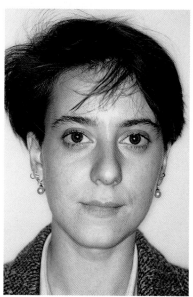 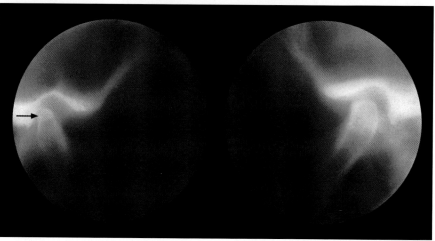

c

d

Fig. 4.**20**   This patient has marked structure alteration leading to a rightward mandibular dislocation in position of maximum tooth intercuspation (**a, b**). As a consequence there is a marked craniofacial asymmetry (**c**) and a posterior displacement of the right condyle (arrow in **d**)

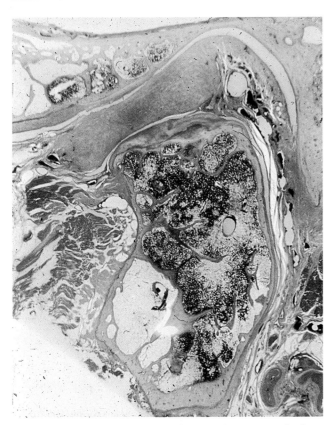

Fig. 4.**21** **Histological specimen of TMJ with posterior displacement of the condyle and consequent compression of the retrodiskal ligament.** Vessel compression and the beginnings of tissue inflammation can be seen. (By courtesy of Professor G. Steinhard, Erlangen)

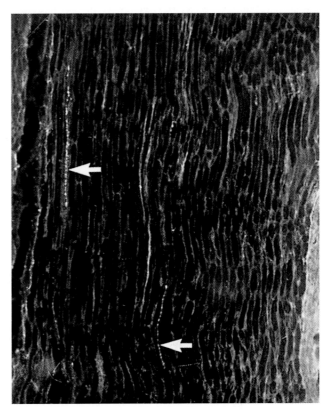

Fig. 4.**22** Histological section of a disk attachment with fluorescent fibers, immunoreactive to substance P. (From Johanson et al., 1986, with permission)

lar disorders and dislocation of the disk (see Chapters 1 and 22).

These situations may provoke pain in several ways. Posterior condylar displacement leads to compression of the retrodiskal pad with blood flow inpingment and possible extravasation and initial inflammatory changes (Fig. 4.**21**). In case of disk displacement, there is a progressive stretching and tearing of the retrodisk ligament. Degenerative joint disease (joint arthrosis) max follow with time. The retrodiskal attachment is rich in nerve endings from the auriculotemporal nerve. In particular, free nociceptor endings are abundant (Dixon, 1962; Thilander, 1964; Keller and Moffett, 1968). Histochemical studies (Johansson et al., 1986) have also shown that substance P is present in the joint tissues (Fig. 4.**22**): substance P is the most important mediator of pain sensations and, as we have seen (Chapter 2), may be a factor of inflammation in the periphery.

All the above-mentioned situations lead to activation of the nociceptors of the retrodiskal attachment and hence to arthrogenous pain. Localized pain during function is a consequence, but in more severe cases it may be constant and spread to the temple and cheek.

References

Bell W.E., *Clinical management of temporomandibular disorders*, Year Book Medical Publishers, Chicago, 1982, 28 – 34.

Bittar G.T., Bibb C.A., Pullinger A.G., *Histologic characteristics of the lateral pterygoid muscle insertion to the temporomandibular joint*, J. Orofac. Pain, 1994, 8 : 243 – 249.

Blackwood H.J.J., *Arthritis of the mandibular joint*, Br. Dent. J., 1963, 115 : 317 – 324.

Blackwood H.J.J., *Pathology of the temporomandibular joint*, J. Am. Dent. Assoc., 1969, 79 : 118 – 124.

Bogduk N., *Headache and the cervical spine. An editorial.*, Cephalalgia, 1984, 4 : 7 – 8.

Bogduk N., *Cervical causes of headache*, Cephalalgia, 1989,10 (9 Suppl.):172 – 3.

Cherrik H.M.,*Pathology*, in: Sarnat B.G., Laskin D.M. (eds.), *The temporomandibular joint*, Charles C. Thomas, Springfield, Ill., 1979, 180 – 204.

Choukas N.C., Sicher H., *The structure of the temporomandibular joint*, Oral Surg., 1960, 13 : 1203 – 1213.

Darlow L.A., Pesco J., Greenberg M.S., *The relationship of posture to myofascial pain dysfunction syndrome*, J. Am. Dent. Assoc., 1987, 114 : 73 – 75.

Dixon A.D., *Structure and functional significance of the intra-articular disc of the human temporomandibular joint*, J. Oral Surg., 1962, 15 : 48.

Fricton J.R., Kroening R., Haley D., et al., *Myofascial pain syndrome of the head and neck: A review of clinical characteristics of 164 patients*, Oral Surg. Oral Med. Oral Pathol., 1985, 60 : 615 – 623.

Gibbs C.H., Messerman T., Reswick J.B., Derda H.J., *Functional movements of the mandible*, J. Prosthet. Dent., 1971, 26 : 601 – 610.

Gibbs C.H., Lundeen H., *Jaw movements and forces during chewing and swallowing and their clinical significance*, in: Gibbs C.H., Lundeen H. (eds.), *Advances in occlusion*, John Wright PSC Inc., Littleton, Mass., 1982, 2 – 32.

Griffin C.J., Sharpe C.J., *The distribution of the synovial membrane and mechanism of its blood supply in the adult human temporomandibular joint*, Aust. Dent. J., 1960, 5 : 367.

Heylings D.J.A., Nielsen I.L., McNeill C., *Lateral pterygoid muscle and the temporomandibular disc.*, J. Orofac. Pain, 1995, 9 : 9 – 16.

Hackey J., Bade D., Clawson A., *Relationship between forward head posture and diagnosed internal derangement of the temporomandibular joint*, J. Orofac. Pain, 1993, 7 : 386 – 390.

Huggare Å., Raustia A.M., *Head posture and cervicovertebral and craniofacial morphology in patients with craniomandibular dysfunction*, Cranio, 1992, 10 : 173 – 179.

Johansson A.S., Isacsson G., Isberg A., Granholm A.C., *Distribution of substance P-like immunoreactive nerve fibers in temporomandibular joint soft tissues of monkey*, Scand. J. Dent. Res. 1986, 94 : 225 – 230,.

Kawamura Y., Fujimoto J., *Some physiologic considerations on measuring rest position of the mandible*, Med. J. Osaka Univ., 1957, 247 – 255.

Keller J.M., Moffett B.C., *Nerve endings in the temporomandibular joint of the Rhesus Macaque*, Anat. Rec., 1968, 160 : 587 – 594.

Kerr FWL, *Central relationships of trigeminal and cervical primary afferents in the spinal cord and medulla*, Brain Res., 1972, 43 : 561 – 572.

Könönen M., *Craniomandibular disorders in psoriatic arthritis. Correlation between subjective symptoms, clinical signs, and radiograghic changes*, Acta Odontol. Scand., 1966, 44 : 369 – 375.

Kreutziger K.L., Mahan P.E., *Temporomandibular degenerative joint disease*, I: *Anatomy pathophysiology and clinical description*, Oral Surg. Oral Med. Oral Pathol., 1975, 40 : 165 – 182.

Lee W.Y., Okeson J.P., Lindroth J., *The relationship between forward head posture and temporomandibular disorderes*, J. Orofac. Pain, 1995, 9 : 161 – 167.

Mahan P.E., *Temporomandibular joint in function and dysfunction*, in: Solberg W.K., Clark G.T. (eds.), *Temporomandibular joint problems*, Quintessence Publishing Co., Chicago, 1980, 33 – 42.

Marbach J.J., Spiera H., *Rheumatoid arthritis of the temporomandibular joint*, Ann. Rheum., Dis., 1967, 26 : 538 – 543.

Möller E., *Computer analysis of electromyographic data in clinical studies of oral function*, Scand. J. Dent. Res., 1970, 78 : 411 – 416.

Mongini F., Tempia-Valenta G., Benvegnu G., *Computer-based assesment of habitual mastication*, J. Prosthet. Dent., 1986, 55 : 638 – 649.

Mongini F., Schmid W., *Craniomandibular and TMJ orthopedics*, Quintessence, Chicago-Berlin, 1989.

Mongini F., Poma M., Bava M., Fabbri G., *Psychosomatic symptoms in different types of headache and facial pain*, Cephalalgia, 1997, 17 : 274 (abs.).

Pöllmann W., Keidel M., Pfaffenrath V., *Headache and the cervical spine: a critical review*, Cephalalgia, 1997, 17 : 801 – 816.

Rasmussen O.C., Bakke M., *Psoriatic arthritis of the temporomandibular joint*, Oral Surg. Oral Med. Oral Pathol., 1982, 53 : 351 – 357.

Rees L.A., *The structure and function of the mandibular joint*, Br. Dent. J., 1954, 96 : 125 – 133.

Ridall A.L., Hayes E.R., Tamburlin J.H., Tabak L.A., Mohl N.D., *Description of elastic fibers in the bilaminar zone*, J. Dent. Res., 1982, 61 : 351 (abs.).

Rocabado M., *The hyoid region*, in: *Head-neck and dentistry manual*, Rocabado Institute, Tacoma, Washington, 1982.

Rocabado M., *Biomechanical relationship of the cranial, cervical, and hyoid regions*, Cranio, 1983, 1 : 61 – 66.

Sarnat B.G., *Developmental facial abnormalities and the temporomandibular joint*, J. Am. Dent. Assoc., 1979, 79 : 108 – 117.

Scapino R.P., *The posterior attachment: Its structure, function, and appearance in TMJ imaging studies. Part. 2*, J. Craniomandib. Disord. Facial Oral Pain, 1991, 5 : 155 – 166.

Simons D.G., Mense, S., *Understanding and measurement of muscle tone as related to clinical muscle pain*, Pain, 1998, 75 : 1 – 17.

Stabrun A.E., *Mandibular morphology and position in juvenile rheumatoid arthritis. A study on postero-anterior radiographs*, Eur. J. Orthodont 985, 7 : 288 – 298.

Stabrun A.E., Höyernall H.M., Larheim T.A., Rösler M., *Temporomandibular joint as a pathogenetic factor to a facial asymmetry in juvenile reumatoid arthritis (J.R.A.), and the clinical significance of skeletal asymmetry*, Scand. J. Reumatol 1984, (Suppl. 53).

Tanaka T.T., *A rational approach to the differential diagnosis of arthritic disorders*, J. Prosthet. Dent., 1986, 8 : 727 – 731.

Tanaka T.T., *An anatomical approach to current controversies*, Proc.: TMJ, State of the art, Paris, 1992.

Thilander B., *Innervation of the temporomandibular disc in man*, Acta Odontol. Scand., 1964, 22 : 152 – 156.

Travell J.G., Simons D.G., *Myofascial pain and dysfunction: The trigger point manual*, Williams & Wilkins, Baltimore, MD, 1983.

Watson D.H., Trott P.H., *Cervical headache: An investigation of natural head posture and upper cervical flexor muscle performance*, Cephalalgia, 1993, 13 : 272 – 284.

Wenneberg B., *Inflammatory involvement of the temporomandibular joint*, Swed. Dent. J., 1983, (Suppl. 20).

Wenneberg B., Kopp S., *Subjective symptoms from the stomatognathic system in ankylosing spondylitis*, Acta Odontol. Scand., 1982, 40 : 215 – 222.

Wenneberg B., Hollender L., Kopp S., *Radiographic changes in the temporomandibular joint in ankylosing spondylitis*, Dentomaxillofac. Radiol., 1983, 12 : 25 – 30.

Wilkes C.H., *Structural and functional alterations of the temporomandibular joint*, North-West Dent., 1978 a, 57 : 287 – 294.

Wilkes C.H., *Arthrography of the temporomandibular joint*, Minn. Med., 1978 b, 61 : 645 – 652.

Wilkinson T.M., *The relationship between the disk and the lateral pterygoid muscle in the human temporomandibular joint*, J. Prosthet. Dent., 1988, 60 : 715 – 724.

Wright V., *Arthritis associated with venereal disease. A comparative study of gonococcal arthritis and Reiter's syndrome*, Ann. Rheum. Dis., 1963, 22 : 77 – 89.

5 Systemic Neurological Factors

Cortical Function

Cortical spontaneous and evoked electrical activity has been investigated in patients with headache and facial pain. Numerous authors have found EEG abnormalities in migraine patients. Such abnormalities include epileptiform activities (Kooi et al., 1965; Kinast et al., 1982; Jay, 1982; Farkas et al., 1993) (Fig. 5.1) and prominent photic driving (Slatter, 1968; Kinast et al., 1982; Simon et al., 1982); generalized or focal slow waves (Slevin et al., 1981; Mariani et al., 1988) (Fig. 5.2); rhythmic high-amplitude slow waves during hyperventilation (Giel et al., 1966); and excessive fast activities (Hughes and Robbins, 1990; van Dijk et al., 1991).

Brain mapping techniques have been used widely for these studies (Facchetti et al., 1990; Hughes and Robbins, 1990; Neufield et al., 1991; Seri et al., 1993; Genco et al., 1994; Valdizan et al., 1994; Asteggiano et al., 1997) (Fig. 5.2). The traditional EEG brain mapping allows better quantification of abnormalities present and is less influenced by the expectations of the investigator.

However, several studies are limited by the lack or inadequacy of control groups, or by the fact that patients were tested while they were undergoing drug treatment (Gronseth and Greenberg, 1995). The most consistent observations seem to relate to prominent driving in response to photic stimulation (Simon et al., 1982, 1983; van Dick et al., 1991; Gronseth and Greenberg, 1995, American Academy of Neurology, 1995), an interhemispheric difference of the alpha rhythm in migraine with aura (Genco et al., 1994; Asteggiano et al., 1997; Vighetti et al., 1997) (Fig. 5.3), or a higher theta/alpha relation (Valdizan et al., 1994).

The relationship between migraine and epilepsy has been studied extensively, since both disorders are characterized by paroxysmal, transient alterations of neurological function (Bazil, 1994). An association between idiopathic epilepsy and migraine is asserted by numerous authors (Basser, 1969; Baier and Doose, 1987; Bladin, 1987; Isler et al., 1987; Sacquegna et al., 1987; Septien et al., 1991; Hughes et al., 1993; Ottman and Lipton, 1994; Lipton et al., 1994). Cases were reported of migraine aura leading to an epileptic seizure (Ehrenberg, 1991) and cases in which headache seemed to be a manifestation of focal epileptic seizures (Jonas, 1966; Swaiman and Frank, 1978; Laplante et al., 1983) or coincided with or followed a childhood epilepsy with occipital paroxysms (Gastaut and Zifkin, 1987; Terzano et al., 1987).

Centrotemporal epilepsy (rolandic epilepsy) has also been associated with migraine in some patients (Bladin, 1987; Septien et al., 1991; Andermann and Zifkin, 1998). This childhood benign epileptic syndrome is characterized by unilateral somatosensory symptoms with preservation of consciousness and slow spikes in the centrotemporal region (Fig. 5.4). Septien et al. (1991), in a retrospective study on 50 patients with centrotemporal epilepsy, found that migraine was present in 63% of the patients. The migraine could last long after the end of the disappearance of the epilepsy. The authors concluded that such association is not chance but is more probably due to a neurochemical alteration common to both diseases.

In summary, a great amount of data, although sometimes contradictory, shows that epilepsy and migraine can coexist or masquerade as each other (Bazil, 1994).

Somatosensory (SEPs), auditory (AEPs) and visual (VEPs) evoked potentials have been studied in headache patients: both stimulus-related potentials (which depend on the physical characteristics of the stimuli), and event-related potentials (which depend on the information content of the stimuli) have been investigated.

A number of authors found latency and amplitude variations of stimulus-related and event-related potentials in migraine patients (Moreira-Filho and Dantos, 1994; Marlowe, 1995; Chayasirisobhon, 1995; Mazzotta et al., 1995; Puca et al., 1996; de Tommaso et al., 1997). However, others could not confirm these findings (Rossi et al., 1996). Significant alterations (with polarity reduction, disappearance of inversion) were found ipsilateral to the visual symptoms in patients with migraine with hemioptic aurea (Tagliati et al., 1995). Schoenen et al. (1995) studied sequential blocks of 50 VEPs calculating mean N1–P1 and P1–N2 amplitude values for each block. They found, in patients with migraine with or without aura, a tendency to a potentiation of the various blocks as compared to the first block. This tendency was in marked contrast with what was observed in normal subjects, which showed a tendency to "habituation," that is, a decrease of mean amplitude values of the blocks following the first block. This effect was partially confirmed by Vighetti et al. (1996) (Fig. 5.5). More recently, Afra et al. (1998) obtained similar results with VEP during long periods (15 min) of pattern-reversal stimulation in migraine patients. A similar phenomenon was also reported for the AEP of migraine patients (Wang et al., 1996). It has been demonstrated by nuclear magnetic resonance spectroscopy studies that in normal subjects habituation counteracts the initial increase of lactate and consequent decrease of pH levels during repetitive light stimulations (Sappey-Marinier et al., 1992). The lack of habituation in migraine patients might favor biochemical alterations that could trigger the migraine attack (Wang et al., 1996; Schoenen, 1998).

Contingent negative variation (CNV), first described by Walter et al. (1964), is another example of cortical activity that has been used in the study of headache patients. CNV is an event-related slow cortical potential that is recorded over the scalp in reaction-time tasks following a warning stimulus and a response stimulus (imperative stimulus). The warning stimulus (S1) is a 1000 Hz frequency noise of 50 ms duration. The imperative stimulus (S2) is a series of light flashes. The subject is asked to interrupt the flash by pressing a button (Schoenen and Timsit-Berthier, 1993). The interstimulus interval can be varied. In most studies an interval of 1 s was used, but the two components of CNV are identifiable with an interval of 3 s or more (Böcker et al., 1990) (Fig. 5.6). The CNV is associated with a number of parameters: expectation, attention, preparation, motivation and readiness (Walter et al., 1964; Rockstroh et al., 1982).

CNV has been studied in psychiatric disorders (Timsit-Berthier, 1976; Timsit-Berthier et al., 1984, 1987, 1989), neurological disorders (Amabile et al., 1986), and, more recently,

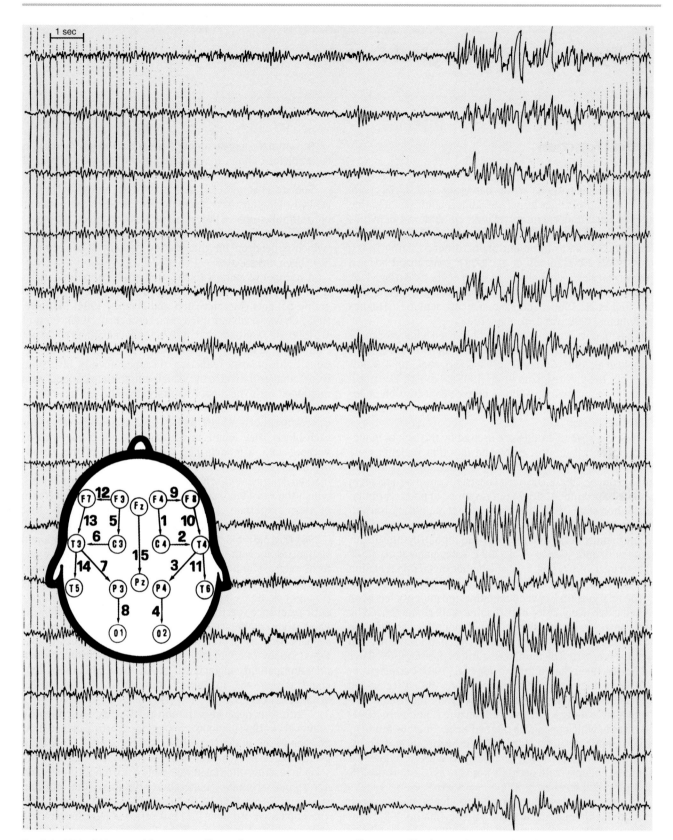

Fig. 5.**1** **EEG of 40-year-old woman suffering from migraine.** Over a well-organized background activity, short bursts of diffused spiky graphoelements appear, prevalently anterior

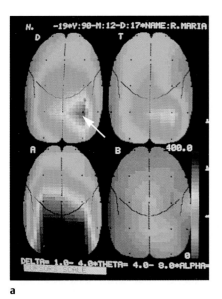 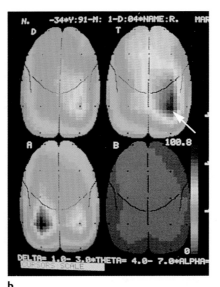 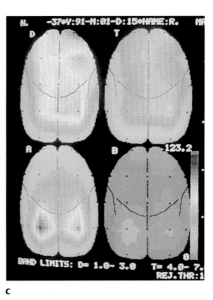

a   b   c

Fig. 5.**2** **Quantitative mapped EEG of a patient, 48 hours (a), 20 days (b), and one month (c) after an attack of migraine with aura.** (**a**) A delta focus is cleary visible (arrow). (**b**) Decrease of delta focus and appearance of theta focus. (**c**) Disappearance of the focus and presence of a diffuse theta-delta power. (By courtesy of Dr. G. Asteggiano, Turin University)

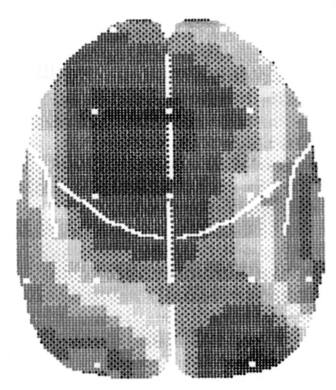

Fig. 5.**3** **Quantitative mapped EEG of a women patient with chronic migraine.** A marked interhemispheric alpha asymmetry is present. (From Vighetti et al., 1997)

in headache patients (Schoenen et al., 1985; Maertens de Noorhout et al., 1986; Kropp and Gerber, 1993, 1995). CNV has been shown to have a high specificity (but moderate sensitivity) in patients suffering from migraine without aura. In such patients during the intercritical period, the average amplitude of CNV is significantly larger than that found in healthy individuals or tension-type headache patients (Schoenen et al., 1985; Maertens de Noordhout et al., 1986; Bpcker et al., 1990; Gerber et al., 1992). Kropp and Gerber (1995) found that CNV

amplitude of patients with migrane without aura in the intercritical period is higher than that of healthy subjects and that of the same patients during an untreated migraine attack (Fig. 5.**7**). After successful treatment of migraine, CNV values return to normal (Schoenen, 1986; Maertens de Noordhout et al., 1987; Schoenen and Timsit-Berthier, 1993) (Fig. 5.**8**). The same significant difference in CNV values was found in a group of children with migraine compared to children with tension-type headache (Besken et al., 1993).

To explain these CNV alterations in patients with migraine without aura, it has been suggested that such alterations might be consequences of hyperreactivity of the catecholaminergic and dopaminergic system (Libet, 1978; Marczynski, 1978; Schoenen and Maertens de Noordhout, 1988; Schoenen et al., 1988; Nagel-Leiby et al., 1990; Timsit-Berthier et al., 1989). Since habituation reflects learned rejection of unwanted stimuli, decreased habituation in migraine patients could be consequent on a disturbance of sensory stimulus modulation and selection (Kropp and Gerber, 1995).

Indeed, a positive correlation was found between CNV amplitude and plasma levels of norepinephrine in a mixed group of headache patients (Schoenen et al., 1984). Additionally, administration of beta-blockers normalizes CNV values (Schoenen, 1986; Maertens de Noordhout et al., 1987; Schoenen and Timsit-Berthier, 1993) (Fig. 5.**8**). Kropp and Gerber (1995) postulate that the migraine attack could be the end of the transitory hyperactive level, with consequent resetting to a normal function: this would explain why the CNV alterations observed during the intercritical period normalize during the attack.

In general, the data from evoked potentials and CNV show the presence in migraine patients during the intercritical period of an altered cortical processing of information. Such alteration could be consequent upon an altered serotoninergic transmission (Wang et al., 1996).

In additional, transcranial magnetic stimulation (TMS) has been employed to study cortical function in migraine patients. By this means Welch et al. (1998) evaluated occipital cortex excitability; they found that the majority of patients with migraine reported phosphenes on occipital cortex

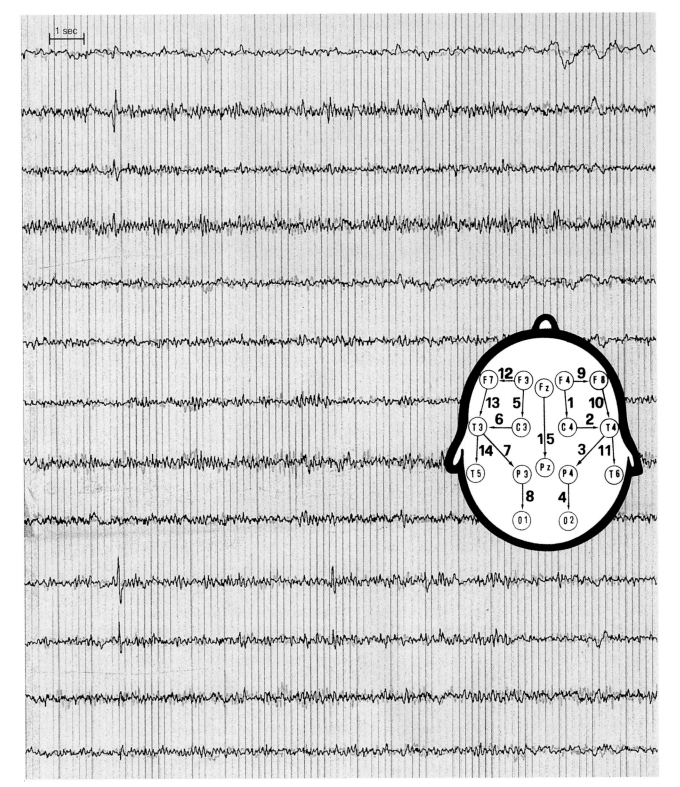

Fig. 5.4 EEG of an 11-year-old girl suffering from migraine attacks. Over a background that is well-organized for her age, high-voltage slow spikes appear in the centrotemporal region of the right hemisphere. The finding is typical for "benign infantile epilepsy" (centrotemporal Roland-type epilepsy). The subject was asymptomatic for epileptic fits

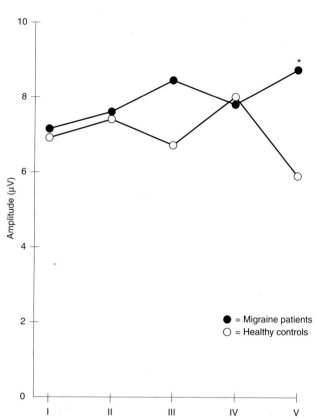

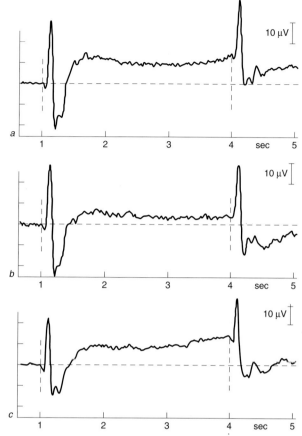

Fig. 5.**5** **Mean amplitude values of visual evoked potentials stimuli examined in 5 consecutive blocks of 50 responses each in a group of migraine patients and in a control group of healthy individuals.** For each block the mean peak-to-peak amplitude N1–P1 was calculated. Habituation was assessed as the amplitude changes in blocks 2–5 compared to block 1. In migraineurs amplitude values significantly higher than those of the normal group are observed in the last block (* P < 0.05). (From Vighetti et al., 1996)

Fig. 5.**7** **Mean contingent negative variation (CNV) in a group of migraine patients in a pain-free interval (a) and during a migraine attack (b).** In (**c**) values of a healthy control group are given. CNV values in (**a**) are significantly higher than in (**b**) and (**c**). (From Kropp and Gerber, 1995, with modifications)

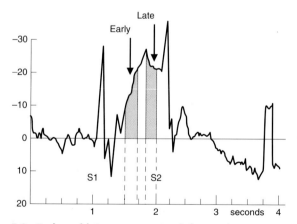

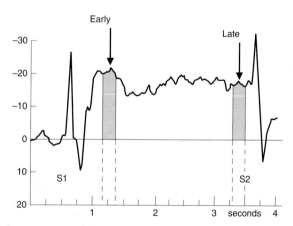

Fig. 5.**6** **Early and late components of the contingent negative variation with interval between the stimuli of 1 s (top) and 3 s (bottom).** With the 1-s interval between stimuli, the mean voltage amplitude is measured during the 200 ms that preceeds the imperative stimuluis (S2). In the case of a 3-s interval between stimuli, the

early component of the contingent variation of negativity is defined by the amplitude of mean voltage measured between 550 and 750 ms after the warning stimulus (S1). The late component is measured as described above. (From Schoenen and Timsit-Berthier, 1993, with modifications)

Before treatment

After treatment

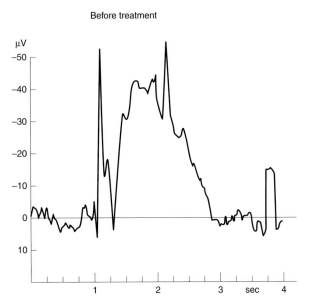

Fig. 5.8 Contingent negative variation in a patient suffering from migraine without aura. The values are high before treatment and return to normal after treatment with propranolol. (From Schoenen and Timsit-Berthier, 1993, with modifications)

stimulation while this phenomenon was reported by only $^3/_{11}$ of the controls. In one patient, TMS triggered a typical aura.

The same authors attempted to trigger migraine attacks in susceptible individuals and to study the earliest moments of the attack through functional MRI. This technique measures relative changes in oxygenation of the brain circulation: the signal intensity is an indirect measure of perfusion that identifies activated brain regions. After repetitive visual stimulations with a colored grid at 9 Hz, headache and visual symptoms occurred in $^8/_{15}$ of the migraine patients and in none of the nine normals tested. Functional MRI showed suppression of neuronal activation before and during the attacks in the eight headache subjects. However, neuronal suppression was accompanied by hyperoxygenation of the occipital cortex during the early minutes of the headache attack. These findings point to a hyperexcitability the occipital cortex in migraine sufferers. Moreover, an activation of the red nucleus and substantia nigra was also observed in these patients during the attack, showing that the cortical event may activate brainstem centers possibly involved in nociception and associated symptoms of the migraine attack (Welch et al., 1998).

The encephalic function has also been studied using positron emission tomography (PET). PET is an imaging technique that detects radioactive tracers and performs a computerized tomographic reconstruction by translating the measured radioactive concentrations into color-coded images. Since only small amounts of short half-life radioligands are administered, PET is not a very invasive methodology. The parameters most frequently investigated are blood flow (analyzed by $H_2{}^{15}O$) (Fig. 5. **9**), glucose catabolism (by ^{18}Fluordeoxyglucose, FGD), and neuroceptors (by specific radioligands) (Sadzot et al., 1995).

Using this methodology, Derbyshire et al. (1994) studied encephalic function in patients with so-called "atypical facial pain" and healthy individuals subjected to painful and nonpainful thermal stimulation. They observed that, compared to controls, the patients had a marked increase in excitation of the cingulate gyrus (Broadman area 24) and a decrease of blood flow in the prefrontal cortex (Fig. 5.**10**). This observation is in agreement with the notion that the anterior cingulate

gyrus plays an important role in the regulation of the attentive-emotional component of pain (Devinsky, 1995): its increased excitation in these patients could be the result of loss of inhibitory activity by the prefrontal cortex. The activation of the right cingulate gyrus was also observed in patients with neuropathic pain (Hsieh et al., 1995) with trigeminal neuralgia (J. C. Hsieh et al., unpublished), and during a nitroglycerine-induced attack of cluster headache (Hsieh et al., 1996) (Fig. 5.**11**).

Finally, some data are indicative of an alteration of the rhythmic organization of the central nervous system in migraine patients (Nappi et al., 1983; Brun et al., 1995). In particular, melatonin, which is produced by the pineal gland with a circadian variation (with high nocturnal and low diurnal

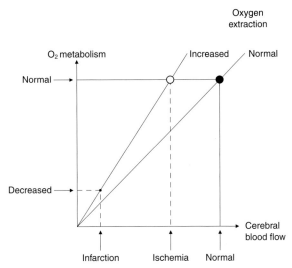

Fig. 5.9 Evaluation of the relation between cerebral blood flow, oxygen extraction and oxygen metabolism using PET. The black dot represents the normal coupling between blood flow and oxygen metabolism. In ischemic conditions a compensatory increase of oxygen extraction takes place that preserves, oxygen metabolism to some degree. After a further decrease of blood flow metabolism decreases and infarction occurs. (From Sadzot et al., 1995, with modifications)

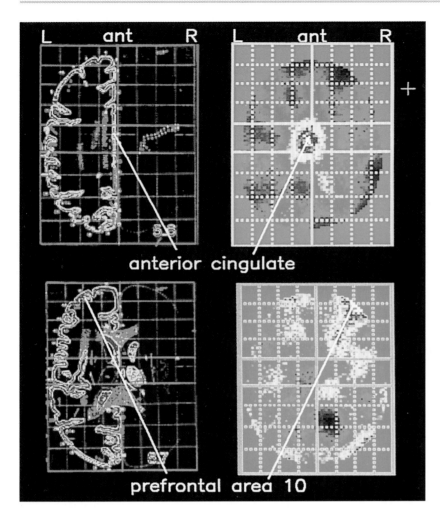

anterior cingulate

prefrontal area 10

Fig. 5.**10** **PET study of the encephalic function in patients with so-called atypical facial pain subjected to thermal stimulation.** Compared to controls, an increased excitation of the cingulate gyrus and decrease exitation of the frontal is observed. (From Derbyshire et al., 1994, with permission)

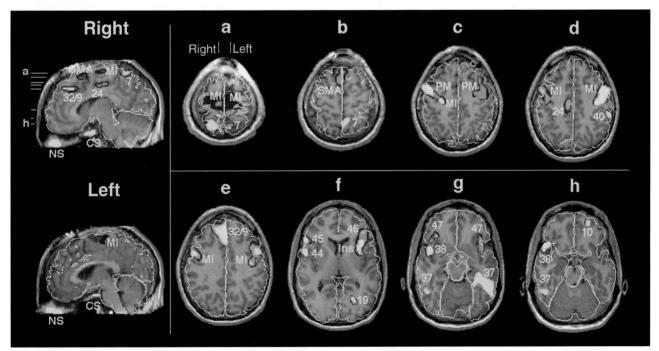

Fig. 5.**11** **Areas with significant changes of cerebral blood flow during attack of cluster headache.** Colored areas indicate four levels of significant change defined as 0.001 P < 0.01 (red, increased blood flow; blue, decreased blood flow) and P < 0.001 (yellow, increased blood flow; light blue, decreased blood flow). The numbers refer to Brodman's nomenclature. Ins, insula; M1, primary motor area; SMA, supplementary motor area; CS, cavernous sinus; NS, nasal sinus. PET images are superimposed on MRI images. (From Hsieh et al., 1995, with permission)

plasma concentrations), in women with migraine shows a nocturnal secretion significantly lower than that in healthy controls (Brun et al., 1995; Murialdo et al., 1994). Similarly, circannual melatonin concentrations in a group of patients with cluster headache were significantly lower than in the control group (Waldenlind et al., 1994).

Alterations of Neurotransmitters

Together the neurotransmitters, serotonin, and norepinephrine play an important role in the pathogenesis of headache and, in particular, of migraine. The association between central serotoninergic transmissions and headache is supported by a number of observations (see review by Marcus, 1995). An increase of serotonin plasma concentrations was found in patients during episodes of tension-type headache (Jensen and Hindberg, 1994). Headache attacks may be induced by substances that lead to release of serotonin, such as reserpine (Bánk, 1991), or by agonists of serotoninergic postsynaptic receptors (Brewerton et al., 1988). In turn, headache may be attenuated by metisergide, a postsaynaptic serotonin antagonist (Bánk, 1991) or by the increase of peripheral circulating serotonin (Kimball et al., 1960; Goadsby and Lance, 1990): this suggests the presence of an autoinhibitory mechanism on the central structures that produce serotonin, such as the raphe dorsal nucleus.

These data may seem to contradict the numerous reports of the inhibitory action in pain modulation of the descending serotoninergic bulbospinal projections (Hutson et al., 1982; Fasmer et al., 1985; Liu et al., 1988; Saito et al., 1990). The integrity of these projections is, at least in part, a factor conditioning the analgesic action of the opioids (Tenen, 1968; Vogt, 1974; Roberts, 1988; Paul et al., 1988; Crisp et al., 1991 a, b). The complexity of the action of serotonin also depends on the presence of numerous serotoninergic subreceptors with variable function (Cesselin et al., 1994; Fields and Basbaum, 1994). Moreover, it has been shown that the action of serotonin applied to biopsy material of the superficial temporal artery removed from the painful side of patients with episodic cluster headache is different from that on biopsy material from the same artery removed from healthy individuals. While in the arteries of healthy subjects serotonin induced a dose-dependent constriction, in arteries from cluster headache patients it systematically triggered rhythmic contractions (Mathiau et al., 1994) (Fig. 5.**12**).

The level of peripheral serotonin is modulated by its release by the platelets, whose function is frequently altered in migraine patients (see Chapter 6). It has also been observed that the expression of 5-HT receptor in monocytes increases during headache induced by isosorbide dinitrate in migraine patients. After relief of headache by sumatriptan or ergotamine administration in these patients, the 5-HT receptor expression increased further (Martelletti et al., 1994 a, b; Martelletti and Giacovazzo, 1995).

The possibility of marking 5-HT receptors by PET opens new perspectives for the analysis of their function during attacks of pain, and of migraine in particular (Sadzot et al., 1995).

A decrease of the plasma levels of nonepinephrine has been observed during migraine attacks (Fog-Moller et al., 1978) as well as an increase of its metabolites (Curran et al., 1965). The question is still open whether such findings are simply due to a reaction to head pain (Marcus, 1995). Nevertheless, the descending noradrenergic pathways play, similarly to the serotoninergic pathways an important role in pain modulation (Proudfit, 1988).

The concept that migraine is, at least in part, the consequence of a central neurotransmission disorder is also supported by the fact that in migraine patients other neurotransmitters show alterations in cerebrospinal fluid levels. In particular, the levels of taurine, glycine, and glutamine were found to be significantly higher in migraine patients than in healthy control subjects (Rothrock et al., 1995).

Endogenous Opioids

Plasma and cerebrospinal fluid levels of endogenous opioids have been investigated extensively in headache sufferers. The problem, which closely relates to the function of the central nervous system, could to some extent also be considered to be hormonal in nature. Indeed, the circulating β-endorphins, together with ACTH and β-lipotropin, are produced almost entirely by the pituitary gland (Krieger and Martin, 1981) and exert a control function on the hypothalamus–pituitary–adrenal axis (Facchinetti and Genazzani, 1988). This control is altered during attacks of premenstrual migraine (Facchinetti et al., 1990). A reduction of the β-endorphin concentration in blood monocytes was also observed in migraine patients and not in tension-type headache patients (Leone et al., 1991, 1992).

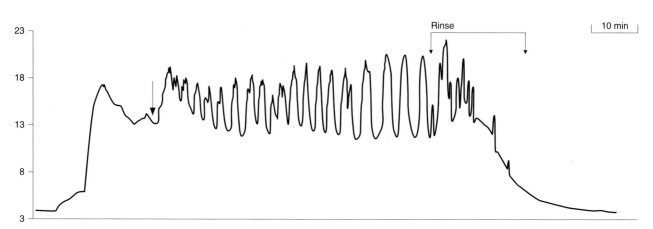

Fig. 5.**12 Constrictions induced by progessively higher serotonin concentrations in a superficial temporal artery from a cluster headache patient.** At a concentration level of 5×10^{-8} nol L^{-1} (arrow) the artery begins to constrict periodically. A rapid, small cyclic activity is superimposed on these slow waves. This cyclic activity stops after removal of serotonin. (From Mathiau et al., 1994, with modifications)

In chronic headache patients a deficiency of the antinociceptive opioid system has been postulated (Sicuteri et al., 1978). One approach to study the activity of this system is to assess neuropeptide concentrations in the cerebrospinal fluid (CSF) on the assumption that these concentrations reflect tissue concentrations in the central nervous system and perhaps synaptic activity (Wood, 1980). Lower β-endorphin levels were found in the CSF of migraine patients (Leppaluoto et al., 1983; Genazzani et al., 1984) and in daily chronic headache patients in whom a chronic tension-type headache and migraine without aura coexist (Martignoni, 1991). The levels correlated inversely with the amount of pain (Facchinetti and Genazzani, 1988). Since CSF levels of adrenocorticotropic hormone (ACTH) were normal in the same patients who had lower β-endorphin levels, it was suggested that specific alterations exist in the neuronal metabolism of pro-opiomelanocortin (POMC), from which both molecules (ACTH and β-endorphin) originate (Genazzani et al., 1984). However, it must be considered that reduced β-endorphin levels were found in other types of chronic pain (such as low back pain) (Panerai, 1987).

Other researchers did not find significant differences of CSF β-endorphin levels in patients with tension-type headache (Bach et al., 1992) or ischemic cerebrovascular headache (Nappi et al., 1985). Higher CSF met-enkephalin immunoreactivity levels were found in patients with chronic tension-type headache (Langemark et al., 1995). These findings may be indicative of an activation of the enkephalinergic antinociceptive system at spinal/trigeminal level consequent upon increased activity of the primary nociceptors (Langemark et al., 1995). Similarly, elevated CSF enkephalin levels were found in fibromyalgia (Vaeroy et al., 1991).

Reflex Responses

Several reflex responses are currently employed as a means to explore the function of pain control systems in normal or painful conditions.

Nociceptive flexion reflexes (NFR) are used to quantify pain threshold in humans (see Sandrini et al., 1993a, for a review) because a close correlation exists between the reflex threshold and the subjective pain threshold (Willer, 1977). NFR can be evoked in both upper limbs (Cambier et al., 1974) and lower limbs (Willer, 1983). In the lower limbs, stimulating surface electrodes are placed in the retromalleolar region, and the flexion response is recorded via surface electrodes placed at the tendon and over the belly of the biceps femoris brevis muscle (Sandrini et al., 1993a) (Fig. 5.**13**). Trains of stimuli are applied (between 20 and 50 ms duration, depending on which reflex component is to be studied) at 300 Hz frequency, with a duration for each stimulus of 1 ms. Two successive components, RII and RIII, are observed (Sandrini et al., 1993). Stimuli eliciting NFR are mainly conveyed along A-delta fibers; however, by applying certain modalities of stimulation, A-alpha and A-beta fibers can also be activated (Willer et al., 1978; Willer and Albe-Fessard, 1983). From the spinal cord, nociceptive stimuli are transmitted to higher centers (mainly through the spinothalamic tract). The response is conditioned by a descending control excercised by the periaqueductal gray, the nucleus of the raphe magnus, and the locus coeruleus. The activity of these centers is modulated by the limbic system and by information from the reticular formation and the lateral branches of the ascending system (Fig. 5.**14**). The reflex is inhibited by stress (Willer and Albe-Fessard, 1980), by morphine (Willer, 1985) and by met-enkephalin analogues (Roby et al., 1983).

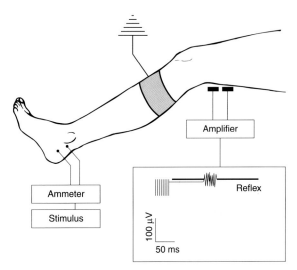

Fig. 5.**13**   Set-up for studying the flexion nociceptive reflex. (From Sandrini et al., 1993a, with modifications)

In headache patients, significant changes of the NFR were found. In patients with chronic daily headache (i.e., migraine and interval headache), decreased thresholds of the NFR were found (Sandrini et al., 1985, 1986). Moreover, such patients exhibited an inverse correlation between headache severity and threshold values (Sandrini et al., 1986). Administration of tryciclic or nontryciclic antidepressants led to a significant increase of the threshold (Nappi et al., 1991). Interestingly enough, an inverse correlation also exists between headache severity and β-endorphin levels in the cerebrospinal fluid (see below). Finally, a lower NFR threshold was also found in tension-type headache patients (Langemark et al., 1993) and in cluster headache patients during the active phase (Sandrini et al., 1992). Similarly, a lower NFR threshold was found on the symptomatic side in patients with chronic paroximal hemicrania and hemicrania continua (Antonaci et al., 1994).

Inhibition reflexes of the masseter and temporal muscles have also been studied. Such "jaw opening" reflexes may be evoked by applying various electric and mechanical stimuli, to the perioral area, the oral cavity and the masseter muscle and, after percussion of the lip, the chin and a single tooth. The reflex is also evoked by interdental contact during chewing movements (Hannam et al., 1968, 1969, 1970; Goldberg and Nakamura, 1968; Griffin and Munro, 1969; Yemm, 1972; Yu et al., 1973; Godaux and Desmedt, 1975; Gillins and Klineberg, 1975; Hannan, 1979; Lund et al., 1983; Di Francesco et al., 1986).

The masseter inhibitory reflex may be evoked by innocuous stimuli and is mediated by A-beta fibers (Cruccu et al., 1989). A prolonged inhibitory response was observed by several authors in patients with muscle and or temporomandibular joint dysfunctions (Balley et al., 1977; Bessette and Shatkin, 1979; Skiba and Laskin, 1981; McCall and Hoffer, 1981; Sharav et al., 1982; Hussein and McCall, 1983, Mongini et al., 1984) (Fig. 5.**15**), whereas it was absent in patients with unilateral masticatory muscle spasm (Cruccu et al., 1993). This difference in response could be due to the different methodologies employed (Türker and Milles, 1993).

Schoenen et al. (1987) found that the inhibitory reflex of the temporal muscles which, following Godaux and Desmedt (1975), they refer to as "esteroceptive suppression of temporal muscle activity," are of diagnostic significance in chronic headache patients. This reflex is evoked by electric stimuli,

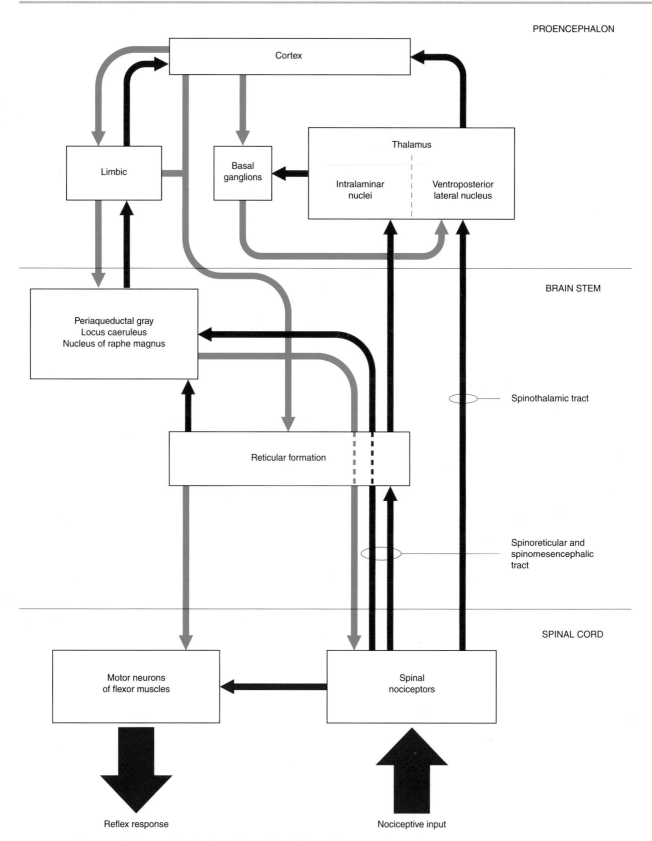

Fig. 5.**14** Schematic of the ascending (red) and descending (blue) pathways regulating the reflex response to nociceptive inputs (From Sandrini et al., 1993 a, with modifications)

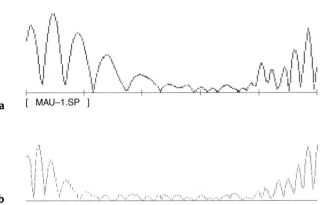

a [MAU–1.SP]

b

Fig. 5.**15 Rectified EMG signal of the silent period evoked in the masseter muscle by chin tapping. a** Silent period in a normal subject. **b** prolonged silent period in patient with dysfunction of the craniofacial muscles. (From Mongini et al., 1984)

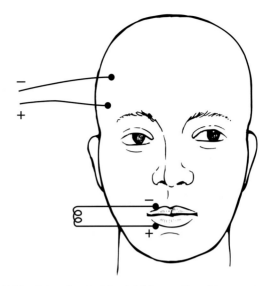

Fig. 5.**16** Set-up for studying inhibitory reflex of temporal muscle. (From Schoenen, 1993, with modifications)

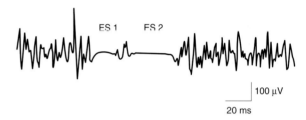

Fig. 5.**17** Early (ES1) and delayed (ES2) suppression period of the temporal muscle. (From Schoenen, 1993, with modifications)

which produce a mild painful stimulation of the skin at innervation sites of the II and III branch of the trigeminal nerve that is recorded with surface electrodes from the temporal muscle while the subject forcefully clenches the teeth (Fig. 5.**16**). Early (ES1) and late (ES2) suppression periods are obtained (Fig. 5.**17**). The pathways leading to the reflex response are not well known, but considering the time of latency, the effect is presumably multisynaptic, and is modulated by the activity of the cortex and of several brain stem structures (Sessle et al., 1976; Sessle and Hu, 1981; Dostrovsky et al., 1982, 1983). The ES2 phase of the reflex has been found to be significantly reduced or absent in chronic tension-type headache patients, but not in migraine patients (Schoenen et al., 1987; Göbel, 1990; Wallasch et al., 1990; Göbel and Weigle, 1991; Keidel et al., 1991; Nakashima and Takahashi, 1991; Wallasch and Reinecke, 1991; Paulus et al., 1992; Wei Wang et al., 1993). This reduction was not correlated with headache intensity. Since psychological factors (and depression in particular) are frequent in chronic tension-type headache patients (see Chapter 8), it is presumed (Schoenen, 1993) that modified inputs from the limbic system to the brain stem centers might account for this finding. However, double blind studies could not confirm these findings (Zwart and Sand, 1995; Bendtsen et al., 1996; Lipchik et al., 1997). Bendtsen et al. (1996), in an accurate blind study on 55 patients with tension-type headache and 55 healthy subjects, did not find significant differences of ES2 between the two groups.

Corneal reflex was also investigated in headache patients. In patients with chronic paroximal hemicrania, the reflex threshold was lower on both sides: this was true for both treated and untreated patients (Antonaci et al., 1994).

The blink reflex is commonly employed to study trigeminal system disorders (Lyon and Van Allen 1972), but was also found to be altered in migraine (Bánk et al., 1992) and in patients with cervicogenic headache (Sand and Zwart, 1994). This reflex is constantly altered in symptomatic trigeminal neuralgia (Fig. 5.**18**) but not in idiopathic trigeminal neuralgia (Cruccu et al., 1990).

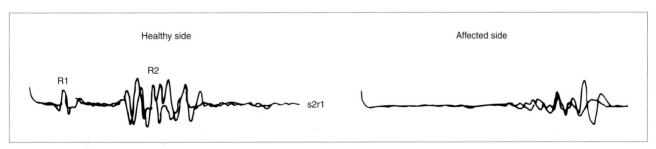

Fig. 5.**18 Early and late wink reflex in a patient suffering from postherpetic neuralgia.** Two recordings are superimposed. Calibration 10 ms/200 μV. On the injured side, R1 is missing and R2 is re- tarded. (From Cruccu et al., 1990, Journal of Neurology, Neurosurgery and Psychiatry, with permission)

Sympathetic System Dysfunction

The sympathetic nervous system, as we have seen (Chapter 2), is directly implicated in certain syndromes characterized by pain in a body segment and local signs of dysautonomy.

There is also much evidence that, in patients suffering from certain types of headache, and in particular from migraine, the autonomic nervous system shows instability (Evers et al., 1998). In such patients the following abnormalities of cardiovascular reflex responses were found in a significantly higher proportion than in a control group: enhanced low-frequency fluctuation during the day and, even more, during the night (Appel et al., 1992); lower diastolic blood pressure changes on orthostatic test and isometric work (Firenze et al., 1989; Mikamo et al., 1989); lower pulse rate variations during normal and deep breathing, during Valsalva maneuver and in orthostatic test (Havanka-Kanniainen et al., 1988; Firenze et al., 1989). Such findings were in general limited to migraine patients (Havanka-Kanniainen et al., 1988) – with or without aura – or to cluster headache patients (Firenze et al., 1989). However, Mikamo et al. (1989) and Pogacnik et al. (1993) found evidence of cardiovascular sympathetic hypofunction also in patients suffering from tension-type headache. Such disturbances seem to be minimal or absent in children (Havanka-Kanniainen et al., 1988; Del Gatto et al., 1989) and to develop gradually with age (Havanka-Kanniainen et al., 1988).

Other signs of sympathetic dysfunction have been observed, including impairment of sweating function (Saunte et al., 1983; Vijayan and Watson, 1982; Lance and Drummond,

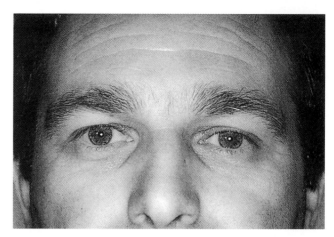

Fig. 5.**19**   **Patient suffering from attacks of frontal and left peri-orbital migraine.** In the intercritical period the Horner syndrome is present on the left (myosis, lid drop, and enophthalmus).

1987) and of retinal arterial reactivity on postural changes (Gomi et al., 1989).

The pupillary function has also been studied rather extensively. The presence of transient or permanent myosis and lid ptosis has been observed in migraine and cluster headache patients (Kunkle and Anderson, 1960; Nieman and Hurwitz, 1961; Drummond, 1988; Riley and Moyer, 1971; Fanciullacci et al., 1982; Salvesen et al., 1987 a, b) (Fig. 5.**19**). Moreover, the symptomatic pupil shows retarded dilatation in darkness (Drummond, 1988 a, b). These observations were confirmed

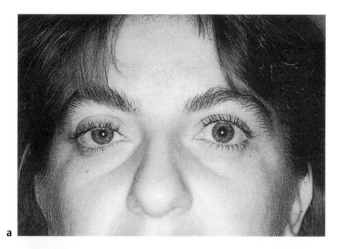

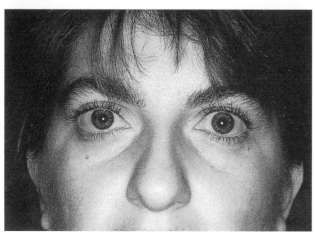

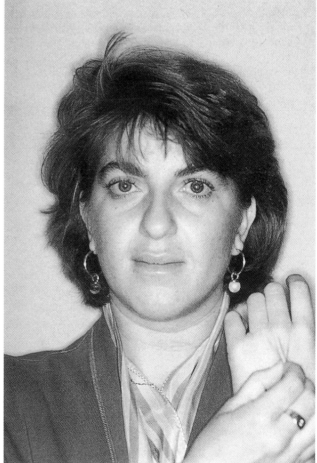

Fig. 5.**20**   Migraine patient with myosis and permanent lid drop of right eye (**a**) which tend to disappear after distant painful stimulation (**b, c**)

by the fact that pupillary dilation in response to tyramine eye-drops in cluster headache patients is less marked on the symptomatic side (Fanciullacci et al., 1982; Salvesen et al., 1987 a) and is symmetrical in those patients in whom attacks were on both sides (Fanciullacci et al., 1982). As opposed to other signs of sympathetic dysfunction discussed above, these findings suggest the presence of a local alteration of postganglion cervical sympathetic fibers. However, in some cases these may be influenced by the general tone of the sympathetic nerve, as was seen in a case observed by Mongini (1993, unpublished) of a migraine patient with permanent unilateral palpebral myosis and ptosis that regressed visibly under stress or after distant painful stimulation (Fig. 5.**20**).

References

Afra J., Cecchini AP, De Pasqua V., Alberta A., Schoenen J., *Visual evoked potentials during long periodsof pattern-reversal stimulation in migraine*, Brain, 1998, 121(pt 2):233–241.

Amabile G., Fattaposta F., Pozzessere G., et al. *Parkinson disease: electrophysiological (CNV) analysis related to pharmacological treatment*, Electroencephalogr. Clin. Neurophysiol., 1986, 64:521.

Andermann F., Zifkin, B., *The benign occipital epilepsies of childhood: an overview of the idiopathic syndromes and of the relationship to migraine*, Epilepsia, 1998, 39(Suppl 4):S9–S23.

American Academy of Neurology, *Practice parameter: The electroencephalogram in the evaluation of headache*, Neurology, 1995, 45:1411–1413.

Antonacci F., Sandrini G., Danilov A., Sand T., *Neurophysiological studies in chronic piaroximal hemicrania and hemicrania continua*, Headache, 1994, 34:479–483.

Appel S., Kuritzky A., Zahavi I., Zigelman M., Akselrod S., *Evidence or instability of the autonomic nervous system in patients with migraine headache*, Headache, 1992, 32:10–17.

Asteggiano G., Bergamasco L., Ciaramitaro P., et al. *Computerized spectral analysis EEG (CSA) in diagnosis of childhood migraine*, It. J. Neurol. Sci., 1997, 18:229.

Bach F.W., Langemark M., Secher N.H., *Cerebrospinal fluid ß-endorphin in chronic tension-type headache*, Pain, 1992, 51:163–168.

Baier W.K., Doose H., *Migraine and petit-mal absence: familial prevalence of migraine and seizures*, in: Andermann F., Lugaresi E. (eds.), *Migraine and epilepsy*, Butterworths, London, 1987, 293–311.

Balley J.O. Jr, McCall W.D. Jr, Ash M.M. Jr, *Electromyographic silent periods and jaw motion parameters: Quantitative measures of temporomandibular joint dysfunction*, J. Dent. Res., 1977, 56:249–253.

Bánk J., *Brainstem auditory evoked potentials in migraine after Rausedyl provocation*, Cephalalgia, 1991, 11:277–279.

Bánk J., Bense E., Király C.S., *The blink reflex in migraine*, Cephalalgia, 1992, 12:289–292.

Basser L.S., *The relation of migraine and epilepsy*, Brain, 1969, 92:285–300.

Bazil C.W., *Migraine and epilepsy*, Neurol. Clin., 1994, 12:115–127.

Bendtsen L., Jensen R., Brennum J., Arendt-Nielsen L., Olesen J., *Exteroceptive suppression of temporal muscle activity is normal in chronic tension-type headache and not related to actual headache state*, Cephalalgia, 1996, 16:251–256.

Besken E., Pothmann R., Sartory G., *Contigent negative variation in childhood migraine*, Cephalalgia, 1993, 13:42–43.

Bessette R.W., Shatkin S.S., *Predicting by electromyography the results of nonsurgical treatment of temporomandibular joint syndrome*, Plast. Reconstr. Surg., 1979, 64:232.

Bladin P.F., *The association of benign rolandic epilepsy with migraine*, in: Andermann F., Lugaresi E. (eds.), *Migraine and epilepsy*, Butterworths, London, 1987, 145–152.

Böcker K.B.E., Timsit-Berthier M., Schoenen J., Brunia C.H.M., *Contingent negative variation in migraine*, Headache, 1990, 30:604–609.

Brewerton T.D., Murphy D.L., Mueller E.A., Jimerson D.C., *Induction of migraine-like headaches by the serotonin agonist m-chlorophenylpiperazine*, Clin. Pharmacol. Ther., 1988, 43:605–609.

Brun J., Claustrat B., Saddier P., Chazot G., *Nocturnal melatonin excretion is decreased in patients with migraine without aura attacks associated with menses*, Cephalalgia, 1995, 15:136–139.

Cambier J., Dehen H., Bathien N., *Upper limb cutaneous polysynaptic reflexes*, J. Neurol. Sci., 1974, 22:39–49.

Cesselin F., Laport A.M., Miquel M.C., Bourgoin S., Hamon M., *Serotonergic mechanisms of pain control*, in: Gebhart G.F., Hammond D.L., Jensen T.S. (eds.), Proceedings of the 7th World Congress on Pain, IASP Press, Seattle, 1994, 669–695.

Chayasirisobhon S., *Somatosensory evoked potentials in acute migraine with sensory aura*, Clin. Electroencephalogr., 1995, 26:65–69.

Crisp T., Stafinsky J.L., Spanos L.J., Uram M., Perni V., Donepudi H.B., *Analgesic effects of serotonin and receptor-selective serotonin agonists in the rat spinal cord*, Gen. Pharmacol., 1991 a, 22:247–251.

Crisp T., Stafinsky J.L., Uram M., Perni V.C., Weaver M.F., Spanos L.J., *Serotonin contributes to the spinal antinociceptive effects of morphine*, Pharmacol. Biochem. Behav., 1991 b, 39:591–595.

Cruccu G., Agostino R., Inghilleri M., Manfredi M., *Ongerboer de Visser BW. The masseter inhibitory reflex is evoked by innocuous stimuli and mediated by A beta afferent fibres*, Exp. Brain Res., 1989, 77:447–450.

Cruccu G. et al, *Idiopathic and symptomatic trigeminal pain*, J. Neurol. Neurosurg. Psychiatry, 1990, 53:1034–1042.

Cruccu G., Pauletti G., Agostino R., Berardelli A., Manfredi M., *Masseter inhibitory reflex in movement disorders. Huntington's chorea, Parkinson's disease, dystonia, and unilateral masticatory spasm*, 1993.

Curran D.A., Hinterberger H., Lance J.W., Total plasma serotonin, 5-hydroxyindoleacetic acid and p-hydroxy-m-methoxymandelic acid excretion in normal and migrainous subjects, Brain, 1965, 88:997–1009.

Del Gatto F., Firenze C., Gallai V., Galati F., *A study of the autonomic nervous system in children with cefalea* (abs.), Cephalalgia, 1989, 9 (Suppl. 10):146.

de Tommaso M., Sciruicchio V., Belloti R., et al., *Discrimination between migraine patients and normal subjects based on steady state visual evoked potentials: discriminant analysis and artificial neural network classifiers*, Funct. Neurol., 1997, 12(6):333–338.

Derbyshire S.W., Jones A.K., Devani P., et al. *Cerebral responses to pain in patients with atypical facial pain measured by positron emission tomography*, J. Neurol. Neurosurg. Psychiatry, 1994, 57:1166–1172.

Devinsky O., Morrel M.J., Vogt B.A., *Contributions of anterior cingulate cortex to behaviour*, Brain, 1995, 118:279–306.

Di Francesco G., Nardone A., Schieppati M., *Inhibition of jaw-closing muscle activity by tactile airjet stimulation of peri- and intra-oral sites in man*, Arch. Oral Biol., 1986, 31:273–278.

Dostrovsky J.O., Hu J.W., Sessle B.J., Sumino R., *Stimulation sites in periaqueductal gray, nucleus raphe magnus and adjacent regions effective in suppressing oral-facial reflexes*, Brain Res., 1982, 252:287–297.

Dostrovsky J.O., Shah Y., Gray B.G., *Descending inhibitory influences from periaqueductal gray, nucleus raphe magnus and adjacent reticular formation, II: Effects on medullary dorsal hom nociceptive and non-nociceptive neurons*, J. Neurophysiol., 1983, 49:948–960.

Drummond P.D., *Autonomic disturbances in cluster headache*, Brain, 1988 a, 111:1199–1209.

Drummond P.D., *Dysfunction of the sympathetic nervous system in cluster headache*, Cephalalgia, 1988 b, 8:181–186.

Ehrenberg B.L., *Unusual clinical manifestations of migraine and the borderland of epilepsy-re-explored*, Semin. Neurol., 1991, 11:118–127.

Evers S., Voss H., Bauer B., Soros P., Husstedt I.W., *Peripheral autonomic potentials in primary headache and drug-induced headache*, Cephalalgia, 1998, 18(4):216–221.

Facchetti D., Marsile C., Faggi L., Donati E., Kokodoko A., Poloni M., *Cerebral mapping in subjects suffering from migraine with aura*, Cephalalgia, 1990, 10:279–284.

Facchinetti F., Genazzani A.R., *Opioids in cerebrospinal fluid and blood of headache sufferers*, in: Olesen J., Edvinsson L. (eds.), *Basic mechanisms of headache*, Elsevier, Amsterdam, 1988, 261–269.

Facchinetti F., Martignoni E., Fioroni L., Sances G., Genazzani A.R., *Opioid control of the hypothalamus-pituitary-adrenal axis cyclically fails in menstrual migraine*, Cephalalgia, 1990, 10:51–56.

Fanciullacci M., Pietrini U., Gatto G., Boccuni M., Sicuteri F., *Latent dysautonomic pupillary lateralization in cluster headache. A pupillometric study*, Cephalalgia, 1982, 2:135–144.

Farkas V., Benninger C., Matthis P., *Computerized analysis of EEG background activity in childhood migraine and generalized epileptic patients* (abs.), Proc. VIth Int. Headache Congress, Paris, Cephalalgia, 1993, 13 (Suppl. 13):215.

Fasmer O.B., Berge O.G., Hole K., *Changes in nociception after lesions of descending serotonergic pathways induced with 5,6-dihydroxytryptamine*, Neuropharmacology, 1985, 24:729–734.

Fields H.L., Basbaum A.I., *Central nervous system mechanisms of pain modulation*, in: Wall P.O., Melzack R. (eds.), *Textbook of pain*, Churchill Livingstone, Edinburgh, 1994, 243–257.

Firenze C., Gallai V., Del Gatto F., Galati F., Bruni A., *Dysfunction of the autonomic nervous system in the cluster headache* (abs.), Cephalalgia, 1989, 9 (Suppl. 10):147.

Fog-Moller F., Genefke I.K., Bryndum B., *Changes in concentration of catecholamines in blood during spontaneous migraine attacks and reserpine-induced attacks*, in: Greene R. (ed.), *Current concepts in migraine research*, Raven Press, New York, 1978, 115 – 119.

Gastaut H., Zifkin B.G., *Benign epilepsy of childhood with occipital spike and wave complexes*, in: Andermann F., Lugaresi E. (eds.), *Migraine and epilepsy*, Butterworths, Boston,1987, 47 – 82.

Genazzani A.R., Nappi G., Facchinetti F., et al. *Progressive impairment of CSFb-EP levels in migraine sufferers*, Pain, 1984, 18 : 127 – 133.

Genco S., de Tommaso M., Prudenzano A.M., Savarese M., Puca F.M., *EEG features in juvenile migraine: topographic analysis of spontaneous and visual evoked brain electrical activity: a comparison with adult migraine*, Cephalalgia, 1994, 14 : 41 – 46.

Gerber W.D., Kropp P., Weber P., *Contingent negative variation (CNV) in migraine: which components differentiate between normals and migraine patients*, in: Ekbom K., Gerber W.D., Henry P., Nappi G. (eds.), European Headache Federation (EHF), 1 st International Conference, Munich, Arcis, 1992.

Giel R., deVlieger M., van Vliet A.G., *Headache and the EEG*, Electroencephalogr. Clin. Neurophysiol., 1966, 21 : 492 – 495.

Gillins B.R.D., Klineberg I.S., *Latency and inhibition of human masticatory muscles following stimuli*, J. Dent. Res., 1975, 54 : 269 – 279.

Goadsby P.J., Lance J.W., *Physiopathology of migraine*, Revue Du Praticien, 1990, 40 : 389 – 393.

Göbel H., *Schmerzmessung. Methodisch-theoretische Grundlagen. Experimentelle und klinische Anwendungen. Habilitationsschrift*, Medizinische Fakultät der Christian-Albrechts-Universität zu Kiel, 1990, 281.

Göbel H., Weigle L., *Exteroceptive suppression periods of temporal muscle in differential diagnosis of headache disorders*, Paneuropean Soc. of Neurol., 2 nd Congress, 1991, 204 (abs.).

Godaux E., Desmedt J.E., *Exteroceptive suppression and motor control of the masseter and temporalis muscles in normal man*, Brain Res., 1975, 85 : 447 – 458.

Goldberg L.J., Nakamura Y., *Lingually induced inhibition of masseteric motoneurons*, Experientia, 1968, 24 : 371 – 373.

Gomi S., Gotoh F., Komatsumoto S., Ishikawa Y., Araki N., Hamada J., *Sweating function and retinal vasomotor reactivity in migraine*, Cephalalgia, 1989, 9 : 179 – 185.

Griffin C.J., Munro R.R., *Electromyography of the jaw closing muscles in the open-close-clench cycle in man*, Arch. Oral Biol., 1969, 14 : 141.

Gronseth G.S., Greenberg M.K., *The utility of the electroencephalogram in the evaluation of patients presenting with headache: A review of the literature*, Neurology, 1995, 45 : 1263 – 1267.

Hannam A.G., *Mastication in man*, in: Bryant P., Gale E., Ruth J. (eds.), *Oral motor behaviour*, NIH Publication, 79 : 1745, 1979.

Hannam A.G., Matthews B., Yemm R., *The unloading reflex in masticatory muscles in man*, Arch. Oral Biol., 1968, 13 : 361.

Hannam A.G., Matthews B., Yemm R., *Changes in the activity of the masseter muscle following tooth contact in man*, Arch. Oral Biol., 1969, 14 : 1401.

Hannam A.G., Matthews B., Yemm R., *Receptors involved in the response of the masseter muscle to tooth contact in man*, Arch. Oral Biol., 1970, 15 : 17.

Havanka-Kanniainen H., Tolonen U., Myllylä, *Autonomic dysfunction in migraine: a survey of 188 patients*, Headache, 1988, 28 : 465 – 470.

Hsieh J.C., Belfrage M., Stond-Elander S., Hansson P., Ingvar M., *Central representation of chronic ongoing neuropathic pain studied by positron emission tomography*, Pain, 1995, 63 : 225 – 236.

Hsieh J.C., Hannerz J., Ingvar M., *Right-lateralised central processing for pain of nitroglycerin-induced cluster headache*, Pain, 1996, 67 : 59 – 68.

Hughes J.R., Robbins L.D., *Brain mapping in migraine*, Clin. Electroencephalogr., 1990, 21 : 14 – 24.

Hughes J., Devinsky O., Feldman E. et al., *Premonitory symptoms in epilepsy*, Seizure, 1993, 2 : 201 – 203.

Hussein S.M., McCall Jr W.D., *Masseteric silent periods electrically evoked in normal subjects and patients with temporomandibular joint dysfunction*, Exp. Neurol., 1983, 81 : 64 – 76.

Hutson P.H., Tricklebank M.D., Curzon G., *Enhancement of foot-shock-induced analgesia by spinal 5,7-dihydroxytryptamine lesions*, Brain Res., 1982, 237 : 367 – 372.

Isler H., Wieser H.G., Egli M., *Hemicrania epileptica: synchronous ipsilateral ictal headache with migraine features*, in: Andermann F., Lugaresi E. (eds.), *Migraine and epilepsy*, Boston, Butterworths, 1987, 249 – 264.

Jay G.W., *Epilepsy, migraine, and EEG abnormalities in children: a review and hypothesis*, Headache, 1982, 22 : 110 – 114.

Jensen R., Hindeberg I., *Plasma serotonin increase during episodes of tension-type headache*, Cephalalgia, 1994, 14 : 219 – 222.

Jonas A.D., *Headaches as seizure equivalents*, Headache, 1966, 6 : 78 – 87.

Keidel M., Reinecke P., Dieter H.C., *Reduced exteroceptive M. temporalis suppression in post-traumatic headache*, Paneuropean Soc. of Neurol., 2 nd Congress, 1991, 78 (abs.).

Kimball R.W., Friedman A.P., Vallejo E., *Effect of serotonin in migraine patients*, Neurology, 1960, 10 : 107 – 111.

Kinast M., Lueders H., Rothner A.D., Erenberg G., *Benign focal epileptiform discharges in childhood migrain (BFEDC)*, Neurology, 1982, 32 : 1309 – 1311.

Kooi K.A., Rajput A.H., DeJong R.N., *Significance of the paraxysmal electroencephalogram in the patient with migraine*, in: Werner E. (ed.), Proc. 6 th Int. Conf. on Electroencephalography and Clinical Neurophysiology, Verlag der Weiner Medizinischen Akademie, Vienna, 1965, 263 – 266.

Krieger D.T., Martin J.B., *Brain peptides*, N. Engl. J. Med., 1981, 304 : 876 – 885.

Kropp P., Gerber W.D., *Contingent negative variation during migraine attack and interval: evidence for normalization of slow cortical potentials during the attack*, Cephalalgia, 1995, 15 : 123 – 128.

Kropp P., Gerber W.D., *Is increased amplitude of contingent negative variation in migraine due to cortical hyperactivity or to reduced habituation?*, Cephalalgia, 1993, 13 : 37 – 41.

Kunkle E.C., Anderson W.B., *Dual mechanisms of eye signs of headache in cluster pattern*, Trans. Am. Neurol. Assoc., 1960, 85 : 75 – 79.

Lance J.W., Drummond P.D., *Horner's syndrome in cluster headache*, in: Clifford Rose F. (ed.), *Current problems in neurology*, vol. 4, Advances in headache research, John Libbey, London, 1987, 169 – 174.

Langemark M., Bach F.W., Ekman R., Olesen J., *Increased cerebrospinal fluid Met-enkephalin immunoreactivity in patients with chronic tension-type headache*, Pain, 1995, 63 : 103 – 107.

Langemark M., Bach Flemming W., Jensen Troels S., Olesen J., *Decreased nociceptive flexion reflex threshold in chronic tension-type headache* (abs.), Proc. VIth Int. Headache Congress, Paris, Cephalalgia, 1993, 13 (Suppl. 13):107.

Laplante P., Saint-Hilaire J.M., Bouvier G., *Headache as an epileptic manifestation*, Neurology, 1983, 33 : 1493 – 1495.

Leone M., Sacerdote P., D'Amico D., et al., *ß-Eendorphin level in lymphocytes of primary headaches patients* (abs.), Cephalalgia, 1991, 11, (Suppl. 11):188.

Leone M., Sacerdote P., D'Amico D., Panerai A.E., Bussone G., *Beta-endorphin concentrations in the peripheral blood mononuclear cells of migraine and tension-type headache patients*, Cephalalgia, 1992, 12 : 155 – 157.

Leppaluoto J., Havanka-Kanniainen H., Myllyla V.V., Hokkanen E., *Secretion of beta-endorphin and pain*, Abstract at the Scandinavian Migraine Meeting, Helsinki, 1983.

Libet B., *Slow postsynaptic responses of sympathetic ganglion cells as models for slow potential changes in the brain*, in: Otto D. (ed.), *Multidisciplinary perspectives in event-related brain potential research*, US Government Printing Office, Washington, 1978, 12 – 19.

Lipchik G.L., Holroyd K.A., Talbot F., Greer M., *Pericranial muscle tenderness and exteroceptive suppression of temporalis muscle activity: a blind study of chronic tension-type headache*, Headache, 1997, 37 : 368 – 376.

Lipton R.B., Ottman R., Ehrenberg B.L., Hauser W.A., *Comorbidity of migraine: the connection between migraine and epilepsy*, Neurology, 1994, 44(10 Suppl 7):S28 –S32.

Liu M.Y., Su C.F., Lin M.T., *The antinociceptive role of bulbospinal serotonergic pathway in the rat brain*, Pain, 1988, 33 : 123 – 129.

Lund J.P., Lamarre Y., Lavigne G., Duquet G., *Human jaw reflexes*, Adv. Neurol., 1983, 39 : 739 – 755.

Lyon L.W., Van Allen M.W., *Orbicularis aculi reflexes. Studies in internuclear ophthalmoplegia and pseudointernuclear ophthalmoplegia*, Arch. Ophthalmol., 1972, 87 : 148 – 154.

McCall Jr W.D., Hoffer M., *Jaw muscle silent periods by tooth tap and chin tap*, J. Oral Rehabil., 1981, 8 : 91 – 96.

Maertens de Noordhout A., Timsit-Berthier M., Timsit M., Schoenen J., *Contingent negative variation in headache*, Ann. Neurol., 1986, 19 : 78 – 80.

Maertens de Noordhout A., Timsit-Berthier M., Timsit M., Schoenen J., *Effects of beta-blockade on continent negative variation in migraine*, Ann. Neurol., 1987, 21 : 111 – 112.

Maertens de Noordhout A., Wang W., Schoenen J., *Clinical neurophysiology and neurotransmitters*, Cephalalgia, 1995, 15 : 301 – 309.

Marcus D.A., *Interrelationships of neurochemicals, estrogen, and recurring headache*, Pain, 1995, 62 : 129 – 139.

Marczynski T.J., *Neurochemical mechanisms in the genesis of slow potentials: a review and some clinical implications*, in: Otto D. (ed.), *Multidisciplinary perspectives in event-related brain potential research*, US Government Printing Office, Washington, 1978, 25 – 35.

Mariani E., Moschini V., Pastorino G., Rizzi F., Severgnini A., Tiengo M., *Pattern-reversal visual evoked potentials and EEG correlations in common migraine patients*, Headache, 1988, 28 : 269 – 271.

Marlowe N., *Somatosensory evoked potentials and headache: a further examination of the central theory*, J. Psychosom. Res., 1995, 39(2):119 – 131.

Martelletti P., Stirparo G., Rinaldi C., Fusco B.M., *Function of the peripheral serotoninergic pathways in migraine: a proposal for an experimental model*, Cephalalgia, 1994 a, 14 : 11 – 15.

Martelletti P., Stirparo G., Rinaldi C., Giacovazzo M., *Upregulated expression of peripheral serotonergic receptors in migraine and cluster headache by sumatriptan*, Int. J. Clin. Pharm. Res., 1994 b, XVI: 167 – 175.

Martelletti P., Giacovazzo M., *Peripheral 5-hydroxytryptaminergic model in headache research*, in: Jes Olesen and Michael A., Moskowitz (eds.), *Experimental headache models*, Lippincott-Raven Publishers, Philadelphia, 1995, 169 – 173.

Martignoni E., *Endogenous opioids in tension-type headache*, 3d Int. Headache Research Seminar, Copenhagen, 1992 (abs.).

Mathiau P., Brochet B., Boulan P., Henry P., Aubineau P., *Spontaneous and 5 HT-induced cyclic contractions in superficial temporal arteries from chronic and episodic cluster headache patients*, Cephalalgia, 1994, 14 : 419 – 429.

Mazzotta G., Alberti A., Santucci A., Gallai V., *The event-related potential P300 during headache-free period and spontaneous attack in adult headache sufferers*, Headache, 1995, 35 : 210 – 215.

Mikamo K., Etsuko A., Takeshima T., Nishikawa S., Takahashi K., *Cardiovascular sympathetic hypofunction in muscle contraction headache and migraine* (abs.), Cephalalgia, 1989, 9 (Suppl. 10):148.

Mongini F., Fabris E., Tempia-Valenta G., *A computer-based system for measuring the masseteric silent period*, Cranio, 1984, 3 : 27 – 30.

Moreira-Filho P.F., Dantas A.M., *Pattern reversal visual evoked potentials in migraine subjects without aura*, Arq. Neuropsiquiatr., 1994, 52 : 484 – 488.

Murialdo G., Fonzi S., Costelli P., et al. *Urinary melatonin excretion throughout the ovarian cycle in menstrually related migraine*, Cephalalgia, 1994, 14 : 205 – 209.

Nagel-Leiby S., Welch K.M.A., D'Andrea G., Grunfeld S., Brown E., *Event-related slow potentials and associated catecholamine function in migraine*, Cephalalgia, 1990, 10 : 317 – 329.

Nakashima K., Takahashi K., *Exteroceptive suppression of the masseter, temporalis and trapezius muscles produced by mental nerve stimulation in patients with chronic headaches*, Cephalalgia, 1991, 11 : 23 – 28.

Nappi G., Micieli G., Sandrini G., Martignoni E., Lottici P., Bono G., *Headache temporal patterns: towards a chronobiological model*, Cephalalgia, 1983, (Suppl. 1):21 – 30.

Nappi G., Facchinetti F., Martignoni E., et al. *Plasma and CSF endorphin levels in primary and symptomatic headaches*, Headache, 1985, 25 : 141 – 144.

Nappi G., Sandrini G., Effects of serotonergic drug administration on nociceptive flexion reflex in daily chronic headache, in: Olesen J., Saxena P. (eds.), *5-Hydroxytryptamine mechanisms in primary headaches*, Raven Press, New York, 1992, 226 – 230.

Neufield M.Y., Treves T.A., Korczyn A.D., *EEG and topographic frequency analysis in common and classic migraine*, Headache, 1991, 31 : 232 – 236.

Nieman E.A., Hurwitz L.J., *Ocular sympathetic palsy in periodic migrainous neuralgia*, J. Neurol. Neurosurg. Psychiatry, 1961, 24 : 369 – 373.

Ottman R., Lipton R.B., *Comorbidity of migraine and epilepsy*, Neurology, 1994, 44(11):2105 – 2110.

Panerai A.E., *Endorfine: 10 anni dopo*, Atti Decimo Congresso AIDS, Delfino, Torino, 1987, 15 – 22.

Paul D., Mana M.J., Pfaus J.G., Pinel J.P.J., *Attenuation of morphine-produced analgesia by serotonin type-2 receptor blockers, pirenperone and ketanserin*, Pharmacol. Biochem. Behav., 1988, 31 : 641 – 647.

Paulus W., Raubüchl O., Strabue A., Schoenen J., *Exteroceptive suppression of temporalis muscle activity in various types of headache*, Headache, 1992, 32 : 41 – 44.

Pogacnik T., Sega S., Mesec A., Kiauta T., *Autonomic function testing in patients with tension-type headache*, Headache 1993, 33 : 63 – 68,.

Proudfit H.K., *Pharmacological evidence for the modulation of nociception by noradrenergic neurons*, in: Fields J.L., Besson J.M. (eds.), *Pain modulation*, Elsevier, Amsterdam, 1988, 357 – 370.

Puca F.M., de Tommaso M., Tota P., Sciruicchio V., *Photic driving in migraine: correlations with clinical features*, Cephalalgia, 1996, 16 : 246 – 250.

Riley F.C., Moyer N.J., *Oculosympathetic paresis associated with cluster headaches*, Am. J. Ophthalmol., 1971, 72 : 763 – 768.

Roberts M.H.T., *Pharmacology of putative neurotransmitters and receptors: 5-hydroxytryptamine*, in: Fields H.L., Besson J.M. (eds.), *Pain mod-ulation*, Elsevier, Amsterdam, 1988, 329 – 338.

Roby A., Willer J.C., Bussel B., *Effect of a synthetic enkephalin analogue on spinal nociceptive messages in humans*, Neuropharmacology, 1983, 22 : 1121 – 1125.

Rockstroh B., Elbert T., Birbaumer N., Lutzenberger W., *Slow brain potentials and behavior*, Urban & Schwarzenberg, Munich, 1982.

Rossi L.N., Pastorino G.C., Bellettini G., Chiodi A., Mariani E., Cortinovis I., *Pattern reversal visual evoked potentials in children with migraine or tension-type headache*, Cephalalgia, 1996, 16 : 104 – 106.

Rothrock J.F., Mar K.R., Yaksh T.L., Golbeck A., Moore A.C., *Cerebrospinal fluid analyses in migraine patients and controls*, Cephalalgia, 1995, 15 : 489 – 493.

Sadzot B., Maquet P., Franck G., *Is positron emission tomography a useful tool for studying migraine?*, Cephalalgia, 1995, 15 : 316 – 322.

Saito Y., Collins J.G., Iwasaki H., *Tonic 5-HT modulation of spinal dorsal horn neuron activity evoked by both noxious and non-noxious stimuli: a source of neuronal plasticity*, Pain, 1990, 40 : 205 – 219.

Salvesen R., Bogucki A., Wysocka-Bakowska M.M., Antonaci F., Fredriksen F., Sjaastad O., *Cluster headache pathogenesis: a pupillometric study*, Cephalalgia, 1987 a, 7 : 273 – 284.

Salvesen R., Fredriksen T.A., Bogucki A., Sjaastad O., *Sweat gland and pupillary responsiveness in Horner's syndrome*, Cephalalgia, 1987 b, 7 : 135 – 146.

Sand T., *EEG in migraine: a review of the literature*, Functional Neurology, 1991, 6(1):7 – 22.

Sand T., Zwart J.A., *The blink reflex in chronic tension-type headache, migraine, and cervicogenic headache*, Cephalalgia, 1994, 14 : 447 – 450.

Sandrini G., Alfonsi E., Sances G., Facchinetti F., Bono G., Nappi G., *Nociceptive flexion reflex threshold in migraine sufferers*, Cephalalgia, 1985, 5 (Suppl. 3):26 – 27.

Sandrini G., Martignoni E., Micieli G., Alfonsi E., Sances G., Nappi G., *Pain reflexes in the clinical assessment of migraine syndromes*, Funct. Neurol., 1986, 1 : 423 – 429.

Sandrini G., Antonaci F., Danilov A., Capararo M., Micieli G., Nappi G., *Nociceptive flexion reflex in cluster headache*, in: Ekbom K., Gerber W.D., Henry P., Nappi G., Pfaffenrath V., Tfelt-Hansen P (eds.), *European Headache Federation (EHF)*, First Int. Conference, Bremen, Arcis Verlag, 1992, 76.

Sandrini G., Arrigo A., Bono G., Nappi G., *The nociceptive flexion reflex as a tool for exploring pain control system in headache and other pain syndromes*, Cephalalgia, 1993 a, 13 : 21 – 27.

Sandrini G., Antonaci F., Capararo M., Micieli G., Danilov A., Nappi G., *Nociceptive flexion reflex in cluster headache* (abs.), Proc. VIth Int. Headache Congress, Paris, Cephalalgia, 1993 b, 13 (Suppl. 13):201.

Sappey-Marinier D., Galabrese G., Fein G., Hugg J.W., Biggins C., Weiner M.W., *Effect of photic stimulation on human visual cortex lactate and phosphates using 1 H and 31 P magnetic resonance spectroscopy*, J. Cereb. Blood Flow Metab., 1992, 12 : 584 – 592.

Saunte C., Russell D., Sjaastad O., *Cluster headache: on the mechanism behind attack-related sweating*, Cephalalgia, 1983, 3 : 175 – 185.

Schoenen J., *Beta-blockers and the central nervous system*, Cephalalgia, 1986, 6 (Suppl. 5):47 – 54.

Schoenen J., *Exteroceptive suppression of temporalis muscle activity: methodological and physiological aspects*, Cephalalgia, 1993, 13 : 3 – 10.

Schoenen J., *Cortical electrophysiology in migraine and possible pathogenetic implications*, Clin. Neurosci., 1998, 5(1):10 – 17.

Schoenen J., Maertens A., Timsit-Berthier M., Timsit M., *Contingent negative variation (CNV) as a diagnostic and physiopathologic tool in headache patients*, in: Clifford Rose (ed.), Migraine, Proc. 5 th Int. Migraine Symp., London, 1984, Karger, Basel, 1985, 17 – 25.

Schoenen J., Maertens de Noordhout A., Timsit-Berthier M., Timsit M., *Contingent negative variation and efficacy of beta-blocking agents in migraine*, Cephalalgia, 1986, 6 : 229 – 233.

Schoenen J., Jamart B., Gerard P., Lenarduzzi P., Delwaide P.J., *Exteroceptive suppression of temporalis muscle activity in chronic headache*, Neurology, 1987,37 : 1834 – 1836.

Schoenen J., Maertens de Nordhout A., *The role of the sympathetic nervous system in migraine and cluster headache*, in: Olesen J., Edvinson L. (eds.), *Basic mechanisms of headache*, Pain research and clinical management, Elsevier, Amsterdam, 1988, 393 – 410.

Schoenen J., Timsit-Berthier M., *Contingent negative variation: methods and potential interest in headache*, Cephalalgia, 1993, 13 : 28 – 32.

Schoenen J., Wang W., Albert A., Delwaide P.J., *Potentiation instead of habituation characterizes visual evoked potentials in migraine patients between attacks*, Eur. J. Neul., 1995, 2 : 115 – 122.

Septien L., Pelletier J.L., Brunotte F., Giroud M., Dumas R., *Migraine in patients with history of centro-temporal epilepsy in childhood: a HmPAO SPECT study*, Cephalalgia, 1991, 11 : 281 – 284.

Seri S., Cerquiglini A., Guidetti V., *Computerized EEG topography in childhood migraine between and during attacks*, Cephalalgia, 1993, 13 : 53 – 56.

Sessle B.J., Dubner R., Greenwood L.F., Lucier G.E., *Descending influences of periaqueductal gray matter and somatosensory cerebral cortex on neurons in trigeminal brain stem, nuclei*, Can. J. Physiol. Pharmacol. 1976, 54:66 –69,.

Sessle B.J., Hu J.W., *Raphe-induced suppression of the jaw-opening reflex and single neurons in trigeminal subnucleus oralis, and influence of naloxone and subnucleus caudalis*, Pain, 1981, 10:19–36.

Sharav Y., McGrath P.A., Dubner R., Brown F., *Masseretic inhibitory periods and sensations evoked by electric tooth-pulp stimulation in patients with oral-facial pain and mandibular dysfunction*, Arch. Oral Biol., 1982, 27:305 –310.

Sicuteri F., Anselmi B., Curradi C., Michelacci S., Sassi A., *Morphine-like factors in CSF of headache patients*, Adv. Biochem. Psychopharmacol., 1978, 18:363–366.

Simon R.H., Zimmerman A.W., Tasman A., Hale M.S., *Spectral analysis of photic stimulation in migraine*, Electroencephalogr. Clin. Neurophysiol., 1982, 53:270–276.

Simon R.H., Zimmerman A.W., Sanderson P., Tasman A., *EEG markers of migraine in children and adults*, Headache, 1983, 23:201–205.

Skiba T.J., Laskin D.M., *Masticatory muscle silent periods in patients with MPD syndrome before and after treatment*, J. Dent. Res., 1981, 60:699.

Slatter K.H., *Some clinical and EEG findings in patients with migraine*, Brain, 1968, 91:85–98.

Slevin J.T., Faught E., Hanna G.R., Lee S.I., *Temporal relationship of EEG abnormalites in migraine to headache and medication*, Headache, 1981, 21:251–254.

Srikiatkhachorn A., Maneesri S., Govitrapong P., Kasantikul V., *Derangement of serotonin system in migranous patients with analgesic abuse headache: clues from platelets*, Headache, 1998 38(1):43–49.

Swaiman K.F., Frank Y., *Seizure headaches in children*, Dev. Med. Child. Neurol., 1978, 20:580–585.

Tagliati M., Sabbadini M., Bernardi G., Silvestrini M., *Multichannel visual evoked potentials in migraine*, Electroencephalogr. Clin. Neurophysiol., 1995, 96:1–5.

Tenen S.S., *Antagonism of the analgesic effect of morphine and other drugs by p-chlorophenylalanine, a serotonin depletor*, Psychopharmacologia, 1968, 12:278–285.

Terzano M.G., Manzoni G.C., Parrino L., *Benign epilepsy with occipital paroxysms and migraine: The question of intercalated attacks*, in: Andermann F., Lugaresi E. (eds.), *Migraine and Epilepsy*, Butterworths, Boston, 1987, 83 –96.

Timsit-Berthier M., *Les potentiels lents liés aux évènements*, Rev. Electroencephalogr. Neurophysiol. Clin., 1976, 6:181–186.

Timsit-Berthier M., Gerono A., Rousseau J.C., Mantanus H., Abraham P., Verhey F., Lamers T., Emonds P., *An international pilot study of CNV in mental illness*, Second Report. Ann. NY Acad. Sci., 1984, 71–77.

Timsit-Berthier M., Mantanus H., Ansseau M., Devoitille J.M., Dal Mas A., Legros J.J., *Contingent negative variation in maior depressive patients*, in: Johnson jr. R., Rohrbaugh J.W., Parasuramen R. (eds.), *Current trends in ERP research* , (EEG Suppl. 40), Elsevier, Amsterdam, 1987, 762–771.

Timsit-Berthier M., Mantanus H., Poncelet M., Marissiaux P., Legros J., *Contingent negative variation as a new method to assess the catecholaminergic system*, in: Gallai V., (ed.), *Maturation of the CNS and evoked potentials*, Oxford, Elsevier, Amsterdam, 1989.

Türker K.S., Miles T.S., *Inhibitory reflexes in human masseter muscle*, in: Van Steenberghe D., De Laat A., editors, *EMG of jaw reflexes in man*, Leuven University Press, 1993, 237–255.

Vaeroy H., Nyberg F., Terenius L., *No evidence for endorphin deficiency in fibromyalgia following investigation of cerebrospinal fluid (CSF) dynorphin A and Met-enkephalin-Arg6-Phe7*, Pain, 1991, 46:139–143.

Valdizan J.R., Andreu C., Almarcegui C., Olivito A., *Quantitative EEG in children with headache*, Headache, 1994, 34:53–55.

van Dijk J.G., Dorresteijn M., Haan J., Ferrari M.D., *Visual evoked potentials and background EEG activity in migraine*, Headache, 1991, 31:392–395.

Vighetti S., Asteggiano G., Mongini F., Bergamasco L., Mattiuzzi M., *Epserps mapping in migraine patients*, It. J. Neurol. Sci., 1997, 18:229–230.

Vijayan N., Watson C., *Evaluation of oculocephalic sympathetic function in vascular headache syndromes, II: Oculocephalic sympathetic function in cluster headache*, Headache, 1982, 22:200–202.

Vogt M., *The effect of lowering the 5-hydroxytryptamine content of the rat spinal cord on analgesia produced by morphine*, Journal of Physiology, 1974, 236:483–498.

Waldenlind E., Ekbom K., Wetterberg L., Fanciullacci M., Marabini S., Sicuteri F., Polleri A., Murialdo G., Filippi U., *Lowered circannual urinary melatonin concentrations in episodic cluster headache*, Cephalalgia, 1994, 14:199–204.

Wallasch T.M., Reinecke M., Langohr H.D., *Exterozeptive Suppression der Temporalismuskelaktivität bei Kopfschmerzen. Seitenvergleich der Dauer der ipsi- und kontralateralen Suppressionsperioden*, Nerveheilkunde, 1990, 9:58 –60.

Wallasch T.M., Reinecke M., *Migräne und Kopfschmerz vom Spannungstyp. Neue Aspekte in der apparativen Diagnostik*, Münch. med. Wschr., 1991, 133:26–31.

Walter W.G., Cooper R., Aldridge V.J., McCallum W.C., Winter A.L., *Contingent negative variation: an electric sign of sensory-motor association and expectancy in the human brain*, Nature, London, 1964, 203:380–394.

Wang W., Timsit-Berthier M., Schoenen J., *Intensity dependence of auditory evoked potentials is pronounced in migraine: An indication of cortical potentiation and low serotonergic neurotransmission?*, Neurology, 1996, 46:1404 –1409.

Wei Wang, Pascale G., Schoenen J., *Reduction of temporalis ES2 after peripheral electrical stimulation is exaggerated in patients with tension-type headache* (abs.), Proc. of the VIth Int. Headache Congress, Paris, Cephalalgia, 1993, 13 (Suppl. 13):147.

Welch K.M.A., Sheena A., Yue C., *Functional MRI, magnetoencephalography and transcranial magnetic stimulation in migraine*. In: Puca F., Bussone G., Gallai V., et al. (eds.), *Le Cefalee*, SISC, Caserta, 1998.

Willer J.C., *Comparative study of perceived pain and nociceptive flexion reflex in man*, Pain, 1977, 3:69–80.

Willer J.C., *Nociceptive flexion reflexes as a tool for pain research in man*, in: Desmedt J.E. (ed.), *Motor control mechanisms in health and disease*, Raven Press, New York, 1983, 809–827.

Willer J.C., *Studies on pain. Effects of morphine on a spinal nociceptive flexion and related pain sensation in man*, Brain Res., 1985, 105–114.

Willer J.C., Boureau F., Albe-Fessar D., *Role of large diameter cutaneous afferents in transmission of nociceptive messages: electrophysiological study in man*, Brain Res., 1978, 152:358–364.

Willer J.C., Albe-Fessard D., *Electrophysiological evidence for a release of endogenous opiates in stress-induced "analgesia" in man*, Brain Res., 1980, 198:419–426.

Willer J.C., Albe-Fessar D., *Further studies on the role of afferent input from relatively large diameter fibers in transmission of nociceptive messages in humans*, Brain Res., 1983, 278:318–321.

Wood J.H., *Neurochemical analysis of cerebrospinal fluid*, Neurology, 1980, 30:645–651.

Yemm R., *Reflex jaw opening following electrical stimulation of oral mucosa membrane in man*, Arch. Oral Biol., 1972, 17:513–523.

Yu S.K., Schmitt A., Sessle B.S., *Inhibitory effects of jaw muscle activity of innocuous and noxious stimulation of facial and intraoral sites on man*, Arch. Oral Biol., 1973, 18:861–870.

Zwart J.A., Sand T., *Exteroceptive suppression of temporalis muscle activity: a blind study of tension-type headache migraine and cervicogenic headache*, Headache, 1995, 35:338–343.

6 Hemodynamic Factors and Platelet Function

Blood Flow Alterations

Extracranial an intracranial blood flow has been widely investigated in headache patients, and in migraine patients in particular. However, owing to the differences in methodology and in the times at which the examinations were performed with respect to the pain attacks, a description of cerebrovascular changes in headache patients can only be based on comparative evaluation of the data. There are essentially two main types of methods for studying cerebral blood flow. In the first category belong angiography and transcranial doppler, which provide information from the large, conductance vessels (arteries and veins). Techniques that provide information on tissue perfusion, such as single-photon emission computed tomography (SPECT), belong to the second category: they retrieve data on regional cerebral blood flow (rCBF), controlled by the resistance vessels, i.e., the arterioles (Friberg, 1996). Blood flow velocity and rCBF are conditioning factors (inverse and direct, respectively) of the degree of vessel dilation.

The presence of rCBF alterations in patients with migraine with area is supported by numerous and consistent data. In patients with migraine with visual aura, using Xe-133 intracarotid injection, Olesen et al. (1981, 1990), Lauritzen et al. (1983), and Skyhøj Olsen et al. (1987) found a reduction of rCBF beginning from the posterior pole of the occipital lobe and spreading anteriorly at a rate of 2 to 3 cm per minute (Fig. 6.1). To some extent, the progressive characteristics of

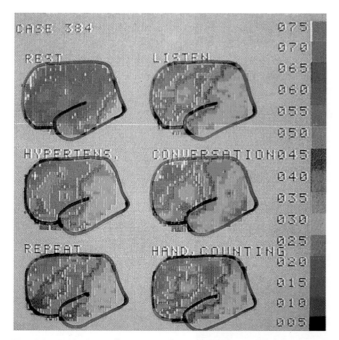

Fig. 6.1 **Patient undergoing migraine aura studied by intra-carotid injection of radioactive xenon.** A zone of progressive oligemia can be seen (blue, from top left to bottom right) which originates from the posterior pole of the occipital lobe and diffuses anteriorly. (From Lauritzen et al., 1983, with permission)

this phenomenon suggest that it is not primarily vascular, but rather due to a neurological factor, similar to *spreading depression,* as described by Leao (1944; Leao and Morrison, 1945) in the experimental animal, as a cortical wave of depolarization followed by repolarization. However, studies of rCBF have shown that, during the aura with scintillating scotoma of a visual half-field, there was a marked reduction of flow in the temporal occipital region of the opposite side (Igarashi et al., 1993).

In patients with migraine with aura, rCBF reduction starts during the aura and continues while headache develops. At a certain point of the headache phase, rCBF increases more than normal: such increase may well persist for a certain time after headache has disappeared (Fig. 6.2). Therefore, rCBF reduction may explain the aura symptoms but may not be strictly related to the migraine pain (Olesen, 1990). Indeed, no reduction or increase in rCBF was observed during attacks of migraine without aura (Lauritzen and Olesen, 1984). Moreover, neither increase of rCBF by acetazolamide injection or CO_2 inhalation, nor reduction of rCBF by administration of indomethacin or hyperventilation cause headache (Friberg, 1996).

On the other hand, as we have seen (Chapter 5), Welch et al. (1998) found an increase in T*-weighted image intensity in the occipital cortex, both in visually activated headache and spontaneous aura subjects. This phenomenon, which indicates an increase in tissue oxygen perfusion, was more widespread than might be expected from the localized nature of visual symptoms.

SPECT studies on migraine patients in the interictal period produced contradictory results. While some authors (Matthew et al., 1976; Sakai and Meyer, 1978), found normal rCBF values, others (Levine et al., 1987; Lagrèze et al., 1988; Schlake et al., 1989, 1992; Mirza et al., 1998) have observed focal alterations. Facco et al. (1996) found that, in the intercritical period, the majority of patients with migraine without aura showed rCBF values higher than the control subjects, while patients with migraine with aura had lower values in the posterior cortical region (Figs. 6.3, 6.4).

Blood flow velocity of the middle cerebral artery, studied by doppler, is decreased on the pain side during attacks of migraine with or without aura (Thie et al., 1990; Friberg et al., 1991; Thomsen et al., 1995). In patients with cluster headache, blood flow velocity of the middle cerebral artery was found to be lower than normal during attacks (Dahl et al., 1990; Micieli et al., 1993, 1994) and higher than normal on the symptomatic side between attacks (Dahl et al., 1990).

After treatment of the headache attack with sumatriptan administration, blood flow velocity of the middle cerebral artery (MCA) becomes normal (Olesen, 1994) (Fig. 6.5). Since, as mentioned, rCBF is not consistently modified during migraine attack, the decrease of blood flow velocity on the symptomatic side is a consequence of dilatation of the middle cerebral artery: presumably, pain of migraine with or without aura is consequent on such vasodilation (Friberg et al., 1991, Friberg, 1996). This hypothesis is also supported by the fact that during experimental headache due to nitroglycerin administration, rCBF does not vary, while blood flow velocity of

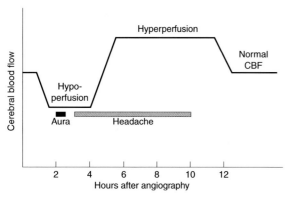

Fig. 6.**2   Changes in cerebral blood flow during attaks of migraine with aura.** There is no correlation between blood flow changes and occurrence of headache. (From Olesen et al., 1990, with modifications)

the middle cerebral artery decreases: as a consequence, this vessel is dilated (Iversen et al., 1991; Tegeler et al., 1996).

The involvement of intracranial vessels in migraine patients is also suggested by angiographic observations. Solomon et al. (1990) report a case of a woman suffering from incapicitating attacks of occipitonuchal migraine, in which cerebral angiography revealed multiple areas of stenosis in the vertebrobasilar and in several cerebral arteries. In reviewing the literature, the same authors found 13 case reports of migraine associated with angiographically demonstrated vascular narrowing. This observation has often been attributed to vasospasm (Ostfeld and Wolff, 1958) that is a consequence of altered sympathetic tonus of the cerebral arteries: these arteries are abundantly innervated by sympathetic fibers of extracranial and intracranial origin (coming respectively from the cervical ganglion and the locus coeruleus or

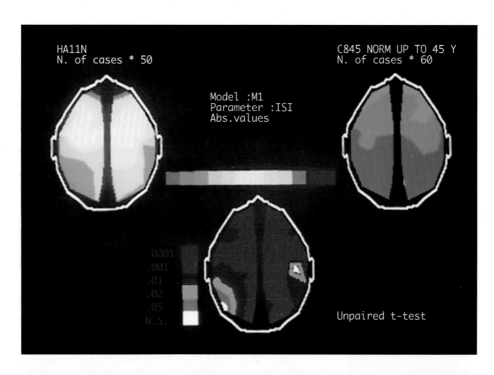

Fig. 6.**3   rCBF maps (**[133]**Xe clearance method) in 50 patients with migraine without aura (left in figure) and 60 healthy subjects (right in figure).** The rCBF is significantly higher than normal in all regions, apart from two small areas in the right temporal and left occipital regions (probability map at the bottom). (From Facco et al., 1996, with permission)

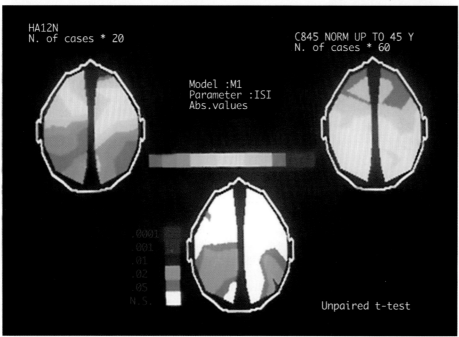

Fig. 6.**4   cCBF maps in 20 patients with migraine with aura (left in figure) and 60 healthy subjects (right in figure).** In the patients with migraine with aura, the rCBF is significantly lower than normal in the posterior regions (probability map at the bottom). (From Facco et al., 1996, with permission)

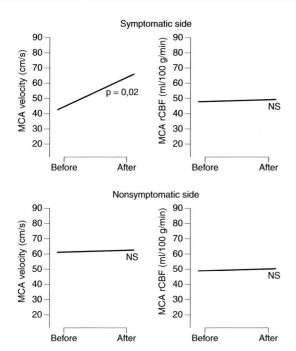

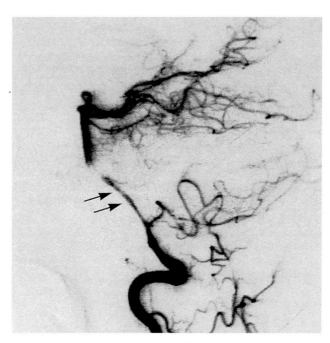

Fig. 6.**5** **Velocity in middle cerebral artery (MCA) and regional cerebral blood flow (rCBF) in the MCA territory during a migraine attack and after treatment with sumatriptan 2 mg i. v.** On the headache side, velocity is low before tretment and normalizes after treatment of the headache attack with sumatriptan. Since rCBF is not consistently modified during migraine attack the decrease of blood flow velocity on the symptomatic side is a consequence of dilatation of the middle cerebral artery that disappears after sumatriptan administration. On the non-headache side the two parameters do not change. (From Olesen et al., 1994, with modifications)

Fig. 6.**6**   Dissecting aneurism (arrows) in patient suffering from migraine. (From Bradac et al., 1981, with permission)

from other nuclei of the cerebral cortex) (Edvinsson and Owman, 1980; Edvinson et al., 1993). However, other mechanisms have been suggested, such as swelling of the vessel wall and consequent stenosis of the intracavernous carotid artery in patients with ophthalmoplegic migraine (Walsh and O'Doherty, 1960), arterial dissection (Bradac et al., 1981; Bousser et al., 1985; Monteiro et al., 1985; Jensen, 1986; Biousse et al., 1994) (Fig. 6.**6**), arteritis (Cupps et al., 1983), and arteriovenous malformations or cavernous angiomas (Monterio et al., 1993).

On the other hand, several findings support the hypothesis of a relation between headache (and migraine in particular) and cerebral alterations in some patients. Migraine is considered a possible etiological factor of cerebral stroke in young patients (Hilton-Jones and Warlow, 1985; Adams et al., 1986; Alvarez et al., 1989; Gautier et al., 1989; Sacquegna et al., 1989; Bogousslavky and Pierre, 1992; Carolei et al., 1993, Welch, 1994; Wöber-Bingöl et al., 1995). Featherstone (1986) reviewed 25 papers reporting individual cases and series of strokes in migraine patients, and concluded that the data suggest that such patients are indeed at increased risk of suffering strokes. Conversely, headache frequently occurs after ischemic stroke (Arboix et al., 1994). Finally, Merkangas et al. (1997), after examining the association between stroke and migraine in an epidemiological study, concluded that this association is not random, especially in young women.

The results of MRI studies in migraine patients, in general, confirm that intracranial vascular alterations that might lead to some brain damage are present in a certain number of patients (Fig. 6.**7**). However, data relating to the frequency differ markedly in the reports of various authors (Kaplan et al.,

1987; Soges et al., 1988; Jacome and Leborgne, 1990; Kuhn and Shekar, 1990; Osborn et al., 1991; Robbins and Friedman, 1992). Fazekas et al. (1992) compared the MRI scans of 38 migraine patients with those of 14 headache-free volunteers of the same age, and found focal areas of hyperintense signals in 39% of the patients and in only 14% of the controls. Moreover, such signal abnormalities were present in 53% of migraine patients with aura, versus 18% of migraine patients without aura. De Benedettis et al. (1993) observed alterations of the

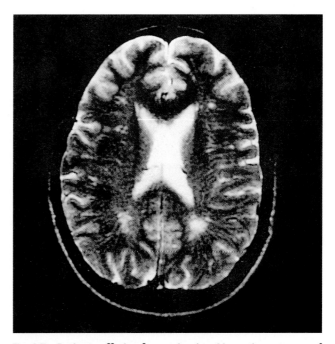

Fig. 6.**7**   **Patient suffering from migraine.** Magnetic resonance of the brain shows diffuse signs of damage to the subcortical white matter. (By courtesy of Professor G. B. Bradac, Director, Institute of Neuroradiology, Turin University)

white matter in 41% of 17 patients suffering from migraine with or without aura.

Epidemiological studies on severe hypertension only demonstrated a statistically significant relationship between this factor and feochromocytoma (Mastrosimone et al., 1987; Granata et al., 1988). However, numerous clinical observations suggest that, in some patients, hypertension has a causal relationship with headache attacks. Some authors (Cugini et al., 1992), through 24-hour blood pressure monitoring, have been able to distinguish between headache patients with high blood pressure in whom headache attacks (in the main with characteristics of migraine) coincided with high blood pressure crises, and others in whom headache episodes were independent of blood pressure. Furthermore, only in the first group of patients did a stress test cause high blood pressure crises and, often, headache. It has also been demonstrated that migraine patients with normal blood pressure do not have normal circadian angiotensin converting enzyme (ACE) serum function and that consequently they find themselves in relatively hyper-ACE-emic conditions in the mornings (Cugini et al., 1988). This fact, together with the demonstrated increased sensitivity of migraine sufferers to stressful stimuli (Boccuni et al., 1987; Martucci et al., 1987), may tend to cause high blood pressure subsequently in these patients. In a study (Cugini et al., 1992) on migraine patients with night attacks, a subgroup of patients with probable cause – effect relationship between migraine crisis and hypertension was distinguished. These patients, normally hypertensive, were found to have a circadian pressure rhythm with acrophase during the night.

The relationship between headache and high blood pressure is also supported by the consideration that, in patients with high blood pressure, alterations of blood platelet function have been described, similar to those found in migraine patients (see later).

The effectiveness of antihypertensive drugs, such as beta-blockers and calcium antagonists, in migraine therapy also supports a close link between the two pathologies even if, as we will see (Chapter 12), this consideration does not hold for all drugs in this category. Propranolol, which is widely used in the preventive treatment of migraine, has effects on the platelet function that can in part explain both its antihypertensive action and its effect against migraine (see later).

At any rate, it is generally accepted that migraine patients present with an abnormal sensitivity and instability of intracranial vessels. Gerber and Fuchs (1991) observed that the peripheral resistance of the temporal artery in conditions of stress was abated in migraine patients, while it increased in normal individuals. Studies by other authors (Thie et al., 1982, 1990; Reinecke et al., 1989; Thomas et al., 1990) suggest that the cerebral vessels in these patients may respond with more fluctuations than normal to various stimuli, such as eye opening, hypercapnia and Valsalva maneuvers. An abnormal response with increase of blood flow velocity was observed at the *cold pressor test* (Micieli et al., 1995) and after adiministration of apomorphine (Piccini et al., 1995). These observations are in agreement with those relative to the different action of serotonin when applied on fragments of temporal artery of migraine patients and normal subjects, respectively (Mathiau et al., 1994, see Chapter 5).

Studies on Platelet Function

Platelet function represents another relevant point in headache patients.

Reports of platelet abnormality in migraine patients are numerous, although rather contradictory (see Malmgren and Hasselmark, 1988, for a review). Nevertheless, most researchers agree that in migraine patients platelet aggregation is increased during headache-free periods (Couch and Hassanein, 1977; Deshmukh and Meyer, 1977; Hanington et al., 1981; Kruglak et al., 1984; Lechner et al., 1985) and during migraine attacks (Kalendovsky and Austin, 1975; Hanington, 1978; O'Neill and Mann, 1978; Gawel et al., 1979). Furthermore, the formation of platelet microaggregates and increased levels of the platelet-secreted proteins β-thromboglobulin and platelet factor 4 have been observed in migraine patients (Gawel et al., 1979; D'Andrea et al., 1982, 1985; Lechner et al., 1985).

Such findings are also typical of hypertensive patients: indeed, in these patients an increase of platelet aggregation (although of variable identity) (Nyrop and Zweifler, 1988), and of β-tromboglobulin plasma levels (Kjelsen et al., 1983) was found, particularly in patients with cerebrovascular disorders (Petralito et al., 1982; Gomi et al., 1988). Also, in these patients, alterations of platelet serotonin uptake and content were reported (Kamal et al., 1984).

Such findings are also typical of patients with ischemic cerebrovascular disorders (Couch and Hassanein, 1976; Al-Mefty et al., 1979), and further support the hypothesis of a predisposition to thrombotic stroke in migraine sufferers.

Since the circulating platelets represent a serotonin reservoir, the problem of platelet dysfunction is closely related to the influence of serotonin in migraine and other headaches. Indeed, as Malmgren and Hasselmark (1988) point out, several similarities can be found between the platelet and the serotoninergic nerve-ending (Fig. 6.**8**).

The relation between platelet function and serotonin and its importance in the pathogenesis of migraine is suggested by studies showing that in migraine patients platelets have a reduced number of imipramine binding sites (Geaney et al., 1984) and of serotonin receptors (Fontes Ribeiro et al., 1990; Govitrapong et al., 1992). Indeed, serotonin metabolism is altered in migraine patients (Ferrari et al., 1989) and such alterations are associated with platelet ultrastructural changes (D'Andrea et al., 1989; Fioroni et al., 1996). Moreover, platelet aggregation is inhibited by Ketanserine, a selective serotonin antagonist (De Clerk et al., 1982). It has been suggested (Govitrapong et al., 1992) that in a situation of impaired serotonin uptake and normal serotonin release, the excessive amount of serotonin accumulated outside the platelets could bring about a downregulation of serotonin receptors.

Propranolol reduces platelet aggregation (Weksler et al., 1977; Vlachakis and Aledort, 1980; Mehta et al., 1983; Siess et al., 1983; Ring et al., 1987) and serotonin release (Bygdeman and Johnsen, 1969; Anfossi et al., 1989) as well as platelet thromboxane production (Bygdeman and Johnson, 1969; Weksler et al., 1977; Vanderhoek and Maurice, 1979; Siess et al., 1983). It also modulates an increase in PGI_2 production (Forster, 1980; Petterson et al., 1991). This prostacyclin inhibits platelet aggregation and has a vasodilatory effect (Moncada and Vane, 1979; Callahan et al., 1985). These actions, as mentioned previously, may explain both antihypertensive and antimigraine drug action.

In their turn, calcium antagonists inhibit all the processes of activation of platelet aggregation: these processes, in fact, require that calcium enter the platelets in order to take place (Han et al., 1983).

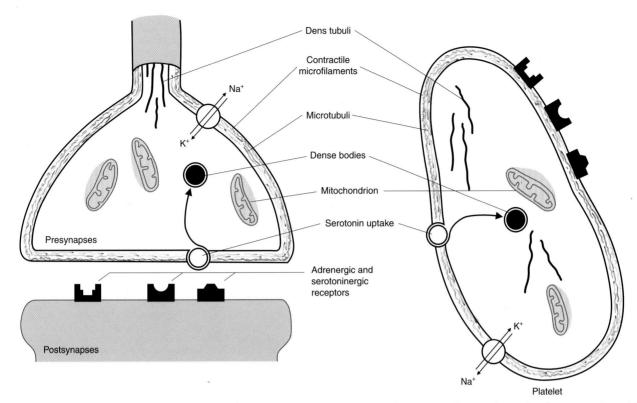

Fig. 6.**8**   Morphofunctional similarity between serotoninergic nerve ending and platelet. (From Malgren and Hasselmark, 1998, with modifications)

References

Adams H.P., Butler M.J., Biller J., *Nonhemorrhagic cerebral infarction in young adults*, Arch. Neurol., 1986, 43 : 793 – 799.

Al-Mefty O., Marano G., Rajaraman S., Nugent G.R., Rodman N., *Transient ischemic attacks due to increased platelet aggregation and adhesiveness*, J. Neurol., 1979 50 : 449 – 453.

Alvarez J., Matius-Guiu J., Sumulla J., et al., *Ischaemic stroke in young adults. I: Analysis of the etiological subgroups*, Acta. Neurol. Scand., 1989, 80 : 28 – 34.

Anfossi G., Trovati M., Mularoni E., Massucco P., Calcamuggi G., Emanuelli G., *Influence of propranolol on platelet aggregation and thromboxane B2 production from platelet rich plasma and whole blood*, Prostaglandins. Leukot. Essent. Fatty Acids., 1989, 36 : 1 – 7.

Arboix A., Massons J., Oliveres M., Arribas M.P., Titus F., *Headache in acute cerebrovascular disease: a prospective clinical study in 240 patients*, Cephalalgia, 1994, 14 : 37 – 40.

Biousse V., D'Anglejan-Chatillon J., Massiou H., Bousser M.G., *Head pain in non-traumatic carotid artery dissection: a series of 65 patients*, Cephalalgia, 1994, 14 : 33 – 36.

Boccuni M., Fusco B.M., Alessandri M., Cangi F., *Arterial hyperreactivity to the alpha-adrenoceptor activation in migraine*, Cephalalgia, 1987, 7, (Suppl. 6):291 – 292.

Bogousslavsky J., Pierre P., *Ischemic stroke in patients under age 45*, Neurol. Clin., 1992, 10 : 113 – 124.

Bousser M.G. Baron J.C., Chiras J., *Ischemic strokes and migraine*, Radiology, 1985, 27 : 583 – 587.

Bradac G.B., Kaernbach A., Bolk-Weischedel D., Finck G.A., *Spontaneous dissecting aneurysm of cervical cerebral arteries*, Neuroradiology, 1981, 21 : 149 – 154.

Bygdeman S., Johnsen O., *Studies on the effects of adrenergic blocking drugs on catecholamine-induced platelet aggregation and uptake of noradrenaline and 5-hydroxytryptamine*, Acta Physiol. Scand., 1969, 75 : 129 – 138.

Callahan K.S., Johnson A.R., Campbell W.B., *Enhancement of the antiaggregatory activity of prostacyclin by propranolol in human platelets*, Circulation, 1985, 71 : 1237 – 1246.

Carolei A., Marini C., Ferranti E., Frontoni M., Principe M., *A prospective study of cerebral ischemia in the young. Analysis of pathogenetic determinants*, Stroke, 1993, 24 : 362 – 367.

Couch J.R., Hassanein F.R., *Platelet aggregation, stroke and transient ischemic attack in middleaged and elderly patients*, Neurology, 1976, 26 : 888 – 895.

Couch J.R., Hassanein R.S., *Platelet aggregability in migraine*, Neurology, 1977, 27 : 843 – 848.

Cugini P., Martelletti P., Letizia C., Granata M., Scavo D., Giacovazzo M., *The non-cyclicity for serum angiotensin-converting-enzyme characterizes the endogenous substrate of migraine patients suggesting a pronociception state*, Schmerz Pain Douleur, 1988, 9 : 32 – 33.

Cugini P., Granata M., Strano S. et al., *Nocturnal headache-hypertension syndrome: a chronobiologic disorder*, Chronobiol. Int., 1992, 9 : 310 – 313.

Cupps T.R., Moore P.M., Fauci A.S., *Isolated angiitis of the central nervous system. Prospective diagnostic and therapeutic experience*, Ann. J. Med., 1983, 74 : 97 – 105.

D'Andrea G., Toldo M., Cortellazzo S., Ferro-Milone F., *Platelet activity in migraine*, Headache, 1982, 22 : 207 – 212.

D'Andrea G., Cananzi A., Toldo M., Ferro-Milone F., *Drugs and platelet activation in migraine and transient ischemic attaks*, Cephalalgia, 1985, 5, (Suppl. 2):103 – 108.

D'Andrea G., Welch M., Riddle J.M., Grunfeld S., Joseph S., *Platelet serotonin metabolism and ultrastructure in migraine*, Arch. Neurol., 1989, 46 : 1187 – 1189.

Dahl A., Russel D., Nyberg-Hansen R., Rostwelt K., *Cluster headache: transcranial doppler ultrasound in CBF studies*, Cephalalgia, 1990, 10 : 87 – 94.

De Benedittis G., Lorenzetti A., Sina C., Bernasconi V., *Magnetic resonance imaging in migraine and tension-type headache* (abs.), Cephalalgia, 1993, 13, (Suppl. 13):154.

De Clerck F., David J.L., Janssen P.A.J., *Inhibition of 5-hydroxytryptamine-induced and - amplified human platelet aggregation by ketanserin (R 41 468), a selective 5-HT2 -receptor antagonist*, Agent Actions, 1982, 12 : 388 – 397.

Deshmukh S.V., Meyer J.S., *Cyclic changes in platelets dynamics and the pathogenesis and prophylaxis of migraine*, Headache, 1977, 17 : 101 – 108.

Edvinsson L., Owman C., *Cerebrovascular nerves and vasomotor receptors*, in: Wilkins R.H. (ed.), *Cerebral arterial spasm*, Williams & Wilkins, Baltimore, 1980, 30 – 36.

Edvinsson L., Gulbenkian S., Jensen I., *Distribution of peptidergic nerves in the human cerebral circulation* (abs.), Cephalalgia, 1993, 13, (Suppl. 13):91.

Facco E., Munari M., Baratto F., et al., *Regional cerebral blood flow (rCBF) in migraine during the interictal period: different rCBF patterns in patients with and without aura*, Cephalalgia, 1996, 16 : 161 – 168.

Fazekas F., Koch M., Schmidt R. et al., *The prevalence of cerebral damage varies with migraine type: a MRI study*, Headache, 1992, 32 : 287 – 291.

Featherstone H., *Clinical features of stroke in migraine: a review*, Headache, 1986, 26 : 128 – 133.

Ferrari M.D., Odink J., Tapparelli C., Van Kempen G.M.J., Pennings E.J.M., Bruyn G.W., *Serotonin metabolism in migraine*, Neurology, 1989, 39 : 1239 – 1242.

Fioroni I. D'Andrea G., Alecci M., Cananzi A., Facchinetti F., *Platelet serotonin pathway in menstrual migraine*, Cephalalgia, 1996, 16 : 427 – 30.

Fontes Ribeiro C.A., Cotrim M.D., Morgadinho M.T., Ramos M.I., Seabra Santos E., Macedo T.R.A., *Migraine, serum serotonin and platelet 5-HT2 receptors*, Cephalalgia, 1990, 10 : 213 – 219.

Forster W., *Effect of various agents on prostaglandin biosynthesis and the antiaggregatory effect*, Acta Med. Scand., 1980, 642, (Suppl.):35 – 46.

Friberg L., *Migraine pathophysiology and its relation to cerebral hemodynamic changes*, in: Clifford Rose F. (ed.), *Towards Migraine 2000*, Elsevier, Amsterdam, 1996, 101 – 109.

Friberg L., Olesen J., Iversen H.K., Sperling B., *Migraine pain associated with middle cerebral artery dilatation: reversal by sumatriptan*, Lancet, 1991, 338 : 13 – 16.

Gautier J.C., Pradat-Diehl P., Loron P., et al. *Accidents vasculaires cerebraux des sujets jeunes: une étude de 133 patients agés de 9 a 45 ans*, Rev. Neurol., 1989, 145 : 437 – 42.

Gawel M., Burkitt M., Clifford Rose F., *The platelet release reaction during migraine attacks*, Headache, 1979, 19 : 323 – 327.

Geaney D.P., Rutterford M.G., Elliot J.M., Schacter M., Peet K.M.S., *Decreased platelet 3 H imipramine binding sites in classical migraine*, J. Neurol. Psychiatry, 1984, 47 : 720 – 723.

Gerber D.W., Fuchs D., *Ultrasonic doppler flow measurements during severe stress induction in migraine patients*, Cephalalgia, 1991, 11, (Suppl. 1):312.

Gomi T., Ikeda T., Yuhara M., et al., *Plasma betathromboglobulin to platelet factor 4 ratios as indices of vascular complications in essential hypertens.*, J. Hypertension, 1988, 6 : 389 – 392.

Govitrapong P., Limthavon C., Srikiatkhachorn A., *5-HT2 serotonin receptor on blood platelet of migraine patients*, Headache, 1992, 32 : 480 – 484.

Granata M., Strano S., Gallo M.F., et al. *Cefalea ed ipertensione, causalità o correlazione, utilità del profilo pressorio delle 24 ore. III Meeting on "Conflicting aspects in the clinical approach to hypertension". Abstract of the italian department of public healt project on blood pressure variability proceedings*, G. Germanò, Montecassino, 1988, 21 – 22, 46 – 47.

Han P., Boatwright C., Ardlie N.G., *Effect of the calcium entry blocking agent nifedipine on activation of human platelets and comparison with verapamil*, Thromb. Haemost., 1983, 50 : 513 – 517.

Hanington E., *Migraine: a blood disorder?*, Lancet, 2 : 501, 1978.

Hanington E., Jones R.J., Amess J.A.L., Wachowicz B., *Migraine: a platelet disorder*, Lancet, 1981, 2 : 720 – 723.

Hilton-Jones D., Warlow C.P., *The causes of stroke in the young*, J. Neurol., 1985, 232 : 137 – 143.

Igarashi H., Sakai F., Kanda T., Saitoh Y., *The reduction of rCBF during aura of migraine in regions corresponding to the cerebral arterial territory* (abs.), Cephalalgia, 1993, 13, (Suppl. 13):18.

Iversen H., Holm S., Friberg L., *Nitroglycerine induced headache and intracranial hemodynamics*, in: Olesen J. (ed.), *Migraine and other headaches: the vascular mechanisms*, Raven Press, New York, 1991, 327 – 330.

Jacome D.E., Leborgne J.L., *MRI studies in basilar artery migraine*, Headache, 1990, 30 : 88 – 90.

Jensen I.W., *Unusual angiographic appearance during attack of hemiplegic migraine*, Headache, 1986, 26 : 295 – 296.

Jensen K., *Headache and extracerebral blood flow*, in: Olesen J., Edvinsson L. (eds.), *Basic mechanisms of headache*, Elsevier, Amsterdam, 1988, 313 – 320.

Kalendovsky Z., Austin J.H., *Complicated migraine: its association with increased platelet aggregability and abnormal plasma coagulation factors*, Headache, 1975, 15 : 18.

Kamal L.A., Quan-Bui K.H.L. Meyer P., *Decrease uptake of 3-H- serotonin and andogenous content of serotonin in blood platelets in hypertensive patients*, Hypertension, 1984, 6 : 568 – 573.

Kaplan R.D., Solomon G.D., Diamond S., Freitag F.G., *The role of MRI in the evaluation of a migraine population. Preliminary data*, Headache, 1987, 27 : 315 – 318.

Kjelsen S., Gjesdal K., Eide I. et al., *Increased beta-thromboglobulin in essential hypertension: interactions between arterial plasma adrenaline, platelet function and blood lipids*, Acta Med. Scand., 1983, 213 : 369 – 573.

Kruglak L., Nathan I., Korczyn A.D., Zolotov Z., Berginer V., Dvilansky A., *Platelet aggregability, disaggregability and serotonin uptake in migraine*, Cephalalgia, 1984, 4 : 221 – 225.

Kuhn M.J., Shekar P.C., *A comparative study of magnetic resonance imaging and computer tomography in the evaluation of migraine*, Comput. Med. Imaging. Graph., 1990, 14 : 149 – 152.

Lagrèze H.L., Dettmers C., Hartmann A., *Abnormalities of interictal cerebral perfusion in classic but not common migraine*, Stroke, 1988, 19 : 1108 – 1111.

Lauritzen M., Skyhoj Olsen T., Lassen N.A., Paulson O.B., *The changes of regional cerebral blood flow during the course of classical migraine attacks*, Ann. Neurol., 1983, 13 : 633 – 641.

Lauritzen M., Olesen J., *Regional cerebral blood flow during migraine attacks by Xenon-133 inhalation and emission tomography*, Brain, 1984, 107 : 447 – 461.

Leao A.A.P., *Spreading depression of activity in cerebral cortex*, J. Neurophysiol., 1944, 7 : 359 – 390.

Leao A.A.P., Morrison R.S., *Propagation of spreading cortical depression*, J. Neurophysiol., 1945, 8 : 33 – 45.

Lechner H., Ott. E., Fazekas F., Pilger E., *Evidence of enhanced platelet aggregation and platelet sensitivity in migraine patients*, Cephalalgia, 1985, 5, (Suppl. 2):89 – 91.

Levine S.R., Welch K.M.A., Ewing J.R., Joseph R., D'Andrea G., *Cerebral blood flow asymmetries in headache-free migraineurs*, Stroke, 1987, 18 : 1164 – 1165.

Malmgren R., Hasselmark L., *The platelet and the neuron: two cells in focus in migraine*, Cephalalgia, 1988, 8 : 7 – 24.

Martucci N., Agnoli A., Manna V., Cerbo R., *Is a migraine patient more sensitive to stressor? A neurophysiological and psychological study*, Cephalalgia, 1987, 7, (Suppl. 6):161 – 163.

Mastrosimone F., Iaccarino C. De Caterina G., *Arterial hypertension as autonomic dysfunction in migraneurs*, Cephalalgia, 1987, 7, (Suppl. 6):293 – 294.

Mathiau P., Brochet B., Boulan P., Henry P., Aubinaeau P., *Spontaneous and 5 HT-induced cyclic contractions in superficial temporal arteries from chronic and episodic cluster headache patients*, Cephalalgia, 1994, 14 : 419 – 429.

Matthew N.T., Hrastnik F., Meyer J.S., *Regional cerebral blood flow in the diagnosis of vascular headache.*, Headache, 1976, 16 : 252 – 260.

Mehta J., Mehta P., Ostrowski N., *Influence of propranolol and 4-hydroxypropranolol on platelet aggregation and thromboxane A2 generation*, Clin. Pharmacol. Ther., 1983, 34 : 559 – 564.

Merikangas K.R., Fenton B.T., Cheng S.H., Stolar M.J., Risch, N., *Association between migraine and stroke in a large-scale epidemiological study of the United States*, Arch. Neurol. 1997, 54(4):362 – 368.

Micieli G., Bosone D., Cavallini A., Tassorelli C., Nappi G., *Cerebral blood velocity changes in cluster headache: evidence for a bilateral asymmetrical impairment* (abs.), Proc. VIth Int. Headache, Congress, Paris, Cephalalgia, 1993, 13, (Suppl. 13):197.

Micieli G., Bosone D., Cavallini A., Rossi F., Pompeo F., Tassorelli C., Nappi G., *Bilateral asymmetry of cerebral blood velocity in cluster headache*, Cephalalgia, 1994, 14 : 346 – 351.

Micieli G., Tassorelli C., Bosone D., Cavallini A., Bellantonio P., Rossi F., Nappi G., *Increased cerebral blood flow velocity induced by cold pressor test in migraine: a possible basis for pathogenesis?*, Cephalalgia, 1995, 15 : 494 – 8.

Milani L., Sanson A., Ambrosio G.B., *Piastrine e ipertensione*, Trombosi & Aterosclerosi, 1993, vol. 4, no. 1.

Mirza M., Tutus A., Erdogan F., et al., *Intercritical SPECT with Tc-99 m HMPAO studies in migraine patients*, Acta Neurol. Belg., 1998, 98(2):190 – 194.

Moncada S., Vane J.R., *Pharmacology and endogenous roles of prostaglandins, endoperoxides and thromboxane A2 and prostacyclin*, Pharmacol. Rev., 1979, 30 : 293 – 331.

Monteiro P., Carneiro L., Lima B., Lopes C., *Migraine and cerebral infarction: three case studies*, Headache, 1985, 25 : 429 – 433.

Monteiro P., Rosas M.J., Correia A.P., Vaz A., *Migraine type headaches and intracranial vascular malformations* (abs.), Cephalalgia, 1993, 13, (Suppl. 13):61.

Nyrop M., Zweifler A.J., *Platelet aggregation in hypertension and the effects of anti-hypertensive treatment*, J. Hypertens. 1988, 6 : 263 – 269.

O'Neill B.P., Mann J.D., *Aspirin prophylaxis in migraine*, Lancet, 1978, 2 : 1179.

Olesen J., *Pathophysiology of human vascular headache*, in: Gebhart G.F., Hammond D.L., Jensen T.S. (eds.), Proceedings of the 7 th World Congress on Pain, Progress in Pain Research and Management, vol. 2, IASP Press, Seattle, 1994, 733 – 3.

Olesen J., Larsen B., Lauritzen M., *Focal hyperemia followed by spreading oligemia and impaired activation of rCBF in classic migraine*, Ann. Neurol., 1981, 9 : 344 – 352.

Olesen J., Friberg L., Skyhøj Olsen T., et al. *Timing and lateralization of cerebral blood flow changes, symptoms and headache during attacks of migraine with aura*, Ann. Neurol., 1990, 28 : 791 – 798.

Osborn R.E., Alder D.C., Mitchell C.S., *MR imaging of the brain in patients with migraine headaches*, AJNR, 1991, 12 : 521 – 524.

Ostfeld A.M., Wolff H.H., *Identification, mechanisms and management of the migraine syndrome*, Med. Clin. North Am., 1958, 42 : 1497 – 1509.

Petralito A., Fiore C.E., Mangiafico R.A. et al., *Beta-thromboglobulin plasma levels in different stages of arterial hypertension*, Thromb. Haemost., 1982, 48 : 241 – 247.

Petterson K., Hansson G., Bjorkman J.A., Ablad B., *Prostacyclin synthesis in relation to sympathoadrenal activation. Effects of ß-blockade*, Circulation, 1991, 84, (Suppl. VI):38 – 43.

Piccini P., Pavese N., Palombo C., Pittella G., Distante A., Bonuccelli U., *Transcranial Doppler ultrasound in migraine and tension-type headache after apomorphine administration: double-blind crossover versus placebo study*, Cephalalgia, 1995, 15 : 399 – 403.

Reinecke M., Wallasch T.M., Langoht H.D., *Abnormal autonomic cerebrovascular reactivity in migraine: clinical experience with a new transcranial doppler method*, Neurology, 1989, 39 (Suppl. 1):324.

Ring M.E., Corrigan J.J., Fanster P.E., *Antiplatelet effects of oral diltiazem, propranolol and their combination*, Clin. Res., 1987, 35 : 116 – 121.

Robbins L., Friedman H., *MRI in migraineurs*, Headache, 1992, 32 : 507 – 508.

Sacquegna T., Andreoli A., Baldrati A., et al. *Ischemic stroke in young adults: the relevance of migrainous infarction*, Cephalalgia, 1989, 9 : 255 – 258.

Sakai F., Meyer J.S., *Regional cerebral hemodynamics during migraine and cluster headaches measured by the 133Xe inhalation method.* Headache, 1978, 18 : 122 – 132.

Schlake H.P., Bottger I.G., Grotemeyer K.H., Husstedt I W , *Brain imaging with 12 I-IMP-Spect in migraine between attacks*, Headache, 1989, 29 : 344 – 349.

Schlake H.P., Bottger I.G., Grotemeyer K.H., Husstedt I.W., Oberwittler C., Schober O., *The influence of acetazolamide on cerebral low-flow regions in migraine-an interictal 99 mTc-HMPAO SPECT study*, Cephalalgia, 1992, 12 : 284 – 288.

Siess W., Lorenz R., Roth P., Weber P.C., *Effects of propranolol in vitro and in vivo on platelet function and thromboxane formation in normal volunteers*, Agents Action, 1983, 13 : 29 – 34.

Skyhøj Olsen T., Friberg L., Lassen N.A., *Ischemia may be the primary cause of the neurological deficits in classic migraine*, Arch. Neurol., 1987, 44 : 156 – 161.

Soges L.J., Cacayorin E.D., Petro G.R., Ramachandran T.S., *Migraine: evaluation by MR*, AJNR, 1988, 9 : 425 – 429.

Solomon S., Lipton R.B., Harris P.Y., *Arterial stenosis in migraine: spasm or arteriopathy?*, Headache, 1990, 30 : 52 – 61.

Tegeler C.H., Davidai G., Gengo F.M., et al., *Middle cerebral velocity correlates with nitroglycerin-induced headache onset.* J. Neuroimaging 1996, 6 : 81 – 86.

Thie A., Spitzer K., Lachenmayer L., Kunze K., *Prolonged vasospasm in migraine detected by noninvasive transcranial doppler ultrasound*, Headache, 1982, 28 : 183 – 186.

Thie A., Fuhlendorf A., Spitzer K., Kunze K., Transcranial doppler evalutation of common and classic migraine, Part 1: Ultrasonic features during the headache free period, Headache, 1990, 30 : 201 – 208.

Thie A., Fuhlendorf A., Spitzer K., Kunze K., *Transcranial doppler evaluation of common and classic migraine*, Part II: *Ultrasonic features during attacks*, Headache, 1990, 30 : 209 – 215.

Thomas D.T., Harpold G.J., Troost B.T., *Cerebrovascular reactivity in migraineurs as measured by transcranial doppler*, Cephalalgia, 1990, 10 : 95 – 99.

Thomsen L.L., Iversen H.K., Olesen J., *Cerebral blood flow velocities are reduced during attacks of unilateral migraine without aura*, Cephalalgia, 1995, 15 : 109 – 116.

Vanderhoek J.Y., Maurice B.F., *Local anesthetics, chlorpromazine and propranolol inhibit stimulus-activation of phospholipase A2 in human platelets*, Mol. Pharmacol., 1979, 16 : 171 – 180.

Vlachakis N.D., Aledort L., *Hypertension and propranolol therapy: effect on blood pressure, plasma catecholamines and platelet aggregation*, Am. J. Cardiol., 1980, 45 : 321 – 325.

Walsh J.P., O'Doherty D.S., *A possible explanation of the mechanism of ophthalmoplegic migraine*, Neurology, 1960, 10 : 1079 – 1084.

Weksler B.B., Gillick M., Pink J., *Effect of propranolol on platelet function*, Blood, 1977, 49 : 185 – 196.

Welch K.M.A., *Relationship of stroke and migraine*, Neurology, 1994, 44 (Suppl. 7):33 – 36.

Welch K.M.A., Sheena A., Yue C., *Functional MRI, magnetoencephalography and transcranial magnetic stimulation in migraine.* In: Puca F., Bussone G., Gallai V., et al. (eds.), *Le Cefalee*, SISC, Caserta, 1998.

Wöber-Bingöl C., Wöber C., Karwautz A., Feucht M., Brandtner S., Scheidinger H., *Migraine and stroke in childhood and adolescence*, Cephalalgia, 1995, 15 : 26 – 30.

7 Hormonal and Immune Factors

Hypothalamo-Pituitary Axis

The hypothalamo-pituitary axis is an important center of hormonal production and regulation: conversely, its activity is modulated by the level of circulating hormones.

An important control function is displayed by the circulating β-endorphins that, together with ACTH and β-lipotropin, are produced almost entirely by the pituitary gland (Krieger and Martin, 1981). Endogenous opioids play an inhibitory action on hypothalamic LH-RH (luteinizing hormone-releasing hormone) neurons. This action is probably modulated by catecholamines (Fioroni et al., 1995) and appears to be reduced during the premenstrual period in women with premenstrual migraine (Facchinetti et al., 1983 a, b) or premenstrual syndrome (Facchinetti et al., 1988). Opioid production from the pituitary gland is stimulated by the hypothalamic corticotropin-releasing hormone (CRH), that, in turn, is potentiated by interleukins (Fagarasan et al., 1989) (Fig. 7.1).

Also the levels of prolactin, which is produced by the adenohypophysis, are frequently altered in women with migraine. A different prolactin response to the assumption of sulpiride was observed by Nappi and co-workers (1981) in women suffering from menstrual migraine. Sulpiride is a dopamine antagonist. Since dopamine inhibits prolactin production, probably at the pituitary level, sulpiride induces an increase of prolactin blood levels. This responae is more marked during the luteal phase (D'Agata, 1980). However, in

migraine patients, this response was present in both phases of the menstrual cycle and was higher than that found in healthy women during the luteal phase. Moreover, women with migraine of post-menopause age show a more marked increase of prolactin than do healthy women of the same age (Polleri et al., 1984).

Other authors (Awaki et al., 1989) tested the presence of prolactin due to simulaneous intravenous injection of thyrotropin-releasing hormone (TRH), LH-RH and insulin, and found that such an increase was significantly higher in migraine patients than in controls. Conversely, Nattero and co-workers (1986) observed that, in migraine sufferers, the inhibition of prolactin secretion consequent on L-dopa administration was lower than normal.

The presence of a dysfunction of the hypothalamo–pituitary axis has also been sugested in cluster headache. In such patients, changes in the 24-hour prolactin secretion pattern have been observed (Polleri et al., 1982), as well as in cortisol, melatonin (Waldenling et al., 1987) and LH (Micieli et al., 1987) secretion. Moreover, a lower thyroid-stimulating hormone (TSH) response to TRH has been observed in cluster headache patients during the cluster period (Bussone et al., 1989) as well as an increase of vasopressin-arginine production (Francescini et al., 1995). It has been assumed that vasopressin, produced by the posterior portion of the pituitary gland, may play an adaptive vasomotor function.

A possible influence of CRH on mastocyte degranulation was observed by Theoharides et al. (1995). These authors have found mastocyte degranulation in the dura of rats undergoing immobilization stress: this effect was completely inhibited in animals pretreated with anti-CRH serum. The authors suggest that stress may induce neurogenic inflammation (see Chapter 2), also through mastocyte degranulation and that this action is modulated by CRH.

Sex Steroid Hormones

The role of sex steroids in headache and migraine in particular is generally accepted. Several clinical observations support this hypothesis, including the higher headache incidence in women, the onset at puberty, the increase during the premenstrual or menstrual phases in many cases, and the fact that a higher proportion of women have fewer or no migraine attacks during pregnancy (Somerville, 1972a; Nattero, 1982; Welch et al., 1984; Edelson, 1985; Martignoni et al., 1987; Bousser et al., 1990; Silberstein and Merriam, 1991; Uknis and Silberstein, 1991; Silberstein, 1996; see review by Welch, 1997).

Moreover, after menopause, migraine tends to improve while tension-type headache tends to worsen (Neri et al., 1993). Differences in mean plasma ovarian steroid levels in migraine patients compared to normal have been reported by several authors (Somerville 1971, 1972a, b, 1975 a, b; Epstein et al., 1975). Somerville (1971, 1972a, 1975a, b) focused his attention on the progesterone and estradiol levels in women subject to premenstrual or menstrual migraine and observed that a drop in estrogen levels seems to be a critical factor pre-

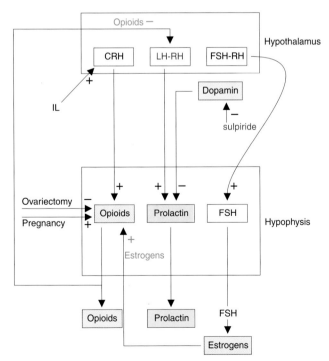

Fig. 7.1 Diagram of the hypothalamus-hypophysis axis and of the activatory (+) and inhibitory (–) influences on production of opioids, prolactin and FSH from the pituitary. Mechanisms that may be enhanced in migraine patients are given in red, those that may be inhibited in blue

cipitating the migraine attack. Several days of estrogen exposure are needed before its withdrawal will provoke headache (Somerville, 1975a). The attack does not occur if the hormone level is kept artificially high by estradiol injections (Somerville, 1975b; De Lignières, 1990). These studies are of interest, but are limited by certain factors (low number of patients enrolled, absence of a control group): this probably explains why other researchers have not been able to replicate these data (Davies et al., 1989). However, other studies (Epstein et al., 1975; Nagel-Leiby et al., 1990) have shown that in women with migraine, plasma estrogen levels are particularly high. As a consequence, in the premenstrual phase these patients have a higher decrement rate of estrogen level. It therefore seems that the extent of estradiol decrement is a critical factor for inducing a migraine attack. Double-blind studies (De Lignières et al., 1986; Dennerstein et al., 1988) have shown that administration of percutaneous estradiol gel is significantly more effective than placebo in preventing menstrual migraine.

With regard to progesterone, while some authors report that progesterone injected (Gray, 1941; Singh et al., 1947) or given orally (Lundberg, 1962) is effective in preventing premenstrual and menstrual migraine, Somerville (1971) disputes this effect.

Testosterone plasma levels have been studied in patients suffering from cluster headache, a type of headache which prevails in men. The results are somewhat contradictory: decreased testosterone plasma levels have been reported in cluster headache patients by some authors (Kudrow, 1977; Micieli et al., 1985; Facchinetti et al., 1986), and only in chronic cluster headache patients by others (Murialdo et al., 1989), while normal values were found by yet other authors (Nelson, 1978; Klimek, 1982).

Different mechanisms have been suggested to explain the relation between hormonal changes and headache. The peculiar prolactin response observed in women suffering from migraine might be related to a different estrogen-dependent modulation of lactotropic cells (Murialdo et al., 1989). Estrogen plasma level could also favour cranial vasoconstriction; Somerville (1975a, b) suggests that estrogen might "prime" such vessels so that they would be more susceptible to other factors possibly implicated in migraine, such as plasma level fluctuation of serotonin. A similar mechanism is suggested by Welch et al. (1984).

Changes in the sex hormones are associated with changes in serotonin levels and serotonin receptors. Estrogen increase leads to higher levels of plasma and platelet serotonin (Guicheney et al., 1988). Decreased peripheral serotonin consequent on decrease of estrogen could be associated with a reduction of an autoinhibitory effect of peripheral serotonin on the serotonin receptors and migraine attacks as a consequence (Marcus, 1995) (see Chapter 5).

The link between hormones and the central nervous system (CNS) is also of importance. Experimental and clinical evidence has been produced that the endogenous opioid system (discussed in Chapter 5) is modulated by sex steroids. Gonadectomy in rats produces a lowering of β-endorphin in the hypothalamus, pituitary and plasma (Petraglia, 1982). This effect is partially corrected by the administration of estradiol or testosterone, respectively, to the castrated female or male rats. This finding has been confirmed in primates by Wehrenberg (1982) and in humans by Shoupe et al. (1985). In women during ovulation and in castrated women, these authors evaluated the endogenous opioid activity as measured by the release of luteinizing hormone after naloxone infusion. In fact, such release correlates with portal plasma β-endorphin levels (Quingley and Yen, 1980; Van Vugt et al., 1982). In castrated women patients it was found that opioid activity was low but increased after administration of estrogens. During pregnancy, an increase of plasma β-endorphin levels is observed that parallels the higher estrogen level (Baldi et al., 1979; Csontos et al., 1979) (Fig. **7.1**). In this way, the sex steroids could directly affect nociception. Indeed, gonadectomy has been shown to decrease the analgesic effect of morphine in rats (Pinsky et al., 1975). In addition, the pain threshold in female rats was found to be higher at the end of pregnancy and returned to normal levels after parturition (Gintzler, 1980).

Some data on the treatment of cluster headache confirm the link between sex steroids and nociception. A reduction of pain in cluster headache patients was demonstrated by Klimek (1985) after testosterone administration, while Sicuteri et al. (1989) obtained a significant reduction of pain with cyproterone, an antiandrogen with progestative action.

Estrogen level is a conditioning factor of the number of dendrites an synapses in the hippocampus (and, in particular, of serotoninergic synapses), hypothalamus and the basal forebrain (Clarke and Goldfarb, 1989; McEwen et al., 1991; Segarra and McEwen, 1991; Wooley and McEwen, 1992). It has also been observed that estrogen injections in the experimental animal may alter the size of the receptive field of the trigeminal mechanoceptors in the rat (Bereiter et al., 1980) as well as the expression of mRNA in the sensory neurons (Soharabji et al., 1994).

Finally, a relation was found between estrogens and catecholamines. Estradiol target sites were found in the locus caeruleus (a structure with high norepinephine levels), and close to catecholamine nerve endings in the midbrain and diencephalon (Heritage et al., 1980).

Very little information exists concerning a possible relation between hormones and facial pain conditions other than headache. However, it has been suggested that here, too, the hormonal changes and their relation to endorphin levels could play an important role (Polleri et al., 1982; Rose, 1984; Facchinetti et al., 1986).

Immune Factors

The relationship between the neuroendocrine system and the immune system is well known (Blalock and Smith, 1985; Weigent and Blalock, 1987; Blalock, 1989; Ferrero, 1996). Thus it is not surprising that research has frequently found alterations of the immune system in headache patients. In the same way as has been found for platelets in migraine patients (see Chapter 6), in the lymphocytes of patients with cluster headache a reduction of the serotonin-binding sites has been found. This reduction has been seen both during cluster periods and in intercritical periods (Martelletti et al., 1987a). Also, in patients with migraine and, to a lesser extent, with tension-type headache, alterations of the interaction of serotonin with lymphocytes and monocytes have been found (Martelletti et al., 1988; Giacovazzo et al., 1990).

As far as the immunopeptidergic side is concerned, an important role in pain modulation, and for cephalic pain in particular, is displayed by cytokines, in particular by interleukin 1 (IL-1) and tumor necrosis factor (TNF). These cytokines are produced by blood monocytes and tissue macrophages and facilitate opioid release by immunocompetent cells (Stein et al., 1994) (see below). Moreover, as mentioned previously, IL-1 stimulates CRH secretion from the hypothalamus. As a consequence, production of opioids and ACTH from the pituitary gland and of cortisone from the suprarenal gland is enhanced (Fig. 7.**2**). Cortisone displays an anti-inflammatory action by inhibiting phospholipase and cytokine gene expression.

Conversely, cytokines, which are also produced at central level, are neurotransmitters or neuromodulators of specific

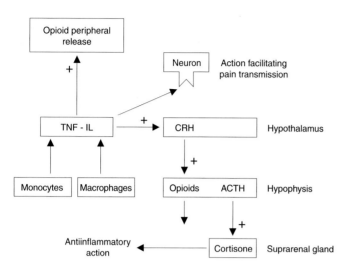

Fig. 7.**2**   Possible inhibiting and facilitating actions on pain transmission of interleukin-1 (IL-1) and tumor necrosis factor (TNF)

receptors and, as such, facilitate pain transmission (Watkins et al., 1995; Walkins, 1996) (Fig. 7.**2**).

In migraine patients an increase in interleukin-1 was observed, both in the active phase and in the intercritical phase (Covelli et al., 1990; Martelletti et al., 1992). The cytotoxic function of the natural killer lymphocytes is also decreased in cluster headache (Martelletti et al., 1987b; Stirparo et al., 1990).

Gallai et al. (1993) have observed, in intercritical periods, a reduction in the chemotactic response in migraine patients and, to a lesser extent, in tension-type headache patients. During attacks, this response increases significantly only in migraine patients. For phagocyte function, the same authors found no difference in migraine patients compared to normal subjects in the intercritical period, but they did find an increase in this response during the attack. They hypothesize that this alteration of the monocyte function is a consequence of the action of one or more mediators that participate in the mechanisms producing neurogenic inflammation.

On the other hand, there is consistent experimental evidence that immunocompetent cells (monocytes, macrophages, T and B lymphocytes) are a peripheral source of opioid release (Sibinga and Goldstein, 1988; Heijnen et al., 1991; Sacerdote et al., 1991; Stein et al., 1990 a, 1993; Przewlocki et al., 1992; Wan Woudenberg et al., 1992; Kilpatrick, 1993; Stein, 1993a). These opioids, β-endorphins and meten-

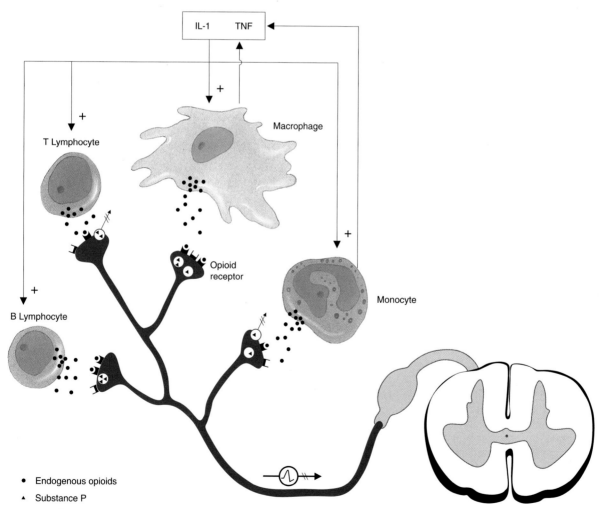

- ● Endogenous opioids
- ▲ Substance P

Fig. 7.**3**   **Release of opioids in peripheral tissues by the immunocompetent cells.** The opioids act on the peripheral receptors, which are preexisting but inactive or which form as a consequence of the inflammatory stimulus, inhibiting both nociceptive signals afferent to the center and the release of substance P. The opioid release in the periphery is enhanced by interleukin-1 (IL-1) and tumor necrosis factor (TNF) produced by monocytes and macrophages (see also Fig. 7.**2**). (From Stein, 1993, with modifications)

cephalins, are found in great quantities in inflamed tissues, whereas they are lacking in noninflamed tissues (Stein, 1993 b). They apparently act on the peripheral receptors of the opioids, whose presence has been shown by many studies (LaMotte et al., 1976; Fields et al., 1980; Ninkovic et al., 1982; Barthò et al., 1990; Stein et al., 1990 a). These receptors might be formed as a consequence of the inflammatory stimulus, and reach the endings by axonal transport (Young et al., 1980; Laduron, 1984). Hassan et al. (1993) have observed an increase of opioid receptors of cutaneous nerve fibers in inflamed tissues. However, such increase took place after about three days, while the antinociceptive effect of exogenous opioid agonists was observed within a short period (minutes to hours): therefore, one would assume that in the inflamed tissues preexisting but inactive opiod receptors are activated (Stein, 1993, 1994). The peripheral effect of the opioids on the nerve endings appears to be doubly inhibitory: on the afferent nociceptive signals to the centre and on the release of substance P (Fig. 7.**3**).

The analgesic effect of the peripheral opioids has been demonstrated through animal studies (Ferreira and Nakumara, 1979; Ferreria et al., 1982; Stein et al., 1988 a, b, 1989; Parsons et al., 1990; Stein et al., 1990 a, b; Taiwo and Levine, 1991). This effect was confirmed in man by the demonstration of the antinociceptive action played by intra-articuar administration of morphine on postoperative pain of patients undergoing knee surgery (Stein et al., 1991; Khoury et al., 1992; Joshi et al., 1993 a, b; Allen et al., 1993; McSwiney et al., 1993; Dalsgaard et al., 1994). The origin of the immunocompetent cell opioids has also been demonstrated by the fact that the analgesic effect disappears if the immune system is blocked by the administration of cyclosporin A or by radiation (Stein et al., 1990 a; Przewlocki et al., 1992).

Moreover, it has been shown that opioid release by immunocompetent cells in the inflamed tissues may be enhanced by cytokines and the CRH (Stein, 1994) (Fig. 7.**2**). The local application of small, systemically inactive, doses of CRH, IL-1, and other cytokines produces potent antinociceptive effects in inflamed, but not in noninflamed, tissues (Czlonkowski et al., 1993). This effect is suppressed by cyclosporin A, by passive immunization with antibodies against endorphins, and by opioid receptor antagonists. Furthermore, CRH and IL-1 induce in vitro the release of endorphine in immune cell suspensions (Stein et al., 1994; Shäfer et al., 1994).

References

Allen G.C., Amand M.A.S., Lui A.C.P., Johnson D.H., Lindsay M.P., *Postarthroscopy analgesia with intra-articular bupivacaine/morphine: a randomized clinical trial*, Anesthesiology, 1993, 79 : 475 – 480.

Awaki E., Takeshima T., Takahashi K., *A neuroendocrinological study in female migraineurs: prolactin and thyroid stimulating hormone responses*, Cephalalgia, 1989, 9 : 187 – 193.

Baldi E., Branconi F., Brocchi F., et al. *Beta-endorphin-like-immunoreactivity (beta-ELI) in pregnancy*, in: Savoldi F., Nappi G. (eds.), Headache, Fidia Research Laboratories, Italy, 1979, 121 – 127.

Barthò L., Stein C., Herz A., *Involvement of capsaicin-sensitive neurones in hyperalgesia and enhanced opioid antinociception in inflammation*, Naunyn Schmiedeberg's Arch. Pharmacol., 1990, 342 : 666 – 670.

Bereiter D.A., Stanford L.R., Barker D.J., *Hormone-induced enlargement of receptive fields in trigeminal mechanoreceptive neurons. II. Possible mechanisms*, Brain Res., 1980, 184 : 411 – 423.

Blalock J.E., *A molecular basis for bidirectional communication between the immune ande neuroendocrine system*, Physiol. Rev., 1989, 69 : 1 – 32.

Blalock J.E., Smith E.M., *A complete regulatory loop between the immune and neuroendocrine systems*, Fed. Proc., 1985, 44 : 108 – 111.

Bousser M.G., Ratinahirna H., Barboix X., *Migraine and pregnancy: a prospective study in 703 women after delivery*, Nerology, 1990, 40(Suppl 1):437.

Bussone G., Leone M., Vescovi A., Peccarisi C., Grazzi L., Parati E.A., *Derangement of the hypothalamo-pituitary axis (HPa) in cluster headache: further considerations*, Cephalalgia, 1989, 9 (Suppl. 10):141.

Clarke W.P., Goldfarb J., *Estrogen enhances a 5-HT1 a response in hippocampal slices from female rats*, Eur. J. Pharmacol., 1989, 160 : 195 – 197.

Covelli V., Maffione A.B., Munno I., Jirillo E., *Alterations of non-specific immunity in patients with common migraine*, J. Clin. Lab. Anal., 1990, 4 : 9 – 15.

Csontos K., Rust M., Hollt V., Mahar W., Kromer W., Teschemacher H.J., *Elevated plasma beta-endorphin levels in pregnant women and their neonates*, Life Sci., 1979, 25 : 835 – 844.

Czlonkowski A., Stein C., Herz A., *Peripheral mechanisms of opioid antinociception in inflammation: involvement of cytokines*, Eur. J. Pharmacol., 1993, 242 : 229 – 235.

D'Agata R., *Estrogens and prolactin release in man*, in: MacLeod R.M., Scapagnini U. (eds.), *Central and peripheral regulation of prolactin function*, Raven Press, New York, 1980, 243 – 251.

Dalsgaard J., Felsby S., Juelsgaard P., Froekjaer J., *Low-dose intra-articular morphine algesia in day-case knee arthroscopy: a randomized, double-blinded, prospective study*, Pain, 1994, 56 : 151 – 154.

Davies P.T.G., Eccles J.K., Steiner T.J., Leathard H.L., Clifford Rose F., *Plasma oestrogen, progesterone and sex-hormone binding globulin levels in the pathogenesis of migraine*, Cephalalgia, 1989, 9 (Suppl. 10):143.

De Lignières B., *La migraine cataméniale*, Rev. Prat., Paris, 1990, 40 : 395 – 398.

De Lignieres B., Vincens M., Mauvais-Jarvis P., Mas J.L., Touboul P.J., Bousser M.G., *Prevention of menstrual migraine by percutaneous oestradiol*, British Medical Journal Clinical Research Ed., 1986, 293 : 1540.

Dennerstein L., Morse C., Burrows G., Oats J., Brown J., Smith M., *Menstrual migraine: a double-blind trial of percutaneous estradiol*, Gynecol. Endocrinol., 1988, 2 : 113 – 120.

Edelson R.N., *Menstrual migraine and other hormonal aspects of migraine*, Headache, 1985, 25 : 376 – 379.

Epstein M.T., Hockaday J.M., Hockaday T.D.R., *Migraine and reproductive hormones throughout the menstrual cycle*, Lancet, 1975, i:543 – 548.

Facchinetti F., Sances G., Volpe A. et al., *Hypothalamus pituitary-ovarian axis in menstrual migraine: effects of dihydroergotamine retard prophylactic treatment*, Cephalalgia, 1983 a, (Suppl. 1):159 – 162.

Facchinetti F., Nappi G., Petraglia F., Volpe A., Genazzani A.R., *Oestradiol/progesterone inbalance and the premenstrual syndrome*, Lancet, 1983 b, ii:1302.

Facchinetti F., Nappi G., Cicoli C. et al., *Reduced testosterone levels in cluster headache: a stress-related phenomenon?* Cephalalgia, 1986, 6 : 29 – 34.

Fagarasan M.O., Eskay R., Axelrod J., *Interleukin-1 potentiates the secretion of ß-endorphin induced by secretagogues in a mouse pituitary cell line (AtT-20)*, Proc. Natl. Acad. Sci., 1989, USA, 86 : 2070 – 2075.

Ferreira S.H., Nakamura M., *Prostaglandin hyperalgesia II: the peripheral analgesic activity of morphine, enkephalins and opioid antagonists*, Prostaglandins, 1979, 18 : 191 – 200.

Ferreira S.H., Molina N., Vettore O., *Prostaglandin hyperalgesia, V: a peripheral analgesic receptor for opiates*, Prostaglandins, 1982, 23 : 53 – 60.

Ferrero M.E., *Interazioni tra sistema neuroendocrino e sistema immunitario (neuroendocrinoimmunomodulazione)*, in: Tiengo M., Benedetti C. (eds.), *Fisiopatologia e terapia del dolore*, Masson, Paris, 1996, 173 – 180.

Fields H.L., Emson P.C., Leigh B.K. et al., *Multiple opiate receptor sites on primary afferent fibres*, Nature, 1980, 284 : 351 – 353.

Fioroni L., Martignoni E., Facchinetti F., *Changes of neuroendocrine axes in patients with menstrual migraine*, Cephalalgia, 1995, 15 : 297 – 300.

Franceschini R., Leandri M., Cataldi A., et al. *Raised plasma arginine vasopressin concentrations during cluster headache attacks*, J. Neurol. Neurosurg. Psychiatry, 1995, 59 : 381 – 383.

Gallai V., Sarchielli P., Trequattrini A., Paciaroni M., *Monocyte chemotactic and phagocytic responses in migraine and tension-type headache patients*, Ital. J. Neurol. Sci., 1993, 14 : 153 – 164.

Giacovazzo M., Bernoni R.M., Di Sabato F., Martelletti P., *Impairment of 5 TH binding to lymphocytes and monocytes from tension-type headache patients*, Headache, 1990, 30 : 220 – 223.

Gintzler A.R., *Endorphin-mediated increases in pain threshold during pregnancy*, Science, 1980, 210 : 193 – 195.

Goadsby P.J., Lance J.W., *Physiopathology of migraine*, Revue Du Praticien, 1990, 40 : 389 – 393.

Gray L.A., *The use of progesterone in nervous tension states*, South Med. J., 1941, 34 : 1004.

Guicheney P., Leger D., Barrat J., et al. *Platelet serotonin content and plasma tryptophan in peri- and postmenopausal women: variations with plasma oestrogen levels and depressive symptoms*, Eur. J. Clin. Invest., 1988, 18 : 297 – 304.

Hassan A.H.S., Ableitner A., Stein C., Herz A., *Inflammation of the rat paw enhances axonal transport of opioid receptors in the sciatic nerve and increases their density in the inflamed tissue*, Neuroscience, 1993, 55 : 185 – 195.

Heijnen C.J., Kavelaars A., Ballieux R.E., *ß-endorphin: cytokine and neuropeptide*, Immunol. Rev., 1991, 119 : 41 – 63.

Heritage A.S., Stumpf W.E., Sar M., Grant L., *Brainstem catecholamine neurons are target sites for sex steroid hormones*, Science, 1980, 207 : 1377 – 1379.

Joshi G.P., McCarroll S.M., Brady O.H., Hurson B.J., Walsh G., *Intra-articular morphine for pain relief after anterior cruciate ligament repair*, Br. J. Anaesth., 1993 a, 70 : 87 – 88.

Joshi G.P., McCarroll S.M., O'Brien T.M., Lenane P., *Intraarticular analgesia following knee arthroscopy*, Anesth. Analg., 1993 b, 76 : 333 – 336.

Khoury G.F., Chen A.C.N., Garland D.E., Stein C., *Intraarticular morphine, bupivacaine, and morphine/bupivacaine for pain control after knee videoarthroscopy*, Anesthesiology, 1992, 77 : 263 – 266.

Kilpatrick D.L., *Opioid peptide expression in peripheral tissues and its functional implications*, in: Herz A. (ed.), *Handbook of experimental pharmacology*, vol. 104/II, *Opioids II*, Springer Verlag, Berlin, 1993, 551 – 570.

Klimek A., *Plasma testosterone levels in patients with cluster headache*, Headache, 1982, 22 : 162 – 164.

Klimek A., *Use of testosterone in the treatment of cluster headache*, Eur. Neurol., 1985, 24 : 53 – 56.

Krieger D.T., Martin J.B., *Brain peptides*, N. Engl. J. Med., 1981, 304 : 876 – 885.

Kudrow L., *Plasma testosterone and LH levels in cluster headache*, Headache, 1977, 17 : 91 – 92.

Laduron P., *Axonal transport of opiate receptors in capsaicin sensitive neurones*, Brain Res., 1984, 294 : 157 – 160.

LaMotte C., Pert C.B., Snyder S.H., *Opiate receptor binding in primate spinal cord: distribution and changes after dorsal root section*, Brain Res., 1976, 112 : 407 – 412.

Lundberg P.O., *Migraine prophylaxis with progestogens*, Acta Endocrinol., 1962, 68 (Suppl. 1).

Marcus D.A., *Interrelationships of neurochemicals, estrogen, and recurring headache*, Pain, 1995, 62 : 129 – 139.

Martelletti P., Alteri E., Pesce A., Rinaldi-Garaci C., Giacovazzo M., *Defect of serotonin binding to mononuclear cells from episodic cluster headache patients*, Headache, 1987 a, 27 : 23 – 26.

Martelletti P., Stirparo G., De Stefano L., Bonmassar E., Giacovazzo M., *Reduced activity of the NK cells from patients with cluster headache and the "in vitro" response to beta-IFN*, Headache, 1987 b, 27 : 548 – 551.

Martelletti P., Alteri E., Pesce A. et al., *In vitro interactions of serotonin (5 TH) with mononuclear cells from migraine patients: alterations related to the phase of the attack*, J. Neuroimmunol., 1988, 18 : 17 – 24.

Martelletti P., Granata M., Rordorf-Adam C., Giacovazzo M., *Lymphokines pattern in cluster headache* (abs.), Proc. 9 th Migraine Trust International Symposium, London, 1992, 56.

Martignoni E., Sances G., Nappi G., *Significance of hormonal changes in migraine and cluster headache*, Gynecol. Endrocrinol., 1987, 1 : 295 – 319.

McEwen B.S., Coirini H., Westlind-Danielsson A., et al. *Steroid hormones as mediators of neural plasticity*, J. Steroid Biochem. Mol. Biol., 1991, 39 : 223 – 232.

McSwiney M.M., Joshi G.P., Kenny P., McCarroll S.M., *Analgesia following arthroscopic knee surgery a controlled study of intra-articular morphine, bupivacaine or both combined*, Anaesth. Intens. Care, 1993, 21 : 201 – 203.

Micieli G., Facchinetti F., Martignoni E., Bono G., Genazzari A.R., Nappi G., *Lowered and phase-delayed 24-h levels of circulating testosterone in cluster headache*, Proc. IId Int. Headache, Congress, Copenhaghen, 1985, 364 – 365.

Micieli G., Facchinetti F., Martignoni E., Manzoni G.C., Cleva M., Nappi G., *Disordered pulsatile LH release in cluster headache*, Cephalalgia, 1987, 7 (Suppl. 6): 79 – 81.

Murialdo G., Fanciullacci M., Nicolodi M., et al. *Cluster headache in the male: sex steroid pattern and gonadotropic response to luteinizing hormone releasing hormone*, Cephalalgia, 1989, 9 : 91 – 98.

Nagel-Leiby S., Welch K.A., Grunfeld S., D'Andrea G., *Ovarian steroid levels in migraine with and without aura*, Cephalalgia, 1990, 10 : 147 – 152.

Nappi G., Martignoni E., Bono G., Savoldi F., Murialdo G., Polleri A., *THDA system function in migraine*, in: Clifford Rose F., Zilkha K.J. (eds.), *Progress in migraine research*, Pitman-Medical, London, 1981, 110 – 123.

Nattero G., *Menstrual headache*, Adv. Neurol., 1982, 33 : 215 – 226.

Nattero G., Corno M., Savi L., Isaia G.C., Priolo C., Mussetta M., *Prolactin and migraine: effect of L-dopa on plasma prolactin levels in migraineurs and normals*, Headache, 1986, 26 : 9 – 12.

Nelson R.F., *Testosterone levels in cluster and noncluster migrainous headache patients*, Headache, 1978, 18 : 265 – 267.

Neri I., Granella F., Nappi R., Manzoni G.C., Facchinetti F., Genazzani A.Z., *Characteristics of headache at menopause: a clinico-epidemiologic study*, Maturitas, 1993, 17 : 31 – 37.

Ninkovic M., Hunt S.P., Gleave J.R.W., *Localization of opiate and histamine H1-receptors in the primary sensory ganglia and spinal cord*, Brain Res., 1982, 241 : 197 – 206.

Parsons C.G., Czlonkowski A., Stein C., Herz A., *Peripheral opioid receptors mediating antinociception in inflammation. Activation by endogenous opioids and role of the pituitary-adrenal axis*, Pain, 1990, 41 : 81 – 93.

Petraglia F., Penalva A., Locatelli V. et al., *Effect of gonadectomy and gonadal steroid replacement on pituitary and plasma beta-endorphin levels in the rat*, Endocrinology, 1982, 111 : 1224 – 1229.

Pinsky C., Koven S.J., Labella F.S., *Evidence for the role of endogenous sex steroids in morphine antinociception*, Life Sci., 1975, 16 : 1785 – 1786.

Polleri A., Nappi G., Murialdo G., Bono G., Martignoni E., Savoldi F., *Changes of the 24-h prolactin pattern in cluster headache*, Cephalalgia, 1982, 2 : 1 – 7.

Polleri A., Nappi G., Murialdo G., et al. *THDA neuron impairment and estrogen receptor modulation in headache*, in: Clifford Rose R. (ed.), *Progress in migraine research*, vol. 2, Pitman, London, 1984, 205 – 214.

Przewlocki R., Hassan A.H.S., Lason W., Epplen C., Herz A., Stein C., *Gene expression and localization of opioid peptides in immune cells of inflamed tissue: functional role in antinociception*, Neuroscience, 1992, 48 : 491 – 500.

Quingley M.E., Yen S.S.C., *The role of endogenous opiates on LH secretion during the menstrual cycle*, J. Clin. Endocrinol. Metab., 1980, 51 : 179.

Rose R.M., *Overview of endocrinology of stress*, in: Brown G.M. Koslow S.H., Reiclin S. (eds.), *Neuro-endocrinology and psychiatric disorders*, Raven Press, New York, 1984, 95 – 122.

Sacerdote P., Rubboli F., Locatelli L., Ciciliato I., Mantegazza P., Panerai, A.E., *Pharmacological modulation of neuropeptides in peripheral mononuclear cells*, J. Neuroimmunol., 1991, 32 : 35 – 41.

Schäfer M., Carter L., Stein C., *Interleukin-b and corticotropin-releasing-factor inhibit pain by releasing opioids from immune cells in inflamed tissue*, Proc. Natl. Acad. Sci. USA, 1994, 91.

Segarra A.C., McEwen B.S., *Estrogen increases spine density in ventromedial hypothalamic neurons of peripubertal rats*, Neuroendocrinology, 1991, 54 : 365 – 372.

Shoupe D., Montz F.J., Lobo R.A., *The effects of estrogen and progestin on endogenous opioid activity in oophorectomized women*, J. Clin. Endocrinol. Metab., 1985, 60 : 178 – 183.

Sibinga N.E.S., Goldstein A., *Opioid peptides and opioid receptors in cells of the immune system*, Annu. Rev. Immunol., 1988, 6 : 219 – 249.

Sicuteri F., Poggioni M., Nicolodi M., Marabini S., Del Bene E., *Sex-pain circuitry in cluster headache*, in: Genazzari A.R., Nappi G., Facchinetti F., Martignoni E. (eds.), *Pain and reproduction*, Parthenon, Park Ridge, N.J., 1989, 155 – 161.

Silberstein S.D., *Sex hormones and headache (1995)*, Towards Migraine 2000, Clifford Rose F. (ed.), Elsevier, Amsterdam, 1996, 201 – 209.

Silberstein S.D., Merriam G.M., *Estrogens, progestins, and headache*, Neurology, 1991, 41 : 786 – 793.

Singh et al., *Progesterone in migraine*, Lancet, 1947, 1 : 745.

Sohrabji F., Miranda R.C., Toran-Allerand C.D., *Estrogen differentially regulates estrogen and nerve growth factor receptor mRNAs in adult sensory neurons*, J. Neurosci., 1994, 14 : 459 – 471.

Somerville B.W., *The role of progesterone in menstrual migraine*, Neurology, 1971, 21 : 853 – 859.

Somerville B.W., *A study of migraine in pregnancy*, Neurology, 1972 a, 22 : 824.

Somerville B.W., *The role of estradiol withdrawal in the etiology of menstrual migraine*, Neurology, 1972 b, 22 : 355.

Somerville B.W., *Estrogen-withdrawal migraine. I. Duration of exposure required and attempted prophylaxis by premenstrual estrogen administration*, Neurology, 1975 a, 25 : 239 – 244.

Somerville B.W., *Estrogen-withdrawal migraine. II. Attempted prophylaxis by continuous estradiol administration*, Neurology, 1975 b, 25 : 245 – 250.

Stein C., *Peripheral mechanisms of opioid analgesia*, Anesth. Analg., 1993 a, 76 : 182 – 191.

Stein C., *Interaction of immune-competent cells and nociceptors*, 7 th World Congress on Pain, IASP Publications, Seattle, 1993 b, 129 (abs.).

Stein C., *Interaction of immune-competent cells and nociceptors*, in: Gebhart G.F., Hammond D.L., Jensen T.S., Proceedings of the 7 th World Congress on Pain, Progress in Pain Research and Management, vol. 2, IASP Press, Seattle, 1994, 285 – 297.

Stein C., Millan M.J., Shippenberg T.S., Herz A., *Peripheral effect of fentanyl upon nociception in inflamed tissue of the rat*, Neurosci. Lett., 1988 a, 84 : 225 – 228.

Stein C., Millan M.J., Yassouridis A., Herz A., *Antinociceptive effects of mu- and kappa-agonists in inflammation are enhanced by a peripheral opioid receptor-specific mechanisms of action*, Euro.J. Pharmacol., 1988 b, 155 : 225 – 264.

Stein C., Millan M.J., Shippenberg T.S. et al., *Peripheral opioid receptors mediating antinociception in inflammation. Evidence for involvement f mu, delta and kappa receptors*, J. Pharmacol. Exp. Ther., 1989, 248 : 1269 – 1275.

Stein C., Hassan A.H.S., Przewlocki R. et al., *Opioids from immunocytes interact with receptors on sensory nerves to inhibit nociception in inflammation*, Proc. Natl. Acad. Sci., USA, 1990, 87 : 5935 – 5939.

Stein C., Gramsch, C., Herz A., *Intrinsic mechanisms of antinociception in inflammation. Local opioid receptors and ß-endorphin*, J. Neurosci., 1990 a, 10 : 1292 – 1298.

Stein C., Gramsch C., Herz A., *Intrinsic mechanisms of antinociception in inflammation. Local opioid receptors and ß-endorphin*, J. Neurosci., 1990 b, 10 : 1292 – 1298.

Stein C., Comisel K., Haimerl E. et al., *Analgesic effect of intraarticular morphine after arthroscopic knee surgery*, N. Engl. J. Med., 1991, 325 : 1123 – 1126.

Stein C., Hassan A.H.S., Lehrberger K., Giefing J., Yassouridis A., *Local analgesic effect of endogenous opioid peptides*, Lancet, 342 : 321 – 324, 1993. Comment in: Lancet, 1993, 342 : 320.

Stein C., Schäfer M., Carter L., Czlonkowski A., Mousa S., Epplen C., *Cytokine-induced antinociception mediated by opioids released from immune cells*, Regul. Pept., 1994, 50:S191-S192.

Stirparo G., Martelletti P., Morrone S., Savares A., Giacovazzo M., *Impaired natural killer activity in PBLs from cluster headache patients is restored by interleukin 2*, Int. J., Immunother., 1990, 6 : 181 – 186.

Taiwo Y.O., Levine J.D., *Kappa- and delta-opioids block sympathetically dependent hyperalgesia*, J. Neurosci., 1991, 11 : 928 – 932.

Theoharides T.C., Spanos C., Pang X., et al. *Stress-induced intracranial mast cell degranulation: a corticotropin-releasing hormone-mediated effect*, Endocrinology, 1995, 136 : 5745 – 5750.

Uknis A., Silbersein S.D., *Migraine and pregnancy*, Headache, 1991, 31 : 372 – 374.

Van Vugt D.A., Vaughn L., Wardlaw S.L., Frantz A.G., Ferin M., *Naloxone's ability to stimulate luteinizing hormone release in the monkey parallels ß-endorphin concentrations in hypophyseal portal blood*, Proc. 64 th Annual Meeting of The Endocrine Society, San Francisco, 1982, (abs.).

Van Woudenberg A.D., Hol. E.M., Wiegant V.M., *Endorphin-like immunoreactivities in uncultured and cultured human peripheral blood mononuclear cells*, Life Sci., 1992, 50 : 705 – 714.

Waldenling E., Gustafsson S.A. Ekbom K.A., Wetterberger L., *Circadian secretion of cortisol and melatonin during active cluster periods and remission*, J. Neurol. Neurosur. Psychiatry., 1987, 50 : 207 – 213.

Watkins L.R. et al., *Pain and the immune system*, Proc. 8 th World Congress. on Pain, IASP Press, 1996, Seattle, 202.

Watkins L.R., Goehler L.E., Relton J., Brewer M.T., Maier S.F., *Mechanisms of tumor necrosis factor-alpha (TNF-alpha) hyperalgesia*, Brain-Res. 1995, 692 : 244 – 250.

Wehrenberg W.B., Wardlaw S.L., Frantz A.G., Ferin M., *Beta-endorphin in hypophyseal portal blood: variations throughout the menstrual cycle*, Endocrinology, 1982, 111 : 879 – 881.

Weigent D.A., Blalock J.E., *Interaction between the neuroendocrine and immune systems: common hormones and receptors*, Immunol. Rev., 1987, 100 : 79 – 87.

Welch K.M.A., Darnely D., Simkins R.T., *The role of estrogen in migraine: a review and hypothesis*, Cephalalgia, 1984, 4 : 227 – 236.

Welch K.M.A., *Migraine and ovarian steroid hormones*, Cephalalgia, 1997, 17(Suppl 20):12 – 16.

Woolley C.S., McEwen B.S., *Estradiol mediates fluctuation in hippocampal synapse density during the estrous cycle in the adult rat*, J. Neurosci., 1992, 12 : 2549 – 2554.

Young III W.S., Wamsley J.K., Zarbin M.A., Kuhar M.J., *Opioid receptors undergo axonal flow*, Science, 1980, 210 : 76 – 77.

8 Psychological Factors

Personality Alterations and Pain

The association between personality changes and chronic pain is well accepted (Sternbach et al., 1973; Schaffer et al., 1980; Blumer and Heilbronn, 1982; Pelz and Merskey, 1982; Reich et al., 1983; France et al., 1984; Dworkin et al., 1985; Katon et al., 1985; Krishnan et al., 1985; Fishbain et al., 1986; Benjamin et al., 1988; Wade et al., 1990; Sullivan et al., 1992). By the use of various psychometric tests, such as the Minnesota Multiphasic Personality Inventory (MMPI), the Hamilton test, the Eysenk Personality Inventory, the Beck depression test, the State-Trait Anxiety Inventory (STAI), and others, depression and anxiety have in general been found to be more elevated in chronic pain populations than in healthy controls (Krishnan et al., 1985; Fishbain et al., 1986; Benjamin et al., 1988; Wade et al., 1990; Mongini et al., 1992; Magni et al., 1994; Rajala et al., 1995; Casten et al., 1995; Smedstad et al., 1995; Ben Debba et al., 1997; Ciccone et al., 1997) (Fig. 8.1). The question whether such personality disorders predispose to pain is still debated, however (Yunus et al., 1991; Ellertsen et al., 1991, 1993; Ellertsen, 1992).

In patients suffering from headache or facial pain, the first question is whether mood or personology disorders, when present, represent a peculiar characteristic of these patients or whether such disorders are simply a consequence of chronic pain. Furthermore, if a relation between head pain and mood or personality disorders exists, the question is whether such relation is unidirectional or bidirectional, that is, whether (1) mood or personality disorders may cause or predispose to headache and facial pain; (2) mood or personality disorders are a consequence of headache and facial pain; or (3) both hypotheses are correct.

Characteristic mood or personality alterations have been reported quite extensively in patients with craniofacial pain and/or headache (Alvarez, 1947; Henryk-Gutt and Ress, 1973; Harrison, 1975; Philips, 1976; Kudrow and Sutkus, 1979;

Schnarch and Hunter, 1979; Sternbach et al., 1980; Cuypers et al., 1981; Dalessio, 1981; Andrasik et al., 1982 a, b; De Domini et al., 1983; Weeks et al., 1983; Eversole et al., 1985; Remick and Blasberg, 1985; Baile and Myers, 1986; Collet et al., 1986; Ellertsen and Klöve, 1987; Ellertsen et al., 1987; Merikangas et al., 1988; Invernizzi et al., 1989; Marchesi et al., 1989; Steward et al., 1989; Brandt et al., 1990; Breslau et al., 1991, 1994; Rasmussen, 1992; Mongini et al., 1992; Keck et al., 1994; Schafer, 1994; Marazziti et al., 1995; Mongini et al., 1997 a, b, c). These findings were also confirmed in children and adolescents (Bille, 1962; Guidetti et al., 1987; Cunningham et al., 1987; Larsson, 1988; Tamminen et al., 1991; Müller et al., 1993).

However, while some authors (Alvarez, 1947; Kudrow and Sutkus, 1979; Andrasik et al., 1982 a; Invernizzi et al., 1989; Brandt et al., 1990; Henry, 1990; Kurman et al., 1991; Puca et al., 1991; Merikangas et al., 1993) maintain that such changes predispose to some types of pain, others (Ellertsen and Klöve, 1987; Ellertsen et al., 1987; Blanchard et al., 1989; Marchesi et al., 1989; Pfaffenrath et al., 1991) reject this hypothesis and believe that psychopathology is rather a consequence of headache or facial pain.

In the majority of investigations concerning migraine, a relation was found between this pathology and mood or personality disorders (see Silberstein et al., 1995, for a review). Using the MMPI in migraine patients, some authors found normal profiles or, at least, a lower scale elevation than in patients with chronic tension-type headache or with migraine and tension type headache superimposed (Kudrow and Sutkus 1979; Andrasik et al., 1982 a, b; De Domini et al., 1983). In contrast, other authors found a marked elevation of several MMPI scales and, in women migraine patients, a typical V configuration of the neurotic triad of the MMPI (with high scores of hypochondria and hysteria, and depression score still high but lower than those of the two other scales) (Ellertsen and Klöve, 1987). Using the Eysenck Personality Questionnaire, higher scores of psychoticism were found (Brandt et atl., 1990). In epidemiological studies, an association was found between migraine and panic attacks (Steward et al., 1989) and between migraine and depression and anxiety or personality disorders (Merikangas et al., 1988; Brandt et al., 1990; Breslau et al., 1991; Rasmussen, 1992; Merikangas et al., 1993; Merikangas, 1994; Breslau and Andreski, 1995). This was confirmed by prospective studies (Merikangas et al., 1990; Breslau and Davis, 1992, Breslau et al., 1994). Mongini et al. in a recent study (1997 a, b) in which 43 women with migraine were examined with MMPI, STAI and history including a checklist of psychosomatic symptoms, found a general elevation of several MMPI scales and STAI scores. According to the different MMPI profiles obtained, the patients could be divided into four different groups: one group had an elevation of the three scales of the neurotic triad (and of depression in particular) and of psychasthenia (indicating anxiety); a second group showed a "conversive V" or "hysterical" configuration of the neurotic triad; a third group ("emotionally overwhelmed") had an elevation of the scales of the neurotic triad and of others relative to psychoticism (paranoia, schizophrenia, mania); and a fourth group had a

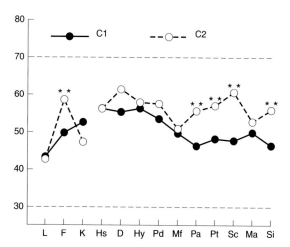

Fig. 8.**1** **MMPI profile of a group of healthy subjects (C1) and of a group of subjects suffering from chronic noncraniofacial pain (C2).** In the patients with pain, the values of numerous scales are elevated. (From Mongini et al., 1992, with modifications). **, P < 0.01.

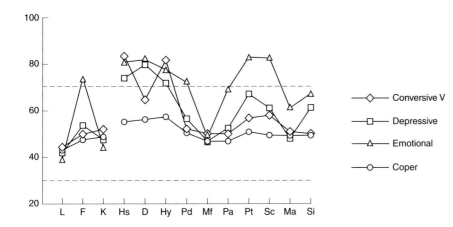

Fig. 8.**2**   The four personality profiles observed with the MMPI in women suffering from migraine. (From Mongini et al., 1997 a)

Table 8.**1**   **Percentage values of prevalence of different symptoms in women with migraine and different personology profiles at the MMPI** (see Fig. 8.**2**). The group with normal personality profile shows the lowest prevalence.

%	Lassitude	Mood changes	Paresthesias	Limb pain	Vertigo	Palpitation	Nail fragility	Menstrual disorders
Conversive V	80	80	80	80	80	90	80	50
Depressive	90	90	70	40	70	100	20	40
Emotional	82	73	55	18	45	64	36	27
Coper	31	38	19	13	19	25	31	0
P =	0.004	0.024	0.009	0.003	0.009	3×10^{-4}	0.031	0.021

normal configuration (the "copers") (Fig. 8.**2**). The majority of the patients had several symptoms, predominantly psychosomatic in nature: however, these symptoms were less prevalent in the group with normal MMPI configuration (Table 8.**1**). Data from a longitudinal study (Breslau et al., 1994) support the hypothesis that the relation between migraine and depression is bidirectional.

Chronic tension-type headache, alone or in conjunction with migraine, is often accompanied by alterations of mood (Kudrow et al., 1979; Sternbach et al., 1980; Andrasik et al., 1982 b; Ellertsen et al., 1987; Blanchard et al., 1989; Mongini et al., 1992, 1994, 1997 b).

This association is even more pronounced in chronic daily headache (CDH), that is for headache present all day or most

of the day, at least six days a week and for at least six months (Langemark et al., 1988; Solomon et al., 1992; Silberstein, 1993). Mongini et al. (1997 b, c) used the MMPI to examine patients with CDH and found that approximately one-third of the patients had a characteristic "conversive V" or "hysterical" configuration while the rest of the patients had elevation of all three neurotic scales (and depression in particular) and of psychasthenia (Fig. 8.**3**). STAI scores were higher in the latter patients, in whom headache chronicity was also higher. Almost all patients had numerous psychosomatic symptoms (Fig. 8.**4**).

Patients with facial pain disorder (so-called *atypical facial pain*) (see Chapter 1) are those in whom the coexistence of the pathology with distinct personality changes seems least de-

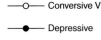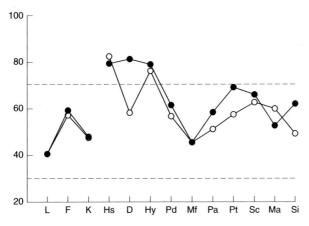

Fig. 8.**3**   The two personality profiles observed with the MMPI in patients with chronic daily headache. (From Mongini et al., 1997 c)

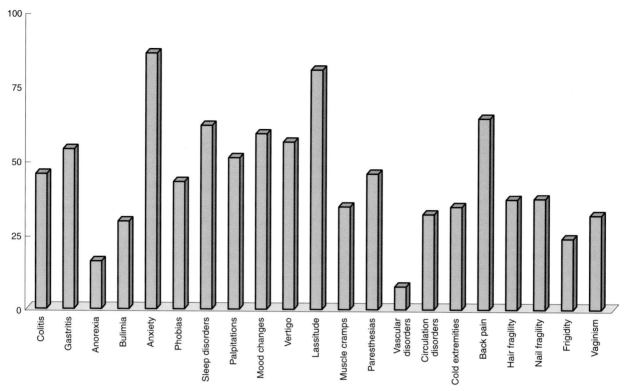

Fig. 8.**4**   Percentage values of prevalence of different symptoms in 37 patients with chronic daily headache. (From Mongini et al., 1997 d)

batable (Sternbach et al., 1973; Eversole et al., 1985; Remick and Blasberg, 1985; Baile and Myers, 1986; Mongini et al., 1992; Brooke and Merskey, 1994). Pain in such patients is usually constant or persistent for most of the day, and is troublesome or poorly defined. At onset, it can be confined to a limited area of the maxilla or the mandible, but it may then spread to a wider area of the face and neck. It is not confined to the distribution of a cranial or cervical nerve root, and no structural source of pain can be identified.

In research using the MMPI to assess personality profiles in patients with different types of headache or facial pain, Mongini et al. (1992) found that the group with facial pain disorder had many scales significantly higher than other groups (Fig. 8.**5**). This finding was independent of the level of pain. Moreover, this was the only group in which all three "neurotic" scales – hypochondria, depression and hysteria – scored

above 70 (clearly above normal values), depression being slightly lower than the other two scales (Fig. 8.**5**).

Thus, a tendency to the already mentioned *hysterical or conversive V configuration* was observed, although in its typical pattern this configuration has the depression score 10 or more points below hypochondria and hysteria scores. Interestingly, a similar tendency to this configuration was also found, as already mentioned, in migraine and CDH, and also in other chronic pain pathologies, such as primary fibromyalgia, in which the psychological factor seems to play an important role (Payne et al., 1982; Ahles et al., 1984; Wolfe et al., 1984; Turk and Flor, 1989; Yunus et al., 1991; Ellertsen et al., 1991, 1993; Magni et al., 1994) (see Chapter 3).

A relation between temporomandibular joint (TMJ) dysfunction and personality changes has also been postulated (Rydd, 1959; Laskin, 1969; Greene, 1979). Indeed, as we have

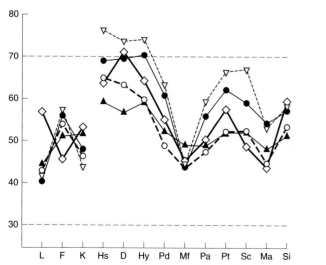

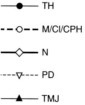

Fig. 8.**5   MMPI profile of subjects with various types of craniofacial pain.** (TH = tension-type headache; M = migraine; Cl = cluster headache; CPH = chronic paroxical hemicrania; N = trigeminal neuralgia; PD = facial pain disorder; TMJ = TMJ dysfunction). The patients with facial pain disorder show a clear elevation of the three neurotic scales (From Mongini et al., 1992, with modifications)

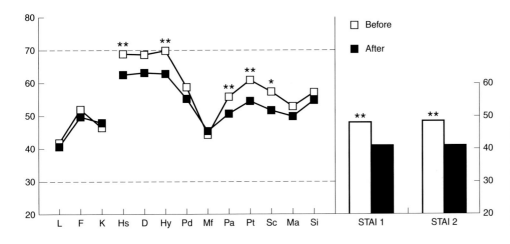

Fig. 8.**6** **MMPI profiles and STAI1 and STAI2 values in a group of patients suffering from headache and/or craniofacial pain.** After treatment, there is an improvement of the personality profile. *, P < 0.016, **, P < 0.001. (From Mongini et al., 1994)

seen (Chapter 1) it is misleading to give a single definition (such as *craniomandibular disorders* or similar terms) to a group of pathologies characterized by chronic or recurrent craniofacial pain that also extends to the preauricular area. Moreover, TMJ disorders may coexist with muscle pain and/or headache (Mongini et al., 1988; Mongini, 1990). Patients with true TMJ intracapsular disorders do not usually show statistically significant personality changes (McCreary et al., 1991; Mongini et al., 1992) (Fig. 8.**5**).

Personality Profiles and Treatment Outcome

The question whether headache and facial pain are associated with mood or personality disorders is related to two additional questions: (1) whether personality profiles before treatment might predict treatment outcome, and (2) whether treatment outcome is proportionally accompanied by an improvement of the personality profile of the patient.

In the first core, some authors (Soto Werder et al., 1981) found that, in headache patients, an elevation of the depression and anxiety scales correlated positively with the biofeedback treatment outcome. However, other authors applying the MMPI conclude that MMPI findings before treatment have no prognostic value of treatment outcome in patients with migraine (Ellertsen et al., 1987; Mongini et al., 1997a) or with different types of headache or facial pain (Mongini et al., 1994, 1997c).

Concerning the second issue, most authors found an improvement of personology profile in headache patients after treatment (Cox and Thomas, 1981; Sovak et al., 1981; Passchier et al., 1985; Blanchard et al., 1986; Ellertsen et al., 1987; Grazzi et al., 1988; Blanchard et al., 1991; Mongini et al., 1994, 1997c). However, this improvement varies conspicuously in the different series, also depending on the pain pathology involved. Mongini et al. (1994) administered MMPI and STAI before and after treatment to 96 patients suffering from different types of headache or craniofacial pain, comparing the data obtained with those concerning improvement in pain after treatment. These authors found a significant reduction in the whole group, after treatment, of numerous MMPI scores (Hs, D, Hy, Pd, Pt, Sc, Si) and of STAI 1 and 2 scores (Fig. 8.**6**). Separate analysis confirmed this trend among women but not among men (Figs. 8.**7**, 8.**8**). Profile improvement was more marked in patients suffering from tension-type headache than in those with migraine or facial pain disorder as somatoform disorder (Figs. 8.**9**, 8.**10**). No relation was found between MMPI and STAI changes before and after treatment and the degree of improvement.

In CDH, the improvement of the personality is related to its characteristics before treatment. In the work above mentioned, Mongini et al. (1997c) found a decrease of several MMPI scales after treatment in CDH patients (Figs. 8.**11**, 8.**12**). However, patients with a conversive V configuration before treatment still showed this configuration after treatment, though at a lower level (Fig. 8.**11**), while several patients with a depressive MMPI profile showed a conversion V after treatment (Fig. 8.**13**). It therefore seems that hysterical traits may be typical of these patients and that they may develop a depressive disorder while headache becomes chronic.

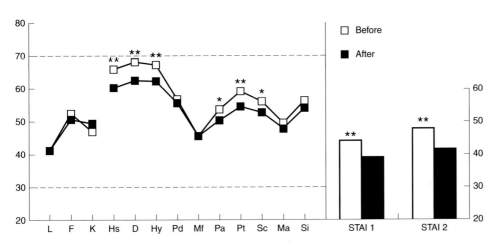

Fig. 8.**7** The group of women with headache and/or craniofacial pain confirms the improvement of the MMPI profile *, P < 0.016; **, P < 0.01. (From Mongini et al., 1994) with modifications)

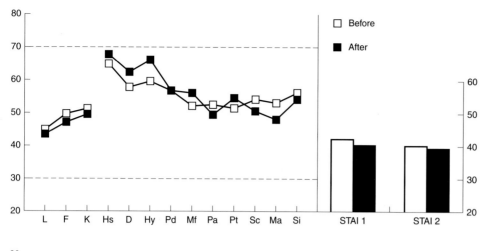

Fig. 8.**8** Improvement of the MMPI profile after therapy is not confirmed in the group of men. (From Mongini et al., 1994)

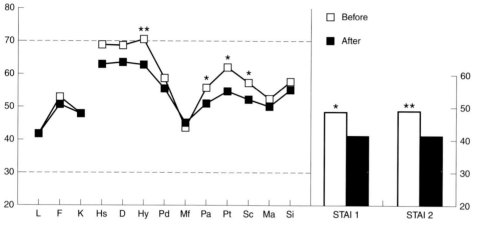

Fig. 8.**9 MMPI profiles and STAI1 and STAI2 values in a group of patients suffering from tension-type haedache.** After treatment, there is a clear improvement of the personality profile. *, P < 0.016; **, P < 0.01. (From Mongini et al., 1994)

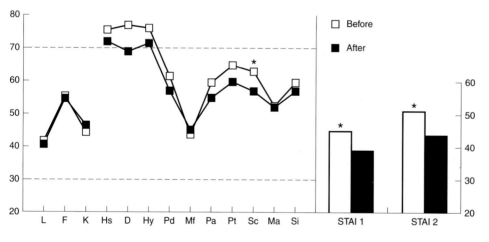

Fig. 8.**10 MMPI profiles and STAI1 and STAI2 values in a group of patients suffering from facial pain disorder.** After treatment, there is a scarce improvement of the personality profile. *, P < 0.016. (From Mongini et al., 1994)

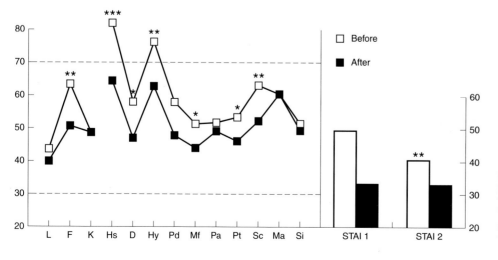

Fig. 8.**11 Patients suffering from chronic daily headache and showing a "hysterical profile" at the MMPI before treatment.** MMPI profiles and STAI1 and STAI2 values before and after treatment are given. After treatment, there is a general and significant decrease of almost all MMPI scales. Nervertheless, the personality profile remains "hysterical" in character. *, P < 0.05; **, P < 0.01; ***, P < 0.001. (From Mongini et al., 1997 c, with modifications)

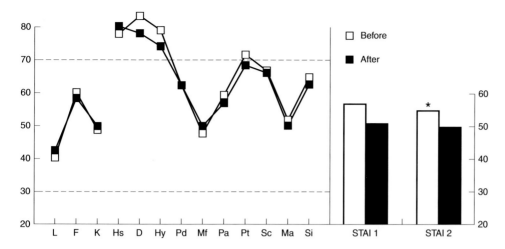

Fig. 8.**12** **Patients suffering from chronic daily headache and showing a "depressive profile" at the MMPI before treatment.** MMPI profiles and STAI1 and STAI2 values before and after treatment are given. After treatment, there is a limited nonsignificant decrease of some MMPI scales. (From Mongini et al., 1997 c, with modifications)

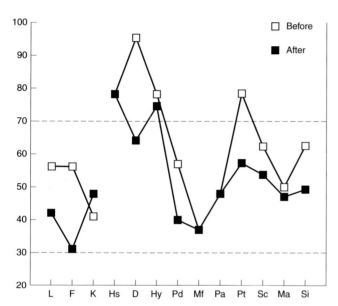

Fig. 8.**13** **Patient suffering from chronic daily headache and showing a "depressive profile" at the MMPI before treatment.** After treatment a "hysterical profile" is observed

The question remains open whether these changes are consequences of symptom improvement or a third variable.

Ellertsen et al. (1987) applied the MMPI test to migraine patients treated with biofeedback, and separated the patients into two subgroups: those who showed most and least improvement. These two groups showed strikingly similar profiles before treatment. However, after treatment, the group that had responded best to therapy, compared to the group that had responded poorly, showed a significant decrease in the values of numerous MMPI scales. In contrast, Blanchard et al. (1986, 1991) found, after treatment, an improvement of the psychological profile of headache patients independent of the treatment outcome. Finally, Mongini et al., in the works mentioned above (1994, 1997 c), did not find any statistical relation between changes in MMPI and STAI before and after treatment and the degree of clinical improvement.

References

Ahles T.A., Yunus M.B., Riley S.D., Bradley J.M., Masi A.T., *Psychological factors associated with primary fibromyalgia syndrome*, Arthritis Rheum., 1984, 27 : 1101 – 1106.

Alvarez W.C., *The migrainous personality and constitution. The essential features of the disease: a study of 500 cases*, Am. J. Med. Sci., 1947, 213 : 1 – 8.

Andrasik F., Blanchard E.B., Arena J.G., Teders S.J., Rodichok L.D., *Cross-validation of the Kudrow-Sutkus MMPI classification system for diagnosis headache type*, Headache, 1982 a, 22 : 2 – 5.

Andrasik F., Blanchard E.B., Arena J.G., et al., *Psychological functioning in headache sufferers*, Psychosom. Med., 1982 b, 44 : 171 – 182.

Baile W.F., Myers D., *Psychological and behavioural dynamics in chronic atypical facial pain*, Anesth. Prog.: 1986, 252 – 257.

Ben Debba M.B., Torgerson W.S., Long D.M., *Personality traits, pain duration and severity functional impairment, and psychological distress in patients with persistent low back pain*, Pain, 1997, 72 : 115 – 125.

Benjamin S., Barnes D., Berger S., Clarke I., Jeacock J., *The relationship of chronic pain, mental illness and organic disorders*, Pain, 1988, 32 : 185 – 195.

Bille B., *Migraine in school children*, Acta Paediatr., 1962, 51 (Suppl. 136).

Blanchard E.B., Andrasik F., Appelbaum K.A., Evans D.D., Myers P., Barron K.D., *Three studies of the psychological changes in chronic headache patients associated with biofeedback and relaxation therapies*, Psychosom. Med., 1986, 48 : 73 – 83.

Blanchard E.B., Kirsch C.A., Appelbaum K.A., Jaccard J., *The role of psychopathology in chronic headache: cause or effect?* Headache, 1989, 29 : 295 – 301.

Blanchard E.B., Steffek B.D., Jaccard J., Nicholson N.L., *Psychological changes accompanying non-pharmacological treatment of chronic headache: the effects of outcome*, Headache, 1991, 31 : 249 – 253.

Blumer D., Heilbronn M., *Chronic pain as a variant of depressive disease. The pain prone disorder*, J. Nerv. Ment. Dis., 1982, 170 : 281 – 406.

Brandt J., Celentano D., Steward W.F., Linet M., Folstein M.F., *Personality and emotional disorders in a community sample of migraine headache sufferes*, Am. J. Psychiatry, 1990, 147 : 303 – 308.

Breslau N., Davis G.C., Andreski P., *Migraine, psychiatric disorders, and suicide attempts: an epidemiologic study of young adults*, Psychiatr. Res., 1991, 37 – 11 – 23.

Breslau N., Davis G.C., *Migraine, major depression and panic disorder: a prospective epidemiologic study of young adults*, Cephalalgia, 1992, 12 : 85 – 90.

Breslau N., Davis G.C., Schultz L.R., Peterson E.L., *Migraine and major depression: a longitudinal study*, Headache, 1994, 34 : 387 – 393.

Breslau N., Merikangas K., Bowden C.L., *Comorbidity of migraine and major affective disorders*, Neurology, 1994, 44(10 Suppl 7):S17 –S22.

Breslau N., Andreski P., *Migraine, personality, and psychiatric comorbidity*, Headache, 1995, 35 : 382 – 386.

Brooke R.I., Merskey H., *Is atypical odontalgia a psychological problem?*, (Letter), Oral Surg. Oral Med. Oral Pathol., 1994, 77 : 2 – 3.

Casten R.J., Parmelee P.A., Kleban M.H., Powell Lawton M. and Katz I.R., *The relationships among anxiety, depression, and pain in a geriatric institutionalized sample*, Pain, 1995, 61 : 271 – 276.

Ciccone D.S., Bandilla E.B., Wu W.H., *Psychological dysfunction in patients with reflex sympathetic dystrophy*, Pain, 1997, 71 : 323 – 333.

Collet L., Cottraux J., Jeunet C., *Tension headaches: relation between MMPI paranoia score and pain and between MMPI hypochondriasis score and frontal EMG*. Headache, 1986, 26 : 365 – 368.

Cox D., Thomas D., *Relationship between headaches and depression*, Headache, 1981, 21 : 261–263.

Cunningham S.J., McGrath P.J., Ferguson H.B., et al. *Personality and behavioural characteristics in pediatric migraine*, Headache, 1987, 27 : 16–20.

Cuypers J., Altenkirch H., Bunge S., *Personality profiles in cluster headache and migraine*, Headache, 21 : 21–24, 1981.

Dalessio D.J., *Some current data on headache research*, Triangle, 1981, 20 : 33–41.

De Domini P., Del Bene E., Gori-Savellini S., et al. *Personality patterns of headache sufferers*, Cephalalgia, Suppl., 1983, 1 : 195–214.

Dworkin R.H., Handlin D.S., Richlin D.M., Brand L., Vannucci C., *Unraveling the effects of compensation, litigation, and employment on treatment response in chronic pain*, Pain, 1985, 23 : 49–59.

Ellertsen B., *Personality factors in recurring and chronic pain*. Cephalalgia, 1992, 12 : 129–132.

Ellertsen B., Klöve H., *MMPI patterns in chronic muscle pain, tension headache, and migraine*, Cephalalgia, 1987, 7 : 65–71.

Ellertsen B., Troland K., Klöve H., *MMPI profiles in migraine before and after biofeedback treatment*, Cephalalgia, 1987, 7 : 101–108.

Ellertsen B., Vaeröy H., Endresen I., Förre O., *MMPI in fibromyalgia and local nonspecific myalgia*, New Trends Exp. Clin. Psychiatry, 1991, 7 : 53–62.

Ellertsen B., Troland K., Vaeröy H., *Psychological assessment of patients with musculoskeletal pain*, in: Vaeröy H., Merskey H., *Progress in fibromyalgia and myofascial pain*, Elsevier, Amsterdam, 1993, 93–99.

Eversole L.R., Stone C.E., Matherson D.W., Kaplan H., *Psychometric profiles and facial pain*, Oral Surg. Med. Oral Pathol., 1985, 60 : 269–274.

Fishbain D.A., Goldberg M., Meacher B.R., Steele R., Rosomoff H.L., *Male and female chronic pain patients categorized by DSM-III psychiatric diagnostic criteria*, Pain, 1986, 26 : 181–197.

France R.D., Houpt J., Skott A., Wallman L.M., Varia I., *The phenomenology of depression in chronic pain*, Proc. 137 th American Psychiatric Association Annual Meeting, Symposium Chronic Pain and Depression, 1984.

Grazzi L., Frediani F., Zappacosta B., Boiardi A., Bussone G., *Psychological assessment in tension headache before and after biofeedback treatment*, Headache, 1988, 28 : 337–338.

Greene C.S., *Myofacial pain dysfunction syndrome: etiology*, in: Sarnat B.G., Laskin D.M. (eds.), *The temporomandibular joint: a biological basis for clinical treatment*, Charles C. Thomas, Springfield, 1979, 289–299.

Guidetti V., Fornara R., Ottaviano S., Petrilli A., Seri S., Cortesi F., *Personality inventory for children and childhood migraine*, Cephalalgia, 1987, 7 : 225–230.

Harrison R.H., *Psychological testing in headache: a review*, Headache, 1975, 13 : 177–185.

Henry P., *Céphalées de tension et céphalées psychogènes*, Rev. Prat., Paris, 1990, 40 : 403–406.

Henryk-Gutt R., Ress W.L., *Psychological aspects of migraine*, J. Psychosom. Res., 1973, 17 : 141–153.

Invernizzi G., Gala C., Buono M., Cittone L., Tavola T., Conte G., *Neurotic traits and disease duration in headache patients*, Cephalalgia, 1989, 9 : 173–178.

Katon W., Egan K., Miller D., *Chronic pain: lifetime psychiatric diagnoses and family history*, Am. J. Psychiatry, 1985, 142 : 1156–1160.

Keck P.E. Jr., Merikangas K.R., McElroy S.L., Strakowski M., *Diagnostic and treatment implications of psychiatric comorbidity with migraine*, Ann. Clin. Psychiatry, 1994, 6 : 165–171.

Krishnan K.R.R., France R.D., Houpt J.L., *Chronic low back pain and depression*, Psychosomatics, 1985, 26 : 299–302.

Kudrow L., Sutkus B.J., *MMPI pattern specificacy in primary headache disorders*, Headache, 1979, 19 : 18–24.

Kurman R., Hursey K., Mathew N., *The utility of the MMPI-2 for discriminating diagnostic headache groups*, Cephalalgia, 1991, 11, Suppl. 11 : 300.

Langemark M., Olesen J., Poulsen D.L., Bech P., *Clinical characterization of patients with chronic tension headache*, Headache, 1988, 28 : 590–596.

Larsson B.S., *The rôle of psychological, health-behaviour and medical factors in adolescent headache*, Dev. Med. Child Neurol., 1988, 30 : 616–625.

Laskin D.M., *Etiology of the pain-dysfunctioning syndrome*, J. Am. Dent. Assoc., 1969, 79 : 147–153.

Magni G., Moreschi C., Rigatti-Luchini S., Merskey H., *Prospective study on the relationship between depressive symptoms and chronic musculoskeletal pain*, Pain, 1994, 56 : 289–297.

Marazziti D., Toni C., Pedri S., et al. *Headache, panic disorder and depression: comorbidity or a spectrum?*, Neuropsychobiology, 1995, 31 : 125–129.

Marchesi C., De Ferri A., Petrolini N., et al. *Prevalence of migraine and muscle tension headache in depressive disorders*, J. Affect. Disord., 1989, 16 : 33–36.

McCreary C., Clark G.T., Merril R.L., Flack V., Oakley M.E., *Psychological distress and diagnostic subgroups of temporomandibular disorder patients*, Pain, 1991, 44 : 29–34.

Merikangas K.R., *Psychopathology and headache syndromes in the community*, Headache, 1994, 34:S17–22.

Merikangas K.R., Risch N.J., Merikangas J.R., Weissman M.M., Kidd K.K., *Migraine and depression: association and familial trasmission*, J. Psychiatr. Res., 1988, 22 : 119–129.

Merikangas K.R., Angst J., Isler H., *Migraine and psychopathology*. Arch Gen Psychiatry, 1990, 47 : 849–853.

Merikangas K.R., Merikangas J.R., Angst J., *Headache syndromes and psychiatric disorders: association and familial transmission*, J. Psychiatr. Res., 1993, 27 : 197–210.

Mongini F., *Assessment of craniofacial pain and dysfunction: a multidisciplinary approach*, Cranio, 1990, 8 : 183–200.

Mongini F., Ventricelli F., Conserva E., *Etiology of craniofacial pain and headache in stomatognathic dysfunction*, in: Dubner R., Gebhart G.F., Bond M.R. (eds.), Proceedings of the Vth World Congress on Pain, Elsevier, Amsterdam, 1988, 512–519.

Mongini F., Ferla E., Maccagnani C., *MMPI profiles in patients with headache or craniofacial pain: a comparative study*, Cephalalgia, 1992, 12 : 91–98.

Mongini F., Ibertis F., Ferla E., *Personality characteristics before and after treatment of different head pain syndromes*, Cephalalgia, 1994, 14 : 368–373.

Mongini F., Ibertis F., Bava M., Negro C., *A psychological profile of migraine in women*, Cephalalgia, 1997 a, 17 : 260 (abs.).

Mongini F., Poma M., Bava M., Fabbri G., *Psychosomatic symptoms in different types of headache and facial pain*, Cephalalgia, 1997 b, 17 : 274 (abs.).

Mongini F., Defilippi N., Negro C., *Chronic daily headache. A clinical and psychological profile before and after treatment*, Headache, 1997 c, 37 : 83–87.

Müller B., Sartory G., Pothmann R., Frankenberg S.V., *Headache, depression and anxiety: results of an epidemiological study in German children and adolescents*, International Headache Seminar Copenhagen, 1993.

Passchier J., Helm-Hylkema H.V.D., Orlebeke J.F., *Lack of concordance between changes and headache activity and in psychophysiological and personality variables following treatment*, Headache, 1985, 25 : 310–316.

Payne T.C., Leavitt F., Garron D.C., Katz R.S., Golden H.E., Glickman P.B., *Vanderplate C: fibrositis and psychological disturbance*, Arthritis Rheum., 1982, 25 : 213–217.

Pelz M., Merskey H., *A description of the psychological effects of chronic painful lesions*, Pain, 1982, 14 : 293–301.

Pfaffenrath V., Hummelsberger J., Pöllmann W., Kaube H., Rath M., *MMPI personality profiles in patients with primary headache syndromes*, Cephalalgia, 1991, 11 : 263–268.

Philips C., *Headache and personality*, J. Psychosom. Res., 1976, 20 : 535–542.

Puca F., Genco S., Savarese M., et al., *Stress, depression and anxiety in primary headache sufferers: evaluation by means of the SCL-90-R*, Cephalalgia, 1991, 11, (Suppl. 11):296.

Rajala U., Keinanan-Kuikaanniemi S., Uusimaki A., Kivela S.L., *Musculoskeletal pains and depression in a middle-aged Finnish population*, Pain, 1995, 61 : 451–457.

Rasmussen B.K., *Migraine and tension-type headache in a general population: psychosocial factors*: Int. J. Epidemiol., 1992, 21 : 1138–1143.

Reich J., Tupen J.P., Abramowitz S.I., *Psychiatric diagnos of chronic pain patients*, Am. J. Psychiatry, 1983, 140 : 149–158.

Remick R.A., Blasberg B., *Psychiatric aspects of atypical facial pain*, Can. Dent. Assoc. J. Dec., 1985, 51 : 913–916.

Ries Merikangas K., Isler H., Angst J., *Comorbidity of migraine and psychiatric disorders: results of a prospective epidemiologic study*, Cephalalgia, 1991, 11, (Suppl. 11):308.

Rydd W.L., *Psychosomatic aspects of temporomandibular joint dysfunction*, J. Am. Dent. Assoc., 1959, 59 : 31.

Schafer M.L., *Typus melancholicus as a personality characteristic of migraine patients*, Eur. Arch. Psychiatry Clin. Neurosci., 1994, 24 : 328–339.

Schaffer C.B., Donlan P.T., Bittle R.M., *Chronic pain and depression: a clinical and family history survey*, Am. J. Psychiatry, 1980, 137 : 118–120.

Schnarch D.M., Hunter J.E., *Personality differences between randomly selected migrainous and non-migrainous people*, Psychother. Theory. Res. Pract., 1979, 16 : 297–309.

Silberstein S.D., *Tension-type and chronic daily headache*, Neurology, 1993, 43 : 1644–1649.

Silberstein S.D., Lipton R.B., Breslau N., *Migraine: association with personality characteristics and psychopathology*, Cephalalgia, 1995, 15:358–369.

Smedstad L.M., Vaglum P., Kvien T.K., Moum T., *The relationship between self-reported pain and sociodemographic variables, anxiety and depressive symptoms in rheumatoid arthritis*, J. Rheumatol., 1995, 22:511–520.

Solomon S., Lipton R.B., Newman L.C., *Clinical features of chronic daily headache*, Headache, 1992, 32:325–329.

Soto Werder D., Sargent J.D., Coyne L., *MMPI profiles of headache patients using self-regulation to control headache activity*, Headache, 1981, 21:164–169.

Sovak N., Kunzel M., Sternback R.A., Dalessio D.J., *Mechanism of the biofeedback theraphy of migraine: volitional manipulation of the psychophysiological background*, Headache, 1981, 21:89–92.

Sternbach R.A., Wolf S.R., Murphy R.W., Akeson W.H., *Traits of pain patients: low-back "loser"*, Psychosomatics, 1973, 14:226–229.

Sternbach R.A., Dalessio D.J., Kunzel M., Bowman G.E., *MMPI patterns in common headache disorders*, Headache, 1980, 19:311–316.

Steward W.F., Linet M.S., Celentano D.D., *Migraine headaches and panic attacks*, Psychosom. Med., 1989, 51:559–569.

Sullivan M.J.L., Reesor K., Mikail S., Fisher R., *The treatment of depression in chronic low back pain: review and recommendations*, Pain, 1992, 50:5–13.

Tamminen T.M., Bredenberg P., Escartin T., et al. *Psychosomatic symptoms in preadolescent children*, Psychother., Psychosom., 1991, 56:70–77.

Turk D.C., Flor H., *Primary fibromyalgia is greater than tender points: toward a multiaxial taxonomy*, J. Rheumatol., 1989, (Suppl. 16):80–86.

Wade J.B., Price D.D., Hamer R.M., Schwartz S.M., Hart R.P., *An emotional component analysis of chronic pain*, Pain, 1990, 40:303–310.

Weeks R., Baskin S., Rapoport A., et al., *A comparison of MMPI personality data frontalis electromyographic readings in migraine and combination headache patients*, Headache, 1983, 23:75–82.

Wolfe F., Cathey M.A., Kleinheksel S.M., et al. *Psychological status in primary fibrositis and fibrositis associated with rheumatoid arthritis*, J. Rheumatol., 1984, 11:500–506.

Yunus M.B., Ahles T.A., Aldag J.C., Mas A.T., *Relationship of clinical features with psychological status in primary fibromyalgia*, Arthritis Rheum., 1991, 34:15–21.

9 Factor Interplay

As mentioned in Chapter 1, the presence of a number of possibly relevant etiological factors in patients with headache or facial pain requires accurate evaluation of their relevance, their temporal sequence and the mechanisms by which they may reciprocally enhance each other. In some patients, two or more factors might have coexisted from very the beginning, while in others a primary factor may subsequently produce others, with consequent aggravation and/or change in symptomatology.

Depending how this *factor interplay* is interpreted, different pathogenetic mechanisms of head pain syndromes may be postulated. A good example is represented by the different theories concerning the relation between tension-type headache and migraine. These headache disorders are considered by some authors as manifestations of the same "continuum" and by others as two separate pathologies. Another example is given by the different relevance attributed to disorders of the cervical column in the pathogenesis of some headaches: on this question also depends whether *cervicogenic headache* should or should not be included in the headache and facial pain classification as a distinct entity. Similarly, as we have seen, there is a discrepancy of opinion on how structure alterations of the maxillary bones and hyperparafunction of the head and neck muscles may cooperate in producing some types of facial pain and temporomandibular joint (TMJ) disorders (see Chapters 3 and 4). Finally, the interplay with psychogenic factors has been investigated in all types of severe and chronic headache (see Chapter 8). These points will now be examined in more detail.

Interplay Between Migraine and Tension-Type Headache

As mentioned, the interplay between migraine and tension-type headache is debated. Various authors accept the hypothesis of a "continuum" between these two types of headache (Waters, 1973; Bakal and Kaganov, 1977, 1979; Drummond and Lance, 1984; Featherstone, 1985; Takeshima and Takahashi, 1988; Marcus, 1992; Leston, 1996). After an analysis of elements of headache history in 50 idiopathic headache patients, Featherstone found that quantitation of symptoms and their characteristics showed a unipolar distribution and that pain severity was directly related to the symptom quantitation score. Takeshima and Takahashi (1988), after quantification analysis of the clinical data of 180 patients with tension-type headache, migraine or combined headache, found a "muscle contraction headache–migraine axis" along which the patients showed diffuse and sequential distribution. To support this theory it is emphasized that, after employing the IHS criteria, a number of headache cases remain difficult to classify (Iversen et al., 1990; Messinger et al., 1991; Pfaffenrath and Isler, 1993; Michel et al., 1993; Sjaastad and Stovner, 1993; Sanin et al., 1994).

The problem of the relation between these two headache types also concerns pericranial muscle function. As mentioned earlier (Chapters 1 and 3), this is considered as a possible etiological factor of tension-type headache (Lange-

mark and Olesen, 1987; International Headache Society, 1988; Hatch et al., 1992; Jensen and Rasmussen, 1996; Jensen et al., 1996; Jensen and Olesen, 1996). However, an increase of muscle tenderness at palpation was also found in migraine patients (Olesen, 1978; Hay, 1979; Tfelt-Hansen et al., 1981; Lous and Olesen, 1982; Jensen and Olesen, 1988). Furthermore, electromyographic studies showed that temporal, masseter, and sternocleidomastoid muscle activity may increase during migraine attacks (Bakke et al., 1982).

In support of the "continuum" theory, it is further objected that some alterations, such as abnormalities in serotonin metabolism, decreased β-endorphin levels, and impaired autonomic function, have been reported in both migraine and tension-type headache (Leston, 1996). This way of thinking supports a *headache severity model* rather than the existence of separate idiopathic headache entities. The characteristics and severity of headache attacks would also depend on the interplay of the above-mentioned factors and on their relevance in the different patients.

Other authors, however, reject this hypothesis and maintain that migraine and tension-type headache are two independent headache models (Olesen, 1978; 1991; Rasmussen, 1996). They suggest that the high prevalence of tension-type headache in a general population may explain the coincidence of the two conditions as a pure chance phenomenon and that a number of factors (hormonal, psychosocial, etc.) seem to have different impacts on the two pathologies (Rasmussen, 1996).

Olesen (1991), although he advocates that a clear distinction between the two headache pathologies be drawn, proposes a "vascular–supraspinal–myogenic" model of migraine and tension-type headache. According to this model, the headache syndrome would result from the interplay of three factors, namely, a myofacial nociceptive input, a vascular nociceptive input, and a supraspinal excitatory or inhibitory control. These inputs would converge on the same neurons (Fig. 9.**1**) and, depending on their prevalence, different types of headache would result. In migraine patients, the primary nociception would be vascular, while in tension-type headache it would be myofacial. In both conditions, the supraspinal facilitation could be large or small, explaining why stress can provoke headache attacks.

Moreover, the superimposition of the different inputs could explain how chronic tension-type headache sufferers may develop migraine episodes and how intravenous injection of histamine, which causes no headache in headache-free subjects, can provoke pulsating headache in migraine sufferers and constant pain in tension-type headache patients (Krabbe and Olesen, 1980).

Mongini et al. (1997 a) examined 717 patients with different types (single or combined) of headache and facial pain (Table 9.**1**). History was taken, which included a semistructured interview with 55 items, and a clinical examination was performed. The group with migraine compared to the tension-type headache group showed a significantly higher prevalence of cholitis, gastritis, digestion problems, tiredness, paresthesias, circulation problems, hair fragility, and chinetosis. In the tension-type headache group, the following symptoms were

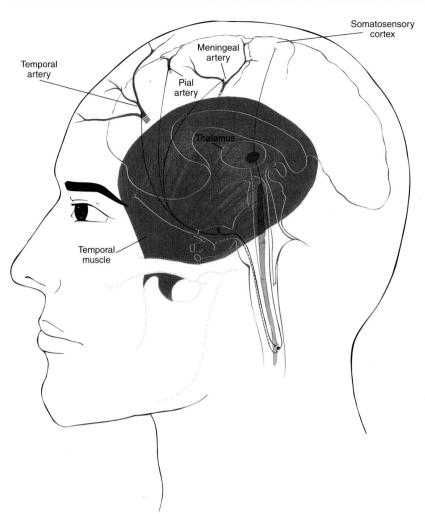

Fig. 9.**1** **Vascular-supraspinal-myogenic model proposed by Olesen for the pathogenesis of migraine and of tension-type headache.** Myofascial and vascular nociceptive inputs and supraspinal inputs converge on the same neurons in the trigeminal sensory nucleus, causing different types of headache according to their prevalence. Further explanation is given in the text. (From Olesen, 1991, with modifications)

Table 9.**1**   Distribution of 717 patients with headache or facial pain according to the different diagnostic groups

	Women					Men					
	N°	%	Mean age		SD	N°	%	Mean age		SD	Tot.
FP	46	90.2	50.2	+/−	12.7	5	9.8	41.2	+/−	9.9	51
TH	44	80.0	34.3	+/−	14.3	11	20.0	34.6	+/−	16.4	55
M	25	78.1	40.7	+/−	12.3	7	21.9	38.7	+/−	20.7	32
MP	196	77.5	38.9	+/−	15.7	57	22.5	35.8	+/−	14.9	253
N	10	58.8	56.9	+/−	15.4	7	41.2	64.4	+/−	12.7	17
TMJ	96	69.1	31.7	+/−	13.7	43	30.9	30.3	+/−	14.2	139
M–TH	29	96.7	39.3	+/−	13.8	1	3.3	31.0	+/−	0.0	30
MP–TH	54	93.1	38.1	+/−	15.5	4	6.9	37.3	+/−	3.6	58
MP–TMJ	65	79.3	34.2	+/−	15.5	17	20.7	20.7	+/−	11.1	82
	565	78.8	38.1		15.6	152	21.2	21.2		15.7	717

From Mongini et al. (1997 a). FP = facial pain disorder (somatoform disorder); TH = tension-type headache; M = migraine; MP = myogenous facial pain; N = neuropathy; TMJ = TMJ dysfunction.

more prevalent: sleep disturbances, muscle parafunction, hypertrophy of the mandible elevator muscles. The group with facial pain disorder as somatoform disorder had higher prevalence of psychosomatic items (bulimia, anxiety, panic attacks, mood changes, phobias, etc.): these symptoms, however, were also found, to a lesser extent, in patients with migraine or tension-type headache (Tables 9.**2**, 9.**3** and Fig. 9.**2**).

Interestingly, when two pathologies were superimposed on the same patient, the prevalence of symptoms was significantly higher compared to that in patients with only one pathology (Table 9.**4**). These data seem to indicate that some factors may play a facilitating role both in tension-type headache and in migraine while others act more specifically in one pathology or the other.

Table 9.**2** Prevalence (%) of symptoms mostly psychosomatic in nature in the different diagnostic groups (see Tab. 9.**1**)

%	Depression	Difficulty in swallowing	Digestion difficulty	Colitis	Gastritis	Bulimia	Anxiety	Phobias	Sleep disorders	Panic attacks	Palpitations	Mood changes	Lassitude	Parafunctions
FP	**60.8**	**23.5**	**47.1**	**47.1**	**43.1**	**43.1**	**43.1**	**54.9**	**70.6**	**49.0**	**64.7**	**72.5**	**66.7**	**68.6**
TH	29.1	16.4	25.5	38.2	29.1	**23.6**	67.3	**41.8**	**50.9**	**32.7**	47.3	50.9	**49.1**	**72.7**
M	**46.9**	**37.5**	**46.9**	**53.1**	**50.0**	28.1	65.6	37.5	46.9	**37.5**	50.0	**62.5**	62.5	50.0
MP	30.4	19.8	30.4	35.6	31.6	16.2	62.1	32.8	44.3	16.6	37.5	48.2	49.4	59.3
N	35.3	11.8	23.5	11.8	17.6	11.8	64.7	41.2	47.1	11.8	47.1	52.9	14.3	29.4
TMJ	15.8	5.8	25.2	25.2	26.6	9.4	51.8	25.9	23.0	15.1	33.8	36.7	34.5	53.2
P =	1.2×10^{-7}	1.3×10^{-4}	1.979×10^{-2}	2.77×10^{-3}	4.42×10^{-2}	4×10^{-6}	3.16×10^{-3}	6.79×10^{-3}	1.2×10^{-7}	2.2×10^{-7}	2.63×10^{-3}	4.5×10^{-4}	2.5×10^{-5}	9.28×10^{-3}

Significant data after chi-square analysis are shown in bold. From Mongini et al. (1997 a).

Table 9.**3** Prevalence (%) of clinical signs in the different diagnostic groups

%	Tenderness of cranial muscles	Tenderness of cranial points	Tenderness of cervical muscles	Posture disorders	Muscle hypertrophy	Joint noises	Restriction of mouth opening
FP	51.0	9.8	45.1	56.9	41.2	25.5	21.6
TH	43.6	**21.8**	**52.7**	**74.5**	**67.3**	56.4	25.5
M	**53.1**	**34.4**	**62.5**	65.6	56.3	50.0	**46.9**
MP	**61.7**	**24.5**	**53.8**	58.5	62.1	47.0	33.6
N	17.6	17.6	11.8	29.4	17.6	41.2	11.8
TMJ	20.9	5.0	25.2	51.8	56.8	**69.8**	43.2
P =	4×10^{-13}	8×10^{-6}	4×10^{-8}	1.1×10^{-2}	8×10^{-4}	1×10^{-6}	5.4×10^{-3}

From Mongini et al. (1997 a). Significant data after chi-square analysis are shown in bold

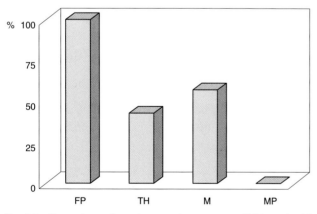

Fig. 9.**2** Percentage of psychosomatic symptoms (14 items) with significantly higher prevalence in patients with facial pain disorder (somatoform disorder) (FP), tension-type headache (TH), migraine (M), and myogenous facial pain (MP). (From Mongini et al., 1997 a)

Table 9.**4** Symptoms with higher prevalence in patients with migraine (M) and tension-type headache (TH) with respect to the patient with one pathology only

%	Parafunctions	Hair fragility	Restriction of mouth opening
TH	72.7	18.2	25.5
M	50.0	**37.5**	**46.9**
M–TH	**83.3**	**40.0**	**60.0**
P =	**0.0131**	**0.0497**	**0.0053**

From Mongini et al. (1997 a).

Chronic daily headache (CDH) is a good model for further studying these problems, since it may represent a development of both migraine and tension-type headache. As previously mentioned (Chapter 1), some authors consider this as an independent headache type, while others maintain that in this case multiple diagnoses are more appropriate (Olesen, 1996).

As we have seen (Chapter 8), Mongini et al. (1997 b) found two distinct MMPI configurations, psychosomatic and depressive, in patients with CDH. Several patients with a depressive MMPI profile before treatment showed a conversive V after treatment (see Fig. 8.**13**). This configuration is also found in numerous women patients with migraine (Mongini et al., 1997 c) (Fig. 8.**2**). Therefore, it seems that there is an initial difference in personality profile and accompanying symptoms between patients with migraine and tension-type headache: this may correspond to a different etiological input. When, with time, headache becomes chronic, the two headache types may converge into CDH.

Interplay with Cervical Problems

The importance of cervical problems as an etiopathogenetic factor of headache is also very much debated. According to some authors, a contraction of the cervical muscles is often prodromic or concomitant with a migraine disorder (Tfelt-Hansen et al. 1981; Boquet et al., 1989; Blau et al., 1994). Other authors maintain that the relationship between migraine and tension-type headache is not chance (Bogduk et al., 1981; Bogduk, 1984; Kidd and Nelson 1993). Moreover, migraine attacks or hemicrania continua consequent on compression of the upper cervical roots by a tumor or prolapsed vertebra disks or spondylotic degeneration have been described (Jansen et al., 1989). The anatomical basis of this relation could consist of a common afference to the caudal portion of the trigeminal spinal nucleus of the trigeminal sensory fibres and of C1, C2 and C3 cervical roots (Fig. 9.3). These roots receive sensory afference from the atlantooccipital and atlantoaxial joints, the vertebral and carotid arteries, the prevertebral, sternocleidomastoid and trapezius muscles, the long muscles of the neck, the posterior cranial fossa and the cerebellar tentorium (Bogduk et al., 1981). Moreover, stimulation in healthy volunteers of the zygapophyseal joint at segment C2–C3 pro-duces pain at characteristic cerviconuchal sites (Dwyer et al. 1990) (Fig. 9.4). These anatomical relations could explain, at least in part, "cervicogenic headache" as described by Sjaastad et al. (1983) as a strictly unilateral noncontinuous headache combined with signs of neck involvement in the form of ipsi-lateral, diffuse pain in the neck, shoulder and arm region and neck movement provoking pain attacks (see Chapter 1).

However, other authors have shown that stimulation of the superior sagittal sinus evokes expression of C-fos type immunoreactivity in the caudal trigeminal nucleus and the upper cervical regions of the dorsal horn (Kaube et al., 1993; Goadsby et al., 1995; Goadsby, 1996) (Fig. 9.5). These authors assert that the migraine attack could stimulate trigeminal nociceptors located in this area and that the common convergence with the upper cervical roots might explain a referred pain in the cervical area even in absence of any alteration of the cervical structures (Goadsby, 1996).

However, alterations of the cervical column may cooperate with other factors, to produce craniofacial pain, and they may be the main source in some cases: in fact, as we have seen (Chapter 4), trigger points are a frequent finding in patients with posture disorders of the cervical column. These trigger points may constitute a source of pain in distant craniofacial areas. Moreover, as already mentioned, disorders of neck posture may lead to muscle hyperfunction and dysfunction, thus expanding the area and increasing the intensity of a tension-type headache. In the aforementioned work, Mongini et al. (1997a) found a significantly high prevalence of posture disorders in patients with tension-type headache (Table 9.3).

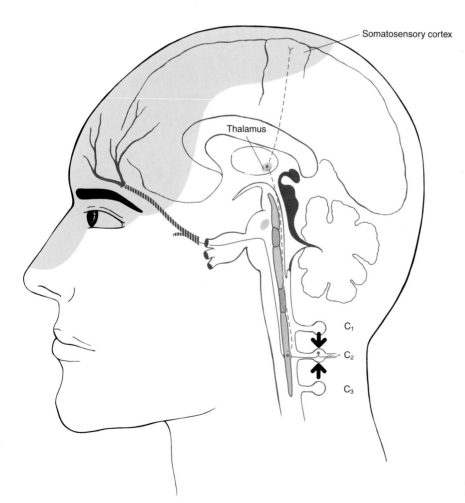

Fig. 9.3 According to Jansen et al., a common afference of cervical and trigeminal nerve fibers to the neurons of the trigeminal sensory nucleus might cause migraine attacks in subjects with compression of the upper cervical roots. (From Jansen et al., 1989, with modifications)

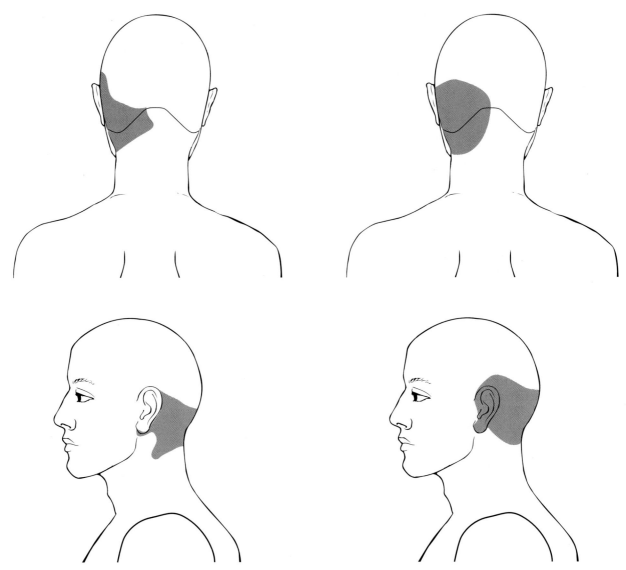

Fig. 9.4 Areas of referred pain after stimulation of the zygapophyseal joints $C^2 – C^3$. (From Dwyer et al., 1990, with modifications)

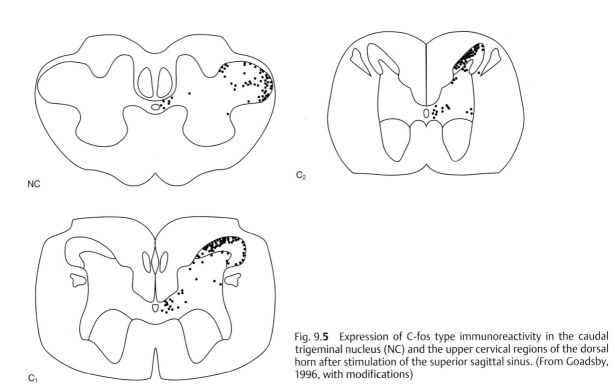

Fig. 9.5 Expression of C-fos type immunoreactivity in the caudal trigeminal nucleus (NC) and the upper cervical regions of the dorsal horn after stimulation of the superior sagittal sinus. (From Goadsby, 1996, with modifications)

Interplay with Psychogenic Factors

Psychogenic factors may variously interact in almost all types of headache and facial pain (see Chapter 8). Obviously, their relevance may vary to a great extent in the different pathologies and different patients. This is of course of primary importance for treatment planning. Both in migraine and in tension-type headache these factors may be highly relevant or less so (Table 9.**2**, Fig. 9.**2**): in the first case, psychotropic drugs, alone or combined with others, are usually the first choice (see Chapter 12). The pathogenetic mechanisms by which psychogenic factors can produce pain may be direct or mediated by other factors. For instance, muscle disorders and psychogenic factors are variously combined in patients with headache and facial pain. One possibility is that psychogenic factors, such as depression and anxiety, may increase the tendency to muscle hyperparafunction, thus leading to muscle fatigue and pain (nociceptive pain) (see Chapters 1 and 3) (Fig. 9.**6**). However, psychogenic factors may lead directly to *somatoform* pain (psychogenic pain), that is, pain mimicking a somatic problem. This mechanism is probably the major source of *facial pain disorder* as a somatoform disorder (Mongini et al., 1988, 1992; Mongini, 1990) (Table 9.**2**, Figs. 9.**2**, 9.**6**), so-called "atypical facial pain", but it may coexist with other factors in patients suffering from tension-type headache, migraine, muscle pain, and, in particular, from chronic daily headache and from two or more associated pathologies (Table 9.**5**). Therefore, it is possible that some patients suffer both from a nociceptive and a psychogenic pain (Fig. 9.**6**).

Table 9.**5** Symptoms with higher prevalence in patients with tension-type headache (TH) and myogenous facial pain (M) with respect to the patient with one pathology only

%	Phobias	Panic attacks	Lassitude	Depression
TH	41.8	**32.7**	49.1	29.1
MP	32.8	16.6	49.4	30.4
MP–TH	**53.4**	**36.2**	**72.4**	**51.7**
P =	**0.0105**	**0.0006**	**0.0055**	**0.0062**

From Mongini et al. (1997 a).

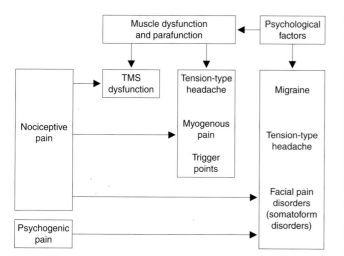

Fig. 9.**6** Mechanisms by which a psychological factor may induce nociceptive and psychogenic facial pain

Interplay with Muscle Dysfunction and Structural Alterations

Muscle dysfunction and structural alterations often coexist in patients with pain due to TMJ disorders. As we have seen (Chapter 4), jaw structure alterations with mandibular displacement in maximum tooth intercuspation are a possible source of TMJ intracapsular derangements. Nevertheless, severe parafunction with prolonged tooth grinding and clenching markedly increases the potentially damaging effect of structural alterations.

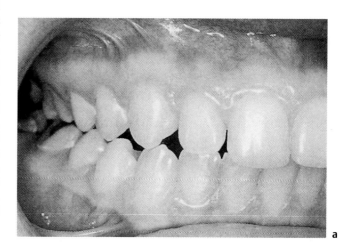

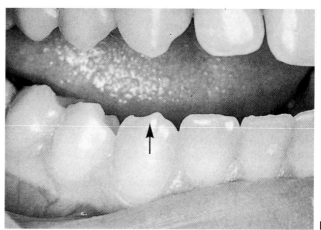

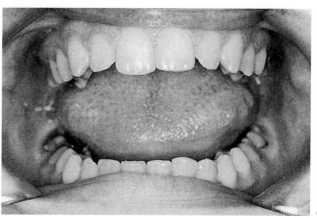

Fig. 9.**7** **Patient with anxiety disorder.** The marked right antero-lateral bruxism movements (**a**), revealed by the characteristic abrasion of the canine (**b**, arrow), produced a disk displacement without reduction of the right TMJ with consequent limitation of mouth opening (**c**)

However, parafunctions with pronounced grinding and excessive protrusive and lateral mandibular movements may produce TMJ intracapsular problems (such as disk displacement with or without reduction) even in the absence of structure alterations (Mongini, 1993 a) (Figs. 9.**6**, 9.**7**). This also explains why tension-type headache, muscle pain and TMJ internal derangement are frequently combined in the same patient. Moreover, parafunctions may, with time, alter tooth occlusion, thus introducing an additional, potentially damaging factor (Fig. 3.**26**). This factor, however, should not be overemphasized.

Since parafunctions may simply be consequences of a mild or moderate stress situation or, in other patients, of a depressive or anxiety disorder (or even a personality disorder in some cases) (Fig. 9.**6**), the interplay between the different factors may vary a great deal, in particular in patients who suffer from more than one type of headache and facial pain.

Interplay with Systemic Factors

In the chapters on systemic factors in headache and facial pain (Chapters 5–8), examples were repeatedly found in which these factors reciprocally influence each other in the same patient. Here, attention will be given to the interplay of hormonal factors with vascular and neurological factors, and between the psychogenic factors and all the others.

To analyse the interplay between these factors in patients with different types of headache and craniofacial pain, Mongini et al. (1993 b) applied a test protocol including history, medical and neurological examination and two psychometric tests (MMPI and STAI) to five groups (n = 30 per group) of healthy subjects and patients with hormonal, vascular, neurological and psychiatric pathologies. Principal component analysis was applied to those signs and symptoms whose different distribution between the groups was statistically significant, to calculate the "weight" of each sign or symptom in the first three components (Fig. 9.**8**). The same procedure was then applied to 101 patients with headache or facial pain, so as to calculate, for each patient and for the groups of patients divided by pathology, and on the basis of the data obtained from the five control groups, the percentage of adherence to normality or to the different categories of systemic disorder. The data obtained are summarized in Fig. 9.**9**. The group of patients with migraine, cluster headache or chronic paroxysmal hemicrania showed a high percentage of vascular factors and an even higher percentage of neurological ones.

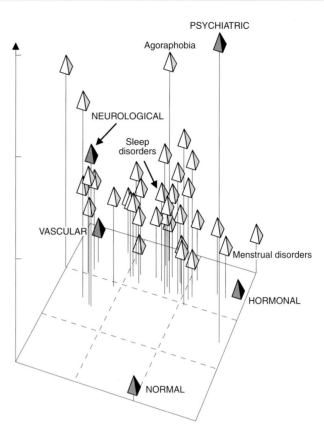

Fig. 9.**8** **Assessment by "principal component analysis"** of the various signs or symptoms compared to a group of normal subjects and to four groups of subjects with specific pathologies. Further explanation is given in the text. (From Monigini et al., 1993 b, with modifications)

The group with atypical facial pain disorder had very high values for the psychiatric factor. The group with tension-type headache was in an intermediate position, with fairly consistent values for all the factors considered (hormonal, vascular, neurological, psychiatric). Lastly, the group with intracapsular TMJ factors had a high normality value; in other words, these patients were relatively healthy from the systemic standpoint. These findings confirm the frequent coexistence and reciprocal influence of more than one systemic factor in most patients with headache and craniofacial pain. Nevertheless, the weight of these factors may vary in the different pathologies.

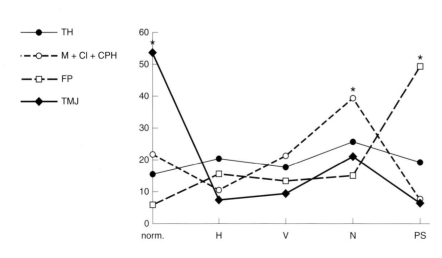

Fig. 9.**9** Percentage of adherence to normality or to different categories of systemic disorders in groups of patients suffering from headache or facial pain of various types. TH = tension-type headache; M = migraine; Cl = cluster headache; CPH = chronic paroxical hemicrania; FP = facial pain disorder; TMJ = TMJ dysfunction; H = hormonal disorders; V = vascular disorders; N = neurological disorders; PS = psychiatric disorders. (From Mongini et al., 1993 b, with modifications)

References

Bakal D.A., Kaganov J.A., *Muscle contraction and migraine headache: psychophysiologic comparison*, Headache, 1977, 17:208–215.

Bakal D.A., Kaganov J.A., *Sympton characteristics of chronic and non chronic headache sufferers*, Headache, 1979, 19:258–259.

Bakke M., Tfelt-Hansen P., Olesen J., Möller E., *Action of some pericranial muscles during provoked attacks of common migraine*, Pain, 1982, 14:121–135.

Blau J.N., Path F.R.C., MacGregor E.A., *Migraine and the neck*, Headache, 1994, 34:88–90.

Bogduk N., *Headaches and the cervical spine. An editorial*, Cephalalgia, 1984, 7–8.

Bogduk N., Lambert G.A., Duckworth J.W., *The anatomy and physiology of the vertebral nerve in relation to cervical migraine*, Cephalalgia, 1981, 1:11–24.

Boquet J., Boismare F., Payenneville G., Leclerc D., Monnier J.C., Moore N., *Lateralization of headache: Possible role of an upper cervical trigger point*, Cephalalgia, 1989, 9:15–24.

Drummond P.D., Lance J.W., *Clinical diagnosis and computer analysis of headache symptoms*, J. Neurol. Neurosurg. Psychiatry, 1984, 47:128–133.

Dwyer A., Aprill C., Bogduk N., *Cervical zygapophyseal joint pain patterns I: A study in normal volunteers*, Spine, 1990, 15:453–457.

Featherstone H.J., *Migraine and muscle contraction headaches: a continuum*, Headache, 1985, 25:194–198.

Fredriksen O., Hovdal H., Sjaastad O., *"Cervicogenic headache": clinical manifestation*, Cephalalgia, 1987, 7:147–160.

Goadsby P.J., *Animal models of migraine: which one and for what?*, in: Clifford Rose F. (ed.), Towards Migraine 2000, 1996 Elsevier, Amsterdam, 85–99.

Goadsby P.J., *Studies of cerebrovascular pain pathways of relevance to migraine*, in: J. Olesen, M. Moskowitz (eds.), *Experimental headache models*, Lippincott-Raven Publishers, Philadelphia, 1995.

Hatch J.P., Moore P.J., Cyr-Provost M., Boutros N.N., Seleshi E., Borcherding S., *The use of electromyography and muscle palpation in the diagnosis of tension-type headache with and without pericranial muscle involvement*, Pain, 1992, 49:175–178.

Hay K.M., *Pain threshold in migraine*, Practitioner, 1979, 222:827–833.

International Headache Society, *Classification and diagnostic criteria for headache disorders, cranial neuralgias and facial pain*, Cephalalgia, 1988, 8(Suppl. 7):1–96.

Iversen H.K., Langemark M., Andersson P.G., Hansen P.E., Olesen J., *Clinical characteristics of migraine and episodic tension-type headache in relation to hold and new diagnostic criteria*, Headache, 1990, 30:514–519.

Jansen J., Markakis E., Rama B., Hildebrandt J., *Hemicranial attacks or permanent hemicrania - a seque of upper cervical root compression*, Cephalalgia, 1989, 9:123–130.

Jensen K., Tuxen C., Olesen J., *Pericranial muscle tenderness and pressure-pain threshold in the temporal region during common migraine*, Pain, 1988, 35:65–70.

Jensen R., Olesen J., *Temporal muscle blood flow in comness and pressure-pain threshold in the temporal region during common migraine*, Pain, 1988, 35:65–70.

Jensen R., Olesen J., *Initiating mechanisms of experimentally induced tension-type headache*, Cephalalgia, 1996, 16:175–182.

Jensen R., Rasmussen B.K., *Muscular disorders in tension-type headache*, Cephalalgia, 1996, 16:97–103.

Kaube H., Keay K., Hoskin K.L., Bandler R., Goadsby P.J., *Expression of c-fos-like immunoreactivity in the trigeminal nucleus caudalis and high cervical cord following stimulation of the sagittal sinus in the cat*, Brain Res., 1993, 629:95–102.

Kidd R.F., Nelson R., *Musculoskeletal dysfunction of the neck in migraine and tension headache*, Headache, 1993, 33:566–569.

Krabbe A.E., Olesen J., *Headache provocation by continuous intravenous infusion of histamine: clinical results and receptor mechanisms*, Pain, 1980, 8:253–259.

Langemark M., Olesen J., *Pericranial tenderness in tension headache*, Cephalalgia, 1987, 7:249–255.

Leston J.A., *Migraine and tension-type headache are not separate disorders*, Cephalalgia, 1996, 16:220–222.

Lous I., Olesen J., *Evaluation of pericranial tenderness and oral function in patients with common migraine, muscle contraction headache and "combination headache"*, Pain, 1982, 12:385–393.

Marcus D.A., *Migraine and tension-type headaches: The questionable validity of current classification systems*, Clin. J. Pain, 1992, 8:28–36.

Messinger H.B., Spierings E.L.H., Vincent A.J.P., *Overlap of migraine and tension-type headache in the International Headache Society Classification*, Cephalalgia, 1991, 11:233–237.

Michel P., Henry P., Letenneur L., Jogeix M., Corson A., Dartigues J.F., *Diagnostic screen for assessment of the IHS criteria for migraine by general practitioners*, Cephalalgia, 1993, 13, (Suppl. 12):54–59.

Mongini F., *Assessment of craniofacial pain and dysfunction: a multidisciplinary approach*, Cranio, 1990, 8:183–200.

Mongini F., Ventricelli F., Conserva E., *Etiology of cranio-facial pain and headache in stomatognathic disfunction*, in: Dubner R., Gebhart G.F., Bond M.R. (eds.), Proceedings of the Vth World Congress on Pain, Elsevier, Amsterdam, 1988, 512–519.

Mongini F., Ferla E., Maccagnani C., *MMPI profiles in patients with headache or craniofacial pain: a comparative study*, Cephalalgia, 1992, 12:91–98.

Mongini F., Rosso C., Gioria A., *Relation between tension-type headache and oromandibular dysfunction*, in: Olesen J. (ed.), *Tension-type headache: classification, mechanisms and treatment*, Raven Press, New York, 1993 a, 237–241.

Mongini F., Rocca R., Gioria A., Carpignano V., Ferla E., *Assessment of systemic factors and personality characteristic in tension-type headache and other types of facial pain*, in: Olesen J., *Tension-type headache: classification, mechanisms and treatment*, Raven Press, New York, 1993 b, 231–236.

Mongini F., Poma M., Bava M., Fabbri G., *Psychosomatic symptoms in different types of headache and facial pain*, Cephalalgia, 1997 a, 17:274 (abs.).

Mongini F., Defilippi N., Negro C., *Chronic daily headache. A clinical and psychological profile before and after treatment*, Headache, 1997 b, 37:83–87.

Mongini F., Ibertis F., Bava M., Negro C., *A psychological profile of migraine in women*, Cephalalgia, 1997 c, 17:260–261.

Olesen J., *Some clinical features of the acute migraine attack. An analysis of 750 patients*, Headache, 1978, 18:268–271.

Olesen J., *Clinical and pathophysiological observations in migraine and tension-type headache explained by integration of vascular, supraspinal and myofascial inputs*, Pain, 1991, 46:125–132.

Olesen J., *The International Headache Society classification and diagnostic criteria are valid and extremely useful*, Cephalalgia, 1996, 16:293–295.

Pfaffenrath V., Isler H., *Evaluation of the nasology of chronic tension-type headache*, Cephalalgia, 1993, 13, (Suppl. 12):60–62.

Rasmussen B.K., *Migraine and tension-type headache are separate disorders*, Cephalalgia, 1996, 217–223.

Sanin L.C., Mathew N.T., Bellmeyer L.R., Ali S., *The International Headache Society (IHS) headache classification as applied to a headache clinic population*, Cephalalgia, 1994, 14:443–446.

Sjaastad O., Stovner L.J., *The IHS classification for common migraine. Is it ideal?*, Headache, 1993, 33:372–375.

Sjaastad O., Saunte C, Hovdahl H., Breivik H., Gronbaek E., *"Cervicogenic" headache. An hypothesis*, Cephalalgia, 1983, 3:249–256.

Takeshima T., Takahashi K., *The relationship between muscle contraction headache and migraine: A multivariate analysis study*, Headache, 1988, 28:272–277.

Tfelt-Hansen P., Lous I, Olesen J., *Prevalence and significance of muscle tenderness during common migraine attacks*, Headache, 1981, 21:63–71.

Waters W.E., *The epidemiological enigma of migraine*, Int. J. Epidemiol., 1973, 2:189–194.

Part II General Clinical Aspects

10 Data Collection

General Principles

As we have seen (Chapters 1, 9), the taxonomic assessment of headache and facial pain is still controversial because different etiological factors, local and/or systemic, may be present in the same patient. Accordingly, data collection must be aimed at quantification and assessment of factors, and detection of their pathogenetic mechanisms: in this way, a correct diagnosis can be obtained.

To this end, two errors should be avoided. The first is to focus the attention mainly on one or only a few possible aspects of the problem and ignore the others. As a consequence, data collection might be very thorough for some aspects and inadequate for others. The criteria may be biased by the operator's own specialty.

The second error is the opposite of this, and consists of having each patient examined by a sequence of specialists and, consequently, of expanding data collection excessively. Moreover, it seems inappropriate to make a sharp dichotomy between patients suffering from headache of different types and patients with facial pain, the borderline between headache and facial pain often being unclear. Numerous patients suffer alternating headache and facial pain; or, both types of pain may be superimposed. And as we have seen in previous chapters, a number of factors may produce both headache and facial pain.

It is desirable that the specialist who deals routinely with patients with headache and/or facial pain should have the capacity to acquire all clinical data that might be of importance for diagnosis and treatment. For this reason, it is important to use a standard examination protocol that is sufficiently exhaustive. This protocol includes history, clinical examination, and the instrumental examinations that may be indicated.

Medical History

A systematic record of medical history is required to elicit all information that might be of diagnostic value. For this purpose we use a questionnaire with different sections, organized so that data can easily be fed into a computer. A yes/no system is largely employed, but space is also provided for comments or description.

The family history (Table 10.1) is particularly indicative in some cases, such as a history of migraine in the family of a headache patient.

The physiological history (and, for women, the gynecological history) (Tables 10.2, 10.3) may elicit information relating to possible systemic disorders or to other interfering factors (trauma at birth, smoking and drinking habits) that might interfere with the etiopathogenetic mechanisms of headache and facial pain.

With the remote and recent medical histories (Tables 10.4, 10.5), useful data are collected that may help in discriminating between the different pathologies. Migraine patients, for instance, frequently report previous acetonemia, kinetosis, cholitis, gastralgia, back pain, and tiredness. A hormone-

Table 10.1 Family history

Headache in family	☐	....
Circulation disorders	☐	....
Diabetes	☐	....
Hereditary diseases	☐	....

Table 10.2 Physiological history

Weight (kg)	....			
Height (cm)	....			
Blood pressure (min mmHg)	....			
Blood pressure (max mmHg)	....			
Born at term	☐	....		
Normal delivery	☐	....		
Breast feeding	☐	....		
Alcohol intake	☐ none	☐ little	☐ moderate	☐ abundant
Cigarettes per day	☐ none	☐ <5	☐ <10	
	☐ <20	☐ >20		

dependent migraine is frequently associated with hair and nail fragility (Mongini et al., 1997 a). Other symptoms, psychosomatic in character, such as anxiety, mood changes, sleep difficulty, bulimia, palpitations, panic attacks, etc., which are indicative of an anxiety or depressive disorder, are often found in patients with facial pain disorder as somatoform disorders, and in patients with chronic daily headache (Mongini et al., 1997 a, b). Parafunctional habits (tooth clenching and bruxing, nail biting, etc.) might be indicative, together with other data that will be collected later, of the presence of a myogenous facial pain (partly, at least).

An accurate history is then taken of past and present drug intake (Table 10.6) in relation to previous diseases and to the patient's actual problems.

With regard to headache or pain history, a section that describes extensively the onset, development and characteristics of symptomatology is preceeded by specific questions (Table 10.7). Further sections examine period of onset, characteristics, frequency, severity and duration of pain symptomatology, first localization and sites of spreading, factors that elicit, aggravate or improve the pain attacks; other symptoms that may precede, accompany or follow the attacks (Tables 10.8 to 10.13). If the patient suffers from headache and another type of facial pain, both questionnaires will be completed. In addition, at the first appointment the patient receives a headache/pain diary to be filled in on a daily basis. In this diary, the patient makes a precise record of times of day when pain is present, its duration and intensity, usage of drugs, and the relation of pain to life events and, in particular, to the menstrual cycle (Fig. 10.1). This diary is extremely important for a precise evaluation of the characteristics of the problem and, subsequently, the results of treatment.

Table 10.**3**   Gynecological history

First menstruation	Age			
Menstrual cycle	Rhythm	regular ☐	irregular ☐	variable ☐
Menstrual cycle	Intensity	scarce ☐	normal ☐	abundant ☐
Cycle duration	Days			
Duration of menses	Days			
Menstrual disorders	....			
Miscarriages	....			
Abortions	....			
Pregnancies at term	....			
Menopause	....			

Table 10.**4**   Remote medical history

Exanthematicus diseases	☐ ....
Acetonemia	☐ ....
Allergies	☐ ....
Rheumatic disease	☐ ....
Craniofacial trauma	☐ ....
Whiplash	☐ ....
Trauma to spinal column	☐ ....
Limb fractures	☐ ....
Hospitalization without surgery	☐ ....
Hospitalization with surgery	☐ ....
Depression	☐ ....
Others	☐ ....
Notes:	
....	
....	

Table 10.**6**   Past and present drug intake

Previous therapy

Benzodiazepines	☐ ....
Antidepressants	☐ ....
Anticonvulsants	☐ ....
Triptans	☐ ....
Other antimigraine drugs	☐ ....
NSAIDs	☐ ....
Cardiovascular	☐ ....
Estrogens/progesterones	☐ ....
Others	☐ ....

Current therapy

Benzodiazepines	☐ ....
Antidepressants	☐ ....
Anticonvulsants	☐ ....
Triptans	☐ ....
Other antimigraine drugs	☐ ....
NSAIDs	☐ ....
Cardiovascular	☐ ....
Estroprogestins	☐ ....
Others	☐ ....

Table 10.**5**   Recent medical history

Colitis	☐ ....
Gastritis	☐ ....
Kinetosis	☐ ....
Swallowing difficulty	☐ ....
Digestive problems	☐ ....
Anorexia	☐ ....
Bulimia	☐ ....
Anxiety	☐ ....
Phobias	☐ ....
Sleep disorders	☐ ....
Palpitation	☐ ....
Panic attacks	☐ ....
Mood changes	☐ ....
Fainting	☐ ....
Vertigo	☐ ....
Lassitude	☐ ....
Parafunctions	☐ ....
Clonus	☐ ....
Cramps	☐ ....
Paresthesias	☐ ....
Back pain	☐ ....
Urination disturbances	☐ ....
Diarrhea or constipation	☐ ....
Hair fragility	☐ ....
Nail fragility	☐ ....
Circulation disorders	☐ ....
Cold limbs	☐ ....
Frequent depressed moods	☐ ....
Other	☐ ....
Notes:	
....	

Female sexual disorders

Frigidity	☐ ....
Vaginism	☐ ....

Male sexual disorders

Impotence	☐ ....
Premature ejaculation	☐ ....

Table 10.**7**   History of headache and/or facial pain

| Time since onset | ☐ <1 month | ☐ >1 month | ☐ >6 months |
| | ☐ >1 year | ☐ >2 years | |

Other: ....

| Initial problem: | ☐ headache | ☐ facial pain |
| ☐ joint crepitation | ☐ mouth opening restriction | |

Other: ....

Symptoms worsening in:	☐ frequency
	☐ intensity
	☐ spreading of painful area

Indicate whether periods of remission occurred: ....

| Symptom changes in: | |
| ☐ quality | ☐ location |

Other associated conditions ☐ ....

Notes: ....
....
....

Tables 10.**8**   Headache characteristics

Age at onset	☐ prepubertal	☐ youth	☐ maturity	☐ presenil–senile (50–70)
Onset	☐ accessional	☐ continuous	☐ combined	☐ long remissions
Frequency of facial pain	☐ <1/month	☐ 1/month	☐ 2/month	
	☐ > 2/month	☐ > 1/week	☐ once or more a day	Notes: ....
Attack duration	☐ < 1 hour	☐ > 1 hour	☐ > 2 hours	
	☐ all day	☐ two or more days	☐ variable	Notes: ....

Attack intensity (score 1–5): ....

Period of presentation	☐ night	☐ day	☐ at awakening	☐ at a fixed time
Quality of pain	☐ piercing	☐ dull	☐ burning	
	☐ pulsing	☐ pressing		

Others: ....   VAS   0├──────────────────────────────┤100

Table 10.**9**   Headache location

Site of origin of pain:

	Right	Left	Unilateral	Bilateral	Unilateral alternating	Unilateral with further spreading
Frontal	☐	☐	☐	☐	☐	☐
Orbital	☐	☐	☐	☐	☐	☐
Parietal	☐	☐	☐	☐	☐	☐
Temporal	☐	☐	☐	☐	☐	☐
Vertex	☐	☐	☐	☐	☐	☐
Facial	☐	☐	☐	☐	☐	☐
Auricular mastoid	☐	☐	☐	☐	☐	☐
Pharyngopalatinal	☐	☐	☐	☐	☐	☐
Occipital	☐	☐	☐	☐	☐	☐

☐ Diffuse

☐ Further spreading ....

Table 10.10   Headache influencing factors

	Worsens	Improves
Standing	☐	☐
Lying	☐	☐
Chewing	☐	☐
Head movements	☐	☐
Sharp movements	☐	☐
Physical fatigue	☐	☐
Mental fatigue	☐	☐
Emotional stress	☐	☐
Working activity	☐	☐
Rest ("Sunday headache")	☐	☐
Cold	☐	☐
Wind	☐	☐
Warmth	☐	☐
Sun exposure	☐	☐
Menses	☐	☐
Pregnancy	☐	☐
Menopause	☐	☐
Diet	☐	☐
Hypertension	☐	☐
Alcohol	☐	☐
Smoking	☐	☐
Enclosed evironment	☐	☐
Sexual intercourse	☐	☐
Other factors	☐	☐

Notes: ....

Table 10.11   Characteristics of migraine aura

Lack of well-being	☐
Dysosmia–hyperosmia	☐
Perceptive distortion	☐
Depression	☐
Excitement	☐
Vertigo	☐
Visual disorders	☐
Scotoma	☐
Insomnia–hyposomnia	☐
Hypersomnia	☐

Table 10.12   Symptoms accompanying or following attacks

Neurovegetative

Nausea	☐
Vomiting	☐
Intestinal hyperperistalsis	☐
Constipation	☐
Polyuria	☐
Oliguria	☐
Insomina	☐
Hyposomnia	☐
Hypersomnia	☐
Sweating	☐
Cold sensation	☐
Shivering	☐
Fever	☐
Bernard–Horner	☐
Paresthesias	☐

Cardiocirculatory

Palpitations	☐
Pulsation and/or dilation of large vessels	☐
Palor	☐
Hypotension	☐
Hypertension	☐
Lacrimation	☐
Rhinorrhea	☐
Epistaxis	☐
Periorbital edema	☐
Conjunctival injection	☐

Sensory and intellective

Tinnitus	☐
Noise hyperesthesia	☐
Light hyperesthesia	☐
Visual disturbances	☐
Hyperosmia	☐
Dysosmia	☐
Movement intolerance	☐
Vertigo	☐
Difficulty in concentrating	☐
Memory disturbance	☐

Phenomena at the end of an attack

Sleep disorders	☐
Urination disorders	☐
Sweating	☐
Diarrhea	☐
Hypotension–lassitude	☐
Unusual appetite	☐

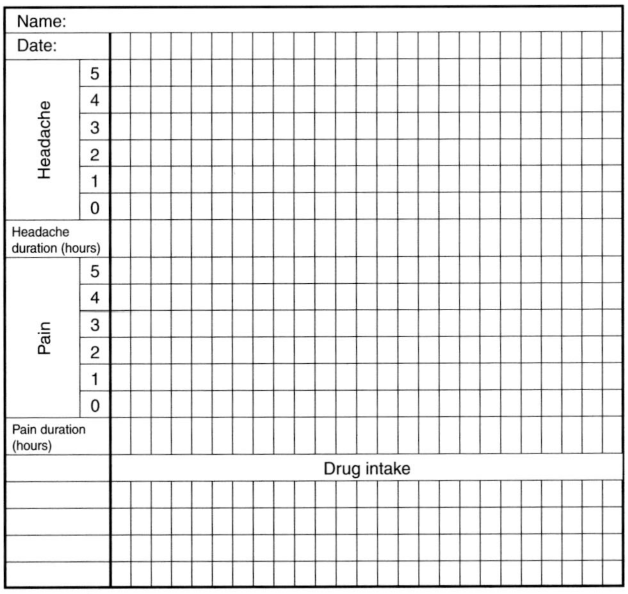

◀ Fig. 10.1   Daily diary of headache and/or pain levels

Table 10.**13**   Characteristics of facial pain

Onset	☐ < 1 month	☐ < 6 months	☐ < 1 year	☐ < 2 years	
	☐ > 2 years				
Location:					
Praeauricular area		☐ initial location	☐ spreading		
Zygomatic and cheek area		☐ initial location	☐ spreading		
Mandibular–submandibular area		☐ initial location	☐ spreading		
Nuchal area		☐ initial location	☐ spreading		
Symptom laterality	☐ unilateral right	☐ unilateral left	☐ bilateral	☐ diffuse	☐ unilateral alternating
Type of pain	☐ pressing	☐ piercing	☐ pulsating	☐ burning	
	☐ dull	☐ lancinating	☐ other		
Intensity of VAS pain	☐ very mild	☐ mild	☐ moderate	☐ severe	☐ excruciating
	0 ├———————————————————————————————┤ 100				
Frequency of facial pain	☐ < 1/month	☐ 1/month	☐ 2/month		
	☐ > 2/month	☐ > 1/week	☐ once or more a day	Notes:	
Duration of facial pain	☐ > 1 hour	☐ > 1 hour	☐ > 2 hours		
	☐ all day	☐ two or more days	☐ variable	Notes:	
Pain during extended mandibular movement		☐ sometimes	☐ often	☐ always	
Chewing pain		☐ sometimes	☐ often	☐ always	
Day period in which pain begins		☐ anytime	☐ after awakening	☐ mornings	

Factors influencing pain

Chewing	☐ worsens	☐ improves
Phonation	☐ worsens	☐ improves
Menses	☐ worsens	☐ improves
Stress	☐ worsens	☐ improves
Cold weather	☐ worsens	☐ improves
Wind	☐ worsens	☐ improves
Warm weather	☐ worsens	☐ improves
Sun exposure	☐ worsens	☐ improves
Other:		

Phenomena accompanying pain

Nausea	☐	Noise hyperesthesia	☐	
Vomiting	☐	Light hyperesthesia	☐	
Lacrimation	☐	Visual disorders	☐	
Conjunctival injection	☐	Other accompanying factors	☐	

Patient Examination

Most patients who turn to a specialist for chronic headache and facial pain have already been examined at regular intervals by their general practitioner. In these cases, the clinical examination will start with inspection of the patient in a standing position (for posture and spinal column disorders) (Fig. 10.**2**), followed by inspection of nutritional state (Fig. 10.**3**), of skin characteristics (Figs. 10.**4**, 10.**5**), of the scalp, of the extremities (Fig. 10.**6**) and of facial expression (Fig. 10.**7**), measurement of pulse and blood pressure. Simple tests will detect any ligament laxity (Fig. 10.**8**). Subsequently, a complete neurological examination should be made, paying great attention to motor and sensory functions of the cranial nerves and to the presence, if any, of Claude Bernard – Horner syndrome. A positive Romberg test (that is, instability on standing with closed eyes) is a relatively common finding in a population of patients suffering from headache or facial pain.

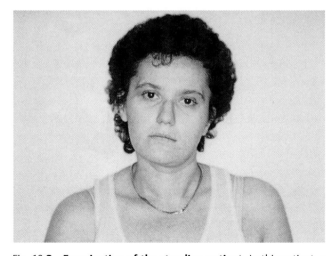

Fig. 10.**2** **Examination of the standing patient.** In this patient, a serious postural defect of the shoulders, neck and head is observed

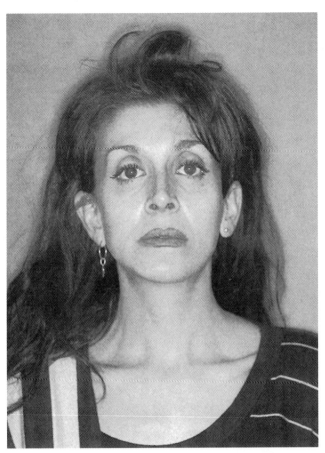

Fig. 10.**3** Ill appearance of patient with a history of anorexia and bulimia

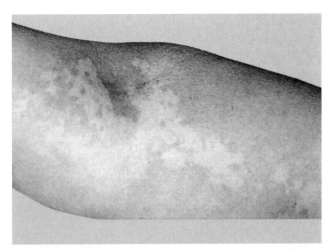

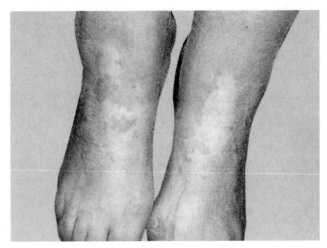

Fig. 10.**4** **Vitiligo which had appeared in a patient during an unwanted pregnancy some years prior to observation.** At the same time, tension-type headache and facial pain disorder appeared

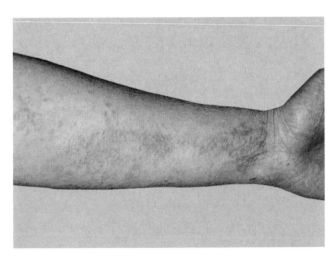

Fig. 10.**5** Bullate dermatitis in a patient suffering from chronic craniofacial pain

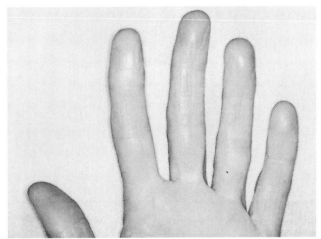

Fig. 10.**6** Typical aspect of the fingers of a patient suffering from rheumatoid arthritis

If positive, this test is repeated, after asking the patient to try to recognize a number traced on his forehead with the finger, while his eyes are closed. An improved stability of posture may indicate that the positive test is of "psychogenic" rather than neurological origin.

Subsequently, craniofacial structures and neck are examined. This consists of inspection, palpation and auscultation. At inspection, the reciprocal position of head, neck, and

shoulders, and the degree of rotation, flection, and antero-postero extension and lateral flexion of the head, are observed (Figs. 10.**9**, 10.**10**).

The patient's face is then examined for any craniofacial asymmetry, swellings and signs of muscle hyperparafunction, such as muscular hypertrophy (Fig. 10.**11**), marked tooth abrasion (Fig. 10.**12**), or scalloped tongue margins (Fig. 10.**13**). A particular type of abrasion is sometimes seen in patients who

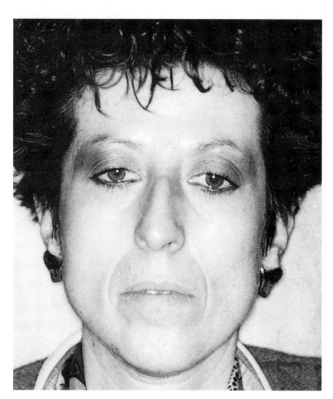

Fig. 10.**7**   Facial expression of a depressed patient

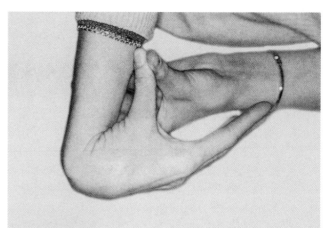

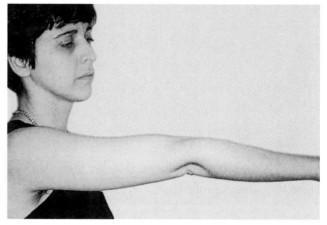

Fig. 10.**8**   Test to detect ligament laxity

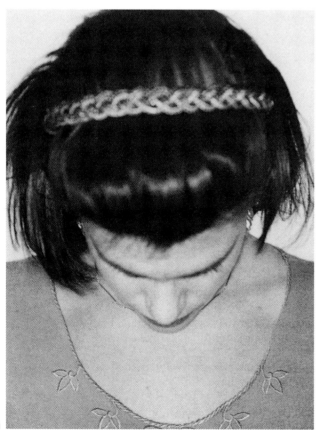

a

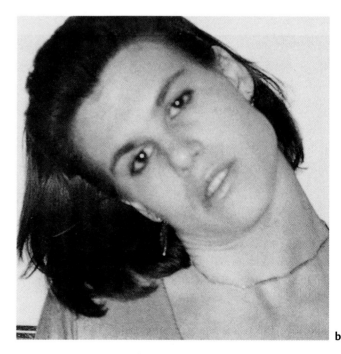

b

Fig. 10.**9**   Examination of free flexion movements of the head forward (**a**) and laterally (**b**)

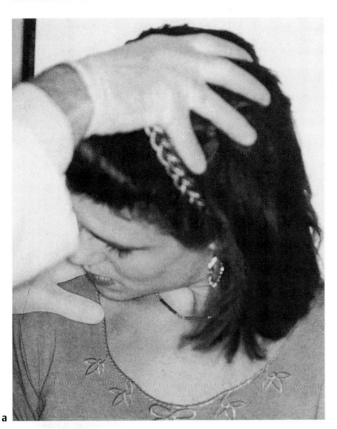
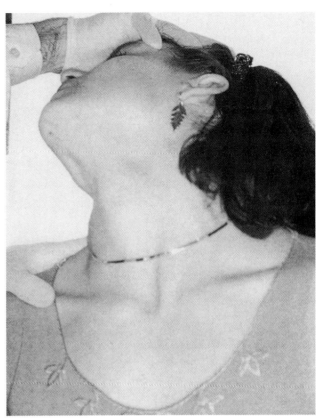

a

b

Fig. 10.**10**   Examination of the degree of maximum rotation of the head at flexion (**a**) and extension (**b**)

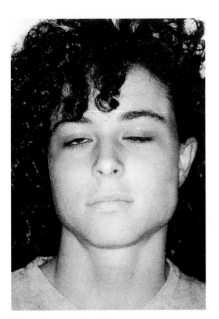
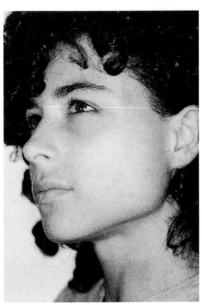

Fig. 10.**11**   Marked unilateral hypertrophy of the left masseter consequent on parafunction in a young woman patient with tension-type headache and myogenous pain

alternate periods of anorexia with periods of bulimia involving frequent vomiting (Fig. 10.**14**).

Extension and characteristics of free jaw movements are then inspected (opening, closing, laterality, and protrusion) (Fig. 10.**15**). The position of the mandible in postural position and at maximum tooth clenching is then examined, to detect any mandibular deviation along the frontal plane from one position to another (Fig. 10.**16**).

By palpation, painful points of cranial nerves are sought where they emerge, at specific points of the cranium, and of craniofacial and neck muscles. The points of nerve emergence

and the cranial points are palpated bilaterally by applying moderate pressure with the tips of the index fingers. For the nerves, the sites examined are: the supraorbital point, the infraorbital foramen and the mental foramen (Fig. 10.**17**) (sites of emergence of the three trigeminal branches); the incisal foramen (emergence of nasopalatine nerve); and the major palatine foramen (where the palatine nerves emerge). The cranial points examined are: the retroauricular point, the lateral poles of the condyle, the posterior zone of the condyle (explored with open mouth) (Fig. 10.**18**), and the external auditory meatus. This last is palpated with the tip of the little finger (Fig. 10.**19**).

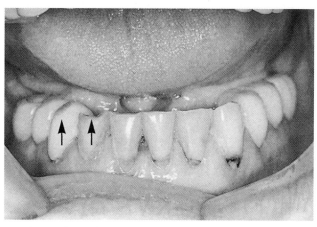

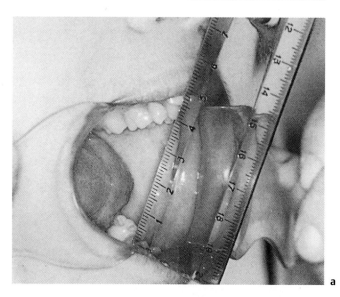

Fig. 10.**12**   The marked asymmetrical abrasion of the teeth (arrows) shows the presence of bruxism movements predominantly on the right side

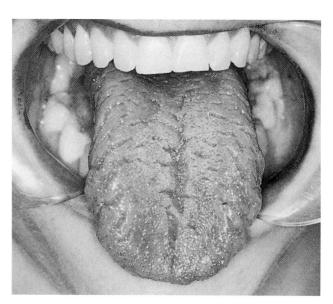

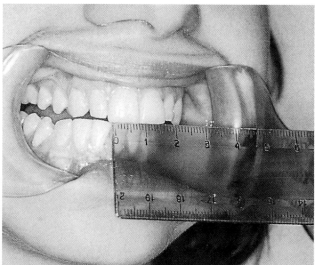

Fig. 10.**13**   Markedly scallopped tongue margins consequent on tongue compression against the teeth at night

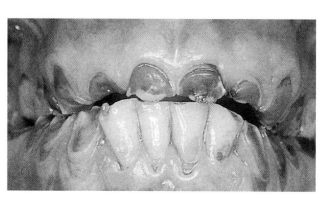

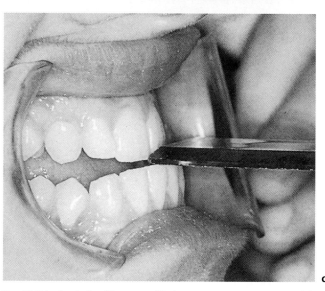

Fig. 10.**14**   **Same patient as Fig. 10.3.** Extreme and characteristic tooth abrasion in patient with prior history of anorexia

Fig. 10.**15**   Analysis of free mandibular movements at opening (**a**), laterally (**b**), and in protrusion (**c**)

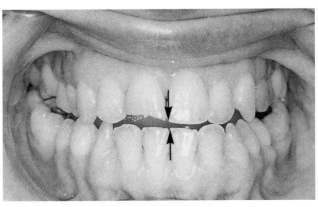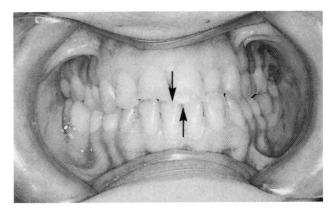

Fig. 10.**16** Marked deviation of the mandible on the frontal plane on closing mouth from the position of initial tooth contact (**a**) to the position of maximum closure (**b**) (arrows)

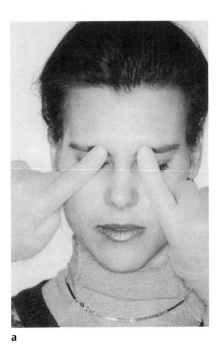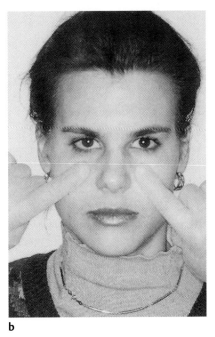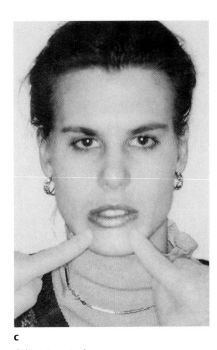

a   b   c

Fig. 10.**17** Palpation of points of emergence of the first (**a**), second (**b**), and third (**c**) branches of the trigeminal nerve

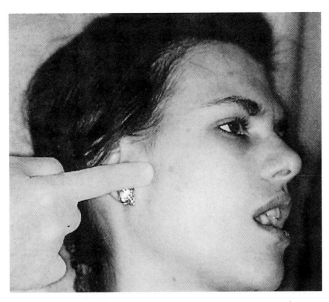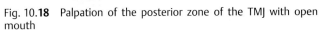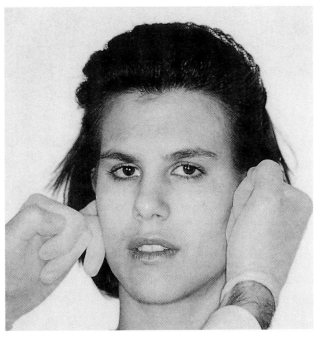

Fig. 10.**18** Palpation of the posterior zone of the TMJ with open mouth

Fig. 10.**19** Palpation of the external auditory meatus

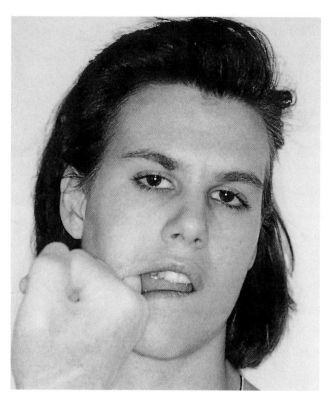

Fig. 10.**20**   Palpation of the lateral pterygoid muscle

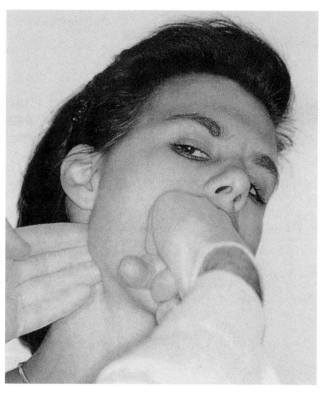

Fig. 10.**21**   Palpation of the medial pterygoid musle

Palpation of the masticatory muscles requires some experience: it must be neither too light nor too energetic. To avoid excessive positive findings, the examiner must consider that palpation, particularly of the intraoral muscles, always causes some discomfort to the patient. The lateral pterygoid muscle is palpated by sliding the little finger upward and backward between the tuber maxillae and the ascending ramus of the mandible (Fig. 10.**20**). Pain provoked by this maneuver provides valuable information, though there is doubt whether, in doing this, the lateral pterygoid muscle is in fact palpated. Palpation of the medial pterygoid muscle is done two-handed: the index finger of one hand is slid inside the mouth toward the corner of the mandible, downward and backward while with the fingers of the other hand slight pressure is applied from outside in the same region (Fig. 10.**21**). Palpation of the masseter muscle is also carried out two-handed. The fingers of both hands are slid in a posteroanterior direction on the mid-zone of the belly of the muscle inside and outside the mouth (Fig. 10.**22**). The patient may then be asked to clench hard on his teeth while his muscles are palpated on either side from outside the mouth (Fig. 10.**23**). The temporal muscle is palpated in two steps: the mandibular head is palpated by running the index upward along the anterior margin of the mandibular ramus toward the muscle's insertion into the coronoid process of the mandible. Ex-

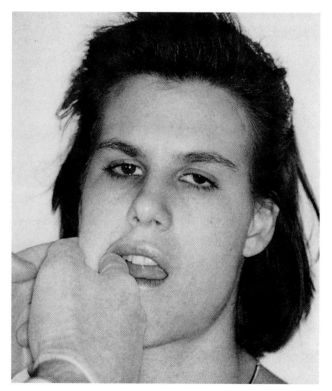

Fig. 10.**22**   Palpation of the masseter muscle

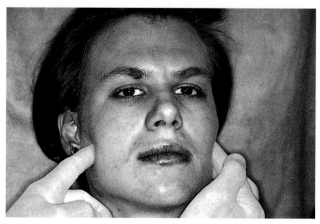

Fig. 10.**23**   Extraoral bilateral palpation of the masseter muscles

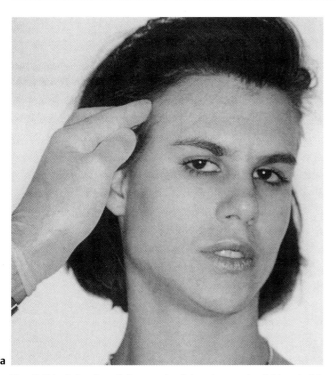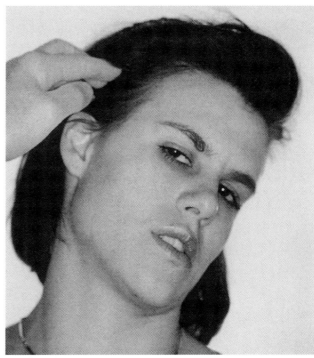

Fig. 10.**24**   Palpation of the anterior (**a**) and posterior (**b**) head of the temporal muscle

tracranial palpation of the anterior, median and posterior heads of the muscle follows, in the cranial insertion zone (Fig. 10.**24**). The muscles of the floor of the mouth are palpated by running the index finger anteroposteriorly along the lower margin of the mandible and at the same time applying light extraoral pressure in the same region with the fingers of the other hand.

Palpation of the cervical muscle is important, particularly if posture problems and trigger points are present. Palpation of the sternocleidomastoid muscle is performed after asking the patient to contract the muscle by rotating his or her head towards the opposite side and slightly upward. If necessary one may ask the patient to exert pressure against the clinician's hand that opposes the head movement. The muscle

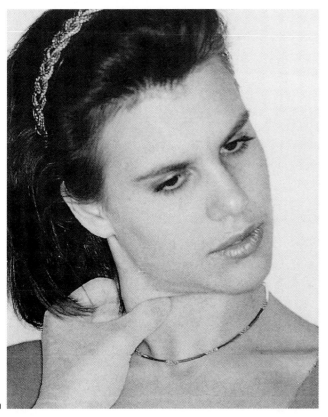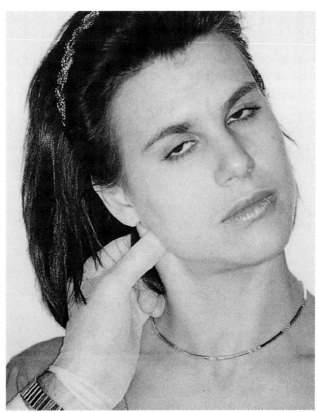

Fig. 10.**25**   Palpation of the belly (**a**) and the cranial insertion (**b**) of the sternocleidomastoid muscle

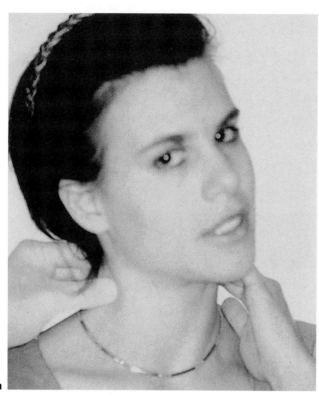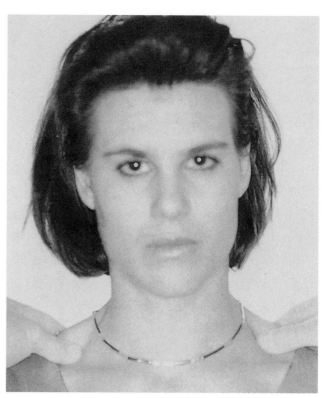

a   b

Fig. 10.**26**   Palpation of the trapezius muscle at the neck (**a**) and at the shoulder (**b**)

belly is palpated by pinching it between the fingers (Fig. 10.**25a**); then the cranial insertion is also palpated (Fig. 10.**25b**). The index finger is then run along the muscle to explore the presence of tender points or taut bands, which are felt as more consistent sites under the skin and are extremely painful at palpation. The patient is asked whether the maneuver causes pain at a distance as well as beneath the finger (referred pain: see Chapter 3). The trapezius muscle is then palpated along the neck and the shoulder (Fig. 10.**26**). Tender or trigger points are often found in this muscle too. Finally the nuchal muscles are palpated simultaneously on both sides, by running the fingers from up to down and exerting moderate pressure on the spinal processes of the vertebrae (Fig. 10.**27**).

Auscultation of articular noises is carried out with a phonendoscope without membrane (Fig. 10.**28**) (to avoid the superimposition of skin noises). The characteristics, intensity and moment of occurrence of articular noises during mouth

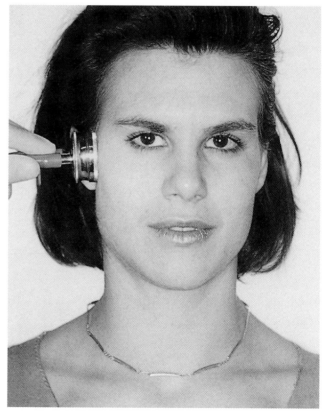

Fig. 10.**27**   Palpation of the nuchal muscles

Fig. 10.**28**   Auscultation of articular noises using a phonendoscope without membrane

opening and closing are noted. Essentially there are three types of articular noise: clicking, popping, and crepitation. The click is a sharp noise, varying in intensity (it may only be audible on auscultation with the phonendoscope or it may be audible at a distance), occurring on one side (more rarely it is bilateral) during mouth opening. Depending on the point at which it occurs, it is classified as early click, mid-opening and late click. It indicates disk displacement with reduction and takes place at the point when the disk suddenly moves backwards from a displaced position into a normal position during mouth opening (see Chapter 22). During closing, there is a second click (reciprocal click) due to the forward displacement of the disk during that movement. This click is in general very much less intense than the opening one, and occurs with the jaw more nearly closed than does the opening click. On inviting the patient to open his mouth and close it in a protruded position, with the incisors edge-to-edge and subsequently to make an opening and closing movement in this position, the click disappears. This is because on opening the mouth the disk returns to the correct position (causing the click) and is then held there by the protruded position of the mandible. The "popping" noise consists of a sequence of small clicking noises of the membraneous type which occur during the entire opening and closing movement, or a good part of it. This noise is produced by changes in shape of the articular heads and of the disk and does not disappear if the opening movement starts from a protruded position. Lastly, the crepitation noise which is produced during opening and closing is practically pathognomonic of arthrotic degeneration of the TMJ tissues.

Instrumental Analysis

After examination of the patient in the way described, the request for further laboratory tests should be evaluated carefully. In the management of chronic pain patients, a source of

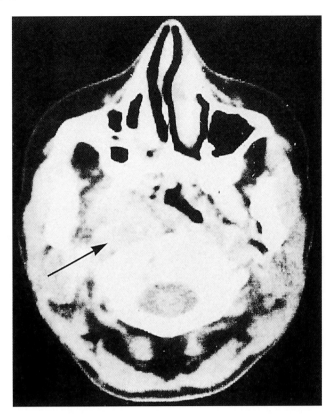

Fig. 10.**29 Young woman patient who had suffered occasional episodes of limited mouth opening.** CT scan showed the presence of a highly invasive craniopharyngioma (arrow)

confusion arises from frequent discrepancy of opinion as to what clinical and laboratory findings are necessary and sufficient (Rudy et al., 1988). This is particularly true for patients with headache and facial pain. Indeed, frequently patients

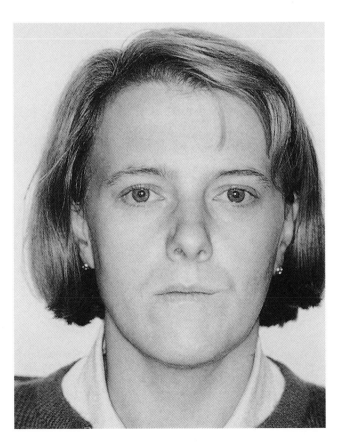

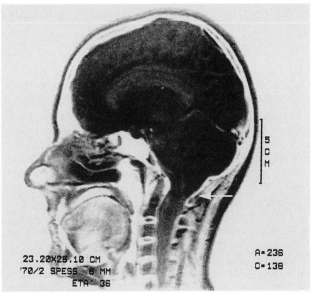

Fig. 10.**30** A patient who presented episodes of **pain of the left hemiface and spasms of the facial muscles** on the same side (**a**). Nuclear magnetic resonance (**b**) revealed an Arnold–Chiari syndrome with impingment of the cerebellar tonsil in the foramen magnum (arrow). Since there were also signs of involvement of the long pathways, it may be presumed that this finding was also responsible for the craniofacial symptomatology (although this is not typical of the syndrome)

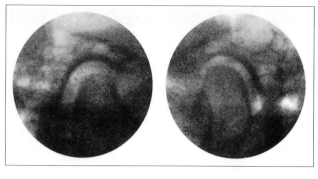

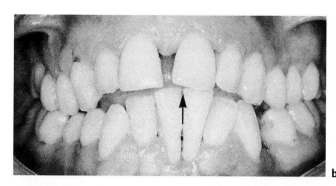

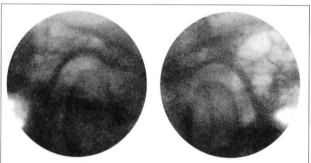

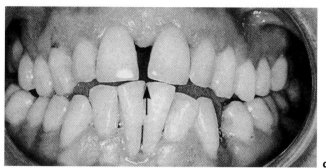

Fig. 10.31 Patient with right TMJ disk displacement without reduction. a Transcranial radiogram of the TMJ. Note that to the left the articular space is reduced. **b** The mandible in closed position appears deviated to the left (arrow). **c** Transcranial radiogram of the TMJ of the same patient after reduction of the disk displacement through manipulation of the mandible: the left articular space is now normal. **d** After reduction of the disk displacement, the mandible position has also changed

with a long history of severe and chronic headache or facial pain are subjected to many complex and costly examinations without obtaining consistent information. In headache patients, although some tests seem to give different results in tension-type headache and migraine (see Chapter 5), no instrumental analysis allows a definite differential diagnosis.

Instrumental tests in these patients will be requested to exclude headache or facial pain being specific pathologies – tumors in particular.

Thus, in a patient with a headache of recent onset, moderate or severe in intensity, especially if positive signs are observed at neurological examination, an EEG should be the examination of first choice, followed by computerized tomography (CT) (Fig. 10.29) and/or MRI, as needed (Fig. 10.30). However, if headache has been present for a long time (years) and neurological examination is completely negative, laboratory tests, if any, may be limited to a routine blood test, often already requested by the general doctor. EEG will also be performed in presence of facial pain with tonic-clonic muscle contraction for which an epilepsy is suspected (see Chapter 21). When a primary muscle disease or a peripheral neuropathy is suspected, appropriate laboratory tests (such as EMG and conduction velocity analysis) will be requested. Specific tests will be also requested for the suspicion that the craniofacial pain might be an expression of a general disease, such as rheumatic fever or autoimmune disease.

If the clinical examination reveals an intracapsular TMJ problem, TMJ radiography will be performed (transcranial plain radiographs and/or tomography or magnetic resonance imaging, MRI) (Figs. 10.31–10.33). Similarly, in the presence of postural disorders with muscle pain and trigger points in the neck and shoulder region, a radiographic examination of the cervical spine will be performed, in anteroposterior,

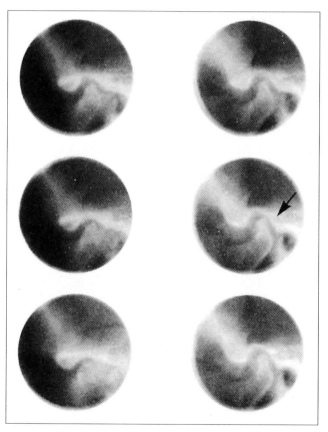

Fig. 10.32 Polytomography of the left temporomandibular joint in a patient with disk displacement without reduction. Note the flattening and concavity of the posterior surface of the condyle (arrow)

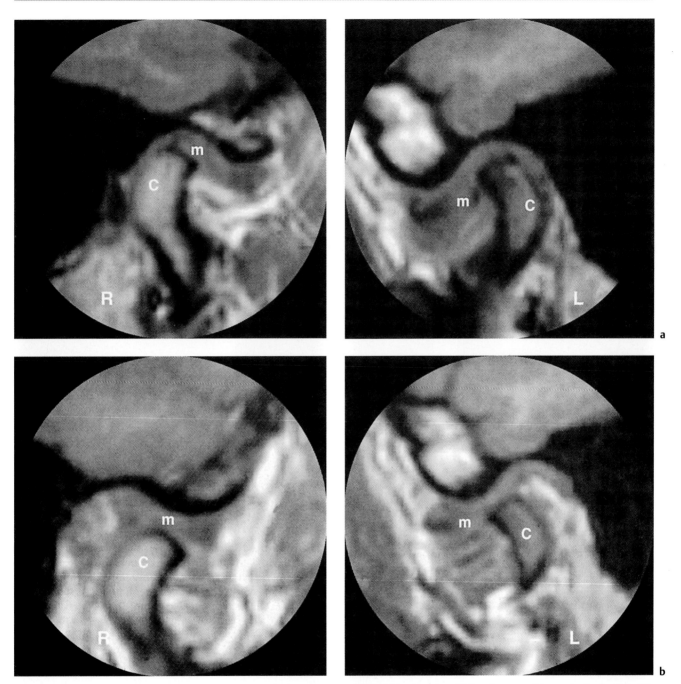

Fig. 10.**33 Nuclear magnetic resonance imaging of the temporomandibular joint with left disk displacement without reduction.** On the left (L) the disc (m) appears displaced forward of the condyle (c) both at closed (**a**) and at open (**b**) mouth. On the right (R), the disk-condyle relationships are normal in both situations

lateral and, possibly, oblique projections (Fig. 10.**34**). In addition, the atlanto-occipital relationship will be evaluated with a radiograph taken with open mouth (Fig. 10.**35**). Attention will be paid to signs of arthrotic degeneration, of disk space and foramen reduction and, in addition, to loss or inversion of the cervical curve, and first or second vertebrae rotation.

As we have seen (Chapters 1 and 8), facial pain in some patients may be conversive and represent only one aspect of a *somatoform disorder.* In such cases the symptomatology is often multifocal and variable in nature and, especially if the patient is a young woman, multiple sclerosis may reasonably be suspected. It is an obvious task of the physician to exclude such a possibility before making the diagnosis of somatoform pain disorder by requesting the appropriate laboratory tests.

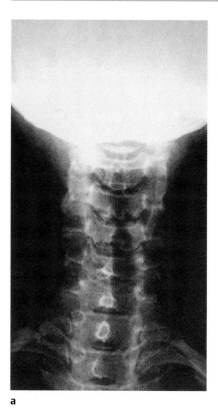
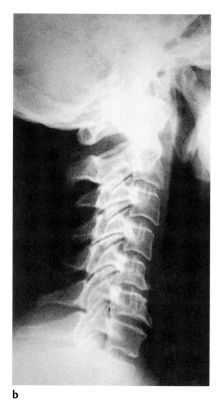
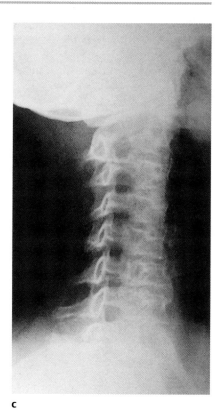

a   b   c

Fig. 10.34 Radiological examination of the cervical spine in anteroposterior (**a**), lateral (**b**), and oblique (**c**) projections. Scoliosis is visible (**a**) as well as loss of lordosis (**b**) and a slight restriction of some intervertebral foramina (**c**)

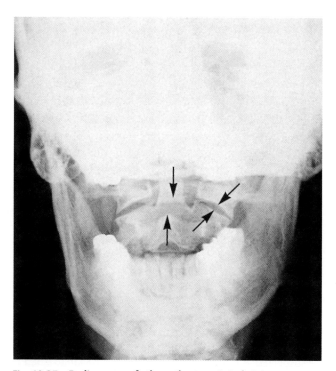

Fig. 10.35 Radiogram of the atlantooccipital joint at open mouth. Note that the tooth of the axis appears eccentric, and the atlantoaxial space is restricted at the left (arrows). This shows an alteration of the reciprocal position of the first two cervical vertebrae

Psychometric Tests and Pain Level Assessment

As already seen (Chapter 8), numerous psychometric tests have been used to assess the personality characteristics in patients with chronic pain (among others the *Beck Depression Inventory,* the *Eysenck Personality Inventory,* the *Hamilton Depression Inventory,* the *Minnesota Multiple Personality Inventory* (MMPI) and the *Spielberg State-Trait Anxiety Inventory* (STAI). A further instrument, the *West Haven – Yale multidimensional Pain Inventory* (MPI) (Kerns et al., 1985; Turk and Rudy, 1988, 1990) aims at multiaxial classification of pain by integrating data relating to psychosocial factors with those obtained from the clinical and instrumental analysis. This system quantifies the patient pain evaluation, the impact of pain on the different aspects of his or her life and the frequency with which specific behavioral strategies are employed as a consequence of pain.

The MMPI (Hathaway and McKinley, 1940) is probably the most widely used instrument in the assessment of personality factors contributing to the experience of chronic pain (Sternbach, 1974; Fordyce, 1976, 1987; Bradley et al., 1978; Armentrout et al., 1982; Bernstein and Garbin, 1983; Mc Gill et al., 1983; Bradley and Van der Heide, 1984; Hart, 1984; McCreary, 1985; Guck et al., 1988). Depending on the answers (true – false) given to a large number of questions, a score is given to three validity scales (L = lie, F = frequency, K = correction or defence) and 10 clinical scales: Hs = hypochondria, D = depression, Hy = hysteria, Pd = psychopathological deviation, Mf = masculinity – femininity, Ps = paranoia, Pt = psychasthenia, Sc = schizophrenia, Ma = hypomania, Si = social introversion.

Various MMPI typologies based on characterizing algorithms have been proposed by several authors (Bradley et al.,

1978; Prokop et al., 1980; Snyder and Power, 1981; Armentrout et al., 1982; Bernstein and Garbin, 1983; McGill et al., 1983; Hart, 1984; McCreary, 1985; Costello et al., 1987; Swimmer et al., 1992). Basically, four types were distinguished in different chronic pain patient populations (Sternbach, 1974; Costello et al., 1987; Wade et al., 1992): one type with the *conversive V* profile (with Hs and Hy above a score of 70 and D being at least 10 points lower) (Fig. 10.**36**); a second type with elevation of the *neurotic triad* (HS, D, Hy) with no other scale being consistently elevated above 70 (Fig. 10.**37**); a third type of *emotionally overwhelmed* patients with scale elevation of the neurotic triad and several other scales (Fig. 10.**38**); and lastly a fourth type (the *coper*) with a normal profile (Fig. 10.**39**). Despite some criticisms having been raised about the adequacy and risks of misinterpretation of some scales (Lienert, 1969, quoted by Franz et al., 1986; Moore et al., 1988),

the MMPI has been used widely to investigate the personality of patients with headache and other types of facial pain.

More recently this instrument has been revised and adapted to accommodate the sociocultural changes and changes of life habits that had made some items obsolete. This new instrument was released as the MMPI-2 (Butcher et al., 1989 a, b; Keller and Butcher, 1991); Butcher et al. (1989 a, b), using the MMPI-2 items have further elaborated 15 *content scales*: anxiety (ANX), fear (FRS), obsessivity (OBS), depression (DEP), health concern (HEA), bizarre ideas (BIZ), anger (ANG), cynism (CYN), antisocial behavior (ASP), hypermotivation, impatience and irritability (TPA), low self-esteem (LSE), social disability (SOD), family problems (FAM), working difficulties (WRK), and treatment difficulty indicators (TRT) (Figs. 10.**40**, 10.**41**). The MMPI-2 was also applied in chronic pain patient populations (Keller and Butcher, 1991).

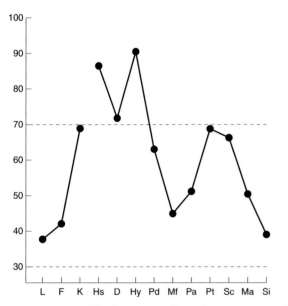

Fig. 10.**36** MMPI profile of a patient suffering from migraine and facial pain disorder. A typical "conversive V" may be seen, with scores for hypochondria (Hs) and hysteria (Hy) above 70 and a point of depression (D) which is high, but lower than the other two neurotic scales

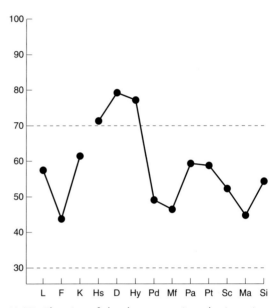

Fig. 10.**37** Elevation of the three neurotic scales in patients with chronic tension-type headache

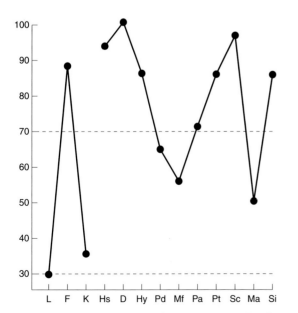

Fig. 10.**38** Elevation of the score of the neurotic triad and numerous other scales in a patient suffering from chronic daily headache

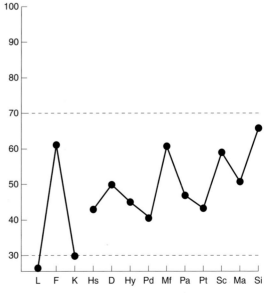

Fig. 10.**39** Normal MMPI profile of a patient suffering from migraine

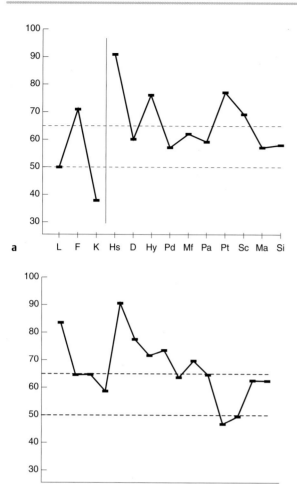

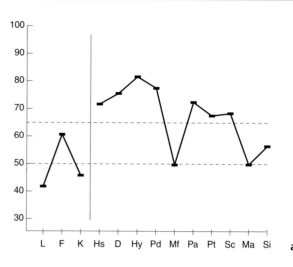

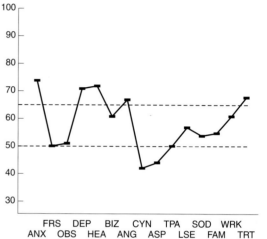

Fig. 10.**40 Woman patient with acute daily migraine attacks and intercritical tension-type headache. a** The MMPI-2 shows a typical conversive V, elevation of the anxiety scale (Pt), and a tendency to autism (Sc). **b** Content scales are high for anxiety (ANX), health concern (HEA), and bizarre ideas (BIZ). Further explanations are given in the text

Fig. 10.**41 Woman patient with constant myogenous pain of the neck. a** The MMPI-2 shows elevation of the majority of the scales. **b** Content scales are high for anxiety (ANX), depression (DEP), health concern (HEA), anger (ANG), and possible treatment difficulties (TRT)

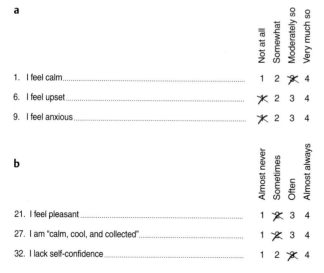

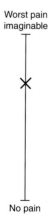

Fig. 10.**42**   Example of STAI items to assess state (**a**) and trait (**b**) anxiety.

Fig. 10.**43**   Visual analogue scale of a patient with craniofacial pain of medium-high intensity

The Spielberg State and Trait Anxiety Inventory (STAI) is also a widely used instrument for assessing the degree of anxiety. This test was originally employed on *normal* subjects, but over time it has come to be employed on different patient populations. It consists of two groups of 20 statements each that describe situations the subject defines as corresponding or not corresponding to his or her own situation, either at the moment when the test is performed (state anxiety) or "usually" (trait) (Spielberg et al., 1970) (Fig. 10.**42**).

Pain measurement techniques may basically be verbal or nonverbal. The most widely used nonverbal technique is the visual analogue scale (VAS). Patients are asked to assess the level of their pain by placing a mark on a vertical or horizontal line 10 cm long at an appropriate distance between the two endpoints (corresponding to no pain and most intense pain imaginable, respectively) (Fig. 10.**43**). This technique has proved to be a valid means of assessing clinical and experimental pain (Woodforde and Merskey, 1972; Joyce et al., 1975; Ohnhaus and Adler, 1975; Revill et al., 1976; Scott and Huskisson, 1976; Aun et al., 1986; Duncan et al., 1989). However, it allows only a one-dimensional assessment of pain, although some modifications have been proposed to distinguish between the sensory and objective components of pain (Price and Harkins, 1987).

Verbal pain assessment techniques aim to quantify pain in more than just the intensity dimension. By far the best-known and most widely employed verbal methodology is the McGill Pain Questionnaire (MPQ) (Melzack, 1975; Dubuisson and Melzack, 1976; Chen and Treede, 1985; Melzack, 1985). This instrument has been used to evaluate various types of facial pain (Grushka and Sessle, 1984; Melzack et al., 1986; Jerome et al., 1988; Harkins et al., 1991; Turp et al., 1997). It consists of 20 sets of qualitative and quantitative verbal descriptions designed to measure the sensory, affective, evaluative and mixed dimensions of pain (Fig. 10.**44**). Two indexes are calculated: the *pain rating index*, which is obtained by summing the values given to each verbal description chosen by the patient and which is calculated for each of the above dimensions, and the present pain intensity, which measures the overall pain intensity on a scale from 0 to 5.

References

Armentrout D.P., Moore J.E., Parker J.C., Hewett J.E., Feltz C., *Pain-patient MMPI subgroups: The psychological dimensions of pain*, J. Behav. Med., 1982, 5; 201–211.

Aun C., Lam Y.M., Collett B., *Evaluation of the use of visual analogue scale in Chinese patients*, Pain, 1986, 25 : 215–222.

Bernstein I., Garbin C., *Hierarchical clustering of pain patients' MMPI profiles: a replication note*, J. Pers. Assess., 1983, 47 : 171–172.

Bradley L.A., Prokop C.K., Margolis R., Gentry W.D., *Multivariate analysis of the MMPI profiles of low back pain patients*, J. Behav. Med., 1978, 1 : 253–272.

Bradley, L.A., Van der Heide L.H., *Pain-related correlates of MMPI profile subgroups among back pain patients*, Health Psychol., 1984, 3 : 157–174.

Butcher J.N., Dahlstrom W.G., Graham J.R., Tellegen A., Kaemmer B., *Manual for the restandardized Minnesota Multiphasic Personality Inventory: MMPI-2. An administrative and interpretive guide*. University of Minnesota Press, Minneapolis, MN, 1989.

Butcher J.N., Graham J.R., Williams C.I., Ben-Porath Y.S., *Development and use of the MMPI-2 content scales*, Minnesota University Press, Minneapolis, MN, 1989 b.

Chen A.C.N., Treede R.-D., *The McGill Pain Questionnaire in the assessment of phasic and tonic experimental pain: behavioral evaluation of the ›pain inhibiting pain' effect*, Pain, 1985, 22 : 67–79.

Costello R.M., Hulsey T.L., Schoenfeld L.S., Ramamurthy S.P-A-I-N: a four-cluster MMPI typology for chronic pain, Pain, 1987, 30 : 199–209.

Dubuisson D., Melzack R., *Classification of clinical pain descriptions by multiple group discriminant analysis*, Exp. Neurol., 1976, 51 : 480–487.

Duncan G.H., Bushnell C., Lavigne G.J., *Comparison of verbal and visual analogue scales for measuring the intensity and unpleasantness of experimental pain*, Pain, 1989, 37 : 295–303.

Fordyce W.E., *Behavioral methods for chronic pain and illness*, Mosby, St Louis, MO, 1976.

Fordyce W.E., *Use of the MMPI with chronic pain patients*, Paper given at the 9 th International Conference on Personality Assessment, Brussel, 1987.

Grushka M., Sessle B.J., *Applicability of the Mc-Gill Pain Questionnaire to the differentiation of ›toothache' pain*, Pain, 1984, 19 : 49–57.

Guck T., Meilman P., Skultery F., Poloni L., *Pain-patient Minnesota Multiphasic Personality Inventory (MMPI) subgroups: evaluation of longterm treatment outcome*, J. Behav. Med., 1988, 11 : 159–169.

Harkins S.W., Bush F.M., Price D.D., Hamer R.M., *Symptom report in orofacial pain patients: relation to chronic pain, experimental pain, illness behavior, and personality*, Clin. J. Pain, 1991, 7 : 102–113.

Hart R., *Chronic pain: replicated multivariate clustering of personality profiles*, J. Clin. Psychol., 1984, 40 : 129–133.

Hathaway S.R., McKinley J.C., *A multiphasic personality schedule (Minnesota): I. Construction of the schedule*, J. Psychol., 1940, 10 : 249–254.

Jerome A., Holroyd K.A., Theofanous A.G., Pingel J.D., Lake A.E., Saper J.R., *Cluster headache pain vs. other vascular headache pain: differences revealed with two approaches to the McGill Pain Questionnaire*, Pain, 1988, 34 : 35–42.

Joyce C.R.B., Zutshi D.W., Hrubes V., Mason R.M., *Comparison of fixed interval and visual analogue scales for rating chronic pain*, Eur. J. Clin. Pharmacol., 1975, 8 : 415–420.

Keller L.S., Butcher J.N., *Assessment of chronic pain patients with the MMPI-2*, University of Minnesota Press, Minneapolis, MN, 1991.

Kerns R.D., Turk D.C., Rudy T.E., *The West Haven-Yale Multidimensional Pain Inventory (WHYMPI)*, Pain, 1985, 23 : 345–356.

1) ☐ Flickering ☐ Quivering ☒ Pulsing ☐ Throbbing ☐ Beating ☐ Pounding	11) ☐ Tiring ☒ Exhausting	
2) ☐ Jumping ☐ Flashing ☒ Shooting	12) ☐ Sickening ☒ Suffocating	
3) ☐ Pricking ☐ Boring ☐ Drilling ☐ Stabbing ☒ Lancinating	13) ☐ Fearful ☒ Frightful ☐ Terrifying	
4) ☐ Sharp ☐ Cutting ☒ Lacerating	14) ☐ Punishing ☐ Gruelling ☒ Cruel	
5) ☐ Pinching ☐ Pressing ☐ Gnawing ☐ Cramping ☒ Crushing	15) ☐ Wretched ☒ Binding	
6) ☐ Tugging ☐ Pulling ☐ Wrenching	16) ☐ Annoying ☐ Troublesome ☐ Miserable ☐ Intense ☒ Unbearable	
7) ☐ Hot ☐ Burning ☐ Scalding ☒ Searing	17) ☐ Spreading ☐ Radiating ☐ Penetrating ☒ Piercing	
8) ☐ Tingling ☐ Itchy ☐ Smarting ☒ Stinging	18) ☐ Tight ☐ Numb ☐ Drawing ☐ Squeezing ☒ Tearing	
9) ☐ Dull ☐ Sore ☐ Hurting ☒ Aching ☐ Heavy	19) ☐ Cool ☒ Cold ☐ Freezing	
10) ☐ Tender ☐ Taut ☐ Rasping ☒ Splitting	20) ☐ Nagging ☐ Nauseating ☐ Agonizing ☐ Dreadful ☒ Torturing	

Fig. 10.**44** Example of compilation of MPQ in a patient with high values of all five dimensions of pain

Lienert G.A., *Testaufbau und Testanalyse*, Belz, Weinheim, 1969. Quoted by Franz C., Paul R., Bautz M., Choroba B., Hildebrandt J., *Psychosomatic aspects of chronic pain: a new way of description based on MMPI items analysis*, Pain, 1986, 26 : 33 – 43.

Lous I., Olesen J., *Evaluation of pericranial tendernes and oral function in patients with common migraine, muscle contraction headache and "combination headache."* Pain, 1982, 12 : 385 – 393.

McCreary C., *Empirically derived MMPI profile clusters and characteristics of low back pain patients*, J. Consult. Clin. Psychol., 1985, 53 : 558 – 560.

McGill J., Lawlis G.E., Selby D., Mooney V., McCoy C.E., *Relationship of Minnesota Multiphasic Personality Inventory (MMPI) profile clusters to pain behaviors*, J. Behav. Med., 1983, 6 : 77 – 92.

Melzack R., *The McGill Pain Questionnaire: major properties and scoring methods*, Pain, 1975, 1 : 277 – 299.

Melzack R., *Discriminative capacity of the McGill Pain Questionnaire (Letter to the Editor)*, Pain, 1985, 23 : 201 – 203.

Melzack R., Terrence C., Fromm G., Amsel R., *Trigeminal neuralgia and atypical facial pain: use of the McGill Pain Questionnaire for discrimination and diagnosis*, Pain, 1986, 27 : 297 – 302.

Mongini F., Poma M., Bava M., Fabbri G., *Psychosomatic symptoms in different types of headache and facial pain*, Cephalalgia, 1997 a, 17 : 274.

Mongini F., Defilippi N., Negro C., *Chronic daily headache. A clinical and psychological profile before and after treatment*, Headache, 1997 b, 37 : 83 – 87.

Moore J.E., McFall M.E., Kivlahan D.R., Capestany F., *Risk of misinterpretation of MMPI schizophrenia scale elevations in chronic pain patients*, Pain, 1988, 32 : 207 – 213.

Ohnhaus E.E., Adler R., *Methodological problems in the measurement of pain: a comparison between the verbal rating scale and the visual analogue scale*, Pain, 1975, 1 : 379 – 384.

Price D.D., Harkins S.W., *Combined use of experimental pain and visual analogue scales in providing standardized measurement of clinical pain*, Clin. J. Pain, 1987, 3 : 1 – 8.

Prokop C.K., Bradley L.A., Margolis R., Gentry W.D., *Multivariate analyses of the MMPI profiles of low back pain patients*, J. Pers. Assess., 1980, 44 : 246 – 252.

Revill S.I., Robinson J.O., Rosen M., Hogg M.I.J., *The reliability of a linear analogue for evaluating pain*, Anaesthesia, 1976, 31 : 1191 – 1198.

Rudy T.E., Turk D.C., Brena S.F., *Differential utility of medical procedures in the assessment of chronic pain patients*, Pain, 1988, 34 : 53 – 60.

Scott J., Huskisson E.C., *Graphic representation of pain*, Pain, 1976, 2 : 174 – 184.

Snyder D., Power D., *Empirical descriptors of unelevated MMPI profiles among chronic pain patients: a typological approach*, J. Clin. Psychol., 1981, 37 : 602 – 607.

Spielberger C.D., Gorsuch R.L., Luschene R.E., *Manual for the State-Trait Anxiety Inventory (Form X: self evalutaion questionnaire)*, Consulting Psychology Press, Palo Alto, 1970.

Sternbach R., *Pain patients: traits and treatment*, Academic Press, New York, 1974.

Swimmer G.I., Robinson M.E., Geisser M.E., *Relationship of MMPI cluster type, pain coping strategy, and treatment outcome*, Clin. J. Pain, 1992, 8 : 131 – 137.

Turk D.C. and Rudy T.E., *Toward an empirically derived taxonomy of chronic pain patents: integration of psychological assessment data*, J. Consult. Clin. Psychol., 1988, 56 : 233 – 238.

Turk D.C. and Rudy T.E., *Robustness of an empirically derived taxonomy of chronic pain patients*, Pain, 1990, 43 : 27 – 36.

Woodforde J.M., Merskey H., *Some relationships between subjective measures of pain*, J. Psychosom. Res., 1972, 16 : 173 – 178.

11 Guidelines for Differential Diagnosis

General Principles

In patients suffering from headache or facial pain, the first problem is to exclude the possibility that pain is the initial symptom of an organic pathology. Then, the diagnostic problem may be to determine a single pathology that produces pain or, frequently, to assess the presence of two or more superimposed pathologies and to quantify their relevance. Moreover, one should evaluate the impact that alterations in system function and personality characteristics may have on the headache/facial pain syndromes.

Concerning the first point, in the presence of a moderate to severe headache – especially if recent in onset and rapidly evolving – one must exclude it being the consequence of an intracranial process, a tumor in particular, and must proceed as indicated in the previous chapter. Multiple sclerosis represents another pathology in which facial pain may be the first symptom. A plaque of demyelinization of the trigeminal nerve may produce typical attacks of trigeminal neuralgia or neuropathic pain (Figs. 2.**9**, 2.**10**). Therefore, if the data from history and clinical examination justify this suspicion, the appropriate instrumental tests (MRI, cerebral fluid examination, evoked potentials, etc.) should be performed to exclude this possibility. Facial pain may also represent the first symptom of a neurome of the acoustic nerve, together with other typical symptoms (such as vertigo, tinnitus, etc.).

Whenever two or more pathologies are superimposed on the same patient, it must be determined whether one disease predominates. For example, a common occurrence is the superimposition of myogenous pain, chronic tension-type headache and TMJ intracapsular dysfunction (Fig. 11.**1**). In these cases, especially when a depressive or anxiety disorder is present, treating the TMJ dysfunction by means of orthopedic splint worn 24 hours a day might worsen the primary problem.

Another example of disease superimposition is the case of a tension type headache superimposed on a migraine. In this case also it must be evaluated which is the primary pathology and whether, consequently, tension-type headache should be treated first (treating the migraine attacks only symptomatically) or whether preventive treatment should be applied for both pathologies. Moreover, in some patients, headache attacks with intercritical periods may also present different features, more migraine-like at some times and more like the tension-type at other times. The question in such cases is whether two diseases are in fact present or whether one disease at times mimics another disease. This problems correlate with that of diagnosis and management of chronic daily headache (see Chapters 1 and 17).

Finally, in a number of cases some systemic disorder (vascular, hormonal, etc.) is present that is not the primary cause of the disease but constitutes an aggravating factor of which account should be taken in the diagnosis and treatment. For example, a migraine may be markedly worsened by menstrual disorders resulting from hormonal dysfunction.

An assessment of whether and how parafunctional habits are consequences of the superimposition of a relevant psychological factor is also of obvious importance. A biofeedback

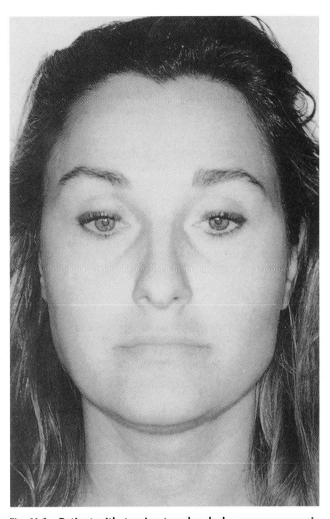

Fig. 11.**1 Patient with, tension-type headache, myogenous pain of the left cheek and mild intracapsular disorder of the left TMJ.** Note the hypertrophy of the left masseter muscle

treatment, to give an example, could be useful in a tension type patient generically "stressed", but my be totally useless, if not actually contraindicated, in patients with mood or personality disorders.

Some diagnostic criteria will now be examined that may help to discriminate between the most frequent pain syndromes (alone or superimposed).

Migraine Versus Tension-Type Headache

In the International Headache Society classification (1988) (see Chapter 1) the previously used terms common and classic migraine have been replaced with the terms *migraine without aura* and *migraine with aura*. Migraine without aura is described as an *idiopathic headache disorder manifesting in attacks lasting 4 – 72 hours. Symptom characteristics are: unilateral location, moderate or severe intensity pulsating quality, aggravation by routine physical activity, nausea and/or vomiting, photopobia and phonophobia.*

Migraine with aura is described as *idiopathic headache disorder manifesting in attacks of neurological symptoms unequivocally localizable to cerebral cortex or brain stem, usually gradually developed over 5–20 minutes and usually lasting no more than 60 minutes. The headache follows the aura with a free interval of no more than 60 minutes (but sometimes it can start before or at the same time as the aura). Pain usually lasts 4–72 hours but may be absent in some cases.*

Tension-type headache is subdivided into episodic and chronic. The episodic form is described as *recurrent episodes of headache lasting minutes or days. The pain is typically pressing/tightening in quality, of mild or moderate intensity,bilateral or variable in location and does not worsen with physical activity. Nausea and photophobia are mild, rare or absent.*

In the chronic form of tension-type headache pain headache is present for more than 15 days a month during at least six months. *The pain is usually pressing/tightening in quality, of mild or moderate severity, bilateral or variable in location and does not worsen with physical activity. Mild nausea, photophobia and phonophobia occur and they may be severe on rare occasions.*

A further distinction is made between tension-type headache associated or not associated with disorders of the pericranial muscles.

While usually the diagnosis of a migraine with aura is easy, discrimination between migraine without aura and tension-type headache may be difficult. Indeed some degree of nausea, phonophobia and, to a greater extent, of photophobia is frequent in attacks of moderate-to-severe headache; a tension-type headache may be unilateral if it is associated with postural and muscle disorders in which the muscle involvement is asymmetrical (Fig. 11.2); the quality of the pain (pulsating or pressing) may be ill-defined by the patient, who may sometimes give both descriptions to define the same headache attack.

In such cases, various other clinical observations may be helpful. In a tension-type headache, cranial muscle palpation usually elicits pain more often and more severely. Typically, prolonged palpation may induce headache. It is imperative, however, that such palpation be carried out systematically (as described in Chapter 10). The tendency of some clinicians to restrict their attention to the frontal and nuchal musculature is a frequent biasing factor. On inspection, signs of muscle hyperfunction and parafunction and of postural disorders are more frequent in tension-type headache patients. A Horner syndrome (Fig. 11.3) or signs of capillary circulation disorders (Fig. 11.4) may be observed in migraine patients, also during intercritical periods.

History is also of great importance: migraine patients have often suffered from frequent acetonemic attacks and kinetosis during childhood and adolescence and more frequently have a family history positive for headache. Moreover, migraine patients are more prone to colitis and gastralgia (Table 9.2). In a hormone-dependent migraine, menstruation disorders and nail and hair fragility are frequently encountered (Mongini et al., 1997).

The distinction between tension-type headache with and without pericranial muscle disorders is questionable on various grounds. Again, accurate palpation is mandatory. Moreover, a facial pain disorder (somatoform) might be misdiagnosed as "tension-type headache without muscle disorders" (see below).

Chronic daily headache (CDH) may present with different characteristics, possibly related to its different origin: transformed migraine, progressively aggravated chronic tension-type headache, or rapid onset headache (see Chapters 1 and

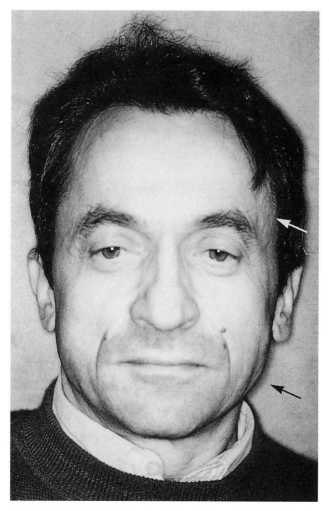

Fig. 11.**2**   Asymmetrical involvement of the craniofacial musculature with hypertrophy of the masseter and temporal muscles (arrows) in a patient suffering from serious tension-type headache with predominant location in the left hemiface

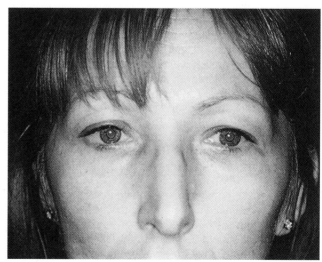

Fig. 11.**3**   Partial Horner syndrome (with lid drop and slight enophthalmus) at left eye in intercritical phase in a patient suffering from migraine attacks predominantly located in the left periorbital region

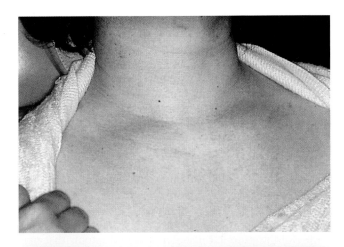

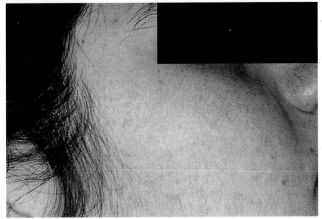

Fig. 11.**4** Signs of alteration of the capillary circulation in a patient suffering from migraine and tension-type headache

17). While the characteristics of frequency and duration of pain attacks may vary in time, different patients may or may not show typical migraine features: pain in some attacks may indeed be severe, pulsating, and be associated with relevant autonomic symptoms and colitis, gastralgia, kinetosis or typical signs of hormonal disturbance (menstruation disorders, hair and nail fragility). Other patients with CDH however, suffer from a constant dull headache without attacks of severe pain. Usually in these cases the accompanying symptoms are more typical of a mood disorder, mainly depressive in nature. Clearly, this is relevant for the treatment plan, which will differ accordingly (see Chapter 17).

Neuralgic Facial Pain. Cluster Headache. Chronic Paroximal Hemicrania

Problems of differential diagnosis may some time arise between trigeminal neuralgia and other diseases characterized by relatively short-lasting, lancinating pain attacks. A classical trigeminal neuralgia consists of attacks of excruciating pain limited to the distribution of one or more branch of the trigeminal nerve (usually the second and/or the third). The quality of pain is like that of electric shock and the duration is limited to a few seconds. Typically pain may be evoked by tactile stimuli at discrete sites of the face (due, for instance, to washing or chewing). The fits of pain may occur many times a day and usually no pain is present during intercritical periods.

In some other cases, or with time, the features of trigeminal neuralgia may be less typical and may justify some doubts

about which is the correct diagnosis. Thus, the intensity and duration of pain attacks may become variable (from slight to severe; from seconds to minutes) and some painful sensation may still be present during the intercritical periods.

Problems of differential diagnosis may arise with SUNCT. This syndrome, which is rare, is characterized by short-lasting neuralgiform pain attacks, moderate to severe in intensity, mainly in the orbital and periorbital area, lasting usually 30–120 seconds. The attacks may be precipitated by minor stimuli. Differential features from trigeminal neuralgia are the localization at the first trigeminal branch (rarely found in trigeminal neuralgia); the presence of sometimes prominent autonomic phenomena (with conjunctival injection, tearing, rhinorrhea and lid ptosis) that are absent in trigeminal neuralgia; and the absence or rarity of pain attacks during night. Both for trigeminal neuralgia and for SUNCT differential diagnosis should be further established with chronic paroxysmal hemicrania (CPH) and cluster headache (CL). These two pathologies have several characteristics in common, which may be summarized as follows: pain is generally unilateral, located in the orbital/periorbital and/or temporal, frontal, or maxillary regions. It is intense and pulsating in character; the pain attacks are always accompanied by autonomic phenomena (conjunctival injection, tearing, rhinorrhea, Horner syndrome); the attacks show a typical "clustering" during certain periods of the year. However they show a different sex ratio (women being more affected than men by chronic paroxysmal hemicrania and less afected than men by cluster headache); the attacks of chronic paroxysmal hemicrania are more frequent but shorter than those of cluster headache (from 5 to 30 minutes in the former, from 15 to 180 minutes in the latter). For differential diagnosis between chronic paroxysmal hemicrania and trigeminal neuralgia, it must be taken into account that during attacks of trigeminal neuralgia some lacrimation may be present, but not myosis or ptosis. Chronic paroxysmal hemicrania or cluster headache attacks are never evoked by tactile stimuli. SUNCT attacks also show a different sex ratio from CPH (males being generally more affected by SUNCT than women) and may be evoked by tactile stimuli.

Lastly, *empirical* criteria are relevant for the differential diagnosis. The classical trigeminal neuralgia shows a good response to GABAergic anticonvulsant drugs, and to carbamazepine in particular, to which SUNCT shows no or very little response and neither do CPH and CL. Indomethacin is highly effective against chronic paroxysmal hemicrania (Sjaastad, 1987), while it has no effect against trigeminal neuralgia. CL attacks respond well to sumatriptan administration, while this drug is totally ineffective against trigeminal neuralgia and SUNCT. Finally, the possibility of rare combined pathologies, such as Cluster–tic and CPH–tic syndromes, should be considered.

Facial Pain Disorder (Somatoform Disorder)

Problems of differential diagnosis may arise with facial pain disorders in which the psychological factor plays a predominant role, defined as *pain disorder*, as a type of *somatoform disorder*, by DSM-IV (American Psychiatric Association, 1994).

This relatively frequent pain syndrome is characterized by a pain that is constant or persistent for most of the day. At onset it may be confined to a limited region of the maxilla or the mandible (sometimes beginning as a "burning sensation" of the gingiva). It may then spread to a wider area of the face and neck or, sometimes, change its site of localization. The quality of pain is ill-defined: it may be described as a slight burning sensation, or as a sensation of swelling or tightening. Intensity is seldom severe: however, it can vary a great deal, and usually during periods when it is more severe the pain is more widely distributed.

The pain syndrome with which it is most often confused on diagnosis is trigeminal neuralgia. A classical trigeminal neuralgia can hardly be misdiagnosed. It differs from the facial pain disorder in its localization (constant and strictly limited to the distribution field of one or more trigeminal branches), the pain characteristics (excruciating and limited to a few seconds), the fact that pain may be evoked by tactile stimuli at discrete sites of the face, and the absence of pain during intercritical periods.

However, as mentioned, in some cases, or with time, the features of trigeminal neuralgia may be less typical and may justify some doubt about which is the correct diagnosis. In these cases the following criteria may be helpful for the differential diagnosis with facial pain disorder. In the latter syndrome pain is not confined to the distribution of the trigeminal branches. In the history, the pain symptomatology will often have appeared during or after a period of intense stress. The psychological involvement may be confirmed by the presence of phobias, obsessive–compulsive behaviour, and other symptoms that are psychosomatic in character (see Chapter 9). Other symptoms are frequently encountered that suggest a general medical condition (such as movement impairment or weakness of one or more limbs, hypoesthesias or paresthesias or diffuse pain in different sites of the body, etc.). If psychometric tests are administered, the psychological profile is always somewhat altered. In particular, the MMPI shows a scale elevation, especially of the "neurotic triad" (Hs–D–Hy), whose scores may often be well above 70. The presence of conversive V (see Chapter 8) (Fig. 11.**5**) may also be observed. The *ex iuvantibus* criteria may also be of help: as mentioned, anticonvulsive drugs (such as carbamezapine and baclofen) are effective against trigeminal neuralgia but are totally ineffective against facial pain disorder.

Another type of pain that should be differentiated from facial pain disorder is neuropathic pain, in particular, sympathetically maintained pain (see Chapter 2). Some characteristics of this pain (continuous, often of burning type) and of the accompanying symptoms (swelling, reddening) may lead to problems in differential diagnosis. However, in this case pain localization to the distribution of a sensory nerve and the *ex iuvantibus* criteria (with improvement of pain after transdermal local application of clonidine) should help in the diagnosis.

Muscle and TMJ Disorders

Patients with contraction of the cranial muscles and those with TMJ intracapsular disorders have symptoms that may appear similar. In both cases, some jaw movement alteration might be observed at inspection and cranial palpation is usually painful. However, the pattern of jaw movement alteration is quite different: in the muscle contraction case, restriction of movement may be severe but can gradually be overcome by applying gradual finger pressure to the jaws, so as to cause a progressive opening of the mouth (Fig. 11.**6**). This maneuver will provoke bilateral pain in the anteroauricular and cheek area at first. Pain usually subsides, at least partially, within some seconds. Lateral movement restriction is usually symmetrical. In the history, movement restriction will not have occurred suddenly, but rather within some hours or days.

In TMJ disk displacement without reduction, movement restriction is usually limited to 28–32 mm of jaw opening, typically with a deviation toward the lesion side (Fig. 11.**7**). Finger pressure will hardly increase the degree of jaw opening and will cause unilateral pain in the TMJ area. In these patients, jaw movement restriction has occurred suddenly and will generally have been preceeded by a period of joint clicking.

Depending on the type of problem, palpation will elicit pain at different points. In cases of muscle contraction, most or all muscles will be painful at palpation while palpation of the intra-auricular point and the retrocondylar aspect will elicit little or no pain. Palpation of the lateral pole of the condyle is also usually painful. This may be erroneously interpreted as a sign of TMJ dysfunction; however, it is often due to the pain projection of a contracted lateral pterygoid muscle (see Chapter 3). Additionally, in these cases, palpation of the neck and shoulder musculature is usually painful and there is often radiographic evidence of partial or total loss of the cervical curve.

Location of pain due to muscle contraction may be different according to the muscles mainly involved: preauricular and cheek areas for the lateral pterygoid and masseter muscles; parietal, temporal, and periorbital areas for the temporal muscle. However, pain may involve different areas, and shift from one to the other at times, so that a distinction from a tension-type headache may be sometimes questionable (Figs. 10.**11**, 11.**1**). During severe attacks, pain may spread to the neck, shoulder and arms, unilaterally or bilaterally.

In cases of TMJ internal derangement, palpation of the intrameatal point and, in particular, of the retrocondylar aspect is particularly painful on the side of the affected joint, and not on the other side.

A clicking noise is usually a sign of TMJ disk displacement with reduction, and a grating noise is diagnostic for a degenerative joint disease. However, it must be kept in mind that slight TMJ noises occur rather frequently in chronic headache/pain cases. They may be the consequence of a lack of

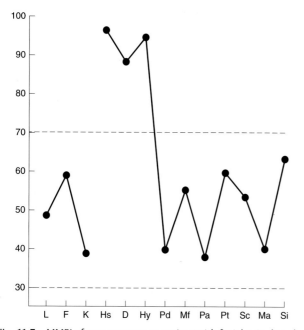

Fig. 11.**5** MMPI of a young woman patient with facial pain disorder, and motory disturbance due to somatoform disorder. A marked *conversive V* may be observed

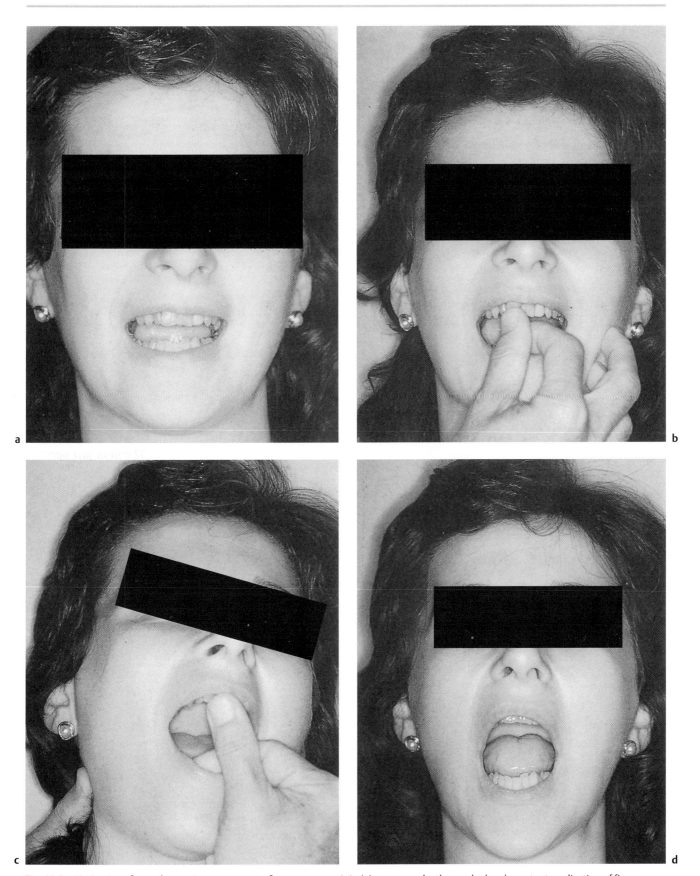

Fig. 11.**6**   Limitation of mouth-opening movement of myogenous origin (**a**) overcome by the gradual and constant application of finger pressure to the two jaws (**b–d**)

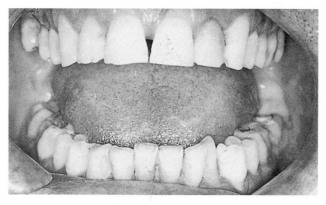

Fig. 11.**7**   Limitation of mouth opening in a patient with disk displacement without reduction in the left TMJ. Opening movement is limited to about 30 mm with deviation towards the lesion side

coordination of the two heads of the lateral pterygoid muscle and/or of an early stage of TMJ disorders in a patient whose main problem may be of a different type.

References

Alhaider A.A., Lei S.Z., Wicox G.L., *Spinal 5-HT3 receptor-mediated antinociception: possible release of GABA*, Journal of Neuroscience, 1991, 11: 1881–1888.

American Psychiatric Association, DSM-IV, *Diagnostic and statistical manual of mental disorders*, 4th ed., Washington, DC, 1994.

International Headache Society, *Classification and diagnostic criteria for headache disorders, cranial neuralgias and facial pain*, Cephalalgia, 1988, 8 (Suppl. 7):1–96.

Mongini F., Poma M., Bava M., Fabbri G., *Psychosomatic symptoms in different types of headache and facial pain*, Cephalalgia, 1997, 17:274.

Sjaastad O., *Chronic paroxysmal hemicrania: clinical aspects and controversies*, in Blau J.N. (ed.), *Migraine. Clinical, therapeutic, conceptual and research aspects*, Chapman and Hall Medical, London, 1987, 135–152.

12 Drug Treatment

General Principles

Since the different types of headache and facial pain may be consequent on numerous etiological factors, it is obvious that the drugs employed in their treatment belong to different groups.

The first decision to take when planning drug treatment is whether it should be symptomatic or preventive. For the first type of treatment, anti-inflammatory drugs (NSAIDs) are often employed: however, as we will see, these drugs may be efficacious for preventive treatment as well. New molecules, the triptans (see later) have been recently introduced for the symptomatic, not preventive, treatment of migraine. Preventive treatment of migraine is obtained through drugs that, besides the antimigraine activity, display other activities and, consequently, are further indicated for other pathologies. The different effects may remain independent (as for the case of some beta-blockers that develop an antihypertensive action and are also useful against migraine). In other cases it is possible that the primary action of a given drug also assists in reducing, at least in part, the head pain. This is the case for antidepressant drugs that, as we will see, are of first choice in patients with chronic headache and depression. We will now examine the drug categories more frequently employed in the treatment of headache and facial pain.

Nonsteroidal Anti-inflammatory Drugs (NSAIDs)

The use of nonsteroidal anti-inflammatory drugs in several forms of chronic or recurrent pain is well established. Most NSAIDs inhibit cyclooxygenase and hence prostaglandin synthesis (Lim et al., 1964; Ferreira et al., 1971; Vane, 1971). Some of them, such as meclofenamate sodium, are also lipooxygenase inhibitors (Siegel et al., 1980; Myers and Siegel, 1983; Perez et al., 1987; Pipitone, 1988) (Fig. 12.1). Prostaglandins are mediators of acute inflammation (Rainsford, 1988); furthermore, some of them behave as endogenous pyrogens

and may increase body temperature at hypothalamic level (Penada, 1990). The anti-inflammatory action of NSAIDs has been interpreted as a consequence of prostaglandin inhibition (Ferreira et al., 1971; Ferreira, 1972; Moncada et al., 1975). However, many other NSAID actions have been demonstrated (Tiengo et al., 1989; Tiengo, 1996) (Table 12.1). In particular, it has been shown that some NSAIDs inhibit polymorphonuclease function and, consequently, superoxide production (Minta and Williams, 1985). Moreover, a possible central analgesic action of NSAIDs, and of aspirin in particular, has been suggested (Shyu et al., 1984; Shyu and Lin., 1985; Catania et al., 1991; Piletta et al., 1991; Vane et al., 1992, Göbel et al., 1992; Vein et al., 1995; Pini et al., 1996, 1997) possibly due to activation of inhibitory serotoninergic and noradrenergic descending pathways (Shyu et al., 1984; Shyu and Lin., 1985). The presence of other mechanisms of action is also demonstrated by the beneficial topical effect of some NSAIDs (DeBenedittis et al., 1992; Steen et al., 1995; De Benedittis and Lorenzetti, 1996). Such local action of NSAIDs is not due to anesthetic effect since it does not alter tactile sensitivity. Moreover, it may be overcome by increasing pain stimulation, which suggests a competitive antinociceptive mechanism (Steen et al., 1995).

Table 12.1 Different actions of NSAIDs

Prostaglandin production
Leukotriene
Superoxide production
Lysomal enzyme release
Neutrophile aggregation and adhesion
Cell membrane function
Enzyme activity (NADPH oxidase/phospholipase)
Anion transmembrane transport
Oxidative phosphorylation
Arachidonate captation
Lymphocytic function
NF-$\varkappa$B activation
Rheumatoid factor production
Cartilage metabolism

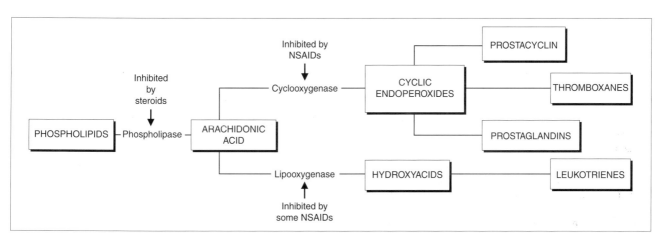

Fig. 12.1 Chain of events leading to the formation of prostacyclin, thromboxanes, prostaglandin, and leukotrienes and the sites of action of anti-inflammatory drugs

Several authors advocate the use of NSAIDs as a drug of first choice in the symptomatic treatment of tension-type headache (Lange and Lentz, 1995; Dahlöf et al., 1996; Schachtel et al., 1996; Steiner et al., 1998) and migraine attacks (Hakkarainen et al., 1978; Wilkinson, 1983, 1990; Pradalier et al., 1985; Johnson et al., 1985; Nestwold et al., 1985, Manzoni et al., 1989; Micieli et al., 1989; Havanka-Kanniainen, 1989; Boureau et al., 1994). Many different types are found on the market (see Racagni et al., 1985; Tiengo et al., 1989; Tiengo, 1996) (Table 12.**2**). In mild or moderate attacks, aspirin or paracetamol may be employed, while in severe attacks, ketoprofen, naproxene, ibuprofen, or thioprofenic acid can be used (Pearce et al., 1983; Havanka-Kanniainen, 1989; Nappi and Manzoni, 1990; Kloster et al., 1992; Lange and Lentz, 1995; Nebe et al., 1995). In acute headache attacks, the use of ketorolac i.v. has been also advocated (Davis et al., 1995; Shrestha et al., 1996).

The use of NSAID has also been advocated in the preventive treatment of headache and facial pain (Graffenried et al., 1980; Sevelius et al., 1980; Diamond, 1983; Peters et al., 1983, Dahlhöf and Jacobs, 1996) and, in particular, of migraine (Anthony and Lance, 1968; Stensrud and Sjaastad, 1974; Peters et al., 1983; Sargent et al., 1985; Welch et al., 1985; Ziegler and Ellis, 1985; Behan and Connelly, 1986). Here their efficacy might also be related to the reduction of platelet aggregation and, consequently, of serotonin release (Masel et al., 1980; Hosman-Benjamisne and Bolhuis, 1986).

Various authors (Wilkinson, 1983; Tfelt-Hansen and Olesen, 1984; Ramswamy and Bapna, 1986; Chabriat et al., 1994; Tfelt-Hansen et al., 1995; Henry et al., 1995) advocate the combination of aspirin and metoclopramide in acute acute migraine. Metoclopramide is a neuroleptic drug and a D_2 receptor antagonist and is particularly efficacious if nausea is present. Moreover, it has the advantage of encouraging gastrointestinal absorption of NSAIDs (Volans, 1975) and reducing their side effects, and, according to some authors, (Ramswamy and Bapna, 1986; Ellis et al., 1993) probably has an analgesic effect on its own.

As mentioned, some NSAIDs also show a topical effect. Topical aspirin administration, in chloroform or diethyl ether suspensions, was effective against herpetic and postherpetic neuralgia (King, 1988; DeBenedittis et al., 1992; De Benedittis and Lorenzetti, 1996).

Indomethacin is the drug of first choice in chronic paroxysmal hemicrania (Sjaastad, 1987) and hemicrania continua (Newman et al., 1994; Pareja and Sjaastad, 1996) (at a daily dosage from 50 to 150 mg) (see Chapter 18). NSAIDs are also useful against muscle or joint pain. In particular, tenoxicam has shown efficacy against musculoskeletal pain in patients with fibromyalgia (Quijada-Carrera et al., 1996).

Plasters for topical slow release of NSAIDs may be used against arthrogenous or myogenous facial pain.

Collateral effects of NSAIDs may be dose-dependent or non-dose-dependent. The most frequent dose-dependent effect is on the gastroduodenal mucosa (Jick, 1981; Silvoso et al., 1979; Lanza et al., 1981; Roth, 1986; Biour et al., 1987; Collins and Du Toit, 1987). To counterbalance this effect, ranitidine may be coadministered. At any rate, NSAIDs are contraindicated in presence of gastroduodenal inflammation or ulcer. Prolonged administration may also provoke a delayed toxicity to the kidneys (Brezin et al., 1979; Ciabattoni et al., 1984; Clive and Stoffi, 1984; Carmichael and Shankel, 1985) and, more rarely, on hemopoiesis (Farid et al., 1971; Böttinger et al., 1979; Heimpel and Heit, 1980; Kornberg and Rachmilewitz, 1982; Lee et al., 1982). Non-dose-dependent collateral effects may be itching or skin rashes, probably due to allergic reaction (Bailin and Matkaluk, 1982).

Benzodiazepines

Benzodiazepines (BZBs) are GABAergic drugs widely used for their anxiolytic, muscle relaxant and anticonvulsant effects. Depending on the type, one of these effects may predominate (Table 12.**3**). BZBs are not specific drugs for pain treatment but may be conveniently employed, for short periods – 4 weeks or less – in acute pain cases with anxiety, insomnia and musle spasm (Greenblatt and Shader, 1974; Lasagna, 1977; Hollister et al., 1981; Monks, 1994). Moreover, they may be used in episodic or chronic tension-type headache and muscle pain in anxious patients, alone or in combination with other drugs or treatment modalities (such as biofeedback). Most of the BZBs

Table 12.**2** Main nonsteroid anti–inflammatory drugs (NSAIDs)

Class	Drug	Mean single dose (mg)	Maximum daily dose	Half-life (h)	Comments
Salicilates	Acetylsalicylic	500–1000	4000	2	
Phenylproprionic acids	Ketoprofen	50–150	300	2	
	Ibuprofen	300–400	1800	2.5	
	Thiaprophenic acid	300	600	2	
	Naproxen	250	1250	10–14	Indicated for chronic pain
	Ketoralac	p.o. 10 i.m. 10 supp. 30	40 90 60	5–60	
Phenylacetic acids	Diclofenac	5–100 (Retard)	150	1.5	
Phenamic acids	Meclophenamate sodium	100	200	3.5	
Oxamic acids	Piroxicam Tenoxicam	20 20	20 20	36–46 60–72	Indicated for chronic pain
Heterocyclic acetic acids	Indomethacine	25–50	150	6	First choice drug in chronic paroxysmal hemicrania
Aniline derivatives	Paracetamol	500	2000	2.5	Not harmful to the stomach, potentially hepatotoxic in case of overdose

Table 12.**3**   Benzodiazepines

Drug	Mean single dose (mg)	Maximum daily dose (mg)	Plasma half-life (h)	Comments
Triazolam	0.125–0.25	0.25	3	Hypnoinducing activity; no active metabolite
Oxazepam	15–30	30–60	3–10	No active metabolite
Flurazepam	15–30	30	2–80	Hypnoinducing; possible accumulation in elderly patients
Clotiazepam	5–10	30	4–6	
Lorazepam	1–2.5	2–5	15	No active metabolite
Alprazolam	0.25–1	4	12–15	Possible antidepressive activity, indicated in panic attacks. Active metabolite: 3-hydroxy-alprazolam
Chlormethyldiazepam	0.5–2	3	10–20	
Bromazepam	1.5–6	6–9	16–20	Sometimes efficacious against trigeminal neuralgia. Active metabolite: 3-hydroxy-bromazepam
Chlordiazepoxide	10–25	30–40	7–28	Active metabolite: nordiazepam, oxazepam
Diazepam	2–5	6–10	20–35	Anxiolytic and muscle-relaxant activity. Active metabolite desmethyldiazepam, oxazepam
Clonazepam	0.5–2	8	25–40	Anticonvulsant activity. Often efficacious against neuropathic pain. No active metabolite
Prazepam	10–20	30	60–80	Active metabolite: desmethyldiazepam, oxazepam

first undergo two metabolic steps before being glucuronidated and eliminated with the urine: these are dealkylation and oxidation. The related metabolites may still have a pharmacological effect (Fig. 12.**2**).

There is a risk of dependency to be taken into account in administering BZBs, which is related to the dosage and the duration of treatment (Marks, 1980; Medical Letter on Drugs, 1981). The minimum effective dose should be applied; this varies from patient to patient and also in relation to the level of his or her psychological involvement. No risk of dependency is present in the short term. Long-term administration may result in diurnal sedation, decreased capacity of coordination and judgment, and other forms of cognitive alterations (Hendler et al., 1980; McNairy et al., 1984). In elderly patients, to avoid accumulation, BZBs with medium or short half-life (such as bromazepam) should be preferred over those with long half-life (such as prazepam). During the use of BZBs no alcohol should be taken, because of possible interaction with the drug. In alcoholics or aged patients with liver deficiency, drugs with no intermediate metabolic steps before glycuronidation (such as oxazepan) should be preferred (Table 12.3, Fig. 12.2).

Some benzodiazepines with pronounced anticonvulsant properties (such as clonazepam) may be used against neuropathic pain (Swerdlow and Cundill, 1981) (see later). Bromazepam has also shown efficacy in some patients with trigeminal neuralgia, although this drug is not usually employed as an anticonvulsant.

Myorelaxants

Myorelaxant agents (Table 12.**4**) are obviously employed when the muscular aspect of pain is prevalent with sites of contraction and trigger points. Traditional myorelaxant drugs (such as cyclobenzadrine, prinidole, colchicoside derivatives, etc.) show often little efficacy against prolonged pain due to contraction of the craniocervicofacial muscles. In general their employment, if any, is limited to the acute phase of pain and contraction in combination with physical therapy and exercises. More efficacy has been shown by tizanidine, which inhibits alpha and gamma motoneuron activity. This drug should be prescribed at night, since a frequent side effect is sleepiness. Otherwise, it is usually a well-tolerated drug and may be prescribed at variable doses between 2 and 6 mg daily for 2–4 weeks.

Antidepressants

The employment of antidepressants in different types of chronic pain is substantiated by an abundant literature (see Magni, 1991, and Onghena and Van Houdenhove, 1992, for a meta-analysis). The drugs are also employed in chronic headache and facial pain patients, alone or in conjunction with other types of drug or non-drug treatment (Lance et al., 1970;

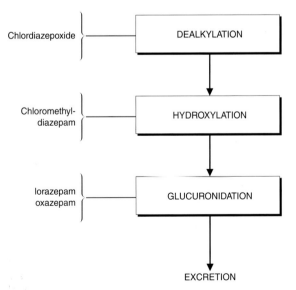

Fig. 12.**2**   Metabolic steps of the main benzodiazepines. Further explanation is given in the text

Table 12.**4**   Central-acting myorelaxants

Drug	Mechanism of action	Method of admini-stration	Dose (mg)	Half-life (h)	Metabolism	Contraindications	Side effects
Tizanidine	α, γ motoneuron activity	p.o.	2–6		Hepatic		Sleepiness
Cyclobenz-aprines	Motoneuron acitivity	p.o.	20–40	24–72	Hepatic	Monoamine oxidase in-hibitors hyperthyroidism; childhood cardiac arryth-mia	Sleepiness, vertigo, dry mouth, urinary retention
Prinidol mesylate	Atropinelike	p.o. i.m. sup.	6–12 2–6 6–12	24	Renal	Glaucoma; prostrate hy-pertrophy; paralytic ileus; tachyarrythmia	Weariness, dry mouth, mindriasis, constipation
Thiocolchicoside	GABA	p.o. i.m.	16–24 8	72	80% hepatic	Flaccid palsy	Diarrhea
Carisoprodol		sup.	1–3 s.	4–6	Hepatic	Granulocytopenia	Insomnia, hemorrhage

Diamond and Baltes, 1971; Gomersall and Stuart, 1973; Couch et al., 1976; Couch and Hassanein, 1976; Holland et al., 1983; Feinmann et al., 1984; Sharav et al., 1987; Nappi et al., 1989, 1990; Bank, 1994; Manna et al., 1994; Saper et al., 1994; Göbel et al., 1994a, b; Foster and Bafaloukos, 1994; Pfaffenrath et al., 1994; Bonuccelli et al., 1996).

They may be classified into tricyclic antidepressants, with a molecular structure similar to phenothiazines (Fig. 12.**3**), and antidepressants of more recent generations, with structures which may vary significantly from one to the other. A distinctive category is represented by monoamine oxidase inhibitors, which are less employed in chronic pain, being drugs with a relatively higher risk of significant side effects.

The action of antidepressants (tricyclic or not) consists mainly in blocking the reuptake of different endogenous amines (norepinephrine, serotonin, dopamine) (Table 12.**5**). However, administration of antidepressants produces other significant effects: in particular, they connect with the receptor sites of a number of neurotransmitters, such as histamine, acetylcholine, norepinephrine, serotonin and dopamine, with different efficacy and selectivity depending on the different molecules. Therefore their effect depends on the interaction between different modulatory systems (serotoninergic, nor-adrenergic, opioid, substance P and histamine) (Vanasia, 1996) (Table 12.**5**).

Even if it may not be excluded that their analgesic efficacy depends partly on their antidepressive action (Paoli, 1960; Lopez Ibor, 1972; Blummer and Heilbronn, 1982), there is evidence that the two actions are essentially separate. In fact, in

the majority of cases the analgesic effect is quicker than the antidepressive effect (3–7 days instead of 2–3 weeks) (Lang-ohr et al., 1982; Hameroff et al., 1984; Smoller, 1984; Monta-struc et al., 1985; Gourlay et al., 1986, Levine et al., 1986; Monks, 1994). Moreover, the analgesic effect may show even in the absence of an antidepressive effect or in non-depressed patients (Couch et al., 1976; Ward et al., 1984; Feinmann et al., 1984; Fogelholm and Murros, 1985; Montastruc et al., 1985; Zeigler et al., 1987; Puttini et al., 1988). The analgesic action is presumably based on the activation of centers and pathways for pain modulation (serotoninergic and adrenergic) at different levels of the central nervous system (Fields and Basmann, 1978; Dubner and Bennet, 1983; Spiegel et al., 1983; Roberts, 1984; Archer, 1993; Eide and Hole, 1993). Recently serotonin receptor subtypes have been identified that are particularly active in nociception control (Alhaider et al., 1991; Archer, 1993; Eide and Hole, 1993).

Antidepressant administration is particularly effective in chronic tension-type headache (CTTH) and chronic daily headache (CDH) (Lance and Curran, 1964; Diamonds and Baltes, 1971; Fogelholm and Murros, 1985; Loldrup et al., 1989; Nappi et al., 1989, 1990; Manna et al., 1994; Saper et al., 1994; Göbel et al., 1994a, b; Foster and Bafaloukos, 1994; Pfaf-fenrath et al., 1994; Bonuccelli et al., 1996; Cerbo et al., 1998), but in migraine patients also good results have been reported (Gomersall and Stuart, 1973; Couch et al., 1976; Ziegler et al., 1987; Bank, 1994; Saper et al., 1994; Steiner et al., 1998). Amitriptyline is the drug of first choice (Lance and Curran, 1964; Diamonds and Baltes, 1971). This is justified by the fact that the antinociceptive efficacy seems to be higher for molecules with a mixed effect (serotoninergic and adrener-gic) than for those having a higher specificity (see meta-analysis by Onghema and Van Houdenhove, 1992). Amitripty-line, in fact, although it has a pronounced action against sero-tonine reuptake (and hence its sedative effect, particularly useful in anxious patients), has a secondary action on the noradrenergic side.

One may start with low doses (15–20 mg at night), gradu-ally increasing until a significant effect is obtained: the corresponding dose will then be maintained for a period of three months or so. Subsequently amitriptyline dosage will be reduced gradually before it is suspended. In case of poor or no result or in presence of severe side effects, antidepressants of a newer generation that produce fewer side effects will be prescribed (Table 12.**5**). Antidepressants of more recent generations will be prescribed as first-choice drugs in

a   Amitryptyline   Imipramine

b

Fig. 12.**3**   **a** Structure of tricyclic antidepressants amitryptiline and imipramine. **b** Structure of phenothiazines

Tab. 12.**5**   Antidepressants (N B. for citalopram and velanfaxine no analgesic action has yet been documented)

Drug	Uptake inhibition			Mean single dose (mg)	Maximum daily dose (mg)	Side effects		
	Na	5HT	Da			Anticholin-ergic	Sedative	Cardio-vascular
Tricyclics								
Amitryptiline	+	+++	–	10 – 30	75	++	+++	++
Nortryptiline	++	+	–	10 – 25	50	+	+	+
Imipramine	+	+++	–	10 – 25	100	++	++	++
Clomipramine	–	+++	–	10 – 25	40 – 75	+	+	++
Desipramine	+++	–	–	10 – 25	75	–	–	+
Nontricyclics								
Mianserin	–	+++	–	10 – 30	60	–	+++	–
Amineptine	–	–	+++	100	200	–	–	–
Trazodone	–	–	+	25 – 100	150	–	+++	+
Latest generation								
Fluoxetine	–	+++	–	20	80	–	–	–
Paroxetine	–	+++	–	20	50	–	–	–
Citalopram	–	+++	–	20	40	–	–	–
Velanfaxine	–	+++	–	37,5	150	–	–	–

N. B. Doses given are those for headache patients

presence of contraindications to the use of tricyclics (see later).

Antidepressants are the first-choice drugs also in patients with facial pain disorder as somatoform disorder (Feinmann and Harris, 1984; Sharav et al., 1987) (see Chapters 1 and 8). Also in this case amitriptyline will be prescribed first and other drugs will then be considered as needed.

Amitriptyline may usefully be combined with neurotropic drugs such as perfenazine (4 – 16 mg/day) (Taub, 1973; Duthie, 1977; Weis et al., 1982). In this case, the two drugs reciprocally enhance their efficacies and the dosage of amitriptyline can be limited to 10 mg twice a day.

Side effects of tricyclic antidepressants are essentially linked to their blocking action, total or partial, of the cholinergic receptors, of the α_1-noradrenergic receptors and of the receptors for histamine H_1 and H_2. Consequently, these drugs may have anticolinergic effects (dry mouth, retention of urine, accommodation disorders, constipation, etc.); sedative effects, due to the action of all three types of receptors; and cardiovascular effects (tachycardia, orthostatic hypotension),

due to the effect on the α-adrenergic receptors. The latter is the most risky effect, especially in elderly patients. In particular, the use of imipramine should be avoided in elderly patients or patients at risk of hypotension (Monks, 1994).

Tricyclic antidepressants are contraindicated in patients with prostate hypertrophy, urine retention, glaucoma (or increase of endophthalmic pressure) and in convalescence after myocardial infarct. Desipramine, nortryptiline and doxepine at low doses fall between the tricyclics with analgesic effects that are more convenient in patients at risk for conduction disturbances (Monks, 1981). During therapy, alcohol consumption must be avoided.

Anticonvulsant Drugs

Anticonvulsant drugs (Table 12.**6**) are essentially employed, alone or in combination with other drugs, in neuralgic and neuropathic pain. Sodium valproate is also employed in preventive treatment of migraine. These drugs have different mechanisms of action: they potentiate the inhibitory action of

Table 12.**6**   Anticonvulsivants in headache and facial pain

Drug	Dose (mg)	Action			Indications	Side effects
		GABAergic	Sodium channel	Antiglut-aminergic		
Carbamazepine	400 – 1200	+			Trigeminal neuralgia	Nausea, drowsiness, lassitude, skin rashes, blood formula alterations
Lamotrigine	150 – 400		+	++	Trigeminal neuralgia	Skin rashes
Baclofen	10 – 25	+			Trigeminal neuralgia	
Sodium valproate	800 – 1600	+			Migraine without area	Hepatic dysfunction
Gabapentin	300 – 1200	+		+	Trigeminal neuralgia Neuropathic pain	
Clonazepam	0.5 – 2	+			Neuropathic pain	Sedation

γ-aminobutirric acid (GABA) on the central nervous system (GABAergic activity), inactivate the sodium channels, and develop an antiglutaminergic activity.

Carbamezapine is one of the GABAergic agents most employed and is the drug of first choice against trigeminal neuralgia. In these patients, it is usually administered at a dose that varies from 400 to 800 mg/day or more. The drug may have several side effects (nausea, drowsiness, skin reactions, etc.) and, if used in the medium–long term, requires regular blood screening, since it may depress hemopoietic activity. According to Fromm et al. (1980, 1984), baclofen is more effective than carbamezapine: the maximum efficacy is obtained with ist L-racemic form (Fromm and Terrence, 1984) (which, however, is not found on the market). Baclofen has also been found effective against muscular spasm (Bergamini et al., 1966), in chronic peripheral neuropathies (Terrence et al., 1985) and in hemifacial spasm (Sandyk, 1984).

Recently, lamotrigine has been marketed, a new anticonvulsant drug which shows a potential for treating carbamazepine-resistant trigeminal neuralgias. Lamotrigine blocks the voltage-dependent sodium channels and, consequently, inhibits the neuronal release of glutamate (Lamb et al., 1985; Millar et al., 1986; Leach et al., 1986; Peck, 1994). It develops a potent antiglutaminergic action and appears to be as effective as carbamazepine, with fewer collateral effects (Meldrum, 1993). Its efficacy against trigeminal neuralgia is supported by clinical reports (Canavero et al., 1995) and by a recent double-blind study (Zakrzewska et al., 1997). It is advisable to begin with a 50 mg dose, and to increase it by 50 mg a day until the minimum efficacious dose is obtained: this may be between 150 and 400 mg depending on the patient. Lamotrigine is not effective against migraine (Steiner et al., 1997). Skin rashes represent the most frequent side effect.

Another anticonvulsant agent than may be employed against trigeminal neuralgia if the above are not successful is sodium valproate (Peiris et al., 1980) in a dosage from 800 to 1600 mg/day, to be reached gradually. Its use should be restricted to a two or three-month period and the liver function should be monitored regularly. As mentioned, sodium valproate or its derivatives have also been indicated for patients with migraine without aura (Sorensen, 1988; Hering and Kuritzky, 1992; Sianard-Gainko et al., 1993; Jensen et al., 1994; Mathew et al. 1995; Lenaerts et al., 1996; Klapper et al., 1997). Moreover, this drug has shown efficacy against chronic daily headache that more typically represents a form of transformed migraine (Rothrock et al., 1994) (see Chapter 1) and against cluster headache (Kuritzky and Hering, 1987). It is not useful in chronic tension-type headache (Rothrock et al., 1994; Vijayan and Spillane, 1995; Lenaerts et al., 1996).

Recently it has been asserted that another anticonvulsant drug, gabapentin, represents a novel class of selective antihyperalgesic agents (Fields et al., 1997). The chemical structure of gabapentin is derived from GABA. Gabapentin increases GABA synthesis and probably decreases glutamate synthesis (Taylor et al., 1998). Good results with the use of gabapentin have been reported in trigeminal neuralgia, both idiopathic (Sist et al., 1997 a) and due to multiple sclerosis (Khan, 1998), and against neuropathic pain (Rosner et al., 1996), in particular of head and neck (Sist et al., 1997 b). One may start with a dose of 300 mg/day, gradually increasing to 900–1200 mg/day or more, as needed.

In case of neuropathic pain, less severe but more persistent than neuralgic pain, clonazepam, a benzodiazepine with anticonvulsant properties, may be efficacious. It may be started at 0.5 mg/day (in one or two doses): in case of partial response, the dose is gradually increased until the minimum effective dose is reached (up to a maximum of 2 mg/day).

Neuroleptics

Neuroleptic drugs may be employed during the acute phase in the treatment of severe migraine attacks (Table 12.**7**). Good results were reported with chloropromazine and prochlorperazine i.v. (Thomas et al., 1994; Herd and Ludwig, 1994; Coppola et al., 1995; Cameron et al., 1995) or with suppositories (Jones et al., 1994). Metoclopramide i.v. is also effective (Cameron et al., 1995).

This drug may be conveniently combined with cortisone derivatives (Saadah, 1994), and, as mentioned, with aspirin. As we have seen previously, neuroleptic drugs may be associated with antidepressants in the preventive treatment of chronic tension-type headache. Combinations of amitriptyline and perfenazine at low doses are marketed for this purpose.

Beta-Blockers

Beta-blockers are the drugs of first choice, particularly in Anglo-Saxon countries, for preventive treatment of migraine (Sjaastad and Stensrud, 1972; Ekbom, 1975; Ekbom and Zetterman, 1977; Weber and Reinmuth, 1977; Prendes, 1980; Diamond et al., 1982; Tfelt-Hansen et al., 1984; Sudilovsky et al., 1987; Kuritzky and Hering, 1987; Carroll et al., 1990). Not all of them are effective against migraine (Table 12.**8**); thus it seems that their efficacy might be independent of their beta-blocking properties. All beta-blockers effective against migraine have in common the absence of any intrinsic sympathetic-mimetic activity (Forssman et al., 1983; Ryan et al., 1983; Fanchamps, 1985; Massiou and Bousser, 1992). Their mechanism of action might be related to a reduction of the cardiac output with a compensatory increase of the peripheral vascular resistance (Man in't Veld and Schalekamp, 1982), an antagonist action on the central serotonin receptors (Fozard, 1982), and perhaps on an anti-platelet aggregation effect (Campbell et al., 1981).

The most widely used beta-blocker and the most effective in migraine prevention is still the first that appeared on the market, namely propranolol. The mean effective dose is 120 mg/day, but 60 mg/day might be sufficient in some cases.

Table 12.**7**   Neuroleptics employed in headache treatment

	Route of administration	Dose (mg)	Comments
Cloropromazine	i.v., rectal	10	
Proclorperazine	i.v., rectal	10–25	
Metoclopramide	p.o.	10	Also in association with aspirin or cortisone
Perphenazine	p.o.	4–16	Also in association with amitryptiline

Table 12.**8** Beta-blockers employed in migraine treatment

Drug	Mean daily dose (mg)	Half-life (h)	Comments
Propranolol	60–120	4	More effective but more side effects. Variable bioavailability
Atenolol	50–100	6.7	Few side effects
Timolol	20	2.7	
Metroprolol	100–200	3.5	
Nadolol	40–160	19	May be administered in single dose because of long half-life

Therefore it is advisable to start with 60 mg/day, gradually increasing until the minimum effective dose is reached. The treatment should last 4–6 months, with regular monitoring of cardiac activity, with gradual dose decrease before suspension.

The most frequent side effects of the beta-blockers are bradycardia, hypotension, vertigo and drowsiness. Contraindications are cardiovascular deficiency, bronchial asthma, diabetes and peripheral vascular diseases. Another contraindication to repetitive treatments with propranolol may be depression. In a prospective study of migraine patients treated with propranolol, Verspeelt et al. (1996) found that patients who had previously been treated with the same drug had a higher incidence (not statistically significant) of depressive episodes than the patients who had not been treated previously with propranolol or had been treated only once (Fig. 12.**4**). It is generally stated that beta-blockers should not be associated with the use of ergot derivatives and monoamine oxidase (MAO) inhibitors. However, good results were

recently reported with atenotol (beta-blocker) and fenelzine (MAO inhibitor) combined in patients with migraine, anxiety, and depression. This drug association seem to produce fewer side effects than the separate administration of the two drugs (Merikangas and Merikangas, 1995).

In a crossover double blind study (Kiaersgard-Rasmussen et al., 1994) on the efficacy of propranolol (40 mg three times a day) compared to that of tolfenamic acid (NSAD) (100 mg three times a day) the two drugs showed a similar efficacy. Drop-outs were due to drowsiness, tiredness and hypotension for propranolol, and to gastrointestinal symptoms for tolfenamic acid. It is clear that one of the most important criteria of choice is the potential impact of the side effects on different patients (see Chapter 14).

Calcium Antagonists

Calcium antagonists are also used extensively in the preventive treatment of migraine (Drillisch and Girke, 1980; Louis, 1981; Amery, 1983; Diamond, 1983; Meyer and Hardenberg, 1983; Frenken and Nuijtten, 1984; Bono et al., 1985 a, b, 1987; Manzoni et al., 1985; Bojaradi et al., 1986; Godfraind et al., 1986; Greenberg, 1986; Sörensen et al., 1986; Vanhoutte and Paoletti, 1987; Agnoli, 1988; Amery, 1988; Lücking et al., 1988; Martínez-Lage, 1988; Spierings and Messinger, 1988; Sorge et al., 1988; Soyka et al., 1988; Fisher and Grotta, 1993; Nuti et al., 1996). One mechanism of calcium antagonists is the inhibition of Ca^{2+} ion influx within the vascular smooth-muscle cell and, consequently of the blokade of the sequence of events leading to muscle contraction (Ca^{2+} release from storage sites in the sarcoplasmic reticulum, its binding to calmodulin, activation of myosinkinase, myosin–actin interaction). Thus, vasoconstriction is avoided (Holmes et al., 1984). Other mechanisms have been suggested: the blockade of platelet serotonin release and aggregation (Solomon and Spaccavento, 1983) and the antagonistic blockade of α_2 and β_2 brain receptors (Glazin and Langer, 1983; Feldman et al., 1985). Some calcium antagonists act selectively on calcium channels activated by norepinephrine receptor activity (receptor operated channels, ROC), others also act on potential-dependent channels (voltage operated channels, VOC) (Godfraind and Miller, 1986; Vanhoutte and Paoletti, 1987). Both types are used in the treatment of migraine (Table 12.**9**).

Verapamil and flunarizine, respectively, are the selective and nonselective calcium antagonists most often employed.

The use of verapamil has gained importance in recent years for the preventive treatment of migraine and, even more, of cluster headache (Solomon et al., 1983; Markley et al., 1984; Molaie et al., 1987; Solomon and Diamond, 1987; Prusinski and Kozubski, 1987; Gabia and Spierings, 1989). Beyond its effect on vascular calcium channels, verapamil induces an α_2 and β_2 receptor blockade (Glazin and Langer,

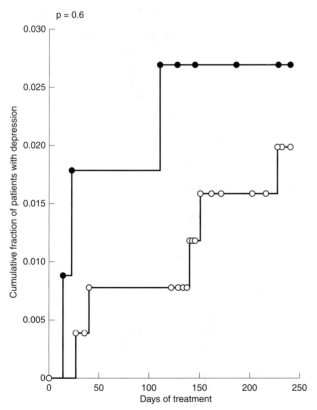

Fig. 12.**4** Influence of previous treatments on the incidence of depression in migraine patients treated with propanolol. ○ = no previous or only one previous treatment with propanolol; ● = more than two previous treatments with propanolol. (From Verspeelt et al., 1996, with modifications)

Table 12.**9**   Calcium antagonists

Drug	Mean daily dose (mg)	Comments
Flunarizine	5 – 10	Single dose at night
Nimodipine	90 – 100	Selective cerebrovascular action, fewer less side effects
Verapamil	240	Also in cluster headache

1983; Feldman et al., 1985). The overall effect of verapamil's alpha blockade is to increase the release of norepinephrine in the hypothalamus (Solomon, 1990). The slow-release preparation is now the most frequently employed (120 mg twice a day). This drug is absolutely contraindicated in cases of heart conduction disorders and, therefore, an electrocardiogram should be performed before its administration. Side effects are mild, abdominal pain and constipation being the most frequent.

Besides its inhibitory effect on transmembrane Ca^{2+} influx, flunarizine blocks dopamine D_2 receptors (Wöber et al., 1994). This action might explain the beneficial effect of flunarizine against nausea and vomiting during migraine attacks (Mitchelson, 1992), while it seems unlikely that it is involved in the antimigraine action of the drug (Piccini et al., 1990; Wöber et al., 1994).

Flunarizine has been used at a dose of 10 mg at night. More recently, however, good results were obtained with only 5 mg at night. Therefore, the actual tendency is to employ the latter dosage, at least as a first choice. Its use should be limited to a 2 to 3-month period. Side effects include increase of weight, drowsiness, and gastric pain. Long-term use should be avoided, since it could result in more severe consequences,

such as Parkinson's disease, tardive dyskinesia, akathisia, and depression (Chouza et al., 1986; Di Rosa et al., 1987; Micheli et al, 1989). It has been shown that patients receiving several flunarizine treatments are more at risk for depression (Verspeelt et al., 1996) (Fig. 12.**5**). Accordingly, the use of flunarizine should be avoided in patients with depression or at risk for depression, in particular if they have already been treated with flunarizine. Side effects are dose-dependent and age-dependent. Therefore, as mentioned, one should always start with 5 mg/day and increase to 10 mg if necessary. Moreover, the use of flunarizine should be avoided in elderly patients.

Another calcium antagonist that is selective for the ROC channels, and whose efficacy in preventing migraine has been studied thoroughly, is nimodipine. This drug is particularly efficacious on the smooth vascular muscles of the cerebral vessels (Towart, 1981; White et al., 1982; Steen et al., 1983; Peroutka et al., 1984) and as a consequence is used to improve intracranial circulation. Its effects in preventing migraine are controversial: whereas some authors (Gelmers, 1983; Havanka-Kanniainen et al., 1985; Bussone et al., 1987; Havanka-Kanniainen et al., 1987; Cavallini et al., 1989) report good results, in other studies the efficacy of nimodipine was lower than that of pizotifene (Gawel, 1987) or comparable to that obtained with a placebo (Ansell et al., 1988). In a recent double blind study on long-term efficacy of flunarizine and nimodipine (Nuti et al., 1996), it was found that flunarizine was more efficacious than nimodipine and had more prolonged effect after drug discontinuation. The use of nimodipine in the symptomatic treatment of migraine crises was not crowned with success (Jensen et al., 1985).

Ergot Derivatives

Ergot derivatives (Table 12.**10**) were the first drugs to be used against migraine. Ergotamine tartrate and mesylate, and dihydroergotamine (DHE) are the compounds actually employed, alone or in combinations with metoclopramide. They are ergopeptides consisting of a natural D-lysergic acid linked to a tricyclic peptide. These molecules inhibit norepinephrine reuptake at the sympathetic nerve terminals and act as agonists of various serotonin receptors (5-HT$_{1A}$, 5-HT$_{1B}$, 5-HT$_{1D}$, 5-HT$_{1F}$) (Peroutka, 1990 a, b; Adhan et al., 1993). They have a vasoconstricting action since they stimulate arterial smooth muscles. This effect is greater for ergotamine tartrate than for DHE (Berde and Stuermer, 1978). They also constrict venous capacitance vessels (Quality Standards Subcommittee of the American Academy of Neurology, 1995). The efficacy of ergotamine tartrate against migraine is demonstrated by numerous studies (Ryan et al., 1970; Adams et al., 1972; Hakkarainen et al., 1978; Blowers et al., 1981; Ala-Hurula, 1982; Bülow et al., 1986; Kinnunen et al., 1988; Friedman et al., 1989). However, frequent adverse effects are reported after using this drug: nausea, vomiting, cramps, paraesthesias, and hypertension. Ergotamine is also employed in combination with caffeine, which enhances its efficacy (Friedman et al.,

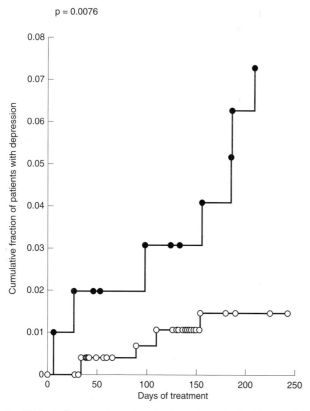

Fig. 12.**5**   Influence of previous treatments on the incidence of depression in migraine patients treated with flunarizine. ○ = no previous or only one previous treatment with propanolol; ● = more than two previous treatments with propanolol. (From Verspeelt et al., 1996, with modifications)

Table 12.**10** Ergot derivatives

Drug	Route of administration	Mean single dose (mg)	Maximum daily dose (mg)	Comments
Ergotamine tartrate	i.v.	0.25	0.5	Acute treatment. Per os with coffeine increases adsorption
	i.m.	0.25	1	
	p.o.	6	10	
	inhalation	0.30×6	12	
Dihydroergotamine				
– Mesilate (slow release)	p.o.	5	10	Symptomatic and preventive treatment. Less toxic than ergotamine but less effective in acute treatment. Efficacious against menstrual migraine
– Tartrate	p.o.	1.3		Symptomatic and preventive treatment of cluster headache during cluster period
	rectal	2		
	i.m.	0.125	10–15	
Lisuride	p.o.	0.025	0.075	Dopaminergic receptor antagonist

1989). Ergotamine tartrate is also employed for treatment of cluster headache (Ekbom, 1947; Friedman and Mikropoulos, 1958; Lance, 1978; Kudrow, 1980; Nappi and Manzoni, 1990). The efficacy of DHE against migraine, transformed migraine, status migrainosus and cluster headache has also been extensively demonstrated (Manzoni, 1987; Silberstein et al., 1990; Ward and Scott, 1991; Silberstein and Silberstein 1992; Robbins and Remmes, 1992; Haugh et al., 1993; Weisz, 1994; Scherl 1995; Winner et al., 1996; Ford and Ford, 1997). In addition, considerably fewer adverse effects are reported with DHE (Silberstein and Young, 1995). This is also true for ergotamine mesylate, whose efficacy and scarcity of adverse effects was also shown in the treatment of childhood migraine (Linder, 1994). These drugs are available for oral, rectal, intramuscular and intravenous administration. A nasal spray preparation is also available, which proved to be efficacious in the acute treatment of migraine (Bousser and Loria, 1985; Paiva et al., 1985; Rohr and Dufresne, 1985; Massiou, 1987; Tulunay et al., 1987; Ziegler et al., 1994; Beubler, 1995; Dihydroergotamine Nasal Spray Multicenter Investigators, 1995).

Ergot derivatives are contraindicated in presence of hypertension, vascular ischemic disorders, liver and kidney diseases, and gastroduodenal ulcer. Manzoni (1987) maintains that migraine with aura is a contraindication to the use of ergotamine. At any rate, chronic intake of ergotamine should be avoided because it increases the risk of severe vascular side effects and of a rebound headache once its use has ceased (Manzoni, 1987; Granella et al., 1987). In particular, ergotamine tartrate, if taken regularly three or more times per week can induce dependency (physiological and psychological) in some patients and lead to a drug abuse headache as a consequence (Saper and Jones, 1986; Saper, 1987, 1988). In this case detoxification is easier if drug discontinuance is rapid (Andersson, 1975, 1988). It is therefore advisable to restrict the use of ergotamine tartrate in the acute treatment of migraine, and to employ DHE in the preventive treatment, which, in any case, should be limited to a three-month period.

Other ergot derivatives employed in the preventive treatment of migraine (and not against migraine attacks) include lisuride and methysergide. Lisuride has an agonist action on the A-dopaminergic receptors and thus is employed against Parkinson disease. Against migraine it is employed at much lower doses (0.025 mg 3 times a day, attained gradually). Herrman et al., 1977, 1978; Somerville and Herrmann, 1978; Manconi et al., 1987).

Metisergide is a serotonin antagonist widely used in the past as first-choice drug against migraine (Sicuteri, 1959; Friedman and Elkind, 1963; Lance et al., 1963; Shekelle and Ostfeld, 1964; Southwell et al., 1964; Pederson and Moller, 1966). The dose is 1 mg three times a day. Chronic use may induce retroperitoneal, cardiac, or pleural fibrosis (Shekelle and Ostfeld, 1964; Southwell et al., 1964). At any rate, the use of lisuride and metisergide is now more limited than in previous times.

Cortisone Derivatives

Cortisone derivatives are not frequently used in craniofacial pain syndromes. In practice, their use is restricted to the preventive treatment of cluster headache (not as first choice, however) and of temporal arteritis (Hortons disease). Of these, the most frequently used drug is prednisone (Jammes, 1975; Couch and Ziegler, 1978; Kudrow, 1978; Prusinski et al., 1987; Nappi and Manzoni, 1990).

The regimen that is usually advocated involves an initial dose of 40 or 50 mg/day for 5–10 days according to the different authors, gradually reduced every three days. When successful, such treatment is effective within a few days. Good results against cluster headache have also been obtained with dexamethazone (16 mg the first day, reducing over the following days) (Prusinski et al., 1987) and with ACTH depot (1 mg i.m. every three days for 12 days) (Nappi and Manzoni, 1990). There are, however, several contraindications: gastroduodenal ulcer, hypertension, diabetes, and cataract. Cortisone derivatives are anti-inflammatory agents in that they are phospholipase inhibitors and hence prevent the formation of arachidonic acid (Fig. 12.**1**). However, it is possible that they interfere with other mechanisms such as regulation of serotonin biosynthesis in the CNS (Nappi and Manzoni, 1990).

Additional Drugs

A variety of other drugs may be employed in the treatment of different types of headache. Among these are two serotoninergic agents, pizotifene (Lance and Anthony, 1968; Ekbom, 1969; Sjaastad and Stensrud, 1969; Arthur and Hornabrook, 1971; Carrol and Maclay, 1975; Heathfield et al., 1977; Lawrence et al., 1977; Capildeo and Clifford Rose, 1982; Louis and Spierings, 1982) and ciproeptadine (Lance et al., 1970; Peroutka and Allen, 1984). They are agonists (at low doses) – antagonists of the 5 HT receptors. Ciproeptadine also has an antihistamine action. Dosages are 0.5–1 mg three times a day for pizotifene, 4 mg three times a day for ciproeptadine (Table 12.**11**).

Table 12.**11**   Agonists of serotonin receptors and serotonin precursors

Drug	Mean daily dose (mg)	Comments
Ciproeptadine	4 – 16	Increases appetite, may induce sleepiness
Pizotifen	1.5 – 3	Increases appetite, may induce sleepiness
Hydroxytryptophan	300 – 600	Antidepressive effect

Tryptophan and 5-hydroxytryptohan, serotonin precursors, are also employed against migraine and cases with superimposition of migraine and tension-type headache. For 5-hydroxytriptophan the dosage is 300 – 600 mg/day (Kamgasniemi et al., 1978; Mathew, 1978; Bono et al., 1982; Titus et al., 1985; Bussone et al., 1987b) (Table 12.**11**). Patients responding well to these drugs seem mainly to be young patients with a tendency to depression. Indeed, these drugs may also be used as antidepressive agents. Moreover, they show a certain sedative action and, therefore, are indicated in patients with sleep disturbances.

The use of magnesium has also been advocated in the preventive treatment of migraine (Swanson, 1988; Weaver, 1990; Mauskop et al., 1993, 1995). Its use is supported by several observations: brain tissue magnesium is reduced during a migraine attack (Ramadan et al., 1989, Welch et al., 1989); and in migraine patients magnesium levels are lower than normal in erythrocytes (Schoenen et al., 1991), serum (Durlach, 1976), and the cerebrospinal fluid (Jain et al., 1985). Reduced magnesium levels might produce thrombin-induced platelet aggregation and consequent serotonin release from platelets (Baudoin-Legros et al., 1986). Controlled studies have given controversial results: positive in menstrual migraine (Facchinetti et al., 1991), but not superior to placebo in a group of migraine patients (Pfaffenrath et al., 1996). At any rate, it seems that magnesium might be conveniently employed, at least in combination with other drugs, in women with migraine and menstrual syndrome. Magnesium is usually administered in a granular preparation, at a dosage of 100 mg twice a day. This treatment may be prolonged for several months if renal dysfunction is absent.

New Generation Serotonine Agonists (Triptans)

Recently molecules have been produced for the symptomatic treatment of migraine attacks that act as selective agonists of specific serotonin receptors (Table 12.**12**). Of these the first and most widely studied is sumatriptan (GR 43 175). Sumatriptan is a selective 5-HT$_{1D}$ receptor agonist and does not interfere with other serotoninergic receptors. Moreover, sumatriptan acts specifically on the 5-HT$_{1D}$ receptors of the cerebral arteries, thus inducing a selective vasoconstriction and reducing perivascular edema (Humphrey and Fenjuk, 1991; Humphrey et al., 1991; Caekebeke et al., 1992; Lance, 1993; Plosker and McTavish, 1994). Another suggested mechanism is the inhibition of the peripheral endings of the trigeminal nerve, with consequent inhibition of neuropeptide release (Buzzi et al., 1990, 1991; Moskowitz, 1992; Huang et al., 1993; Kaube et al., 1993; Goadsby, 1993; Humphrey and Goadsby, 1994). This hypothesis is supported by the fact that sumatriptan blocks plasma extravasation due to neurogenic inflammation after electrical stimulation of the trigeminal ganglion (Buzzi and Moskowitz, 1991) (see Chapter 2).

The efficacy of sumatriptan in the acute treatment of migraine attacks is now supported by a great number of studies. Sumatriptan proved to be more effective than other drugs and, in particular, than ergotamine derivatives (Dahlöf et al., 1989; Ferrari et al., 1989; Krabbe, 1989; Tfelt-Hansen et al., 1989; Cady et al., 1991; Ekbom, 1991; Ensink, 1991; The Multinational Oral Sumatriptan and Caffergot Comparative Study Group, 1991; The Subcutaneous Sumatriptan International Study Group, 1991; Brennum et al., 1992; Dahlöf et al., 1992; Saxena and Ferrari, 1992; Ferrari and Saxena, 1993; Tansey et al., 1993; Plosker and McTavish, 1994; Nappi et al., 1994; Pilgrim, 1994; Rederich et al., 1995; Boureau et al., 1995; Russell et al., 1995; Sargent et al., 1995; Winner et al., 1996; Pini et al., 1995; Touchon et al., 1996). A number of clinical studies has shown that sumatriptan is also effective against cluster headache attacks (Plosker and McTavish, 1994; Moreno et al., 1995; Monstad et al., 1995; Stovner et al., 1995; Centonze et al., 1996).

Sumatriptan is available for oral administration (at doses of 50 or 100 mg), for subcutaneous administration (6 mg), as nasal spray and as suppositories (25 mg). Because it has been shown that a 50 mg oral dose is highly effective and shows reduced adverse effects (Sargent et al., 1995; Frediani et al., 1995; Vallaperta, 1995; Cutler et al., 1995; Moschiano et al., 1996), it is advisable to start with this dose and apply a 100 mg dose only in case of partial response. Subcutaneous sumatriptan administration has the advantage of a very rapid response (usually within 15 minutes) (Scott, 1994; Plosker and McTavish, 1994) and is particularly indicated in cluster head-

Table 12.**12**   Serotonin agonists of the new generation (triptans)

Drug	Dose (mg)	5HT receptor activity	
		1B	1D
Sumatriptan	p.o. 50 – 100 rectal 25 s.c. 6		×
Zolmitriptan	2.5	×	×
Naratriptan	2.5	×	×
Elitriptan	5		×
Rizatriptan	5	×	×
Alniditan	1.4	×	×

ache attacks (Goadsby, 1994; Dahlöf et al., 1994; Alberca et al., 1994, Plosker and McTavish, 1994).

Although this drug has no indication for preventive treatment it may, in some cases, prevent or reduce headache recurrence (Ferrari et al., 1994; Pini et al., 1995; Rappaport et al., 1995; Winner et al., 1996). The side effect most frequently reported is chest constriction (Brown et al., 1991; Tansey et al., 1993; Lloyd, 1994; Wilkinson et al., 1995; Visser et al., 1996a, b). Since sumatriptan might facilitate coronary spasm (Peters et al., 1994; Kelly, 1995; Mueller et al., 1996) its use is contraindicated in patients with cardiac ischemia, angina pectoris, previous cardiac infarct and uncontrolled hypertension. In all other patients this drug is usually well tolerated and side effects, if they occur, are temporary and mild. Its use in combination with antidepressants does not lead to particular problems (Blier and Bergeron, 1995). Sumatriptan is not effective against chronic paroxysmal hemicrania and hemicrania continua (Antonacci et al., 1998), nor against the attacks of tension-type headache (Brennum et al., 1996): this may serve as an additional criterion for differential diagnosis.

Current pharmacological research aims to elaborate molecules that are at least as effective as sumatriptan but have fewer side effects. New "triptans" are now available. Elitriptan is a partial and selective agonist of 5-HT_{1D} receptors whose absorption is rapid and complete (Morgan et al., 1997). This drug seems to have a comparable effect to sumatriptan on the blood flow of the carotid artery but a more limited effect on the blood flow of the femoral artery and on the diameter of the coronary arteries (Gupta et al., 1996). Hence the drug should be better tolerated by the cardiovascular system (Diener, 1997; Milton et al., 1997).

Zolmitriptan is a selective agonist of H-HT_{1B} and 5-HT_{1D} receptors. This should allow action on both peripheral and central sites of the trigeminal vascular system. Moreover, while sumatriptan crosses the blood – brain barrier after it has been altered by the migraine attack (Humphrey and Feniuk, 1991; Kaube et al., 1993), zolmitriptan seems cross it while it is still unaltered. Its efficacy was established by a number of studies on animals and man (Dalhöf, et al., 1995; Thomsen et al., 1996; Martin, 1997; Dixon and Warander, 1997; Dixon et al., 1997; Dowson, 1997; Ferrari, 1997; Schoenen and Sawer, 1997).

Also naratriptan, rizatriptan and alniditan are selective agonists of 5-HT_{1B} and 5-HT_{1D} receptors and, as such, should present similar advantages in efficacy and tolerability (Goldstein et al., 1996; Connor et al., 1997; Kempsford et al., 1997a, b; Diener and de Beukelaar, 1997; Dahlof and de Beukelaar, 1997; Bomhof et al., 1998).

Topical Applications

Topical applications, alone or combined with other forms of drug administration, may be useful in some cases of craniofacial pain.

As already discussed, NSAIDs may be administered in slow-release transdermal applications on sites of muscle or joint pain or as topical aspirin administration, in chloroform or diethyl ether suspensions, against acute herpetic neuralgia and postherpetic neuralgia (King, 1988; DeBenedittis et al., 1992; De Benedittis and Lorenzetti, 1996).

Slow-release transdermal application of clonidine showed some efficacy in the preventive treatment of cluster headache (D'Andrea et al., 1995).

Clonidine is an α_2-adrenergic presynaptic agonist and, as such, regulates the sympathetic tone in the central nervous system by reducing the synaptic catecholamine outflow: consequently, clonidine has a potent antihypertensive effect. Its use in the preventive treatment of migraine was not satisfactory (Mylecharane et al., 1993). A further indication for clonidine topical administration is represented by sympathetically maintained pain (Davis et al., 1991) or by any superficial pain in the head and neck regions with signs of autonomic involvement (flaring, swelling, dermographism, etc.). Preparations are found on the market that release 0.2 mg clonidine a day for one week. This treatment is obviously contraindicated in patients with hypotension.

Topical applications of capsaicin have also been advocated for the treatment of neuropathic pain. Capsaicin is a neurotoxin, selectively active on the unmyelinated C-fibers, that increases the release and inhibits the reuptake of substance P and other neuroactive peptides from these fibers (Bernstein, 1983; Fitzgerald, 1983; Lynn, 1990). The block of substance P axonal transport and levels explains the capacity of capsaicin to desensitize nociceptive C-fiber endings. Positive effects were described after topical administration of capsaicin in cases of postherpetic neuralgia (Bernstein et al., 1989), diabetic neuropathy (Ross and Varipapa, 1989), neuropathic orofacial pain (Epstein and Marcoe, 1994), traumatic dysesthesia of the trigeminal nerve (Canavan et al., 1994), and cervical chronic pain (Mathias et al., 1995). Capsaicin extracts are available in a 0.25 % and a 0.75 % preparation. However, these preparations may produce an intense burning, thus inducing the patient to discontinue their use (Watson et al., 1988).

References

Adams M., Addis-Jones C.D., Aikman P.M. et al., *Treatment of migraine*, Practitioner, 1972, 206: 551 – 554.

Adham N., Kao H.T., Schechter L.E. et al., *Cloning of another human serotonin receptor (5-HT1 F): a fifth 5-HT1 receptor subtype coupled to the inhibition of adenylate cyclase*, Neurobiology, 1993, 90: 408 – 412.

Agnoli A., *The classification of calcium antagonists by the WHO expert committee: relevance in neurology*, Cephalalgia, 1988, 8, (Suppl. 8): 7 – 10.

Ala-Hurula V., *Bioavailability and antimigraine efficacy of effervescent ergotamine*, Headache, 1982, 22: 167 – 170.

Alberca R., Lopez J.M., Aguilera J.M., et al. *Chronic cluster headache: course and outcome of treatment*, Neurologia, 1994, 9: 379 – 386.

Alhaider A.A., Lei S.Z., Wilcox G.L., *Spinal 5-HT3, receptor mediated antinociception. Possible release of GABA*, Journal of Neuroscience 1991, 11: 1881 – 1888.

Amery W.K., *Flunarizine, a calcium channel blocker: a new prophylactic drug in migraine*, Headache, 1983, 23: 70 – 74.

Amery W.K., *Onset of action of various migraine prophylactics*, Cephalalgia, 1988, 8 (Suppl. 8): 11 – 13.

Andersson P.G., *Ergotamine headache*, Headache, 1975, 15: 118 – 121.

Andersson P.G., *Ergotism-the clinical picture*, in: Diener H.C., Wilkinson M. (eds.), *Drug-induced headache*, Berlin, Springer-Verlag, 1988, 16 – 19.

Ansell E., Fazzone T., Festenstein R., et al. *Nimodipine in migraine prophylaxis*, Cephalalgia, 1988, 8: 269 – 272.

Anthony M., Lance J.W., *Indomethacin in migraine*, Med. J. Aust., 1968, 1: 56 – 57.

Antonacci F., Pareja J.A., Caminero A.B., Sjaastad O., *Chronic paroxysmal hemicrania and hemicrania continua: lack of efficacy of sumatriptan*, Headache, 1998, 38(3): 197 – 200.

Archer T., *The antinociceptive efficacy of typical and atypical antidepressant compounds. Further evidence of serotonergic function in analgesia*, Nord J. Psychiatry, 1993, 47: 343 – 349.

Arthur G.P., Hornabrook R.W., *The treatment of migraine with BC 105 (Pizotifen): a double blind trial*, N.Z. Med. J., 1971, 73: 5 – 9.

Bailin P.L., Matkaluk R.M., *Cutaneous reactions to rheumatological drugs*, Clin. Rheum. Dis., 1982, 8: 493.

Bank J., *A comparative study of amitriptyline and fluvoxamine in migraine prophylaxis*, Headache, 1994, 34: 476 – 478.

Baudouin-Legros M., Dard B., Guichency P., *Hyperreactivity of platelets from spontaneously hypertensive rats. Role of external magnesium*, Hypertension, 1986, 8: 694 – 699.

Behan P.O., Connelly K., *Prophylaxis of migraine: a comparison between naproxen sodium and pizotifen*, Headache, 1986, 26:237–239.

Berde B., Stuermer E., *Introduction to the pharmacology of ergot alkaloids and related compounds as a basis of their therapeutic application*, in: Berde B., Schild H.O. (eds.), *Ergot alkaloids and related compounds*, Berlin, Springer-Verlag, 1978, 1–28.

Bergamini L., Riccio A., Bergamasco B., *Un farmaco ad azione antispastica della muscolatura striata*, Minerva Medica, 1966, 57:2723–2729.

Bernstein J.E., *Neuropeptides and the skin*, in: Goldsmith L.A. (ed.), *Biochemistry and physiology of the skin*, Oxford University Press, New York, 1983, 1217–1232.

Bernstein J.E., Korman N.J., Bickers D.R., Dahl M.V., Millikan L.E., *Topical capsaicin treatment of chronic postherpetic neuralgia*, J. Am. Acad. Dermatol., 1989, 21:265–270.

Beubler E., *Migraine: dihydroergotamine nasal spray—an alternative*, Wien. Med. Wochenschr., 1995, 145:326–31.

Biour M., Blanquart A., Moore N., et al. *Incidence of NSAID–related, severe gastrointestinal bleeding*, Lancet, 1987, 1:340–341.

Blier P., Bergeron R., *The safety of concomitant use of sumatriptan and antidepressant*, J. Clin. Psychopharmacol., 1995, 15:106–109.

Blowers A.J., Cameron E.G., Lawrence E.R., *Effervescent ergotamine tartrate (Effergot) in the treatment of the acute migraine attack*, Br J. Clin. Pract., 1981, 35:188–190.

Blumer D., Heilbronn M., *Chronic pain as a variant of depressive disease. The pain-prone disorder*, J. Nerv. Ment. Dis., 1982, 170:381–394.

Bojardi A., Gemma M., Porta E., Peccarisi C., Bussone G., *Calcium entry blocker: treatment in acute pain in cluster headache*, Ital. J. Neurol. Sci., 1986, 7:531–534.

Bomhof M.A.M., Heywood J., Pradalier A., Enahoro H., Winter P., Hassani H., on behalf of the Naratriptan Long-term Study Group, *Tolerability and efficacy of naratriptan tablets with long-term treatment (6 months)*, Cephalalgia, 1998, 18:33–37.

Bono G., Criscuoli M., Martignoni E., Salmon S., Nappi G., *Serotonin precursors in migraine prophylaxis*, in: Critchley M. et al. (ed.), *Advances in Neurology*, vol. 33, Raven Press, New York, 1982, 357–363.

Bono G., Micieli G., Manzoni G.C., Trucco M., Martucci N., Nappi G., *Calcium entry blockers in headache treatment: pathophysiological and pharmacological implications*, J. Neurol., 1985 a, 232, (Suppl.):218.

Bono G., Manzoni G.C., Martucci N., et al., *Flunarizine in common migraine: Italian cooperative trial, II: Long-term follow up*, Cephalalgia, 1985 b, (Suppl. 2):155–158.

Bono G., Manzoni G.C., Martucci N., et al., *Calcium entry blockers in migraine syndromes: therapeutic profile of flunarizine*, New Trends Clin. Neuropharmacol., 1987, 1:49–54.

Bonuccelli U., Nuti A., Lucetti C., Pavese N., Dell'Agnello G., Muratorio A., *Amitriptyline and dexamethasone combined treatment in drug-induced headache*, Cephalalgia, 1996, 16:197–200.

Böttinger L.E., *Phenylbutazone, oxyphenibutazone and aplastic anaemia*, Br. Med. J., 1979, 2:265.

Böttinger L.E., Furhoff A.K., Holmber L., *Drug induced blood dyscrasias*, Acta Med. Scand., 1979, 205:457–461.

Boureau F., Joubert J.M., Lasserre V., Prum B., Delecoeuillerie G., *Double-blind comparison of an acetaminophen 400 mg-codeine 25 mg combination versus aspirin 100 mg and placebo in acute migraine attack*, Cephalalgia, 1994, 14:156–161.

Boureau F., Chazot G., Emile J., Bertin L., D'Allens H., *Comparison of subcutaneous sumatriptan with usual acute treatments for migraine. French Sumatriptan Study Group*, Eur. Neurol., 1995, 35:264–269.

Bousser M.G., Loria Y., *Efficacy of dihydroergotamine nasal spray in the acute treatment of migraine attacks*, Cephalalgia, 1985, 5 (Suppl. 3):554–555.

Brennum J., Kjeldsen M., Olesen J., *The 5-HT1-like agonist sumatriptan has a significant effect in chronic tension-type headache*, Cephalalgia, 1992, 12:375–379.

Brennum J., Brinck T., Schriver L., et al. *Sumatriptan has no clinically relevant effect in the treatment of episodic tension-type headache*, Eur. J. Neurol., 1996, 3:23–28.

Brezin J., Kats S.M., Swartz A.B., Chinitz J.L., *Reversible renal failure and nephrotic syndrome associated with non steroidal anti-inflammatory drugs*, N. Engl. J. Med., 1979, 301:1271–1273.

Brown E.G., Endersby C.A., Smith R.N., Talbot J.C.C., *The safety and tolerability of sumatriptan: an overview*, Eur. Neurol., 1991, 31:339–344.

Bülow P., Ibraheem J.J., Paalzow L., Tfelt-Hansen P., *Ergotamine tartrate, 1 mg rectally, is biologically active despite unmeasurable plasma levels*, Cephalalgia, 1986, 6:107–111.

Bussone G., Baldini S. D'Andrea G., et al. *Nimodipine versus flunarizine in common migraine: a controlled pilot trial*, Headache, 1987 a, 27:76–79.

Bussone G., Frediani F., Lampeti L., Boiardi A., *5-HTP in migraine headache treatment: actual views and perspectives*, Cephalalgia, 1987 b, 7, (Suppl. 6):514–516.

Buzzi M.G., Moskowitz M.A., *The antimigraine drug, sumatriptan (GR43175), selectively blocks neurogenic plasma extravasation from blood vessels in dura mater*, Br. J. Pharmacol., 1990, 99:202–206.

Buzzi M.G., Carter W.B., Shimizu T., Heath H., Moskowitz M.A., *Dihydroergotamine and sumatriptan attenuate levels of CGRP in plasma in rat superior sagittal sinus during electrical stimulation of the trigeminal ganglion*, Neuropharmacology, 1991 a, 30:1193–1200.

Buzzi M.G., Moskowitz M.A., *Evidence for 5-HT1B/1D receptors mediating the antimigraine effect of sumatriptan and dihydroergotamine*, Cephalalgia, 1991 b, 11:165–168.

Cady R.K., Wendt J.K., Kirchner J.R., Sargent J.D., Rothrock J.F., Skaggs H., *Treatment of acute migraine with subcutaneous sumatriptan*, JAMA, 1991, 265:2831–2835.

Caekebeke J.F.V., Ferrari M.D., Zwetsloot C.P., Jansen J., Saxena P.R., *Antimigraine drug sumatriptan increases blood flow velocity in large cerebral arteries during migraine attacks*, Neurology, 1992, 42:1522–1526.

Cameron J.D., Lane P.L., Speechley M., *Intravenous chlorpromazine vs intravenous metoclopramide in acute migraine headache*, Acad. Emerg. Med., 1995, 2:597–602.

Campbell W.B., Johnson A.R., Callahan K.S., Graham R.M., *Anti-platelet activity of beta-andrenergic antagonists: inhibition of thromboxane synthesis and platelet aggregation in patients receiving long-term propranolol treatment*, Lancet, 1981, 2:1382–1384.

Canavan D., Graff-Radford S.B., Gratt B.M., *Traumatic dysesthesia of the trigeminal nerve*, J. Orofac. Pain, 1994, 8(4):391–396.

Canavero S., Bonicalzi V., Ferroli P., et al., *Lamotrigine control of idiopathic trigeminal neuralgia*, JNNP, 1995, 59.

Capildeo R., Clifford Rose F., *Single-dose pizotifen, 1,5 mg nocte: a new approach in the prophylaxis of migraine*, Headache, 1982, 22:272–275.

Carmichael J., Shankel S.W., *Effects of nonsteroidal anti-inflammatory drugs on prostaglandins and renal function*, Am. J. Med., 1985, 78:992.

Carroll J.D., Maclay W.P., *Pizotifen (BC 105) in migraine prophylaxis*, Curr. Med. Res. Opin., 1975, 3:68–71.

Carroll J.D., Reidy M., Savundra P.A., Cleave N., McAinsh J., *Long-acting propranolol in the prophylaxis of migraine: a comparative study of two doses*, Cephalalgia, 1990, 10:101–105.

Catania A., Arnold J., Macaluso A., *Inhibition of acute inflammation in the periphery by central action of salicyclates*, Proc. Natl. Acad. Sci., 1991, 88:8544–8547.

Cavallini A., Micieli G., Iannacchero R., Tassorelli C., Coppola F., *Nimodipine versus pizotifene nell'emicrania comune: efficacia clinica e tollerabilità*, in: Richichi I., Nappi G. (eds.), *Cefalee di Interesse Cardiovascolare*, Confinia Cephalalgica, vol. 7, Cluster Press, Milan, 1989, 191–198.

Centonze V., Polito B.M., Attolini E., et al. *Use of high sumatriptan dosages during episodic cluster headache: three clinical cases*, Headache, 1996, 36:389–391.

Cerbo R., Barbanti P., Fabbrini, G., Pascali M.P., Catarci T., *Amitriptyline is effective in chronic but not in episodic tension-type headache: pathogenetic implications*, Headache, 1998, 28(6):453–457.

Chabriat H., Joire J.E., Danchot J., Grippon P., Bousser M.G., *Combined oral lysine acetylsalicylate and metoclopramide in the acute treatment of migraine: a multicentre double-blind placebo-controlled study*, Cephalalgia, 1994, 14:297–300.

Chouza C., Scarameli A., Caama[ntilde]o J.L., De Medina O., Alijanati R., Romero S., *Parkinsonism, tardive dyskinesia, akathisia and depression induced by flunarizine*, Lancet, 1986, 1:1303–1304.

Ciabattoni G., Cinotti G.A., Pierucci A., et al. *Effects of sulindac and ibuprofen in patients with chronic glomerular disease. Evidence for the dependence of renal function on prostacyclin*, N. Engl. J. Med., 1984, 310:279–283.

Clive D.M., Stoffi J.S., *Renal syndromes associated with nonsteroidal anti-inflammatory drugs*, N. Engl. J. Med., 1984, 310:563–572.

Collins A.J., Du Toit J.A., *Upper gastrointestinal findings and faecal occult blood in patients with rheumatic disease taking nonsteroidal antiinflammatory drugs*, Br. J. Rheumatol., 1987, 26:295–298.

Connor H.E., Feniuk W., Beattie D.T., et al. *Naratriptan: biological profile in animal models relevant to migraine*, Cephalalgia, 1997, 17:145–52.

Coppola M., Yealy D.M., Leibold R.A., *Randomized, placebo-controlled evaluation of prochlorperazine versus metoclopramide for emergency department treatment of migraine headache*, Ann. Emerg. Med., 1995, 26:541–546.

Couch J.R., Hassanein R.S., *Migraine and depression: effect of amitriptyline prophylaxis*, Trans. Am. Neurol. Assoc., 1976, 101:1–4.

Couch J.R., Ziegler D.K., Hassanein R., *Amitriptyline in the prophylaxis of migraine. Effectiveness and relationship of antimigraine and anti-depressant effects*, Neurology, 1976, 26 : 121 – 127.

Couch J.R., Ziegler D.K., *Prednisone therapy for cluster headache*, Headache, 1978, 18 : 219 – 221.

Cutler N., Mushet G.R., Davis R., Clements B., Whitcher L., *Oral sumatriptan for the acute treatment of migraine: evaluation of three dosage strengths*, Neurology, 1995, 45 (Suppl. 7):S5 – 9.

D'Andrea G., Perini F., Granella F., Cananzi A., Sergi A., *Efficacy of transdermal clonidine in short-term treatment of cluster headache: a pilot study*, Cephalalgia, 1995, 15 : 430 – 433.

Dahlöf C., Winter P., Ludlow S., *Oral GR43 175, a 5 HTI-like antagonist, for the treatment of the acute migraine attack: an international study. Preliminary results*, Cephalalgia, 1989, 9, (Suppl. 10):351 – 352.

Dahlöf C., Edwards C., Toth A.L., *Sumatriptan injection is superior to placebo in the acute treatment of migraine-with regard to both efficacy and general well-being*, Cephalalgia, 1992, 12 : 214 – 220.

Dahlöf C., Ekbom K., Persson L., *Clinical experiences from Sweden on the use of subcutaneously administered sumatriptan in migraine and cluster headache*, Arch. Neurol., 1994, 51 : 1256 – 1261.

Dahlöf C.G.H., Jacobs L.D., *Ketoprofen, paracetamol and placebo in the treatment of episodic tension-type headache*, Cephalalgia, 1996, 16 : 117 – 123.

Dahlöf C., Diener H.C., Goadsby P., et al. *A multicentre double-blind, placebo-controlled, dose-range finding study to investigate the efficacy and safety of oral doses of 311 C90 in the acute treatment of migraine*, Headache, 1995, 35 : 292.

Dahlöf C., Jacobs L.D., *Ketoprofen, paracetamol and placebo in the treatment of episodic tension-type headache*, Cephalalgia, 1996, 16 : 117 – 123.

Dahlöf C., de Beukelaar F., *An alniditan (PasmigrenR) trial (ALN-INT-12*) re-assessed using a more stringent efficacy end-point: 24 h pain-free*, Migränkliniken, Cephalalgia, 1997, 17, 428.

Davis C.P., Torre P.R., Williams C., et al. *Ketorolac versus meperidine-plus-promethazine treatment of migraine headache: evaluations by patients*, Am. J. Emerg. Med., 1995, 13 : 146 – 150.

Davis K.D., Treede R.D., Raja S.N., Meyer R.A., Campbell J.N., *Topical application of clonidine relieves hyperalgesia in patients with sympathetically maintained pain*, Pain, 1991, 47 : 309 – 317.

De Benedittis G., Besana F., Lorenzetti A., *A new topical treatment for acute herpetic neuralgia and post-herpetic neuralgia: the aspirin/diethyl ether mixture. An open label study plus a double-blind controlled study*, Pain, 1992, 48 : 383 – 390.

De Benedittis G., Lorenzetti A., *Topical aspirin/diethyl ether mixture versus indomethacin and diclofenac/diethyl ether mixtures for acute herpetic neuralgia and postherpetic neuralgia: a double-blind crossover placebo-controlled study*, Pain, 1996, 65 : 45 – 51.

Diamond S., *Ibuprofen versus aspirin and placebo in the treatment of muscle-contraction headache*, Headache, 1983, 23 : 206 – 208.

Diamond S., Baltes B.J., *Chronic tension headache treated with amitriptyline – a double study*, Headache, 1971, 11 : 110 – 116.

Diamond S., Kudrow L., Stevens J., Shapiro D.B., *Long-term study of propranolol in the treatment of migraine*, Headache, 1982, 22 : 268 – 271.

Dihydroergotamine Nasal Spray Multicenter Investigators, *Efficacy, safety, and tolerability of dihydroergotamine nasal spray as monotherapy in the treatment of acute migraine*, Headache, 1995, 35 : 177 – 184.

Di Rosa A.E., Morgante L., Meduri M., et al., *Parkinson-like side effects during prolonged treatment with flunarizine*, Funct. Neurol., 1987, 1 : 47 – 50.

Diener H.C., *Evidence for the improved efficacy and safety of eletriptan compared with sumatriptan*, Cephalalgia, 1997, 17 : 477.

Diener H.C., de Beukelaar F., *A placebo controlled comparison of SC alniditan (PasmigrenR) with SC sumatriptan in the acute treatment of migraine*, Cephalalgia, 1997, 428.

Di Magni G., *The use of antidepressant in the treatment of chronic pain. A review of the current evidence*, Drugs, 1991, 42 : 730 – 748.

Dixon R., Gillotin C., Gibbens M., Posner J., Peck R.W., *The pharmacokinetics and effects on blood pressure of multiple doses of the novel anti-migraine drug zolmitriptan (311 C90) in healthy volunteers*, Br. J. Clin. Pharmacol., 1997, 43 : 273 – 281.

Dixon R., Warrander A., *The clinical pharmacokinetics of zolmitriptan*, Cephalalgia, 1997, 17 (Suppl. 18):15 – 20.

Dowson A.J., *311 C90: Patient profiles and typical case histories of migraine management*, Neurology, 1997, 48 (3 Suppl. 3):S29-S33.

Drillisch C., Girke W., *Ergebnisse der Behandlung von Migraene Patienten mit Cinnarizin und Flunarizin*, Med. Welt., 1980, 31 : 1870 – 1872.

Dubner R., Bennet G.J., *Spinal and trigeminal mechanisms of nociception*, Annu. Rev. Neurosci., 1983, 6 : 381 – 418.

Durlach J., *Neurological manifestations of magnesium imballance*, Handbk Clin. Neurol., 1976, 8 : 545 – 79.

Duthie A.M., *The use of phenothiazines and tricyclic antidepressants in the treatment of intractable pain*, S. Afr. Med. J., 1977, 51 : 246 – 247.

Eide P.K., Hole K., *The role of 5-hydroxytryptamine (5-HT) receptor subtypes and plasticity in the 5-HT systems in the regulation of nociceptive sensitivity*, Cephalalgia, 1993, 13 : 75 – 85.

Ekbom K.A., *Ergotamine tartrate orally in Horton's "histaminic cephalgia" (also called Harri's "ciliary neurologia")*, Acta Psychiatr. Scand., 1947, 46 (Suppl.):106 – 113.

Ekbom K.A., *Prophylactic treatment of cluster headache with a new serotonine antagonist BC 105*, Acta Neurol. Scand., 1969, 45 : 601 – 610.

Ekbom K.A., *Alprenolol for migraine prophylaxis*, Headache, 1975, 15 : 129 – 132.

Ekbom K.A., *For the sumatriptan cluster headache study group. Treatment of acute cluster headache with sumatriptan in cluster headache*, N. Engl. J. Med., 1991, 325 : 322 – 326.

Ekbom K.A., *Treatment of cluster headache: clinical trials, design and results*, Cephalalgia, 1995, 15 (Suppl 15): 33 – 36.

Ekbom K.A., Zetterman M., *Oxprenolol in the treatment of migraine*, Acta Neurol. Scand., 1977, 56 : 181 – 184.

Ellis G.L., Delaney J., De Hart D.A., Owens A., *The efficacy of metoclopramide in the treatment of migraine headache*, Ann. Emerg. Med., 1993, 22 : 191 – 5.

Ensink F.B.M., *For the sumatriptan international study group. Subcutaneous sumatriptan in the acute treatment of migraine*, Neurology, 1991, 238 : 66 – 69.

Epstein J.B., Marcoe J.H., *Topical application of capsaicin for treatment of oral neuropathic pain and trigeminal neuralgia*, Oral Surg. Oral Med. Oral Pathol., 1994, 77 : 135 – 140.

Facchinetti F., Sances G., Borella P., Genazzani A.R., Nappi G., *Magnesium prophylaxis of menstrual migraine: effects on intracellular magnesium*, Headache, 1991, 31 : 298 – 310.

Fanchamps A., *Why do not all beta-blockers prevent migraine?* Headache, 1985, 25 : 61 – 62.

Farid N.R., Johnson R.J., Low W.T., *Haemolytic reaction to mefenamic acid*, Lancet, 1971, 2 : 382.

Feinmann C., Harris M., Cawley R., *Psychogenic facial pain: presentation and treatment*, Br. Med. J., 1984, 288 : 436 – 438.

Feinmann C., Harris M. et al., *Psychogenic facial pain: presentation and treatment*, Br. Med. J., 1984, 288 : 436 – 438.

Feldman R., Park G., Lai C., *The interaction of verapamil and norverapamil with B-adrenergic receptors*, Circulation, 1985, 72 : 547 – 554.

Ferrari M.D., *311 C90: Increasing the options for therapy with effective acute antimigraine 5 HT receptor agonists1 B/1 D*, Neurology, 1997, 48 (3 Suppl. 3):S21-S24.

Ferrari M.D., Bayliss E.M., Luslow S., Pilgrim A.J., *Subcutaneous GR43 175 in the treatment of acute migraine: an international study*, Cephalalgia, 1989, 9, (Suppl. 10):348.

Ferrari M.D., Saxena P.R., *Clinical and experimental effects of sumatriptan in humans*, Trends Pharmacol. Sci., 1993, 14 : 129 – 133.

Ferrari M.D., James M.H., Bates D., et al. *Oral sumatriptan: effect of a second dose, and incidence and treatment of headache recurrences*, Cephalagia, 1994, 14 : 330 – 8.

Ferreira S.H., *Prostaglandins, aspirin-like drugs and analgesia*, Nature, 1972, 240 : 200 – 203.

Ferreira S.H., Moncada S., Vane J.R., *Indomethacin and aspirin abolish prostaglandin release from the spleen*, Nature, 1971, 231 : 237 – 239.

Field M.J., Oles R.J., Lewis A.S., McCleary S., Hughes J., Singh L., *Gabapentin (neurontin) and S-(+)-3-isobutylgaba represent a novel class of selective antihyperalgesic agents*, Br. J. Pharmacol., 1997, 121(8):1513 – 1522.

Fields H.L., *Peripheral neuropathic pain: an approach to management*, in: Wall P.D., Melzack R. (eds.), *Textbook of Pain*, Churchill Livingstone, Edinburgh, 1994, 991 – 996.

Fields H.L., Basbaum A., *Brain-stem control of spinal pain transmission neurons*, Annu. Rev. Physiol., 1978, 40 : 193.

Fisher M., Grotta J., *New uses for calcium channel blockers. Therapeutic implications*, Drugs, 1993, 46(6):961 – 975.

Fitzgerald M., *Capsaicin and sensory neurons. A review*, Pain, 1983, 15 : 109 – 130.

Fogelholm R., Murros K., *Maprotyline in chronic tension headaches: a double blind crossover study*, Headache, 1985, 25 : 273 – 275.

Ford R.G., Ford K.T., *Continuous intravenous dihydroergotamine in the treatment of intractable headache*, Headache, 1997, 37 : 129 – 136.

Forssman B., Lindblad C.J., Zbornikova V., *Atenolol for migraine prophylaxis*, Headache, 1983, 23 : 188 – 190.

Foster C.A., Bafaloukos I., *Paroxetine in the treatment of chronic daily headache*, Headache, 1994, 34 : 587 – 589.

Fozard J.R., *Basic mechanism of antimigraine drugs*, in: Critchley M., Friedman A.P., Gorini S. and Sicuteri F. (eds.), *Headache: Physiopathological and clinical concepts, Advances in Neurology*, vol. 33, Raven Press, New York, 1982, 295 – 307.

Frediani F., Cavazzuti I., Patruno G., Novi C., *Sumatriptan: esperienza clinica con l'impiego di dosaggi differenti*, Masson, 1995, vol. 4, suppl. to no. 2, 4–7.

Frenken C.W.G.M., Nuijten S.T.M., *Flunarizine, a new preventive approach to migraine. A double-blind comparison with placebo*, Clin. Neurol. Neurosurg., 1984, 86 : 17–20.

Friedman A.P., Mikropoulos H.E., *Cluster headaches*, Neurology, 1958, 8 : 653–663.

Friedman A.P., Elkind A.H., *Appraisal of methysergide in treatment of vascular headaches of migraine type*, J. Am. Med. Assoc., 1963, 184 : 125–128.

Friedman A.P., DiSerio F.J., Hwang D.S., *Symptomatic relief of migraine: multicenter comparison of Cafergot PB, Cafergot, and placebo*, Clin. Ther., 1989, 11 : 170–182.

Fromm G.H., Terrence C.F., Chattha A.S., Glass J.D., *Baclofen in trigeminal neurologia. Its effect on the spinal trigeminal nucleus: a pilot study*, Arch. Neurol., 1980, 37 : 768–771.

Fromm G.H., Terrence C.F., Chattha A.S., *Baclofen in the treatment of trigeminal neuralgia: double-blind study and long-term follow-up*, Ann. Neurol., 1984, 15 : 240–244.

Fromm G.H., Terrence C.F., *Comparison of L-baclofen and racemic baclofen in trigeminal neuralgia*, Neurology, 1987, 37 : 1725–1728.

Gabia T.J., Spierings E.L.H., *Prophylactic treatment of cluster headache with verapamil*, Headache, 1989, 29 : 167–168.

Gawel M., *A double-blind, cross over study of nimodipine versus pizotyline in common and classical migraine*, Cephalalgia, 1987, 7, (Suppl. 6):453–454.

Gelmers H.J., *Nimodipine, a new calcium antagonist in the prophylactic treatment of migraine*, Headache, 1983, 23 : 106–109.

Glazin A.M., Langer S.Z., *Presynaptic alpha 2-adrenoceptor antagonism by verapamil but not by dictiazem in rabbit hypothalamic slices*, Br. J. Pharmacol., 1983, 78 : 571–577.

Goadsby P.J., *The clinical profile of sumatriptan: cluster headache*, Eur. Neurol., 1994, 34 (Suppl. 2):35–39.

Göbel H., Ernst M., Jeschke, Keil R., Weigle I., *Acetylsalicylic acid activates antinociceptive brain stem reflex activity in headache patients and in healthy subjects*, Pain, 1992, 48 : 187–196.

Göbel H., Hamouz V., Hansen C., et al. *Amitriptyline in therapy of chronic tension headache*, Nervenarzt, 1994 a, 65 : 670–679.

Göbel H., Hamouz V., Hansen C., et al. *Chronic tension-type headache: amitriptyline reduces clinical headache-duration and experimental pain sensitivity but does not alter pericranial muscle activity readings*, Pain, 1994 b, 59 : 241–249.

Godfraind T., Miller E., Wibo M., *Calcium Antagonism and calcium entry-blockade*, Pharmacol. Reviews, 1986, 38 : 321–416.

Goldstein J., Dahlöf C.G.H., Diener H.C., et al. *Alniditan in the acute treatment of migraine attacks: a subcutaneous dose-finding study*, Cephalalgia, 1996, 16 : 497–502.

Gomersall J.D., Stuart A., *Amitriptyline in migraine prophylaxis, Changes in pattern of attacks during a controlled clinical trial*, J. Neurol. Neurosurg. Psychiatry, 1973, 36 : 684–690.

Gourlay G.K., Cherry D.A., Cousins M.F., Love B.L., Graham J.R., McLachlan M.O., *A controlled study of a serotonin reuptake blocker, zimelidine, in the treatment of chronic pain*, Pain, 1986, 25 : 35–52.

Graffenried B.V., Hill R.C., Nuesch E., *Headache as a model for assessing mild analgesic drugs*, J. Clin. Pharmacol., 1980, 20 : 131–144.

Granella F., Farina S., Malferrari G., Manzoni G.C., *Drug abuse in chronic headache: a clinic-epidemiologic study*, Cephalalgia, 1987, 7 : 15–19.

Greenberg D.A., *Calcium channel antagonists and the treatment of migraine*, Clin. Neuropharmacol., 1986, 9 : 311–328.

Greenblatt D.J., Shader R.I., *Benzodiazepines, Parts I and II*, N. Engl. J. Med., 1974, 291 : 1011–1015, 1239–1243.

Gupta P., Scatchard J., Shepperson N.B. et al., *In vitro pharmacology of eletriptan (UK-116,044) at the ›5-HT10-like' receptor in the dog saphenous vein*, Cephalalgia, 1996, 16.386.

Hakkarainen H., Gustafsson B., Stockman O., *A comparative trial of ergotamine tartrate, acetyl salicylic acid and a dextropropoxyphene compound in acute migraine attacks*, Headache, 1978, 18 : 35–39.

Hameroff S.R., Weiss J.L., Lerman J.C. et al., *Doxepin effects on chronic pain and depression: a controlled study*, J. Clin. Psychiatry, 1984, 45 : 45–52.

Haugh M.J., Lavander L., Jensen L.A., Thaler H., Giuliano R., *Dihydroergotamine (DHE) versus DHE and metoclopramide in the office treatment of intractable acute migraine headache* (abs.), Proc. VIth Int. Headache Congress, Paris, Cephalalgia, 1993, 13, Suppl. 13 : 101.

Havanka-Kannaiainen H., *Treatment of acute migraine attack: ibuprofen and placebo compared*, Headache, 1989, 29 : 507–509.

Havanka-Kannaiainen H., Hokkanen E., Myllyla V.V., *Efficacy of nimodipine in the prophylaxis of migraine*, Cephalalgia, 1985, 5 : 39–43.

Havanka-Kannaiainen H., Hokkanen E., Myllya V.V., *Efficacy of nimodipine in comparison with pizotifen in the prophylaxis of migraine*, Cephalalgia, 1987, 7 : 7–13.

Heathfield K.W.G., Stone P., Crowder P., *Pizotifen in the treatment of migraine*, Practitioner, 1977, 218 : 428–4307.

Heimpel H., Heit W., *Drug induced aplastic anaemia. Clinical aspects*, Clin. Haematol., 1980, 9 : 641–662.

Hendler N., Cimini A., Terence M.A., Long D., *A comparison of cognitive impairment due to benzodiazepines and to narcotics*, Am. J. Psychiatry, 1980, 137 : 828–830.

Henry P., Hiesse Provost O., Dillenschneider A., Ganry H., Insuasty J., *Efficacy and tolerance of an effervescent aspirin-metoclopramide combination in the treatment of a migraine attack. Randomized double-blind study using a placebo*, Presse Medicale, 1995, 24 : 254–258.

Herd A., Ludwig L., *Relief of posttraumatic headache by intravenous chlorpromazine*, J. Emerg. Med., 1994, 12 : 849–851.

Hering R., Kuritzky A., *Sodium valproate in the prophylactic treatment of migraine: a double-blind study versus placebo*, Cephalalgia, 1992, 12 : 81–84.

Herrmann W.M., Horowski R., Dannehl K., Kramer U., Lurati K., *Clinical effectiveness of lisuride hydrogen maleate: a double blind trial versus methysergide*, Headache, 1977, 17 : 54–60.

Herrmann W.M., Kristof M., Hernandez M.S.Y., *Preventive treatment of migraine headache with a new isoergolenyl derivate*, J. Int. Med. Res., 1978, 6 : 476–482.

Holland J., Holland C., Kudrow L., *Low-dose amitriptilyne prophylaxis in chronic scalp muscle contraction headache*, in: Proceedings of the First International Headache Congress, Munich, 1983.

Hollister L.E., Conley F.K., Britt R.H., Shuer L., *Long-term use of diazepam*, J. Am. Med. Assoc., 1981, 246 : 1568–1570.

Holmes B., Brogden R.N., Heel R.C., Speight T.M., Avery G.S., *Flunarizine: a review of its pharmacodynamic and pharmakokinetic properties and therapeutic use*, Drugs, 1984, 27 : 6–44.

Hosman-Benjamisne S.L., Bolhuis P.A., *Migraine and platelet aggregation in patients treated with low dose acetylsalicyclic acid*, Headache, 1986, 26 : 282–284.

Huang Z., Byun B., Matsubara T., Moskowitz M., *Time-dependent blockade of neurogenic plasma extravasation in dura mater by 511 T1 B/ D agonists and endopeptidase 24.11*, Br. J. Pharmacol., 1993, 108 : 331 –335.

Humphrey P.P.A., Feniuk W., *Mode of action of the anti-migraine drug sumatriptan*, Trends Pharmacol. Sci., 1991, 12 : 444–445.

Humphrey P.P.A., Feniuk W., Motevalian M., Parsons A.A., Whalley E.T., *The vasoconstrictor action of sumatriptan on human isolated dura mater*, in: Fozard J.R., Saxena P.R. (eds.), *Serotonin: molecular biology, receptors and functional effects*, Birkhauser Verlag, Basel,1991, 421–429.

Humphrey P.P.A., Goadsby P.J., *The mode of action of sumatriptan is vascular? A debate*, Cephalalgia, 1994, 14 : 401–410.

Jain A.C., Sethi N.C., Balbar P.K., *A clinical electroencephalographic and trace element study with special reference to zinc, copper and magnesium in serum and cerebrospinal fluid (CSF) in cases of migraine*, J. Neurol., 1985, 232 : 161.

Jammes J.L., *The treatment of cluster headache with prednisone*, Dis. Nerv. Syst., 1975, 36 : 375–376.

Jensen R., Brinck T., Olesen J., *Sodium valproate has a prophylactic effect in migraine without aura: a triple-bind, placebo-controlled crossover study*, Neurology, 1994, 44 : 647–651.

Jensen R., Brinck T., Olesen J., *Sodium valproate has a prophylactic effect in migraine without aura*, Neurology, 1994, 44 : 647–651.

Jensen K., Tfelt-Hansen P., Lauritzen M., Olesen J., *Clinical trial of nimodipine for single attacks of classic migraine*, Cephalalgia, 1985, 5 : 125–131.

Jick H., *Effects of aspirin and acetaminophen in gastrointestinal hemorrhage*, Arch. Intern. Med., 1981, 141 : 316–321.

Johnson E.S., Ratcliffe D.M., Wilkinson M., *Naproxen sodium in the treatment of migraine*, Cephalalgia, 1985, 5 : 5–10.

Jones E.B., Gonzales E.R., Boggs J.G., Grillo J.A., Elswick R.K. Jr., *Safety and efficacy of rectal prochlorperazine for the treatment of migraine in the emergency department [published erratum appears in Ann. Emerg. Med. 1994, 24: 618 [see comments]*, Ann. Emerg. Med., 1994, 24 : 237–241.

Kamgasniemi P., Falck B., Langvik V., Hyyppa M.T., *Levotryptophan treatment in migraine*, Headache, 1978, 18 : 161–166.

Kaube H., Hoskin K.L., Goadsby P.J., *Inhibition by sumatriptan of central trigeminal neurones only after blood brain barrier disruption*, Br. J. Pharmacol., 1993, 109 (Suppl. 3):788–792.

Kelly K.M., *Cardiac arrest following use of sumatriptan*, Neurology, 1995, 45 : 1211–1213.

Kempsford R.D., Baille P., Fuseau E., *Oral naratriptan tablets (2.5 – 10 mg) exhibit dose-proportional pharmacokinetics*, Cephalalgia, 1997 a (abs.), 17 : 408.

Kempsford R.D., Fuseau E., Snell P., Crisp A., Noble J.M., Ford G.A., *Oral naratriptan pharmacokinetics are predictable in subjects with impaired renal function*, Cephalalgia, 1997 b (abs.), 17 : 408.

Khan O.A., *Gabapentin relieves trigeminal neuralgia in multiple sclerosis patients*, Neurology, 1998, 51(2):611 – 614.

Kiaersgard-Rasmussen M.J., Holt Larsen B., Borg L., Soelberg-Sorensen P., Hansen P.E., *Tolfenamic acid versus propanolol in the prophylactic treatment of migraine*, Acta. Neurol. Scand., 1994, 89(6):446 – 450.

King R.B., *Concerning the management of pain associated with herpes zoster and of postherpetic neuralgia*, Pain, 1988, 33 : 73 – 78.

Kinnunen E., Erkinjuntti T., Färkkilä M. et al., *Placebo-controlled double-blind trial of pirprofen and an ergotamine tartrate compound in migraine attacks*, Cephalalgia, 1988, 8 : 175 – 179.

Klapper J., *Divalproex sodium in migraine prophylaxis: a dose-controlled study*, Cephalalgia, 1997, 17 : 103 – 108.

Kloster R., Nestvold K., Vilming S.T., *A double blind study of ibuprofen verus placebo in the treatment of acute migraine attacks*, Cephalalgia, 1992, 12 : 169 – 171.

Kornberg A., Rachmilewitz E.A., *Aplastic anaemia prolonged ingestion of indomethacin*, Acta Haematol., 1982, 67 : 136 – 138.

Krabbe A., *Early clinical experience with subcutaneous GR43175 in acute cluster headache attacks*, Cephalalgia, 1989, 9(Suppl. 10):406.

Kudrow L., *Comparative results of prednisone, methysergide, and lithium therapy in cluster headache*, in: Greene R. (ed.), *Current concepts in migraine research*, Raven Press, New York, 1978, 159 – 163.

Kudrow L., *Cluster headache. Mechanisms and management*, Oxford University Press, New York, 1980.

Kuritzky A., Hering R., *Prophylactic treatment of migraine with long-active propranolol*, Cephalalgia, 1987, 7 (Suppl. 6):457 – 458.

Lamb R.J., Leach M.J., Miller A.A., Wheatley P.L., *Anticonvulsant profile in mice of lamotrigine, a novel anticonvulsant*, Br J. Pharmacol., 1985, 85 (Suppl):235.

Lance J.W., *Mechanism and management of headache*, Butterworths, London, 1978.

Lance J.W., *The pathogenesis of migraine*, in: *The mechanism and management of headache*, 5 th ed., Oxford, Butterworth Heinemann, 1993, 111 – 121.

Lance J.W., Fine R.D., Curran D.A., *An evaluation of methysergide in the prevention of migraine and other vascular headaches*, Med. J. Aust., 1963, 1 : 814 – 818.

Lance J.W., Curran D.A., *Treatment of chronic tension headache*, Lancet, 1964, 1 : 1236 – 1239.

Lance J.W., Anthony M., *Clinical trial of a new serotonin antagonist BC 105, in the prevention of migraine*, Med. J. Aust., 1968, 1 : 54 – 55.

Lance J.W., Anthony M., Somerville B., *Comparative trial of serotonin antagonists in the management of migraine*, Br. Med. J., 1970, 2 : 327 – 330.

Lange R., Lentz R., *Comparison of ketoprofen, ibuprofen and naproxen sodium in the treatment of tension-type headache*, Drugs Under Experimental and Clinical Research, 1995, 21 : 89 – 96.

Langohr H.D., Stöhr M., Petruch F., *An open and double-blind cross-over study on the efficacy of clomipramine (Anafranil) in patients with painful mono-and polyneuropathies*, European Neurology, 1982, 2 : 309 – 317.

Lanza F.L., Royer G.L. Jr., Nelson R.S., et al., *A comparative endoscopic evaluation of the damaging effects of non steroidal anti-inflammatory agents on the gastric and duodenal mucosa*, Am. J. Gastroenterol., 1981, 75 : 17.

Lasagna L., *The role of benzodiazepines in nonpsychiatric medical practice*, Am. J. Psychiatry, 1977, 134 : 656 – 658.

Lawrence E.R., Hossain M., Littlestone W., *Sandomigran for migraine prophylaxis; controlled multicenter trial in general practice*, Headache, 1977, 17 : 109 – 112.

Leach M.J., Marden C.M., Miller A.A., *Pharmacological studies on lamotrigine, a novel potential antiepileptic drug. II Neurochemical studies on the mechanism of action*, Epilepsia, 1986, 27 : 490 – 497.

Lee S.H., Fawlett V., Preece J.M., *Aplastic anaemia associated with piroxicam*, Lancet, 1982, 1 : 1186.

Lenaerts M., Bastings E., Sianard J., Schoenen J., *Sodium valproate in severe migraine and tension-type headache: an open study of long-term efficacy and correlation with blood levels*, Acta Neurol. Belg., 1996, 96 : 126 – 129.

Levine J.D., Gordon N.C., Smith R., McBryde R., *Desipramine enhances opiate postoperative analgesia*, Pain, 1986, 27 – 45 – 49.

Lim R.K.S., Guzman F., Rodgers D.W., et al. Arch. Int. Pharmacodyn. Ther., 1964, 152 : 25.

Linder S.L., *Treatment of childhood headache with dihydroergotamine mesylate*, Headache, 1994, 34 : 578 – 580.

Lloyd K., *The clinical profile of sumatriptan: safety and tolerability*, Eur. Neurol., 1994, 34 (Suppl. 2):40 – 43.

Loldrup D., Langemark M., Hansen H.J., Olesen J., Bech P., *Clomipramine and mianserin in chronic idiopathic pain syndrome*, Psychopharmacology, 1989, 99 : 1 – 7.

Lopez Ibor J.J., *Masked depressions*, Br. J. Psychiatry, 1972, 120 : 245 – 257.

Louis P., *A double-blind placebo-controlled prophylactic study of flunarizine (Sibelium) in migraine*, Headache, 1981, 21 : 235 – 239.

Louis P., Spierings E.L., *Comparison of flunarizine (Sibelium) and pizotifen (Sandomigran) in migraine treatment: a double blind study*, Cephalalgia, 1982, 2 : 197 – 203.

Lücking C.H., Oestreich W., Schmidt R., Soyka D., *Flunarizine vs. propranolol in the prophylaxis of migraine*, Cephalalgia, 1988, 8(Suppl. 8):21 – 6.

Lynn B., *Capsaicin: actions on nociceptive C-fibres and therapeutic potential*, Pain, 1990, 41 : 61 – 69.

Man in't Veld A.J., Schalekamp M.A.D.H., *How intrinsic sympathomimetic activity modulates the haemodynamic responses to ß-adrenoceptor antagonists. A clue to the nature of their antihypertensive mechanism*, Br. J. Clin. Pharmacol, 1982, 13 : 245 – 257.

Manconi F.M., Zuddas A., Pedditzi M., Del Zompo M., Corsini G.U., *Importanza del sistema dopaminergico nella cefalea catameniale*, in: Manzoni G.C. et al. (eds.), *Le Cefalee*, CIC Edizioni Internazionali, Roma, 1987, 179 – 185.

Manna V., Bolino F., Di Cicco L., *Chronic tension-type headache, mood depression and serotonin: therapeutic effects of fluvoxamine and mianserine*, Headache, 1994, 34 : 44 – 49.

Manzoni G.C., *Use, misuse and abuse of ergotamine and its derivatives in migraine treatment*, in: Nappi G. et al. (eds.), *Neurotoxicology. Basic and clinical research*, CIC Edizioni Internazionali, Roma, 1987, 64.

Manzoni G.C., Bono G., Sacquegna T., et al. *Flunarizine in common migraine: Italian cooperative trial, I: Short-term results and responders definition*, Cephalalgia, 1985, 5(Suppl. 2):155 – 158.

Manzoni G.C., Zanferrari C., Granella F., et al., *Piroxicam-beta-ciclodestrina nel trattamento sintomatico delle cefalee primarie*, Meeting interdisciplinare di Cardiologia e Neurologia, Selecta Neurologica, 1989, 449 – 453.

Markley H.G., Cheronis J.C.D., Piepho R.W., *Verapamil in prophylactic therapy of migraine*, Neurology, 1984, 34 : 973 – 976.

Marks J., *The benzodiazepines—use and abuse*, Arzneimittel Forschung/Drug Res., 1980, 30 : 889 – 891.

Martin G.R., *Pre-clinical pharmacology of zolmitriptan (ZomigTM, formerly 311 C90), a centrally and peripherally acting 5 HT1 B/1 D agonist for migraine*, Cephalalgia, 1997, 17 (Suppl. 18):4 – 14.

Martínez-Lage J.M., *Flunarizine (Sibelium) in the prophylaxis of migraine. An open, long-term, multicenter trial*, Cephalalgia, 1988, 8 (Suppl. 8):15 – 20.

Masel B.E., Chesson A.L., Peters B.H., Levin H.S., Alperin J.B., *Platelet antagonists in migraine prophylaxis. A clinical trial using aspirin and dipyridamole*, Headache, 1980, 20 : 13 – 18.

Massiou H., *Dihydroergotamine nasal spray in prevention and treatment of migraine attacks: two controlled trials versus placebo*, Cephalalgia, 1987, 7 (Suppl. 6):440 – 441.

Massiou H., Bousser M.J., *Bêta-bloquants et migraine*, Pathologie et Biologie, 1992, 40 : 373 – 380.

Mathew N.T., *5-hydroxy/tryptophane in the prophylaxis of migraine: a double blind study*, Headache, 1978, 18 : 111.

Mathew N.T., Saper J.R., Silberstein S.D., et al. *Migraine prophylaxis with divalproex [see comments]*, Arch. Neurol., 1995, 52 : 281 – 286.

Mathias B.J., Dillingham T.R., Zeigler D.N., Chang A.S., Belandres P.V., *Topical capsaicin for chronic neck pain. A pilot study*, Am. J. Phys. Med. Rehabil., 1995, 74 : 39 – 44.

Mauskop A., Altura B.T., Cracco R.Q., Altura B.M., *Deficiency in serum ionized magnesium but not total magnesium in patients with migraines. Possible role of ICa2 +/Imag2 + ratio*, Headache, 1993, 33 : 135 – 138.

Mauskop A., Altura B.T., Cracco R.Q., Altura B.M., *Intravenous magnesium sulphate relieves migraine attacks in patients with low serum ionized magnesium levels: a pilot study*, Clin. Sci. Colch., 1995, 89 : 633 – 636.

Mauskop A., Altura B.T., Cracco R.Q., Altura B.M., *Intravenous magnesium sulfate relieves cluster headaches in patients with low serum ionized magnesium levels*, Headache, 1995, 35 : 597 – 600.

McNairy S.L., Maruta T., Ivnik R.J., Swanson D.W., Ilstrup D.M., *Prescription medication dependence and neuropsychologic function*, Pain, 1984, 18 : 169 – 178.

Medical Letter on Drugs and Therapeutics Choice of benzodiazepines, 1981, 23 : 41 – 42.

Meldrum B.S., *Pharmacology and mechanisms of action of lamotrigine*, in: Reynolds E.M., *Lamotriginem—a new advance in the treatment of epilepsy*. RSMS international congress and symposium series No 204, Royal Society of Medicine Services, London, 1993.

Merikangas K.R., Merikangas J.R., *Combination monoamine oxidase inhibitor and beta-blocker treatment of migraine, with anxiety and depression*, Biol. Psychiatry., 1995, 38 : 603 – 610.

Meyer J.S., Hardenberg J., *Clinical effectiveness of calcium entry blockers in prophylactic treatment of migraine and cluster headaches*, Headache, 1983, 23 : 266 – 277.

Micheli F., Pardal M.F., Giannaula R., et al., *Movement disorders and depression due to flunarizine and cinnarizine*, Mov. Disord., 1989, 4 : 139 – 146.

Micieli G., Iannacchero R., Tassorelli C., Russano G., Sibilla L., Nappi G., *Effetto antalgico del complesso piroxicam-beta-ciclodextrina nel trattamento dell'emicrania comune. Studio controllato vs naprossene sodico a dosaggio elevato (550 mg)*, Giornale di Neuropsicofarmacol., 1989, 4 : 170 – 173.

Millar A.A., Wheatley P., Sawyer D.A. et al., *Pharmacological studies on lamotrigine, a novel potential antiepileptic drug.* I Anticonvulsant profile in mice and rats, Epilepsia, 1986, 27 : 483 – 489.

Milton K.A., Allen M.J., Abel S., et al. *The safety, tolerability, pharmacokinetics and pharmacodynamics of oral and intravenous eletriptan, a potent and selective "5 HT1 D-like" receptor partial agonist*, Cephalalgia, 1997, 17 : 414.

Minta J.O., Williams M.D., *Some nonsteroidal antiinflammatory drugs inhibit the generation of superoxide anions by activated polymorphs by blocking ligand-receptor interactions*, J. Rheumatol., 1985, 12 : 751 – 757.

Mitchelson F., *Pharmacological agents effecting emesis*, A review (Part. II), Drugs, 1992, 43 : 443 – 63.

Molaie M., Olson C.M., Koch J., *The effects of intravenous verapamil on acute migraine headache*, Headache, 1987, 27 : 51 – 53.

Moncada S., Ferreira S.H., Vane J.R., *Inhibition of prostaglandin biosynthesis as the mechanism of analgesia of aspirin-like drugs in the dog knee-joint*, Eur. J. Pharmacol., 1975, 31 : 250 – 260.

Monks R.C., *Psychotropic drugs*, in: Wall P.D., Melzack R. (eds.), *Textbook of Pain*, Churchill Livingstone, Edinburgh, 1994, 963 : 989.

Monks R.C., *Psychopharmacological management of post myocardial depression and anxiety*, Can. Fam. Physician, 1981, 27 : 1117 – 1121.

Monstad I., Krabbe A., Micieli G., et al. *Preemptive oral treatment with sumatriptan during a cluster period*, Headache, 1995, 35 : 607 – 613.

Montastruc J.L., Tran M.A., Blanc M. et al., *Measurement of plasma levels of clomipramine in the treatment of chronic pain*, Clin. Neuropharmacol., 1985, 8 : 78 – 82.

Moreno A., Serrano V., Casado J.L., Arenas C., Alberca R., *Sumatriptan and cluster headache*, Neurologia, 1995, 10 : 76 – 80.

Morgan P., Rance D., James G., Mitchell R., Milton A., *Comparative absorption and elimination of eletriptan in rat, dog and human*, Cephalalgia, 1997, 17 : 414.

Moschiano F., D'Amico D., Grazzi L., Leone M., Bussone G., *Sumatriptan nel trattamento acuto dell'emicrania senza aura: efficacia della dose di 50 mg*, Suppl. JAMA ed. it., 1996, 8 : 1 – 3.

Moskowitz M.A., *Neurogenic vs vascular mechanisms of sumatriptan and ergot alkaloids in migraine*, Trends Pharmacol. Sci., 1992, 13 : 307 – 311.

Mueller L., Gallagher R.M., Ciervo C.A., *Vasospasm-induced myocardial infarction with sumatriptan*, Headache, 1996, 36 : 329 – 331.

Myers R.F., Siegel M.I., *Differential effects of antinflammatory drugs on lipoxigenase and cyclox ygenase activities of neutrophils from a reverse passive Arthurs reaction*, Biochem. Biopys. Res. Commun., 1983, 112 : 586 – 594.

Mylecharane E.J., Tfelt-Hansen P., *Migraine, miscellaneous drugs*, in: Olesen J., Tfelt-Hansen P., Welch K.M.A. (eds.), *The headaches*, New York, Raven Press, 1993, 397 – 402.

Nappi G., Granella G., Sandrini G., et al. *Effectiveness of ritanserin, a selective serotonin-S2 receptor antagonist in the treatment of chronic headache with dysthymic disorder*, Cephalalgia, 1989, 9, (Suppl. 10):371 – 372.

Nappi G., Manzoni G.C., *Manuale delle cefalee*, Cluster Press, Milano, 1990.

Nappi G., Sicuteri F., Byrne M., Roncolato M., Zerbini O., *Oral sumatriptan compared with placebo in the acute treatment of migraine*, J. Neurol., 1994, 241 : 138 – 144.

Nappi G., Sandrini G., Granella F. et al., *A new 5-HT2 antagonist (ritanserin) in the treatment of chronic headache with depression. A double-blind study vs amitriptyline*, Headache, 1990, 30 : 439 – 444.

Nebe J., Heier M., Diener H.C., *Low-dose ibuprofen in self-medication of mild to moderate headache: a comparison with acetylsalicylic acid and placebo*, Cephalalgia, 1995, 15 : 531 – 535.

Nestwold K., Kloster R., Partinen M., Sulkava R., *Treatment of acute migraine attack: naproxen and placebo compared*, Cephalalgia, 1985, 5 : 115 – 119.

Newman L.C., Lipton R.B., Solomon S., *Hemicrania continua: ten new cases and a review of the literature*, Neurology, 1994, 44 : 2111 – 2114.

Nuti A., Lucetti C., Pavese N., Dell'Agnello G., Rossi G., Bonuccelli U., *Long-term follow-up after flunarizine or nimodipine discontinuation in migraine patients*, Cephalalgia, 1996, 16 : 337 – 340.

Onghena P., Van Houdenhove B., *Antidepressant-induced analgesia in chronic non-malignant pain: a meta-analysis of 39 placebo-controlled studies*, Pain, 1992, 49 : 205 – 219.

Paiva T., Esperanca P., Marcelino L., Assis G., *A double-blind trial with dihydroergotamine spray in migraine crisis*, Cephalalgia, 1985, 5 (Suppl. 3):140 – 141.

Paoli F., Darcourt G., Cossa P., *Note préliminaire sur l'action de l'imipramine dans les états douloureux*, Rev. Neurol., Paris, 1960, 102 : 503 – 504.

Pareja J., Sjaastad O., *Chronic paroxysmal hemicrania and hemicrania continua. Interval between indomethacin administration and response*, Headache, 1996, 36 : 20 – 23.

Pearce I., Frank G.I., Pearce J.M.S., *Ibuprofen compared with paracetamol in migraine*, Practitioner, 1983, 227 : 465 – 467.

Peck A.W., *Lamotrigine: historical background*, Rev. Contemp, Pharmacother., 1994, 5 : 95 – 105.

Pedersen E., Moller C.E., *Methysergide in the migraine prophylaxis*, Clin. Pharmacol. Ther., 1966, 7 : 520 – 526.

Peiris J.B., Perera G.L.S., Devendra S.V., Lionel N.D.W., *Sodium valproate in trigeminal neuralgia*, Med. J. Aust., 1980, 2 : 278.

Penada G., *Chimica farmaceutica e tossicologica*, 2 d ed. Libreria Progetto, 1990, 1 : 409, 433.

Perez H.D., Elfman F., Marder S., *Meclofenamate sodium monohydrate inhibits chemotactic factor-induced human polymorphonuclear leukocyte function. A possible explanation for its antiinflammatory effect*, Arthritis Rheum., 1987, 30 : 1023 – 1031.

Peroutka S.J., *Developments in 5-hydroxytryptamine receptor pharmacology in migraine*, Neurol. Clin., 1990 a, 8 : 829 – 838.

Peroutka S.J., *The pharmacology of current anti-migraine drugs*, Headache, 1990 b, 30 (Suppl. 1):12.

Peroutka S.J., Allen G.S., *The calcium antagonist properties of cyproheptadine: implications for anti-migraine action*, Neurology, 1984, 34 : 304 – 309.

Peroutka S.J., Banghart S.B., Allen G.S., *Relative potency and selectivity of calcium antagonists used in the treatment of migraine*, Headache, 1984, 24 : 55 – 58.

Peters B.H., Fraim C.J., Masel B.E., *Comparison of 650 mg aspirin and 1000 mg acetaminophen with each other, and with placebo in moderately severe headache*, Am. J. Med., 1983, 74 : 36 – 42.

Peters B.H., Meyburg H.W., Westendorp P.H., Westerhof P.W., *Use of sumatriptan (Imigran) in a female patient with coronary spasm*, Ned. Tijdschr. Geneskd., 1994, 138(10):1872 – 1874.

Pfaffenrath V., Diener H.C., Isler H., et al. *Efficacy and tolerability of amitriptylinoxide in the treatment of chronic tension-type headache: a multi-centre controlled study*, Cephalalgia, 1994, 14 : 149 – 55.

Pfaffenrath V., Wessely P., Meyer C., et al. *Magnesium in the prophylaxis of migraine-a double-blind, placebo-controlled study*, Cephalalgia, 1996, 16 : 436 – 440.

Piccini P., Nuti A., Paoletti A.M., Napolitano A., Melis G.B., Bonucelli U., *Possible involvement of dopaminergic mechanisms in the antimigraine action of flumarizine*, Cephalalgia, 1990, 10 : 3 – 8.

Piletta P., Porchet H.C., Dayea P., *Central analgesic effect of acetominophen but not of aspirin*, Clin. Pharmacol. Ther., 1991, 49 : 350 – 354.

Pilgrim A.J., *The clinical profile of sumatriptan: efficacy in migraine*, Eur. Neurol., 1994, 34 (Suppl. 2):26 – 34.

Pini L.A., Sandrini M., Vitale G., *The antinociceptive action of paracetamol is associated with changes in the serotonergic system in the rat brain*, Eur. J. Pharmacol., 1996, 308 : 31 – 40.

Pini L.A., Sternieri E., Fabbri L., Zerbini O., Bamfi F., *High efficacy and low frequency of headache recurrence after oral sumatriptan. The Oral Sumatriptan Italian Study Group*, J. Int. Med. Res., 1995, 23 : 96 – 105.

Pini L.A., Vitale G., Sandrini M., *Serotonin and opiate involvement in the antinociceptive effect of acetylsalicylic acid*, Pharmacology, 1997, 54 : 84 – 91.

Pipitone V., *I farmaci antiflogistici non steroidei*, Riv. Medico Pratico-Reumatol., 1988, 5 : 55.

Plosker G.L., McTavish D., *Sumatriptan. A reappraisal of its pharmacology and therapeutic efficacy in the acute treatment of migraine and cluster headache*, Drugs, 1994, 47 : 622 – 651.

Pradalier A., Rancurel G., Verdure L., Rascol A., Dry J., *Acute migraine attack theraphy — comparison of naproxen sodium and an ergotamine tartrate compound*, Cephalalgia, 1985, 5 : 107 – 113.

Prendes J.L., *Considerations on the use of propranolol in complicated migraine*, Headache, 1980, 20 : 93 – 95.

Prusinski A., Kozubski W., *Use of verapamil in the treatment of migraine*, Wiad Lek, 1987, 1 : 734 – 738.

Prusinski A., Kozubski W., Szule-Kuberska J., *Steroid treatment in the interruption of clusters in cluster headache patients*, Cephalalgia, 1987, 7: 332–333.

Puttini P.S., Cazzola M., Bocassini L. et al., *A comparison of dothiepin versus placebo in the treatment of pain in rheumatoid arthritis and the association of pain with depression*, J. Int. Med. Res., 1988, 16: 331–337.

Quality Standards Subcommittee of the American Academy of Neurology, *Practice parameter: Appropriate use of ergotamine tartrate and dihydroergotamine in the treatment of migraine and status migrainosus (Summary statement)*, Neurology, 1995, 45: 585–587.

Quijada-Carrera J., Valenzuela-Castano A., Poredano-Gomez J., et al., *Comparison of tenoxicam and bromazepan in the treatment of fibromyalgia: a ramdomized, double-blind, placebo-controlled trial*, Pain, 1996, 65: 221–225.

Racagni G., Nobili G., Tiengo M., *Farmaci nella terapia del dolore*, Edi-Ermes, Milano, 1985.

Rainsford K.D., in: Curtis-Prior C.P. (ed.), *Hand book of prostaglandins and related eicosanoids*, Churchill Livingstone, Edinburgh, 1988, 52.

Ramadan N.M., Halvorson H., Vande-Linde A., Levine S., Helpern J.A., Welch K.M.A., *Low brain magnesium in migraine*, Headache, 1989, 29: 590–593.

Ramswamy S. Bapna J.S., *Analgesic effect of metoclopramide and its mechanism*, Life Sci., 1986, 38: 1289–1292.

Rappaport A.M., Visser W.H., Cutler N.R., et al. *Oral sumatriptan in preventing headache recurrence after treatment of migraine attacks with subcutaneous sumatriptan*, Neurology, 1995, 45: 1505–1509.

Rederich G., Rappaport A.M., Cutler N., Hazelrigg R., Jamerson B., *Oral sumatriptan for the long-term treatment of migraine: clinical findings*, Neurology, 1995, 45 (Suppl. 7):S15–20.

Robbins L., Remmes A., *Outpatient repetitive intravenous dehydroergotamine.* Headache, 1992, 32: 455–458.

Roberts M.H.T., *5-Hydroxytryptamine and antinociception*, Neuropharmacology, 1984, 23: 1529–1536.

Rohr J., Dufresne J.J., *Dihydroergotamine nasal spray for the treatment of migraine attacks: a comparative double-blind crossover study with placebo*, Cephalalgia, 1985, 5 (Suppl. 3):142–143.

Rosner H., Rubin L., Kestenbaum A., *Gabapentin adjunctive therapy in neuropathic pain states*, Clin J. Pain, 1996, 12(1):56–58.

Ross D.R., Varipapa R.J., *Treatment of painful diabetic neuropathy with topical capsaicin*, N. Engl. J. Med., 1989, 321: 474–475.

Roth S.H., *Non steroidal anti-inflammatory drug gastropathy*, Arch. Intern. Med., 1986, 146: 1075–1076.

Rothrock J.F., Kelly N.M., Brody M.L., Golbeck A., *A differential response to treatment with divalproex sodium in patients with intractable headache*, Cephalalgia, 1994, 14: 241–244.

Russell M.B., Holm-Thomsen-O.E., Nielsen M.R., Cleal A., Pilgrim A.J., Olesen J., *Sumatriptan treatment of migraine in general practice. A randomized, double-blind, placebo-controlled cross-over study*, Ugeskr-Laeger, 1995, 157(17):2320–2323.

Ryan R.E., *Double-blind clinical evaluation of the efficacy and safety of ergostine-caffeine and placebo in migraine headache*, Headache, 1970, 9: 212–220.

Ryan R.E. sr., Ryan R.E. Jr., Sudilovsky A., *Nadolol: its use in the prophylactic treatment of migraine*, Headache, 1983, 23: 26–31.

Saadah H.A., *Abortive migraine therapy in the office with dexamethasone and prochlorperazine*, Headache, 1994, 34: 366–370.

Sandyk R., *Baclofen in hemifacial spasm*, Eur. Neurol., 1984, 23: 163–165.

Saper J.R., *Ergotamine dependency – a review*, Headache, 1987, 27: 435–438.

Saper J.R., *Ergotamine tartrate dependency: possible mechanisms*, in: Diener H.C., Wilkinson M. (eds.), *Drug-induced headache*, Springer Verlag, Berlin, 1988, 117–124.

Saper J.R., Jones J.M., *Ergotamine tartrate dependency: features and possible mechanisms*, Clin. Neuropharmacol., 1986, 9: 244–256.

Saper J.R., Silberstein S.D., Lake A.E. 3 rd, Winters M.E., *Double-blind trial of fluoxetine: chronic daily headache and migraine [see comments]*, Headache, 1994, 34: 497–502.

Sargent J., Kirchner J.R., Davis R., Kirkhart B., *Oral sumatriptan is effective and well tolerated for the acute treatment of migraine: results of a multicenter study*, Neurology, 1995, 45 (Suppl. 7):S10–14.

Sargent J., Solbach P., Damasio H., et al., *A comparison of naproxen sodium to propranolol hydrochloride and a placebo control for the prophylaxis of migraine headache*, Headache, 1985, 25: 320–324.

Saxena P.R., Ferrari M.D., *From serotonin receptor classification to the antimigraine drug sumatriptan*, Cephalalgia, 1992, 12: 187–196.

Scherl E.R., Wilson J.F., *Comparison of dihydroergotamine with metoclopramide versus meperidine with promethazine in the treatment of acute migraine*, Headache, 1995, 35: 256–259.

Schachtel B.P., Furey S.A., Thoden W.R., *Nonprescription ibuprofen and acetaminophen in the treatment of tension-type headache*, J. Clin. Pharmacol., 1996, 36: 1120–1125.

Schoenen J., Sianard-Gainko J., Lenaerts M., *Blood magnesium levels in migraine*, Cephalalgia, 1991, 11: 97–99.

Schoenen J., Sawyer J., *Zolmitriptan (ZomigTM, 311 C90), a novel dual central and peripheral 5HT1B/1D agonist: an overview of efficacy*, Cephalalgia, 1997, 17 (Suppl. 18):28–40.

Scott A.K., *Sumatriptan clinical pharmacokinetics*, Clin. Pharmacokinet, 1994, 27: 337–344.

Sevelius H., Segre E., Bursick K., *Comparative analgesic effects of naproxen sodium, aspirin and placebo*, J. Clin. Pharm., 1980, 20: 480–485.

Sharav Y., Singer E., Schmidt E., Dionne R.A., Dubner R., *The analgesic effect of amitriptyline on chronic facial pain*, Pain, 1987, 31: 199–209.

Shekelle R.B., Ostfeld A.M., *Methysergide in the migraine syndrome*, Clin. Pharmacol. Ther., 1964, 5: 201–204.

Shrestha M., Singh R., Moreden J., Hayes J.E., *Ketorolac vs chlorpromazine in the treatment of acute migraine without aura. A prospective, randomized, double-blind trial*, Arch. Intern. Med., 1996, 156: 1725–1728.

Shyu K.W., Lin M.T., Wu T.C., *Central serotoninergie neurons, their possible role in the development of dental pain and aspirin induced analgesia in monkyes*, Exp. Neurol., 1984, 84: 179–187.

Shyu K.W., Lin M.T., *Hypothalamic monoaminergic mechanism of aspirin-induced analgesia in monkeys*, J. Neural. Transm., 1985, 62: 285–293.

Sianard-Gainko J., Lenaerts M., Bastings E., Schoenen J., *Sodium valproate in severe migraine and tension-type headache: clinical efficacy and correlations with blood levels* (abs.), Proc. VIth Int. Headache Congress, Paris, Cephalalgia, 1993, 13(Suppl. 13):252.

Sicuteri F., *Prophylactic and therapeutic properties of 1-methyl-lysergic acid butanolamide in migraine*, Int. Arch. Allergy., 1959, 15: 300–307.

Siegel M.I., McConnel, Porter N.A., *Aspirin-like drugs inhibit arachidonic acid metabolism via lipoxygenase and ciclo-oxygenase in rat neutrophils from carragenin pleural exudates.* Biochem. Biophys. Res. Commun., 1980, 92: 688.

Silberstein S.D., Schulman E.A., Hopkins M.M., *Repetitive in travenous DHE in the treatment of refractory headache*, Headache, 1990, 30: 334–339.

Silberstein S.D., Silberstein J.R., *Chronic daily headache long-term prognosis following inpatient treatment with repetitive IV DHE*, Headache, 1992, 32: 439–445.

Silberstein S.D., Young W.B., *Safety and efficacy of ergotamine tartrate and dihydroergotamine in the treatment of migraine and status migrainosus. Working Panel of the Headache and Facial Pain Section of the American Academy of Neurology*, Neurology, 1995, 45: 577–584.

Silvoso G.R., Ivey K.J., Butt J.H., et al., *Incidence of gastric lesions in patients with rheumatic disease on chronic aspirin therapy*, Ann. Intern. Med., 1979, 91: 517–520.

Sist T.C., Filadora V., Miner M., Lema, M., *Gabapentin for idiopathic trigeminal neuralgia: report of two cases*, Neurology, 1997a, 48(5):1467.

Sist T.C., Filadora V.A. 2 nd, Miner M., Lema, M., *Experience with gabapentin for neuropathic pain in the head and neck: report of ten cases*, Reg Anesth, 1997b, 22: 473–478.

Sjaastad O., *Chronic paroxysmal hemicrania: clinical aspects and controversies*, in: Blau J.N. (ed.), *Migraine. Clinical, therapeutic, conceptual and research aspects*, Chapman and Hall Medical, London, 1987, 135–152.

Sjaastad O., Stensrud P., *Appraisal of BC 105 in migraine prophylaxis*, Acta Neurol. Scand., 1969, 45: 594–600.

Sjaastad O., Stensrud S., *Clinical trial of a beta-receptor blocking agent (LB46) in migraine prophylaxis*, Acta Neurol. Scand., 1972, 48: 124–128.

Smoller B., *The use of dexamethasone suppression test as a marker of efficacy in the treatment of a myofascial syndrome with amitriptyline*, Pain, 1984, (Suppl.) 2:S250.

Solomon G.D., *Pharmacology and use of headache medications*, Journal of Medicine, 1990, 57: 627–635.

Solomon G.D., Spaccavento L.J., *Verapamil prophylaxis of migraine: A double-blind, placebo-controlled trial*, JAMA, 1983, 250: 2500–2502.

Solomon G.D., Diamond S., *Verapamil in migraine prophylaxis; comparison of dosages*, Clin. Pharmacol. Ther., 1987, 41: 202.

Somerville B.W., Herrmann W.M., *Migraine prophylaxis with lisuride hydrogen maleate. A double blind study of lisuride versus placebo*, Headache, 1978, 18: 75–79.

Sorensen K.V., *Valproate, a new drug in migraine prophylaxis*, Acta Neurol. Scand., 1988, 78: 346–348.

Sorensen P.S., Hansen K., Olesen J., *A placebo-controlled, double-blind, cross-over trial of flunarizine in common migraine*, Cephalalgia, 1986, 6: 7–14.

Sorge F., De Simone R., Marano E., Nolano M., Orefice G., Carrieri P., *Flunarizine in prophylaxis of childhood migraine. A double-blind, placebo-controlled, crossover study*, Cephalalgia, 1988, 8: 1–6.

Southwell N., Williams J.D., Mackenzie I., *Methysergide in the prophylaxis of migraine*, Lancet, 1964, 1 : 523 – 524.

Soyka D., Taneri Z., Oestreich W., Schmidt R., *Flunarizine i. v. in the acute treatment of the migraine attack. A double-blind placebo-controlled study*, Cephalalgia, 1988, 8(Suppl. 8):35 – 40.

Spiegel K., Kalb R., Pasternak G.W., *Analgesic activity of tricyclic antidepressant*, Ann. Neurol., 1983, 13 : 462 – 465.

Spierings E.L.H., Messinger H.B., *Flunarizine vs. pizotifen in migraine prophylaxis: a review of comparative studies*, Cephalalgia, 1988, 8(Suppl. 8):27 – 30.

Steen P.A., Newberg L.A., Milde J.H., Michenfelder J.D., *Nimodipine improves cerebral ischemia in the dog*, J. Cereb. Blood Flow Metab., 1983, 1 : 38 – 43.

Steen K.H., Reeh P.W., Kreysel H.W., *Topical acetylsalicylic, salicylic, acid and indomethacin suppress pain from experimental tissue acidosis in human skin*, Pain, 1995, 62 : 339, 347.

Steiner T.J., Lange R., *Ketoprofen (25 mg) in the symptomatic treatment of episodic tension-type headache: double-blind placebo-controlled comparison with acetaminophen (1000 mg)*, Cephalalgia, 1998, 18 : 38 – 43.

Steiner T.J., Findley L.J., Yuen A.W.C., *Lamotrigine versus placebo in the prophylaxis of migraine with and without aura*, Cephalalgia, 1997, 17 : 109 – 12.

Steiner T.J., Ahmed F., Findley L.J., MacGregor E.A., Wilkinson M., *S-Fluoxetine in the prophylaxis of migraine: a phase II double-blind randomized placebo-controlled study*, Cephalalgia, 1998, 18 : 283 – 286.

Stensrud P., Sjaastad O., *Clinical trial of a new antibradykinin anti-inflammatory drug, ketoprofen (19.583 R.P.) in migraine prophylaxis*, Headache, 1974, 14 : 96 – 100.

Stovner L.J., Sjaastad O., *Treatment of cluster headache and its variants*, Curr. Opin. Neurol., 1995, 8 : 243 – 7.

Sudilovsky A., Elkind A.H., Ryan R.E., Saper J.R., Stern M.A., Meyer J.H., *Comparative efficacy of nadolol and propranolol in the management of migraine*, Headache, 1987, 27 : 421 – 426.

Swanson D.R., *Migraine and magnesium: eleven neglected connections*, Perspect. Biol. Med., 1988, 31(4):526 – 557.

Swerdlow M., Cundill J.C., *Anticonvulsant drugs used in the treatment of lancinating pain*, A comparison, Anaesthesia, 1981, 36 : 1129 – 1132.

Tansey M.J.B., Pilgrim A.J., Lloyd K., *Sumatriptan in the acute treatment of migraine*. J. Neurol. Sci., 1993, 114 : 109 – 116.

Taub A., *Relief of post herpetic neuralgia with psychotropic drugs*, J. Neurosurg., 1973, 39 : 235 – 239.

Taylor C.P., Gee N.S., Su T.Z. et al., *A summary of mechanistic hypotheses of gabapentin pharmacology*, Epilepsy Res., 1998, 3 : 233 – 249.

Terrence C.F., Fromm G.H., Tenicela R., *Baclofen as an analgesic in chronic peripheral nerve disease*, Eur. Neurol., 1985, 24 : 380 – 385.

Tfelt-Hansen P., Standnes B., Kangasniemi P., Hakkarainen H., Olesen J., *Timolol vs propranolol vs placebo in common migraine prophylaxis: a double-blind multicenter trial*, Acta Neurol. Scand., 1984, 69 : 1 – 8.

Tfelt-Hansen P., Olesen J., *Effervescent metoclopramide and aspirin (Migravess) versus effervescent aspirin or placebo for migraine attacks: a double-blind study*, Cephalalgia, 1984, 4 : 107 – 111.

Tfelt-Hansen P., Brand J., Dano P., et al. *Early clinical experience with subcutaneous GR43 175 in acute migraine: an overview*, Cephalalgia, 1989, 9(Suppl. 9):73 – 77.

Tfelt-Hansen P., Henry P., Mulder L.J., Scheldewaert R.G., Schoenen J., Chazot G., *The effectiveness of combined oral lysine acetylsalicylate and metoclopramide compared with oral sumatriptan for migraine*, Lancet, 1995, 346 : 923 – 926.

The Multinational Oral Sumatriptan and Cafergot Comparative Study Group, *A randomized, double-blind comparison of sumatriptan and Cafergot in the acute treatment of migraine*, Eur. Neurol., 1991, 31 : 314 – 22.

The Subcutaneous Sumatriptan International Study Group (Ferrari M.D., Melamed E., Gawel M.J. et al.), *Treatment of migraine attacks with sumatriptan*, N. Engl. J. Med., 1991, 325 : 316 – 321.

Thomas S.H., Stone C.K., Ray V.G., Whitley T.W., *Intravenous versus rectal prochlorperazine in the treatment of benign vascular or tension headache: a randomized, prospective, double-bind trial*, Ann. Emerg. Med., 1994, 24 : 923 – 7.

Thomsen L.L., Dixon R., Lassen L.H., et al. *311 C90 (Zolmitriptan), a novel centrally and peripheral acting oral 5-hydroxytryptamine-1 D agonist: a comparison of its absorption during a migraine attack and in a migraine-free period* , Cephalalgia, 1996, 16 : 270 – 275.

Tiengo C., *I fans*, in: Tiengo M., Benedetti C., *Fisiopatologia e terapia del dolore*, Masson, Paris,1996, 149 – 163.

Tiengo M., Ungaro R., Salaffi F., *Il dolore: aspetti diagnostici e terapeutici*, Fogliazza, Milano, 1989.

Titus F., Davalos A., Codina A., *5-hydroxytrythophan versus methysergide in the prophylaxis of migraine: a randomized clinical trial*, Cephalalgia, 1985, 5(Suppl. 3):518 – 519.

Touchon J., Bertin L., Pilgrim A.J., Phil D., Ashford E., Bès A., *A comparison of subcutaneous sumatriptan and dihydroergotamine nasal spray in the acute treatment of migraine*, Neurology, 1996, 47 : 361 – 365.

Towart R., *The selective inhibition of serotonin-induced contractions of rabbit cerebral vascular smooth muscle by calcium antagonistic dihydropyridines. An investigation of the mechanism of action of Nimodipine*, Circ. Res., 1981, 5 : 650 – 657.

Tulunay F.C., Karan O., Aydin N., Culcuoglu A., Guvener A., *Dihydroergotamine nasal spray during migraine attacks: a double-blind crossover study with placebo*, Cephalalgia, 1987, 7 : 131 – 133.

Vanasia M., *Gli antidepressivi nel trattamento del dolore*, in: Tiengo M., Benedetti C., *Fisiopatologia e terapia del dolore*, Masson, Paris, 1996, 173 – 180.

Vallaperta P., *Terapia dell'emicrania: la migrazione spontanea dalla dose piena alla mezza dose. Risultati di un'indagine sulla pratica clinica con Sumatriptan del medico specialista e del medico di base*, 1995, vol. 4, suppl. to no. 2, 4 – 7.

Vane J.R., *Inibition of Prostaglandin Synthesis as a mechanism of action for aspirin-like drugs*, Nature, 1971, 231 : 232 – 235.

Vane J.R., Botting R.M., *Analgesic action of aspirin*, in: Vane J.R., Botting R.M. (ed.), *Aspirin and other salicylates*, Chapman and Hall, London, 1992, 166 – 212.

Vanhoutte P.M., Paoletti R., *The WHO classification of calcium antagonists*, TIPS, 1987, 8 : 4 – 5.

Vein A., Voznesenskaya T., Danilov A., *The effects of aspirin on the CNV in healthy individuals*, Cephalalgia, 1995, 15 : 129 – 31.

Verspeelt J., De Locht P., Amery W.K., *Post-marketing cohort study comparing the safety and efficacy of flunarizine and propranolol in the prophylaxis of migraine*, Cephalalgia, 1996, 16 : 328 – 336.

Veys E.M., *20 years' experience with ketoprofen*, Scand. J. Rheumatol., 1991, (Suppl 90):3 – 44.

Vijayan N., *Headache following removal of acoustic neuroma*, Headache, 1995, 35 : 639.

Vijayan N., Spillane T., *Valproic acid treatment of chronic daily headache*, Headache, 1995, 35 : 540 – 543.

Visser W.H., De Vriend R.H.M., Jaspers N.M.W.H., Ferrari M.D., *Sumatriptan in clinical practice: A 2-year review of 453 migraine patients*, Neurology, 1996 a, 47 : 46 – 51.

Visser W.H., Jaspers N.M.W.H., De Vriend R.H.M., Ferrari M.D., *Chest symptoms after sumatriptan: a two-year clinical practice review in 735 consecutive migraine patients*, Cephalalgia, 1996 b, 16 : 554 – 559.

Volans G.N., *The effect of metoclopramide of the absorption of effervescent aspirin in migraine*, Br. J. Clin. Pharmacol., 1975, 2 : 63 – 67.

Ward T.N., Bokan J.A., Phillips M., Benedetti C., Butler S., Splengler D., *Antidepressants in concomitant chronic back pain and depression: doxepin and desipramine compared*, J. Clin. Psychiatry, 1984, 45 : 54 – 59.

Ward T.N., Scott G., *Dihydroergotamine suppositories in a headache clinic*, Headache, 1991, 31 : 465 – 466.

Watson C.P.N., Evans R.J., Watt V.R., *Post-herpetic neuralgia and topical capsaicin*, Pain, 1988,33 : 333 – 340.

Weaver K., *Magnesium and migraine*, (Letter to the editor), Headache, 1990, 30 : 168.

Weber R.B., Reinmuth O.M., *The treatment of migraine with propranolol*, Neurology, 1977, 22 : 33 – 45.

Weis O., Sriwatanakul K., Weintraub M., *Treatment of post-herpetic neuralgia and acute herpetic pain with amitriptyline and perphenazine*, S. Afr. Med. J., 1982, 62 : 274 – 275.

Weisz M.A., El-Raheb-M., Blumenthal H.j., *Home administration of intramuscular DHE for the treatment of acute migraine headache*, Headache, 1994, 34 : 371 – 373.

Welch K.M.A., Ellis D.J., Keenan P.A., *Successful migraine prophylaxis with naproxen sodium*, Neurology, 1985, 35 : 1304 – 1310.

Welch K.M.A., Levine S.R., D'Andrea G., Schultz L., Helpern J.A., *Preliminary observations on brain energy metabolism in migraine studied by in vivo 31-phosphorus spectroscopy*, Neurology, 1989, 39 : 538 – 541.

White R.P., Cunningham M.P., Robertson J.T., *Effect of the calcium antagonist Nimodipine on contractile responses of isolated canine basilar arteries induced by serotonin, prostaglandin F2 alfa, thrombin, and whole blood*, Neurosurgery, 1982, 3 : 344 – 348.

Wilkinson M., *Treatment of the acute migraine attack-current status*, Cephalalgia, 1983, 3 : 61 – 67.

Wilkinson M., *Treatment of the acute migraine: the British experience*, Headache, 1990, 30 : 545 – 549.

Wilkinson M., Pfaffenrath V., Schoenen J., Diener H.C., Steiner T.J., *Migraine and cluster headache—their management with sumatriptan: a critical review of the current clinical experience*, Cephalalgia, 1995, 15 : 337 – 357.

Winner P., Ricalde O., Le Force B., Saper J., Margul B., *A double-blind study of subcutaneous dihydroergotamine vs subcutaneous sumatriptan in the treatment of acute migraine*, Arch. Neurol., 1996, 53 : 180 – 184.

Wöber C., Brücke T., Wöber-Bingöl C., Asenbaum S., Wessely P., Podreka I., *Dopamine D2 receptor blockade and antimigraine action of flunarizine*, Cephalalgia, 1994, 14 : 235 – 240.

Zakrzewska J.M., Chaudhry Z., Nurmikko T.J., Patton D.W., Mullens E.L., *Lamotrigine (Lamictal) in refractory trigeminal neuralgia: results from a double-blind placebo controlled crossover trial*, Pain, 1997, 73 : 223 – 230.

Ziegler D.K., Ellis D.J., *Naproxen in prophylaxis of migraine*, Arch. Neurol., 1985, 42 : 582 – 584.

Zeigler D.K., Hurwitz A., Hassanein R.S., Kodanaz H.A., Preskorn S.H., Mason J., *Migraine prophylaxis. A comparison of popranoloe and amitriptyline*, Arch. Neurol., 1987, 44 : 486 – 489.

Ziegler D.K., Ford R., Kriegler J., et al. *Dihydroergotamine nasal spray for the acute treatment of migraine [see comments]*, Neurology, 1994, 44 : 447 – 453.

13 Nonpharmacological Treatment

Biofeedback

Biofeedback is the most widely employed means of "cognitive treatment," that is, of a treatment whose aim is to make the patient aware of his or her problem. The principle of biofeedback is to give the patient constant information about an organic function that is normally totally or partially outside his or her consciousness. The technique may be applied to different functions, such as the degree of muscle relaxation or activity, skin temperature, heart rate, blood pressure, galvanic skin response, or electrical brain activity (Paskewitz, 1975): a biofeedback device records the level of these functions and provides the patient with acoustic and/or visual information representing that level. The patient uses this information to learn how to keep the level of that function within normal limits.

Biofeedback therapy has been indicated for anxiety, phobias, drug dependency and insomnia (Budzynski, 1973), back pain (Gentry et al., 1977; Flor et al., 1983, 1986; Biederman et al., 1989), and Raynaud disease (Freedman, 1985; 1991), among others. Biofeedback is also recommended in physiotherapy for muscular rehabilitation (Blanchard and Yong, 1974).

In treating headache and facial pain, electromyographic biofeedback is the instrument that is most often used. It gives the patient information about the activity and degree of relaxation of the masticatory or craniofacial muscles, thus facilitating relaxation training of these muscle groups through subjective control of the contraction and the parafunctional habits by the patient.

Although no direct relationship between pain and electromyographic activity has been found (Anderson and Franks, 1981), nor between clinical improvement and the reduction of electromyographic activity (Phillips and Hunter, 1981), numerous authors have reported success through biofeedback therapy in cases of muscle pain (Solberg and Rugh, 1972; Budzynski and Stoyva, 1973; Heller and Strang, 1973; Gessel and Harrison, 1974; Rugh and Solberg, 1975; Rappaport et al., 1975; Dohrman and Laskin, 1976; Butler et al., 1976; Rugh, 1976; Kardachi and Clarke, 1977; Berry and Wilmot, 1977; Beemsterboer et al., 1978; Kardachi et al., 1978) and tension-type headache (Budzinsky et al., 1973; Adler and Adler, 1976; Montgomery and Ehrisman, 1976; Bruhn et al., 1979; Cott et al., 1981; Blanchard et al., 1982 a, b; Biondi and Guerani, 1983; Diamond and Montrose, 1984; Brazzi et al., 1988, 1993; Arena et al., 1988; Matusevicius and Pauza, 1993; Pauza and Matusevicius, 1993). In migraine treatment also good results were obtained after treatment with thermic or electromyographic biofeedback (Gauthier et al., 1988, 1991, 1994; Kim and Blanchard, 1992; Grazzi et al., 1993; Marcus et al., 1998). This treatment is also indicated for muscle hyperfunction and parafunction (such as bruxism – see Chapter 3) (Solberg and Rugh, 1972, 1973; Rappaport et al., 1975). However, it appears to be less effective in depressed patients (Blanchard et al., 1982 a, b; Levine, 1984).

Many biofeedback devices with different technical characteristics are found on the market. The simpler ones have only one channel and record electromyographic activity of one side or of both sides cumulatively, depending on the mode of ap-

plication of the surface electrodes (Fig. 13.**1**). More sophisticated devices record the muscular activity of both sides separately. The type of the feedback signal varies in different devices; the acoustic signal may be a continuous tone of varying intensity or a series of brief, sharp sounds of varying frequency. Visual feedback may be a meter readout or a luminous panel numerical display on which the microvoltage corresponding to the electrical muscular activity is given (Fig. 13.**2**). The more sophisticated devices may also be connected to a chart recorder; thus a graphic record of the data

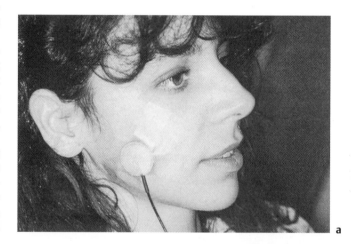

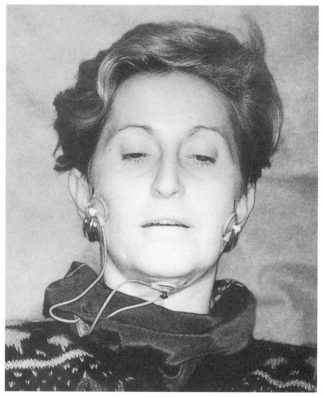

Fig. 13.**1** Unilateral (**a**) and bilateral (**b**) application of the electrodes of a single-channel biofeedback appliance

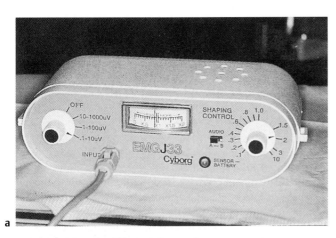

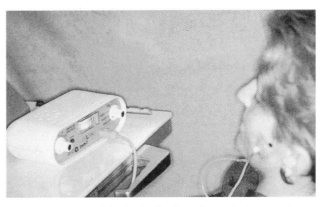

Fig. 13.**4** Position of the biofeedback appliance during a session

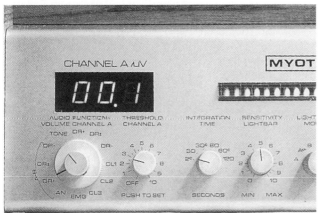

Fig. 13.**2** Visual feedback with millimetre scale (**a**) and with luminous panel (**b**) in two types of biofeedback appliance

Single-channel devices normally have three electrodes, one of them being neutral (the "earth"). In cases of unilateral pain in the cheek or temple regions, the two active electrodes are applied on the belly of the masseter and temporal muscles of the same side; otherwise they are applied bilaterally (Fig. 13.**1 b**). The earth electrode may be applied either on the postauricular area or below the chin. With a two-channel device, electrodes may be applied bilaterally (Fig. 13.**5**) or to different muscle groups, for example, masseter and temporal muscles. Bilateral application of the electrodes on the frontal muscles is particularly indicated in cases of tension-type headache in this area.

If the electrodes are placed on the elevator muscles, at the beginning of the session the patient is asked to clench the teeth and relax several times to become familiarized with the visual and acoustic signals induced by doing so. Then the patient is asked to relax the mouth and the level is sought at which the device stays silent. In patients with parafunctions, this level is usually higher than normal. The device is then brought to a "normal" level: this usually produces an intense signal. It is therefore easy to make the patient aware of the fact that, even when believing himself or herself to relax, the muscle are active well above normal and may therefore become fatigued and painful. The threshold suited to the patient is then again determined and the device is adjusted to a slightly lower level. The patient is asked to relax until the device stays silent and the visual signal is negative. To facilitate the relaxation of the masseter and temporal muscles, it may be useful to invite the patient to let the jaw drop as though he or she had fallen asleep sitting down. If the patient is a quick learner, the threshold is promptly lowered. The patient is then left alone to proceed with the exercise for 15–20 minutes: during this time patients may ajust the threshold level themselves, if necessary. Nevertheless, it is advisable, at least during the first sessions, that the clinician checks the results obtained two or three times during the session. In subsequent sessions, progressively advanced "goals" will be established

may be provided for clinical or research purposes (Fig. 13.**3**). It is usually possible to vary the threshold beyond which the acoustic signal is given as required. Thus, the training may be initiated with a relatively high threshold, which then may be reduced progressively.

Before starting the training session, the patient should be informed briefly about the characteristics of this type of treatment. Emphasis should be laid particularly on the fact that the treatment is absolutely innocuous. Furthermore, it should be stressed that this treatment involves the patient's will in a process of learning and self-control, which must also continue between sessions. The patient is then asked to lie down on a chair in a reclining position. The room must be as quiet as possible and the light should not be too bright. The biofeedback device must be located so that the patient may easily see it without moving his or her head (Fig. 13.**4**). After removal of the skin fat by energetic scrubbing with cotton soaked in alcohol, the surface electrodes are applied. The point of application depends on the type of device and patient's symptoms.

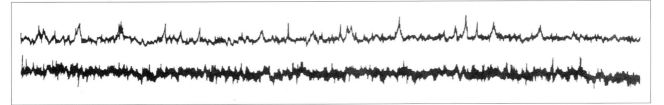

Fig. 13.**3** Graphic recording of the integrated EMG signal from the right (upper part) and left masseter (lower part) during a biofeedback session. Note the gradual slow decrease of mean voltage

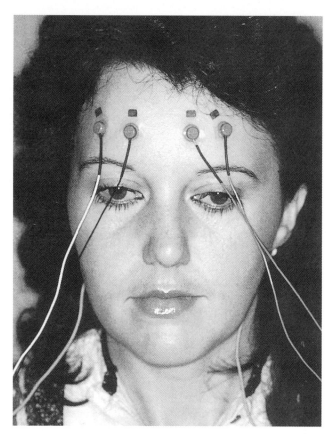

Fig. 13.**5** Application of the electrodes of a dual-channel biofeedback appliance to the frontal muscles

by adjusting the threshold to increasingly lower levels. The patient is asked to memorize and repeat the relaxation training at home once a day, for about 15 minutes, without the device. To aid relaxations, warm pads may be applied on the cheeks and the neck: these pads should be placed so that patients need not hold them in place with their hands. The same state of relaxation should be achievable automatically each time that the patient finds himself or herself with clenched teeth or other parafunctional habits during the day. To this end, a visual reminder may be useful, such as colored labels placed at strategic points where the patient's glance may fall during the day.

It is advisable to carry out six to ten sessions, weekly or, preferably, twice weekly. Follow-up sessions may be carried out after some time. However, it is important to emphasize that aim of the sessions is to learn a technique that should be further practiced at home: without that practice no significant result can be expected.

The patient's response to biofeedback treatment may vary from very good to poor. The treatment should be interrupted if the response is negative or paradoxical, with increase of anxiety and pain: the latter is very rare, but might occur in particularly depressed patients.

TENS

Among the many modalities of physical treatment used in facial pain and headache syndromes, transcutaneous electrical nerve stimulation (TENS) is one of the most widely employed. The use of TENS is based on the gate theory of pain (Melzack and Wall, 1965) and on the observation that coincident activity of large-diameter low-threshold mechanoceptors inhibits the response of dorsal horn cells to nociceptive inputs (Wall

and Cronly Dillon, 1960; Wall, 1964; Hongo et al., 1968). TENS application to somatic receptive fields probably activates large-diameter, myelinated neurons. Such excitation influences the activity of dorsal horn neurons by reducing spontaneous firing (Garrison and Foreman, 1994) and the firing resulting from input from thin myelinated and unmyelinated nociceptors, thus inhibiting the transmission of the nociceptive information to supraspinal levels (Sjølund et al., 1990; Nelson and Currier, 1991; Garrison and Foreman, 1994). It has also been found that TENS increases the blood opioid level (Sjølund and Eriksson, 1979), modulates the autonomic responses, causing an increase in skin temperature (Owens et al., 1979; Abram et al., 1980), and reduces the secondary hyperalgesia (Sluka et al., 1998).

In contrast to acupuncture, TENS application requires the generation of a nonpainful paresthesia in the painful area. The pulses produced by TENS may be of various configurations (Woolf and Thompson, 1944) (Fig. 13.**6**), but in practice rectangular pulses are usually employed. Pulse frequency (Fig. 13.**7**) and intensity may also vary. Conventional TENS is usually employed at a frequency between 70 and 100 Hz.

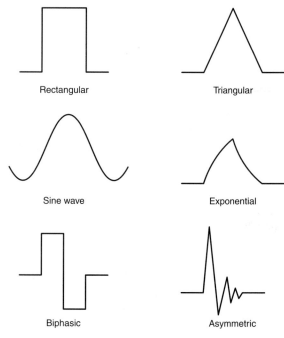

Fig. 13.**6** **Different configurations of pulses that may be generated by electrical pulse generators.** During TENS applications, rectangular pulses are usually employed. (From Woolf and Thomson, 1994, with modifications)

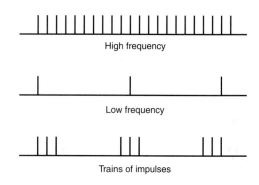

Fig. 13.**7** Different patterns of pulse generation used in TENS. (From Woolf and Thomson, 1994, with modifications)

Pulse intensity should be such as to induce a nonpainful tingling sensation and is usually 10–30 mA (Thompson and Filshie, 1993). Intensity may be higher using short trains of high-frequency (100 Hz) bursts repeated at low frequency (3 Hz) (Fig. 13.**7**). Thus, the stimulus intensity may be increased to 15–50 mA (Eriksson, 1979). This "acupuncture-like TENS" is advocated by some authors (Eriksson and Sjølund, 1976; Eriksson et al., 1979; Lehmann et al., 1986), at least in cases in which conventional TENS is scarcely effective. Finally, low-frequency trains of low-intensity pulses may also be used (pulsed TENS) (Thompson and Filshie, 1993).

As mentioned, the use of TENS has been described in a great variety of acute and chronic pain conditions (Fox and Melzack, 1976; Coan et al., 1980; Melzack et al., 1983; Woolf and Thompson, 1994): postoperative pain (Hymes et al., 1974; Cooperman et al., 1977; Pike, 1978; Ali et al., 1981; Smith et al., 1986); neuropathic pain, as in sympathetic reflex dystrophy, deafferentiation, entrapment, causalgia, and postherpetic neuralgia (Meyer and Fields, 1972; Nathan and Wall, 1974; Loeser et al., 1975; Györy and Caine, 1977); back and myogenous pain (Lehman et al., 1986; Willer, 1988; Arroyo and Cohen, 1993; Herman et al., 1994); cancer and ischemic pain (Tsang et al., 1994); and menstrual pain (Kaplan et al., 1994). In chronic pain conditions, long-terme use of TENS is associated with a significant reduction in the use of pain medication and physical/occupational therapy (Chabal et al., 1998).

In the craniofacial region, the use of TENS has been advocated not only for tension-type headache and trigeminal neuralgia, but also against muscle and TMJ pain (Ihalainen and Perkki, 1978; Hay, 1982; Hansson and Ekblom, 1983; Graff-Radford et al., 1989; Murphy, 1990; Laczny et al., 1994). In these patients, TENS may usefully be combined with other means of treatment. In muscle contraction pain, TENS application may preceed biofeedback sessions.

Electrode placement depends on the site of the pain. One electrode may be placed over the site of maximum pain and the second one over the site of emergence of the corresponding trigeminal branch (Fig. 13.**8**). In the treatment of cervical muscle contracture and pain associated with trigger points, electrodes are placed over the muscle belly in correspondence to the trigger points (Fig. 13.**9**). TENS application may be extended to several hours a day, especially if the patient employs a portable device at home. Otherwise, sessions should last for a minimum of 60 minutes, at least three times a week. In the majority of patients, the analgesic effect takes place 10–15 minutes after the beginning of the session. The duration of this effect after stimulation may vary greatly in different patients (from minutes to hours). With time, the patient may develop a certain degree of tolerance and the analgesic efficacy may consequently be reduced. Long-term studies have shown that this reduction is a consequence of the rapid reduction of the placebo effect, while the therapeutic efficacy of TENS tends to decrease more slowly until a stable long-term success rate of 20–30% is achieved (Woolf and Thompson, 1994) (Fig. 13.**10**).

TENS is usually free from side effects, apart from occasional and mild skin irritation at the site of stimulation that can be avoided by a correct and sufficient application of electrolyte gel and may be treated with the application of an anti-inflammatory cream preparation. TENS is contraindicated in patients with pacemakers and during pregnancy. The electrodes should not be applied in the anterior cervical region, to avoid the risk of stimulating the nerves of the laryngeal muscles and so causing a laryngeal spasm.

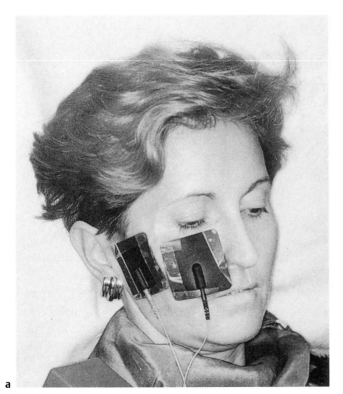

a

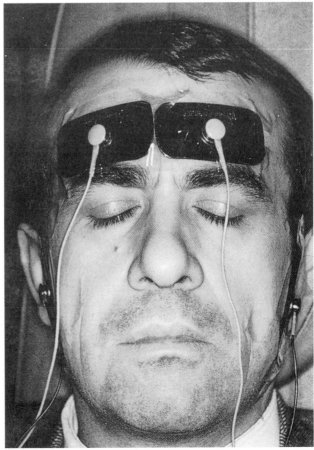

b

Fig. 13.**8**   Application of the electrodes of a TENS appliance in a case of pain of TMJ and right cheek (**a**) and of frontal and periorbital pain (**b**)

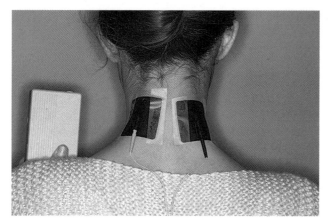

Fig. 13.**9**   Application of TENS electrodes in a case of cervical pain

Other Types of Physical Treatment

Soft laser therapy (Fig. 13.**11**) is another type of physical treatment which may conveniently be employed in some cases, usually in association with other modalities. It has not yet been shown that soft laser radiation can penetrate deep struc-

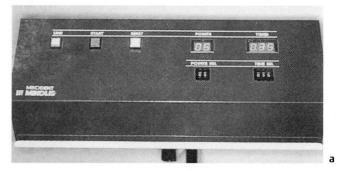

a

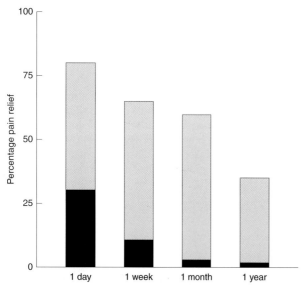

Fig. 13.**10**   **Histogram indicating TENS efficacy with time in controlling chronic pain.** The black area represents the contribution of the placebo effect, the grey area represents the contribution made by TENS. (From Woolf and Thomson, 1994, with modifications)

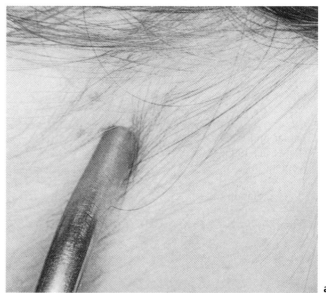

a

Fig. 13.**11**   Soft laser radiation (**a**) and its application to a cervical trigger point (**b**)

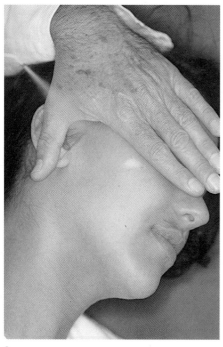

a

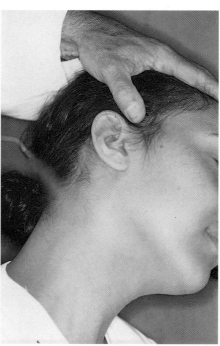

b

Fig. 13.**12**   Application of a cold spray to the masseter region (**a**) and the sternocleidomastoid muscle (**b**)

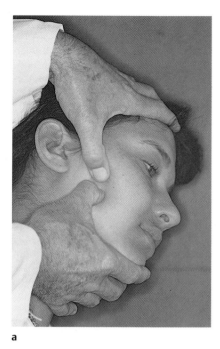
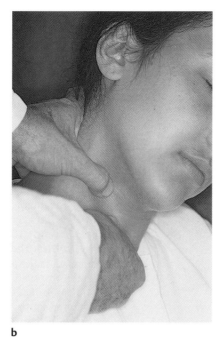
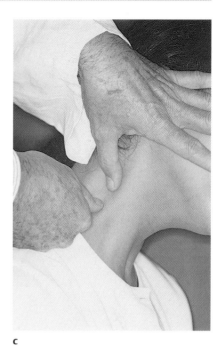

a   b   c

Fig. 13.**13** Technique of digital pressure and strech for trigger points in the masseter (**a**), the sternocleidomastoid (**b**), and the trapezius muscle (**c**)

tures, and the results of treatment with this technique for muscular and skeletal pain are controversial (Walker, 1983; Baxter et al., 1993; Gam et al., 1993). Nevertheless, an improvement has been reported using this technique in TMJ and muscle pain (Bezuur et al., 1988; Bertolucci and Grey, 1995).

Laser radiation may be also useful against trigger points, alone or combined with anesthetic injections (see later).

Application of *cold* or *heat* is a useful therapeutic tool against contraction of the craniofacial muscles. Local cold sprays of ethyl chloride or fluoromethane are indicated in acute situations with muscular spasms and sharp pain (Travell and Simons, 1983). The spray should be applied with back-and-forth movements along the main direction of the muscle fibers (Fig. 13.**12**) and should be interrupted as soon as the patient reports an intense cold sensation. When applied on trigger points, cold application may be followed by digital pressure on and stretching of the site (Fig. 13.**13**).

Applications of heat (humid or dry) may be employed by the patient at home, on a regular basis. The source of heat should be applied bilaterally on the cheeks and the articular

or cervical areas for at least 15–20 minutes once or twice daily. The patient should sit in a reclined position and, at the same time, try to relax his or her muscles as much as possible. Application of heat may be usefully combined with biofeedback treatment.

Anesthetic injections (Fig. 13.**14**) are useful in treating trigger points (Travell and Simons, 1983). The anesthetic employed may be procaine, lidocaine without epinephrine, or bupivacaine. Carlson et al. (1993) have observed that trigger point injection in the trapezius muscle may reduce the EMG activity of the masseter.

Exercises for the Elevator Muscles and the TMJ

A number of exercises have been described to improve coordination of mandibular movements in the presence of elevator muscle contracture. Yavelow et al. (1973) advocate brief *opening and closing movements* from the mandibular postural position: the movement should be less than 5 mm, should not involve any mandibular forward or side-to-side deviation, and should be performed with minimal muscle contraction. During the closing movement, the teeth should never come into contact. The patient is asked to perform this exercise for about one minute several times each day. Mouth opening and closing exercises may be performed in the mirror so that mandibular deviation is avoided.

Another similar exercise consists of rhythmical opening and closing movements performed while the tip of the tongue is placed against the palate (Fig. 13.**15**).

Counter-resistance exercises are indicated against muscle contracture and disk displacement with reduction at initial stages, in particular when it is produced by bruxing habits. The patient performs brief opening movements from the postural position, while at the same time a strong resistance is exerted with the first applied under the chin (Fig. 13.**16a**). The exercise may last for some seconds and should be repeated several times, alternating with brief relaxation periods. This

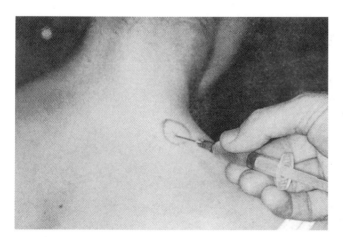

Fig. 13.**14** Infiltration of anesthetic at a cervical trigger point

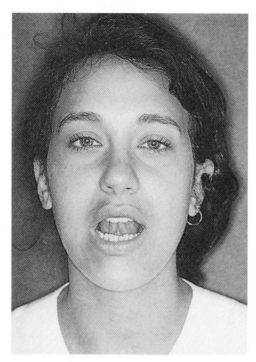

Fig. 13.**15** Exercise of rhythmical opening and closing with the tongue tip on the patate

exercise is based on the principle that strong contraction of a muscle group (the mandibular depressors in this case) may induce relaxation of the antagonist muscles (the mandibular elevators). Additionally, in case of disk displacement the exercise may stabilize the disk – condyle relationships, provided it is performed when the disk is in a correct position with re-

spect to the condyle. This may be assured by asking the patient to first open his mouth until the clicking noise is produced (indicating that the disk has gone into a normal position), and then to bring the mandible into a position of moderate opening in protrusion, to avoid further disk displacement. After the counter-resistance exercise has been performed, the patient should open the mouth fully: if no clicking noise occurs, the exercise has been performed correctly; the occurrence of a joint noise indicates that the exercise was not performed correctly, that is, that the disk was out of its normal place while the exercise was being performed. It should be emphasized that, if correctly performed, this exercise may be beneficial for the articular function (and sometimes may lead to improvement or disappearance of the clicking noise); however, if it is not performed correctly, further TMJ damage could occur. The exercise may be repeated laterally (Fig. 13.**16b**). The response may be variable in different patients and the exercise should be suspended if no improvement is observed.

In cases of disk compression or dislocation, *articular distraction* exercises are also useful. Downward pressure is exerted with the thumb applied to the occlusal surface of the molars of the lesion side. It is advisable to use the ipsilateral hand, so that, while the thumb is placed on the molars of the same side, the inferior mandibular margin of the other side is taken from the outside with the other fingers: while pivoting on these fingers, moderate pressure is exerted with the thumb on the molars of the opposite side for some seconds (Fig. 13.**17**). This exercise is repeated several times alternating with relaxation periods.

Counter-resistance and traction exercises should be performed several times during the day.

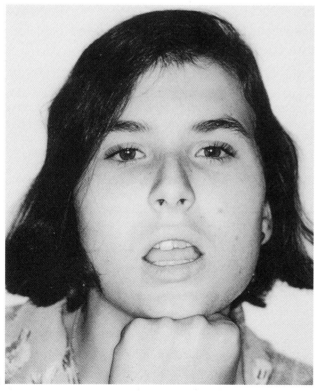
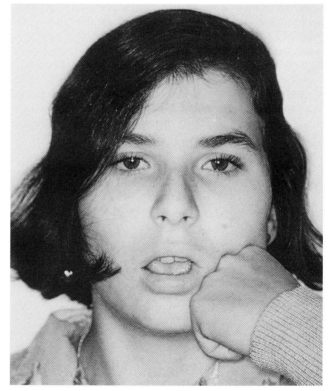

a   b

Fig. 13.**16** Counter-resistance exercises on opening (**a**) and laterally (**b**)

It is obvious that if severe orthopedic deviations are present, especially in the growing or young patient, he or she should be referred to a specialist in orthopedics or to a physiotherapist for diagnosis and treatment. Nevertheless, the exercises that are described here are, from our experience, useful and easy to perform: they are taken, in part or whole, from those described by Rocabado (1982, 1992).

A preliminary exercise to improve shoulder posture is performed in an erect position with the ankles, the hips, and the nape against the wall. While the rest of the body does not move, the shoulders are brought into contact with the wall and released, rhythmically (Fig. 13.**18**). Then, while the body is kept against the wall, horizontal movements of the head are made, forwards and backwards (Fig. 13.**19**). To perform a third

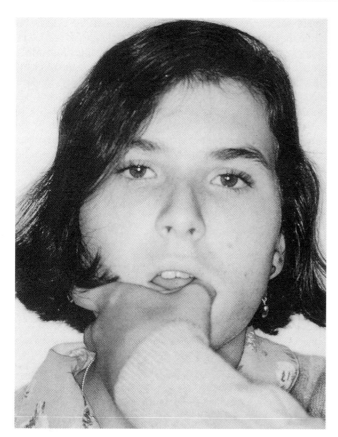

Fig. 13.**17**   Finger distraction excercise of the left TMJ

Posture Exercise

As we have seen (Chapter 4), the baricenter of the skull is located ahead of the craniovertebral fulcrum, that is, of the occipital condyles, and therefore the force of gravity must be counterbalanced by the action of the posterior neck muscles. A frequent cause of alteration of head and neck posture is the failure of the posterior neck muscles to counteract the skull's weight. As a consequence, the cervical curvature is lost or inverted: this phenomenon may be exacerbated by the tendency of some individuals under stress to contract and stiffen the cervical muscles. Such alterations result in a relative displacement of the hyoid bone and, consequently, may result in alterations of the mandibular postural position (Figs. 4.**6**, 4.**7**). Posture alterations on the frontal plane are also frequent: of the head with respect to the neck, and of the neck with respect to the shoulders. They are frequently the consequence of a misalignment of the shoulders (Fig. 13.**18a**) (see Chapter 4).

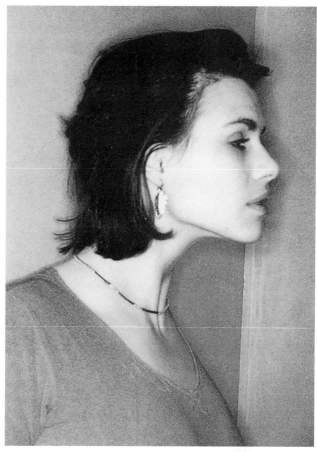

Fig. 13.**19**   Exercise for the cervical column. With the body against the wall, horizontal movements of the head are made, forward and backward

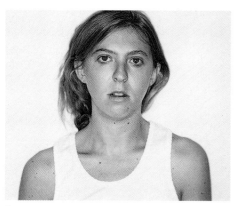

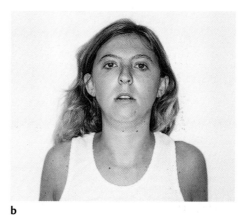

a   b

Fig. 13.**18**   **Excercise to improve shoulder posture.** In an erect position with the body against the wall (**a**) the shoulders are brought into contact with the wall (**b**) and released, rhythmically. Note that the patient shows a definite shoulder misalignment with the right shoulder lower than the left (**a**). The misalignment disappears while the exercise is performed (**b**)

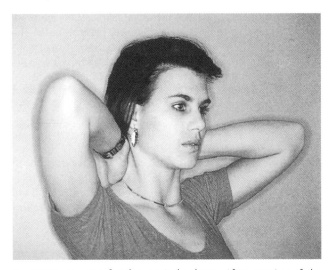

Fig. 13.**20** Exercise for the cervical column. After cupping of the hands behind the neck, stretching movements of the head are performed backward, with forward counterpressure from the hands, for a duration of a few seconds

exercise, the patient, after cupping the hands behind the neck, performs stretching movements of the head backward, with forward counterpressure from the hands (Fig. 13.**20**). When a loss of the cervical curve is present, one may initially prescribe these three exercises, each of them to be performed 7–10 times every two or three hours during the day. If too many exercises are prescribed from the beginning, the probability that they will be performed regularly and correctly is markedly reduced. It is advisable each time the patient is reexamined to emphasize the importance of performing them frequently and correctly, reminding the patient that they require very little time; moreover, the clinician should check personally whether they are performed correctly.

Later, especially if cervical pain and head–neck posture alterations are present, the following exercise may be also prescribed: the head is tilted about 15–20° on one side and the long and middle fingers are placed on the temple on the op-posite side; then the head is pushed to a straight position while the fingers exert a gentle counter-resistance (Fig. 13.**21**). This exercise should be performed rhythmically, alternating with brief relaxation periods. It may then be repeated after inclining the head sideways, backward and slightly upward (Fig. 13.**22**). This exercise provides for a rhythmical contraction of the straight and oblique posterior neck muscles.

Another exercise is useful in presence of postural problems on the frontal plane: the upper limb is raised upward and backward while the head is brought sideways toward the raised limb (Fig. 13.**23**).

References

Abram S.E., Asiddao C.B., Reynolds A.C., *Increased skin temperature during TENS*, Anesth. Analg., 1980, 59:22–25.

Adler C.S., Adler S.M., *Biofeedback psychotherapy for the treatment of beadaches: A 5-years follow-up*, Headache, 1976, 16:189–191.

Ali J.A., Yaffee C.S., Serretti C., *The effect of transcutaneous electric nerve stimulation of postoperative pain and pulmonary function*, Surgery, 1981, 89:507–512.

Andersen C.D., Franks R.D., *Migraine and tension headache, is there a physiological difference?*, Headache, 1981, 21:63–71.

Arena J.G., Hightower N.E., Chong G.C., *Relaxation therapy for tension headache in the elderly: a prospective study*, Psychol. Aging, 1988, 3:96–98.

Arroyo J.F., Cohen M.I., *Abnormal responses to electrocutaneous stimulation in fibromyalgia*, J. Rhematol., 1993, 20:1925–31.

Baxter G.D., Mokhtar B., Bell A.J., Allen J.M., Walsh D.M., *A double blind placebo controlled investigation of the hypoalgesic effects of combined phototherapy and low intensity laser therapy upon experimental ischaemic pain*, (abs.), 7 th World Congress on Pain, IASP Publications, Seattle, 1993, 402.

Beemsterboer P.L., Clark G.T., Rugh J.D., *Treatment of bruxism using nocturnal biofeedback with an arousal task*, J. Dent. Res., 1978, 57 (Special Issue A):366.

Berry D.C., Wilmot G., *The use of a biofeedback technique in the treatment of mandibular dysfunction pain*, J. Oral Rehabil., 1977, 4:255–260.

Bertolucci L.E., Grey T., *Clinical analysis of mid-laser versus placebo treatment of arthralgic TMJ degenerative joints*, Cranio, 1995, 13(1):26–29.

Bezuur N.J., Habets L.L., Hansson T.L., *The effect of therapeutic laser treatment in patients with craniomandibular disorders*, J. Craniomandib. Disord., 1988, 2:83–86.

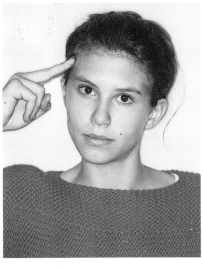

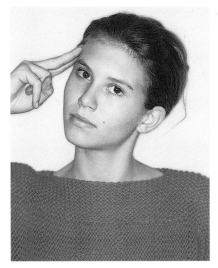

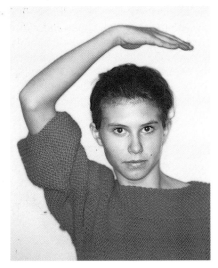

Fig. 13.**21**   Fig. 13.**22**   Fig. 13.**23**

Fig. 13.**21**   Counter resistance exercise for the recti posterior muscles of the neck

Fig. 13.**22**   Counter resistance exercise for the oblique posterior muscles of the neck

Fig. 13.**23**   Exercise to improve posture of head and neck on the frontal plane

Biedermann H.J., Inglis J., Monga T.N., Shanks G.L., *Differential treatment responses on somatic pain indicators after EMG biofeedback training in back pain patients*, Int. J. Psychosom., 1989, 36 : 53 – 57.

Biondi M., Guerani G., *Il trattamento non farmacologico della cefalea da tensione muscolare*, Medicina Psicosomatica, 1983, 28 : 187 – 210.

Blanchard E.B., Yong L.D., *Clinical applications of biofeedback training. A review of evidence*, Arch. Gen. Psychiatry, 1974, 30 : 573 – 589.

Blanchard E.B., Andrasik F., Neff D.F., et al., *Biofeedback and relaxation training with three kinds of headache: treatment effects and their predictions*, J. Consult. Clin. Psychol., 1982 a, 562 – 575.

Blanchard E.B., Andrasik F., Neff D.F., et al., *Sequential comparisons of relaxation training and biofeedback in the treatment of three kinds of chronic headache or the machines may by necessary some of the time*, Behavioural Research and Therapy, 1982 b, 20 : 469 – 481.

Bruhn P., Olesen J., Melgaard B., *Controlled trial of EMG feedback in muscle contraction headache*, Ann. Neurol., 1979, 6 : 34 – 36.

Budzynski T.H., *Biofeedback procedures in the clinic*, Semin. Psychiatry., 1973, 5 : 537 – 547.

Budzynski T.H., Stoyva J.A., Adler C.S., Mullaney D.J., *E.M.G. biofeedback and tension headache: a controlled outcome study*, Psychosom. Med., 1973, 35 : 484 – 496.

Budzynski T.H., Stoyva J., *An electromyographic feedback technique for teaching voluntary relaxation of the masseter muscle*, J. Dent., 1973, 52 : 116.

Butler J.H., Abbott B.M., Bush E.M., *Biofeedback as a method of controlling bruxism. IADR*, J. Dent. Res., 1976, 55:B310.

Carlson C.R., Okeson J.P., Falace D.A., Nitz A.J., Lindroth E., *Reduction of pain and EMG activity in the masseter region by trapezius trigger point injection*, Pain, 1993, 55 : 397 – 400.

Chabal C., Fishbain D.A., Weaver M., Heine L.W., *Long-term transcutaneous electrical nerve stimulation (TENS) use: impact on medication utilization and physical therapy costs*, Clin. J. Pain, 1998, 14(1):66 – 73.

Coan R.M., Wong G., Ku S.L., Chan Y.C., Wang L., Ozer F.T., Coan P.L., *The acupuncture treatment of low back pain: a raandomized controlled study*, Am. J. Clin. Med., 1980, 8 : 181 – 189.

Cooperman A.M., Hall B., Mikalacki K., Hardy R., Sadar E., *Use of transcutaneous electrical stimulationin control of postoperative pain-results of a prospective, randomized, controlled study*, Am. J. Surg., 1977, 133 : 185 – 187.

Cott A., Goldman J.A., Pavloski R.P., Kirschberg G.J., Fabich M., *The long term therapeutic significance of the addition of electromyographic biofeedback to relaxation training in the treatment of tension headaches*, Behav. Ther., 1981, 12:556 – 559.

Diamond S., Montrose D., *The value of biofeedback in the treatment of chronic headache: a four-year retrospective study*, Headache, 1984, 24 : 5 – 18.

Dohrmann R.J., Laskin D.M., *Treatment of myofascial pain-dysfunction syndrome with EMG biofeedback*, J. Dent. Res., 1976 (abs.), 55, (Spec. Issue B):249.

Eriksson M.B.E., Sjølund B.H, *Acupuncture-like electroanalgesia in TNS-resistant chronic pain*, in: Zotterman Y. (ed.), *Sensory functions of the skin*, Pergamon Press, Oxford, 1976, 575 – 581.

Eriksson M.B.E., Sjølund B.H., Nielzén S., *Long term results of peripheral conditioning stimulation as an analgesic measure in chronic pain*, Pain, 1979, 6 : 335 – 347.

Flor H., Haag G., Turk D.C., Köhler H., *Efficacy of EMG biofeedback, pseudotherapy and medical treatment for chronic rheumatic back pain*, Pain, 1983, 17 : 21 – 31.

Flor H., Haag G., Turk D.C., *Long-term efficacy of EMG biofeedback for chronic rheumatic back pain*, Pain, 1986, 27 : 195 – 202.

Fox E.J., Melzack R., *Comparison of transcutaneous electrical stimulation and acupuncture in the treatment of chronic pain*, in: Bonica J.J., Albe-Fessard D. (eds.), *Advances in pain research and therapy*, Raven Press, New York, 1976, 797 – 801.

Freedman R.R., *Behavioral treatment of Raynaud's disease and phenomenon*, Adv. Microcirc., 1985, 12 : 138 – 156.

Freedman R.R., *Physiological mechanisms of temperature biofeedback*, Biofeedback Self-Regul., 1991, 16 : 95 – 114.

Gam A.N., Thorsen H., Lönnberg F., *The effect of low-level laser therapy on musculoskeletal pain: a meta-analysis*, Pain, 1993, 52 : 63 – 66.

Garrison D.W., Foreman R.D., *Research reports. Decreased activity of spontaneous and noxiously evoked dorsal horn cells during transcutaneous electrical nerve stimulation (TENS)*, Pain, 1994, 58 : 309 – 315.

Gauthier J.G., Fradet C., Roberge C., *The differential effects of biofeedback in the treatment of classical and common migraine*, Headache, 1988, 28 : 39 – 46.

Gauthier J.G., Fournier A., Roberge C., *The differential effects of biofeedback in the treatment of menstrual and nonmenstrual migraine*, Headache, 1991, 31 : 82 – 90.

Gauthier J.G., Core G., French D., *The role of home practice in the termal biofeedback treatment of migraine headacle*, J. Consult Clin. Psychol., 1994, 62(1):180 – 4.

Gentry W.D., Bernal G.A.A., *Chronic pain*, in: Williams R.B., Gentry W.D. (eds.), *Behavioral approaches to medical treatment*, Ballinger, Cambridge (MA.), 1977, 173 – 182.

Gessel A.H., Harrison S., *Bilateral electromyographic feedback treatment of chronic mandibular dislocation*, Proceedings of the Biofeedback Research Society, 5 th Annual Meeting, Colorado Springs, CO, 1974.

Graff-Radford S.B., Reeves J.L., Baker R.L., Chiu D., *Effects of transcutaneous electrical nerve stimulation on myofascial pain and trigger point sensitivity*, Pain, 1989, 37 : 1 – 5.

Grazzi L., Frediani F., Zappacosta B., Boiardi A., Bussone G., *Psychological assessment in tension headache before and after biofeedback treatment*, Headache, 1988, 28 : 337 – 338.

Grazzi L., D'Amico D., Bussone G., *Controlled study of electromyographic-biofeedback treatment efficacy for tension-type headache in children and adolescents* (abs.), 7 th World Congress on Pain, IASP Publications, Seattle, 1993, 230.

Györy A.N., Caine D.C., *Electric pain control of a painful forearm amputation stump*, Med. J. Aust., 1977, 2 : 156 – 158.

Hansson P., Ekblom A., *Transcutaneous electrical nerve stimulation (TENS) as compared to placebo (TENS) for the relief of acute oro-facial pain*, Pain, 1983, 15 : 157 – 165.

Hay K.M., *Control of head pain in migraine using transcutaneous electrical nerve stimulation*, Practitioner, 1982, 226:771 – 775.

Heller R.F., Strang H.R., *Controlling bruxism through automated aversive conditioning*, Behav. Res. Ther., 1973, 11 : 327.

Herman E., William R., Stratford P., Fargas-Babjak A., Trott M., *A randomized controlled trial of transcutaneous electrical nerve stimulation (CODETRON) to determine its benefits in a rehabilitation program for acute occupational low back pain*, Spine, 1994, 19 : 561 – 56.

Hongo T., Jankowska E., Lundberg A., *Postsynaptic excitation and inhibition from primary afferents in neurons of the spinocervical tract*, J. Physiol., 1968, 199 : 569 – 592.

Hymes A.C., Raab D.E., Yonchiro E.G., Nelson G.D., Drintz A.L., *Acute pain control by electrostimulation: a preliminary report*, in: Bonica J.J. (ed.), *Advances in neurology 4*, Raven Press, New York, 1974, 761 – 773.

Ihalainen U., Perkki K., *The effect of transcutaneous nerve stimulation (TNS) on chronic facial pain*, Proc. Finn. Dent. Soc., 1978, 74 : 86 – 90.

Kaplan B., Peled Y., Pardo J., et al. *Transcutaneous electrical nerve stimulation (TENS) as a relief for dysmenorrhea*, Clin. Exp. Obstet. Gynecol., 1994, 21 : 87 – 90.

Kardachi B.J., Clarke N.G., *The use of biofeedback to control bruxism*, J. Periodontol., 1977, 48 : 639 – 642.

Kardachi B.J., Bailley J.O. Jr, Ash M.M. Jr., *A comparison of biofeedback and occlusal adjustment on bruxism*, J. Periodontol., 1978, 49 : 367 – 372.

Kim M., Blanchard E.B., *Two studies of the non-pharmacological treatment of menstrually-related migraine headaches*, Headache, 1992, 32 : 197 – 202.

Laczny J.L., Hockers T., Legrand R., *Approche neuromusculaire du syndrome algo-dysfonctionnel de l'articulation temporomandibulaire*, Rev. Med. Liège, 1994, 49 : 375 – 381.

Lehmann T.R., Russell D.W., Spratt K.F. et al., *Efficacy of electroacupuncture and TENS in the rehabilitation of chronic low back pain patients*, Pain, 1986, 26:277 – 290.

Levine B.A., *Effects of depression and headache type on biofeedback for muscle contraction headaches*, Behav. Psychother., 1984, 12 : 300 – 307.

Loeser J.D., Black R.G., Christman R.M., *Relief of pain by transcutaneous stimulation*, J. Neurosurg., 1975, 42 : 308 – 314.

Marcus D.A., Scharff L., Mercer S., Turk D.C., *Nonpharmacological treatment for migraine: incremental utility of physical therapy with relaxation and thermal biofeedback*, Cephalalgia, 1998 18(5):266 – 272.

Matusevicius D., Pauza V., *Comparative study of combined migraine and tension type headache treatment*, (abs.), 7 th World Congress on Pain, IASP Publications, Seattle, 1993, 410.

Melzack R., Vetere P., Finch L., *Transcutaneous electrical nerve stimulation for low back pain. A comparison of TENS and massage for pain and range of motion*, Phys. Ther., 1983, 63 : 489 – 493.

Melzack R., Wall P., *Pain mechanisms: new theory*, Science, 1965, 150 : 971 – 979.

Meyer G.A., Fields H.L., *Causalgia treated by selective large fibre stimulation of peripheral nerves*, Brain, 1972, 95 : 163 – 167.

Montgomery P.S., Ehrisman W.J., *Biofeedback-alleviated headaches: a follow-up*, Headache, 1976, 16 : 64 – 67.

Murphy G.J., *Utilization of transcutaneous electrical nerve stimulation in managing craniofacial pain*, Clin. J. Pain, 1990, 6 : 64 – 69.

Nathan P.W., Wall P.D., *Treatment of post-herpetic neuralgia by prolonged electric stimulation*, Br. Med. J., 1974, 3 : 645 – 647.

Nelson R.M., Currier D.P., *Clinical Electrotherapy*, 2 d ed., Appleton and Lange, Stamford, USA, 1991.

Owens S., Atkinson R., Lees D.E., *Thermographic evidence of reduced sympathetic tone with TENS*, Anesthesiology, 1979, 50 : 62 – 65.

Paskewitz D.A., *Biofeedback instrumentation: soldering closed the loop*, Am. Psychol., 1975, 30 : 371 – 378.

Pauza V., Matusevicius D., *The assessment of treatment tension-type headache combined with panic attacks using biofeedback*, (abs.), 7 th World Congress on Pain, IASP Publications, Seattle, 1993, 410.

Phillips C., Hunter M., *The treatment of tension headache, I: Muscular abnormality and bio-feedback*, Behav. Res. Ther., 1981, 19 : 485 – 498.

Pike P.M., *Transcutaneous electrical stimulation: its use in management of postoperative pain*, Anaesthesia, 1978, 33 : 165 – 171.

Rappaport A.F., Cammer L., Cannistraci A., Gelb A., Strong D., *EMG feedback for the treatment of bruxism: A stress control program*, Proc. Biofeedback Res. Society, 6 th Annual Meeting, Monterey, 1975.

Rocabado M., *Head-Neck and dentistry manual*, Rocabado Institute, Tacoma, Washington, 1982.

Rugh J.D., *A behavioral approach to the diagnosis and treatment of functional oral disorders: Biofeedback and self control techniques*, in: Rugh J., Perlis D.B., Disraeli R.I. (eds.), *Biofeedback in dentistry: research and clinical applications*, Semantodontics, Phoenix, 1976.

Rugh J.D., Solberg W.K., *Electromyographic studies of bruxist behavior before and during treatment*, J. Calif. Dent. Assoc., 1975, 3 : 56 – 59.

Sjølund B.H., Eriksson B.E., *Endorphins and analgesia produced by peripheral conditioning stimulation*, in: Bonica J.J., Liebeskind J.C., Albe-Fessard D.G. (eds.), *Advances in pain research and therapy*, Raven Press, New York, 1979, 3 : 585 – 592.

Sjølund B.H. et al., *Transcutaneous and implanted electrical stimulation of peripheral nerves*, in: Bonica J.J. (ed.), *The management of pain*, vol. 2, 2 nd edn., Lea and Febinger, Philadelphia, 1990, 1852 – 1858.

Sluka K.A., Bailey K., Bogush J., Olson R., Ricketts A., *Treatment with either high or low frequency TENS reduces the secondary hyperalgesia observed after injection of kaolin and carrageenan into the knee joint*, Pain, 1998, 77 : 97 – 102.

Smith C.M., Guralnick M.S., Gelfund M.M., Jeans M.E., *The effects of transcutaneous nerve stimulation on post-Cesarian pain*, Pain, 1986, 27 : 181 – 194.

Solberg W.K., Rugh J.D., *The use of biofeedback devices in the treatment of bruxism*, J. Calif. Dent. Assoc., 1972, 40 : 852.

Solberg W.K., Rugh J.D., *Biofeedback induced muscle relaxation used in the treatment of bruxism*, J. Dent. Res., 1973, 52:(Spec. Issue), 73 (abs.).

Thompson J.W., Filshie J., *Transcutaneous electrical nerve stimulation (TENS) and acupuncture*, in: Doyle D., Hanks G., MacDonald N. (eds.), *Oxford textbook of palliative medicine*, Oxford University Press, Oxford, 1993, 229 – 244.

Travell J.G., Simons D.G., *Myofascial pain and dysfunction: a trigger point manual*, vol. 15, Williams and Wilkins, Baltimore, MD, 1983, 46 – 50, 67 – 86, 183 – 190, 194 – 196.

Tsang G.M., Green M.A., Crow A.J., et al. *Chronic muscle stimulation improves ischremic muscle performace in patients with peripheral vascular disease*, Eur. J. Vasc. Surg., 1994, 8 : 419 – 422.

Walker J.B., *Relief from chronic pain by low power laser irradiation*, Neurosci. Lett., 1983, 43 : 339 – 344.

Wall P.D., *Presynaptic control of impulses at the first central synapse in the cutaneous pathway*, in: *Physiology of spinal neurons*. Progress in Brain Research, vol. 12, Elsevier, Amsterdam, 1964, 92 – 118.

Wall P.D., Cronly Dillon J.R., *Pain, itch and vibration*, Arch. Neurol., 1960, 2 : 365 – 375.

Willer J.C., *Relieving effect of TENS on painful muscle contraction produced by an impairment of reciprocal innervation: an electrophysiological analysis*, Pain, 1988, 32 : 271 – 274.

Woolf C.J., Thompson J.W., *Stimulation-induced analgesia: transcutaneous electrical nerve stimulation (TENS) and vibration*, in: Wall P.D., Melzack R. (eds.), *Texbook of pain*, Churchill, Linvingstone, Edinburgh, 1994, 1191 – 1208.

Yavelow I., Forster I., Wininger M., *Mandibular relearning*, Oral Surg., 1973, 36 : 632.

14 Criteria for Choice of Treatment and Treatment Planning

General Principles

The treatment plan of each patient obviously depends on which diagnosis was made and on which answer was given to three fundamental questions:

1. Does the patient suffer from one pathology or from more than one pathologies superimposed?
2. In the latter case, does one pathology predominate?
3. Is there a dysfunction of one or more systems that may provoke or facilitate the patient's syndrome?

Once these questions have been answered, the different treatment options may be evaluated. It is important not to allow one's medical specialty to induce an a priori bia toward a particular type of treatment. Any excessive schematisation should also be avoided. We have seen that different etiological factors may be present in the pathologies characterized by headache and/or facial pain; accordingly, the treatment plan may be different even for patients in which the same primary diagnosis has been made. This difference may relate to the pharmacological treatment, to the nonpharmacological treatment or to a combined treatment of both types.

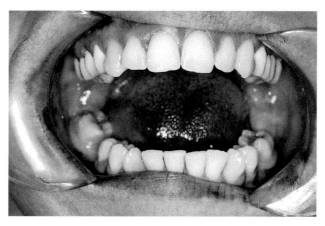

Fig. 14.**1** **Disk displacement without reduction of the left TMJ.** Mouth opening is limited and slightly deviated toward the lesion side

In addition, the temporal sequence of the different types of treatment must be carefully evaluated in each different case. For instance, in a case of mild tension-type headache with muscle contraction, the treatment of first choice may be bio-

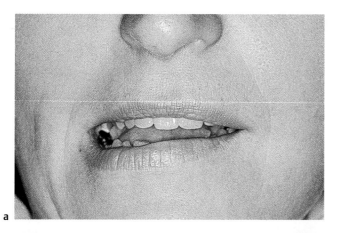
a

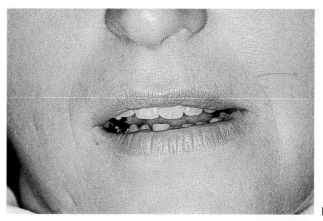
b

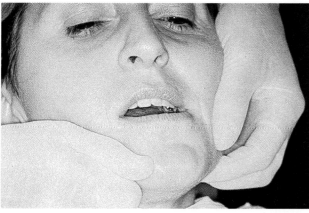
c

d

Fig. 14.**2** **Manipulation of the TMJ in disk displacement. a, b** Stage one: the patients is invited to make numerous rhythmic lateral movements to right and left. **c** Stage two: gentle finger pressure is applied on both sides of the mandible concomitantly with the lateral

movements performed by the patient. **d** Stage three: the mandible is suddenly pushed towards the side opposite the lesion, applying strong manual pressure at the corner of the mandible while the patient performs a sideways movement toward the same direction

feedback, occasionally combined, when needed, with short-term administration of minor tranquilizers. In contrast, in cases of moderate or severe headache or facial pain in a patient with pronounced anxiety or depressive disorder, psychotropic drugs will be the drugs of first choice. When two equally relevant pathologies are present, they will be treated together in the most appropriate way. For example, in a case of disk displacement without reduction associated with a severe tension-type headache, treatment of the intracapsular TMJ lesion will be by a mandibular manipulation to restore a better disk–condyle relation (Figs 14.**1**–14.**3**) and an orthopedic splint will be inserted (Fig. 14.**4**), while for the management of the headache problem biofeedback sessions and drug treatment might be programmed as needed.

However, when one pathology clearly predominates, this will be treated first. Thus, no invasive orthopedic treatment

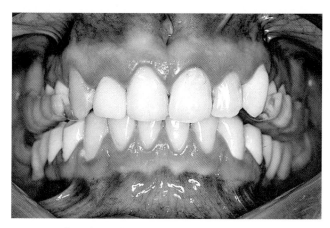

Fig. 14.**5**   Flat splint to be worn mainly at night

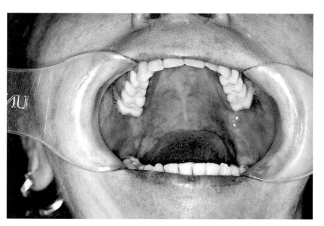

Fig. 14.**3**   Sudden and marked increase of mouth opening capacity after manipulation

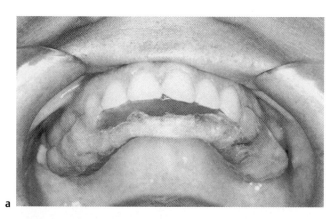

a

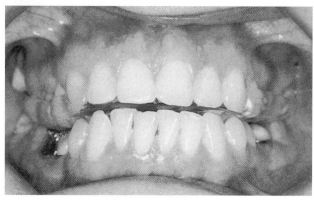

b

Fig. 14.**4**   Orthopedic splint (**a**) to keep the mandible in the correct closing position (**b**)

will be performed in a patient with chronic headache or facial pain who subsequently develops a mild TMJ dysfunction. In such cases, the treatment of the articular problem may be limited to prescription of exercises and physical therapy. If headache or myogenous pain are still present at awakening in a patient with pronounced nightly parafunctions, a flat maxillary splint (Fig. 14. **5**) may be applied subsequently during the night. The efficacy of this course, often overenthusiastically evaluated in particular by odontologists, is variable and limited. Consequently, it should be removed promptly in case of no or negative result. An any rate, it is advisable to recommend the patient to remove the splint whenever he or she perceives it as irritating or invasive.

Evaluation of treatment should be as objective as possible. When treating headache and facial pain, one should consider that the placebo effect is particularly relevant and may account for approximately 30% of symptom improvement. The use of pain diaries by patients facilitates the evaluation of the improvement and of the efficacy of the different therapeutic modalities (Fig. 14.**6**).

Drug Treatment Planning

The choice of drug from among all those indicated for the disease that has been diagnosed depends on the following questions:

Is the drug indicated only for the pain or disease diagnosed or does it have other indications?
What are its side effects?
What are the features of the patient's hormonal, vascular, and nervous system functioning and of the patient's personality?
And, in particular:
Did the clinical and instrumental analysis indicate a dysfunction of one or more systems or the presence of a mood or personality disorder?

Almost all drugs employed against headache and facial pain are used in other fields of medicine. Benzodiazepines, antidepressants and neuroleptics are used in neurology and psychiatry; beta-blockers are prescribed against hypertension and paroxysmal tachycardia; calcium antagonists (flunarizine in particular) are currently employed by otologists against vertigo; and NSAIDs and cortisone derivatives are widely employed in many different diseases.

Thus, a comparative analysis of indications and contraindications of the different drugs with the patient's data will help in the choice of the drug (Fig. 14.**7**).

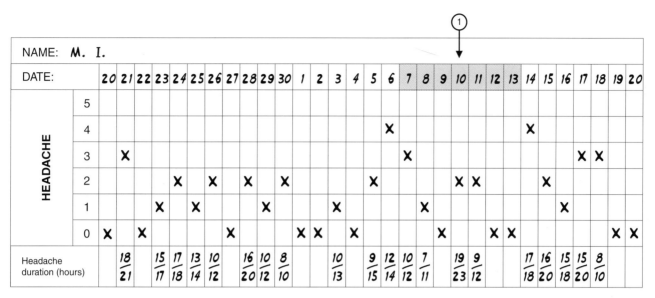

① = Reduction of disk displacement and insertion of orthopedic splint

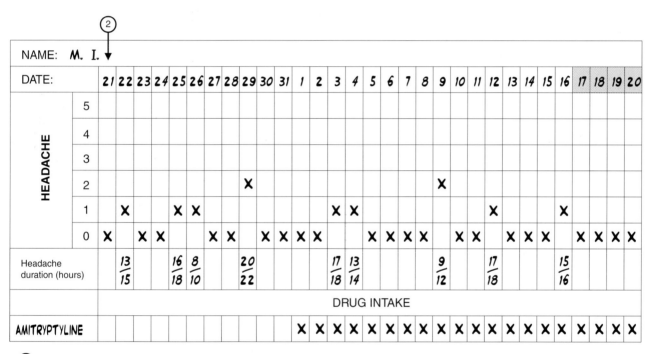

② = Biofeedback sessions start

Fig. 14.6 Headache diary of a young woman suffering from chronic tension type headache and disk displacement without reduction of left TMJ. The mandible manipulation, carried out successfully, had no influence on the headache, which improved significantly after biofeedback treatment and taking of amitryptiline

In migraine patients, propranolol is the drug of first choice if blood pressure tends to be high and if episodes of paroxysmal tachycardia and functional arhythmia occur. In such cases calcium antagonists (and verapamil in particular) are also indicated. Conversely, with low blood pressure, ergot derivatives or dopaminergic agents might be preferred. If there is a severe concomitant vertigo, flunarizine is the most appropriate drug, while metoclopramide might be prescribed when nausea and vomiting are relevant features.

In cases of concomitant depression, serotonin precursors might be effective against both migraine and depression, but the use of beta-blockers and flunarizine is to be avoided.

Another question concerns the choice between preventive, symptomatic, or combined treatment. If no contraindica-

tion is present, the new-generation serotonin agonists (the triptans) are the first-choice drugs in the symptomatic treatment of migraine attacks and, as such, may also be useful as an *empirical* means to differentiate these attacks from attacks of tension-type headache, moderate or severe. On the other hand, the patient may suffer from frequent headache attacks with different characteristics, some typical of migraine and others typical of tension-type headache. In this case, benzodiazepines may be prescribed if moderate anxiety is present; however, if anxiety is a symptom of a masked depressive disorder, antidepressants must be prescribed alone or in combination with neuroleptics. In these cases the triptans will be employed only against the acute migraine attacks (Fig. 14.**8**). However, if the headache diary still shows the presence of

	Beta-blockers	Verapamil	Flunarizine	NSAIDs	Ergot derivatives	Triptans	Amitryp-tiline	New generation anti-depressants	BZP
Hypertension	△△	△△	–	–	●●	●●	–	–	–
Hypotension	●●	●●	–	–	△△	●	●	–	●
Tachycardia	△△	–	–	–	–	–	●	–	–
Bradycardia	●●	●●	–	–	–	●	–	–	–
Heart conduction disorders	△△	●●	–	–	–	–	●●	–	–
Peripheral vasoconstriction	△△	–	△△	–	●●	●	–	–	–
Venous circulation disorders	●	●	–	–	△△	–	–	–	–
Cerebral circulation disorders	–	–	–	–	–	–	–	–	●
Depression	●	–	●●	–	–	–	△△	△△	–
Anxiety disorder	△△	–	●	–	–	–	–	●	△△
Loss of libido	●	●	●	–	–	–	●	●	●
Parkinsonism	–	–	●●	–	–	–	–	–	–
Glaucoma	–	–	–	–	●●	–	●●	–	–
Asthma	●●	–	–	–	–	–	–	–	–
Vertigo	–	–	△△	–	●	–	–	–	●
Peptic ulcer	–	–	–	●●	–	–	–	–	–
Prostate hypertrophy	–	–	–	–	–	–	●●	–	●
Pregnancy	●	–	–	–	●●	–	–	–	●●
Breast feeding	–	–	–	–	●●	–	–	–	●●
Car driving	–	–	●	–	–	–	●	–	●

Fig. 14.7 Indications and contraindications of the drugs frequently used in the treatment of migraine and other headaches. △△ = indicated, ● = partially contraindicated, ●● = totally contraindicated

NAME: D. R.																														
DATE:		15	16	17	18	19	20	21	22	23	24	25	26	27	28	29	30	31	1	2	3	4	5	6	7	8	9	10	11	12	13	14

HEADACHE

	5	X				X		X								X															
	4			X	X					X																					X	
	3		X									X												X				X			
	2													X								X			X					
	1																													
	0					X		X		X		X		X		X	X	X	X		X		X		X		X			

| Headache duration (hours) | 3 | | | 7 | | | 7 | | | 3 | | 9 | | | | | | 6 | | 2 | 3 | | | | | 7 | |

PAIN

	5		X			X						X	X	X												X	
	4				X		X	X																			
	3		X						X														X				
	2						X											X								
	1													X												
	0	X		X		X			X	X			X	X	X		X	X	X	X	X	X		X			

| Pain duration (hours) | 10 | 2 | | 2 | | 3 | 4 | 4 | 2 | 5 | | 4 | 8 | 2 | | | 2 | | | | | 3 | 12 | |

DRUG INTAKE																															
NSAID		X		X			X																							X
PROPHENAZONE											X																	
DIPYRONE				X							X																

Fig. 14.**8 a**

NAME: D. R.

b

DATE:	14	15	16	17	18	19	20	21	22	23	24	25	26	27	28	29	1	2	3	4	5	6	7	8	9	10	11	12	13	14	15
HEADACHE 5						X	X	X	X	X																					
4					X							X	X	X		X	X	X												X	X
3	X			X																											
2															X																
1																															
0		X	X								X									X	X	X	X	X	X	X	X	X	X	X	X
Headache duration (hours)	6			9	6	8					6	8	5	2	5	6	4													7	6
PAIN 5						X	X	X	X																						X
4											X	X	X																		
3					X																										
2																															
1																															
0	X	X	X	X	X						X							X	X	X	X	X	X	X	X	X	X	X	X	X	X
Pain duration (hours)						4	12	10	15	16		10	13	15																	20

DRUG INTAKE

NSAID						X	X	X	X	X	X		X	X	X																
ERGOTAMINE MESYLATE	X	X	X	X	X	X	X	X	X	X	X	X	X	X	X	X	X	X	X	X	X	X	X	X	X	X	X	X	X	X	X
AMITRYPTILINE + PERPHENAZINE	X	X	X	X	X	X	X	X	X	X	X	X	X	X	X	X	X	X	X	X	X	X	X	X	X	X	X	X	X	X	X
ZOLPIDEM	X	X	X	X	X	X	X	X	X	X	X	X	X	X	X	X	X	X	X	X	X	X	X	X	X	X	X	X	X	X	X

NAME: D. R.

c

DATE:	16	17	18	19	20	21	22	23	24	25	26	27	28	29	30	31	1	2	3	4	5	6	7	8	9	10	11	12	13	14	15
HEADACHE 5									X																						
4																															
3							X	X			X																			X	
2						X																						X			
1										X																					
0	X	X	X	X	X					X			X	X	X	X	X	X	X	X	X	X	X	X	X	X	X		X	X	X
Headache duration (hours)							6	8	4	5		3	4																3		5
PAIN 5																												X			
4																													X		
3									X																						
2																															
1																															
0	X	X	X	X	X	X	X	X		X		X	X	X	X	X	X	X	X	X	X	X	X	X					X	X	X
Pain duration (hours)									6																				7	3	

DRUG INTAKE

NSAID									X																						
ERGOTAMINE MESYLATE	X	X	X	X	X	X	X	X	X	X	X	X	X	X	X	X	X	X	X	X	X	X	X	X	X	X	X	X	X	X	X
AMITRYPTILINE + PERPHENAZINE	X	X	X	X	X	X	X	X	X	X	X	X	X	X	X	X	X	X	X	X	X	X	X	X	X	X	X	X	X	X	X
ZOLPIDEM	X	X	X	X	X	X	X	X	X	X	X		X		X					X	X	X						X			

Fig. 14.**8** **a** Headache and pain diary of a young woman suffering from migraine, tension-type headache, and myogenous cervico-facial pain. **b, c** The results of a combined pharmacological and nonpharmacological treatment are satisfactory. Episodic migraine attacks are still present. Sumatriptan was prescribed after suspending the intake of ergot derivatives

frequent migraine attacks, a specific treatment for migraine will be combined with the antidepressive therapy.

Antidepressants are also the drugs of first choice in patients with facial pain disorder as somatoform disorder. In this case, an antimigraine treatment will be also be associated as needed.

Particular care should given to the use of anticonvulsant drugs in neuropathic pain. Carbamazepine still is the first-choice drug in classical cases of trigeminal neuralgia. If the response is not satisfactory, other anticonvulsant drugs may be employed (see Chapter 12). However, a tendency to indiscriminate use of carbamezapine as a first-choice drug even in non-neuralgic pain syndromes is unjustified.

In the presence of orofacial pain not easily distinguishable between facial pain disorder and neuropathic pain, one might appropriately prescribe amitriptyline first and then associate or replace it with clonazepam or gabapentin if there is only partial or no response.

Topically applied drugs should be considered in localized facial pain syndromes. Topical administration offers the advantage of a more selective action and of fewer side effects. It may be associated with other modalities of drug administra-

tion: however, the concurrent administration of drugs that have the same side effects should be avoided (for instance, topical and nontopical NSAIDs, or topical administration of clonidine associated with oral administration of beta-blockers).

Planning of Nonpharmacological Treatment

The relevance of nonpharmacological treatment depends on the type of pain and its severity. In general, more consideration should be given to nonpharmacological treatment than is usually given by many clinicians. It may promote resolution in a number of cases of headache and facial pain and may be adjuvant to drug treatment in other cases by increasing the drug's efficacy and reducing minimal effective dose.

Nonpharmacological treatment is the first, and often the sole, treatment modality in patients with episodic tension-type headache in absence of evident signs of anxiety or depression. In these cases a program of biofeedback sessions and relaxation exercises at home, on a daily basis, might be

a — NAME: C. G.

HEADACHE	11	12	13	14	15	16	17	18	19	20	21	22	23	24	25	26	27	28	29	30	31	1	2	3	4	5	6	7	8	9	10
5																															
4																X															
3			X																							X	X				
2	X						X	X					X				X	X		X	X			X	X						
1																															
0		X		X	X	X			X	X	X	X		X	X				X			X	X					X	X	X	X
Headache duration (hours)	13/16		12/15				13/17	14/15					10/16			16/18	8/16	8/12		8/10	12/16			8/20	13/17	8/20	8/20				

b — NAME: C. G.

HEADACHE	17	18	19	20	21	22	23	24	25	26	27	28	29	30	31	1	2	3	4	5	6	7	8	9	10	11	12	13	14	15	16
5																															
4																															
3				X																											
2			X		X								X						X												
1																															
0	X	X				X	X	X	X	X	X	X		X	X	X	X	X		X	X	X	X	X	X	X	X	X	X	X	X
Headache duration (hours)			13/15	13/15	8/10								10/12						10/12												

DRUG INTAKE

SUMATRIPTAN	17	18	19	20	21	22	23	24	25	26	27	28	29	30	31	1	2	3	4	5	6	7	8	9	10	11	12	13	14	15	16
				X																											

Fig. 14.**9** **a Headache diary of a 35-year-old woman suffering from headache attacks of tension-type and pulsating. b, c** After a nonpharmacological treatment the tension-type headache has almost disappeared. Episodic migraine attacks are fully managed with oral sumatriptan 50 mg

planned. This can be combined with regular physical activity or sports practice and the use of a visual reminder, such as colored labels, to limit daily parafunction.

In myogenous pain, TENS sessions and application of warm pads may be added to the above program. The simple posture exercises described in Chapter 13 will be prescribed additionally if postural problems are also present, as is often the case.

The problems mentioned above are often associated with signs of mild TMJ dysfunction, such as a clicking noise and occasional joint pain. In these cases, specific exercises (traction and counter-resistance) will also be prescribed (see Chapter 13).

A problem that may arise with nonpharmacological treatment is that of a poor compliance by patients, because they underestimate the potential of the treatment or because it requires more time and discipline than a pharmacological treatment. The clinician should emphasize its advantages, including reduction of drug use, provided it is performed regularly and correctly. It is advisable to prescribe few exercises initially and, once the clinician has checked that they are performed correctly, add others later as needed.

Pharmacological and Nonpharmacological Treatment Association

The association of the two types of treatment is convenient in numerous cases. In patients for whom drugs should be prescribed but who show clear signs of muscle hyperparafunction, nonpharmacological treatment described above should be applied.

The response of patients to this association may vary conspicuously, depending on the extent of their apprehension of the non-pharmacologial treatment and their discipline in carrying it out. The combination of biofeedback sessions and relaxation exercises at home may give excellent results in patients in whom the cognitive aspect of the treatment is particularly efficacious: these are typically patients who undertake the prescribed program enthusiastically, stating that they "feel safer" because they can often succeed in blocking or reducing the intensity of the pain attack (for instance of a tension-type headache) whenever they perceive its onset. In these patients it is often possible to reduce the dosage of the psychotropic drugs, if they have been prescribed, particularly if the patient performs physical or sporting activity on a regular basis. Other patients may show a paradoxical response to biofeedback sessions, with increased anxiety: in these cases the treatment must be promptly suspended.

Likewise, appropriate exercises will be prescribed in patients with headache or facial pain that needs pharmacological treatment and shows associated signs of TMJ dysfunction. Sometimes a patient is excessively concerned about these signs and fears that a block of mouth movement might develop. The clinician should reassure the patient about the real nature of the problem entity and explain that with all probability it will be conveniently managed with the prescribed exercises, and also explain the nature of the head pain that represents the patient's substantive problem. Patients often tend to consider the joint symptom, for example, the clicking noise, as the cause of their pain syndrome rather than a secondary consequence, as is often the case. This might also be due to previous incorrect diagnoses.

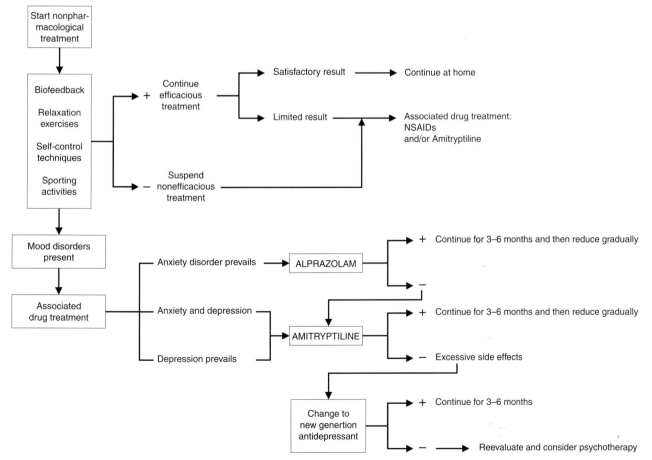

Fig. 14.**10** Algorithm for the management of tension-type headache (TTH). +, positive result, –, negative or limited result

The association of pharmacological and nonpharmacological treatment may also be indicated in neuropathic pain. In addition to the pharmacological treatment discussed, one may conveniently test the response obtained after one or two TENS sessions and plan a session program if the response is positive. The same applies in cases of acute and localized myogenous pain. Figures 14.**10**–14.**12** give algorithms for the management of some of the more frequent headache–pain syndromes.

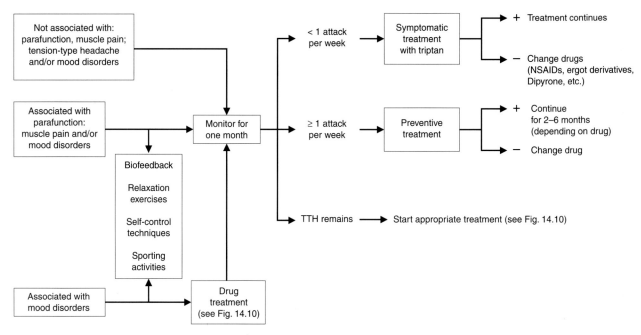

Fig. 14.**11**   **Algorithm for the management of migraine**

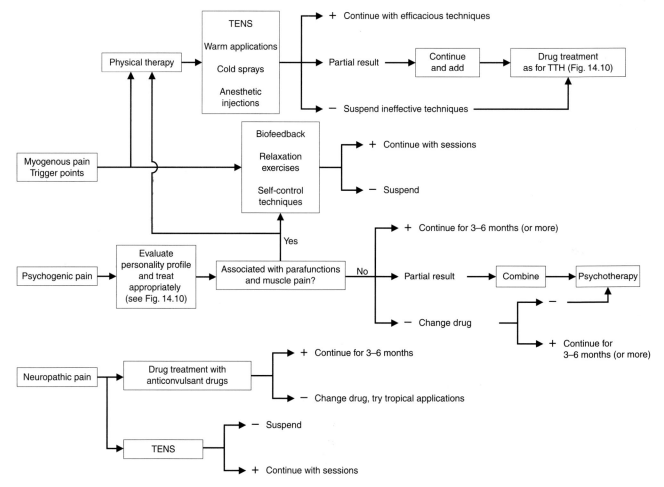

Fig. 14.**12**   Algorithm for the management of myogenous, neuropathic, and psychogenic pain

Part III Diagnosis and Therapy of Headache

15 Tension-Type Headache

General Characteristics. Aetiological and Triggering Factors

The tension-type headache (TTH) is the most common type of headache. According to an epidemiological study (Rasmussen et al., 1991), its prevalence over the lifetime is 69% in men and 88% in women, while the annual prevalence is 63 % in men and 88% in women. As seen in Chapter 1, the IHS classification (1988) distinguishes between "episodic" (ETTH) and "chronic" (CTTH) cases of TTH. This distinction is essentially based on frequency: less than 15 days a month for ETTH, at least 15 days a month for at least six months for CTTH. The diagnostic criteria that distinguish TTH from other types of headache, particularly migraine, are clinical and pertain to quality, intensity, location and duration of the pain, in addition to the absence of autonomic symptoms. The IHS classification suggests the following criteria for ETTH:

Headache lasts from 30 minutes to 7 days and has at least two of the following pain characteristics:

1. Pressing/tightening (non-pulsating) quality
2. Mild or moderate intensity (may inhibit, but does not prohibit activities)
3. Bilateral or variable location (more than just symmetric side shifts)
4. No aggravation by physical activity. No nausea or vomiting. Phonophobia and photophobia may occur, though not simultaneously.
    CTTH pain has the same characteristics. No vomiting occurs. Either nausea, phonophobia, or photophobia may occur.

Both ETTH and CTTH are further classified by the IHS as tension-type headaches associated or not associated with disorder of pericranial muscles depending upon whether headache is associated with increased levels of tenderness and/or EMG activity of pericranial muscles.

Although at least two of the reported characteristics must be present, as stated earlier, it is advisable to consider that both somewhat frequently involve exceptions (Blau, 1993). A pressing, heavy, tightening pain may also occur in migraine (Olesen, 1978), the pain can be unilateral in TTH and bilateral in migraine, and TTH may involve a certain degree of nausea associated with photophobia or phonophobia. The diagnosis is made by an integrated evaluation of medical history and clinical data (inspection, palpation, etc.). In this regard it should be noted, as seen in Chapter 1, that several authors advise a separate analysis of each symptom and the introduction of a symptom degree criterion to distinguish diagnostically between TTH and migraine (Michel et al., 1993; Pfaffenrath and Isler, 1993).

The relationship between TTH and psychological problems is controversial (see Chapter 8). In CTTH, whether simple or associated with migraine, the frequent association of mood disorders has been reported (Kudrow et al., 1979; Sternbach et al., 1980; Andrasik et al., 1982; Ellertsen et al., 1987; Blanchard et al., 1989; Mongini et al., 1992, 1994, 1997). On some MMPI scales patients with CTTH had higher scores than healthy con-

trol subjects (Mongini et al., 1992; De Benedittis and Lorenzetti, 1992 a). These scores tended to normalize after therapy (Mongini et al., 1994). Moreover, CTTH was associated with stressful life events (Invernizzi et al., 1985; Nattero et al., 1986; Sternbach et al., 1986; De Benedittis et al., 1990; De Benedittis and Lorenzetti, 1992 b). It was therefore hypothesized that mood disorders may intervene as a third variable in the relationship between chronic headache and stressors (De Benedittis and Lorenzetti, 1992 a).

The relationship between parafunctions, craniofacial muscle fatigue and tension-type headaches is, as seen in Chapter 3, still under debate. In fact, although there is not always a relationship between the muscle tenderness and the degree of headache, tension-type headache sufferers have more tenderness in their pericranial muscles than do non-sufferers (Langemark and Olesen, 1987; Hatch et al., 1992; Jensen et al., 1993; Mongini et al., 1997) and tenderness increases during headache attacks (Jensen and Olesen, 1996). It

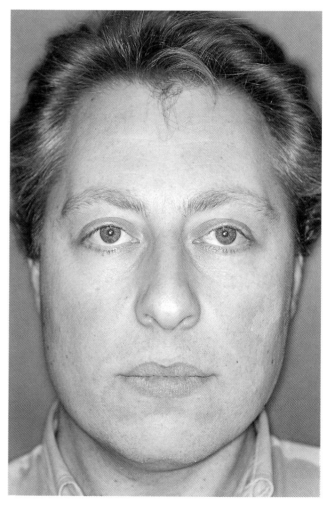

Fig. 15.**1** **Patient with tension-type headache predominantly located in the frontal and left temporal region.** Note the greater degree of hypertrophy of the masseter and temporal area on that side

is advisable to palpate not only some of the muscular heads but to palpate all over and systematically (see Chapter 10).

Episodic Tension-Type Headache (ETTH)

As mentioned earlier, the distinction between ETTH and CTTH is based on the frequency of the episodes. In ETTH the anamnestic data most commonly show that stressful events are a major triggering factor. Under clinical examination, signs of muscular hyperparafunction may be observed (muscular hypertrophy, scalloped tongue edges, discernible dental abrasion, etc.) (Figs. 15.**1**, 15.**2**). Palpation of the muscles often causes a certain degree of pain. Anxiety symptoms are frequently observed, but by and large there are no actual mood disorders (Figs. 15.**3** – 15.**6**).

In these cases, a nondrug therapy is usually quite effective. During the examination the patient should be reassured that the problem is minor and easily managed. A series of biofeedback sessions should be scheduled, along with relaxation exercises to be done at home every day by the patient. Posture correction and physical exercises should be prescribed when appropriate. If there are areas of a muscle that are aching particularly, a series of physical therapy sessions can be scheduled. If the patient grinds his or her teeth at night, a flat splint can be used at night. Pharmaceuticals can be avoided or

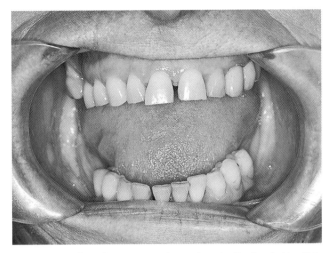

Fig. 15.**2** Scalloped tongue margins and markedly abraded teeth in a patients with tension-type headache

limited to low doses of benzodiazepine or amitriptyline once a day in the evening for a brief period (a few weeks). This program produces good to excellent results within a few months (Figs. 15.**7** – 15.**10**).

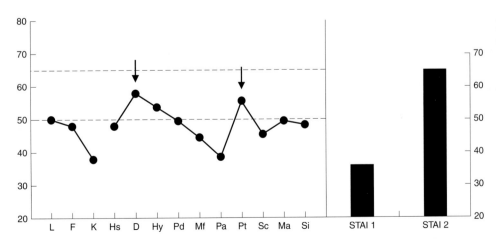

NAME:	**R. R.**																																
DATE:		*1*	*2*	*3*	*4*	*5*	*6*	*7*	*8*	*9*	*10*	*11*	*12*	*13*	*14*	*15*	*16*	*17*	*18*	*19*	*20*	*21*	*22*	*23*	*24*	*25*	*26*	*27*	*28*	*29*	*30*	*31*
HEADACHE	5																															
	4																															
	3																															
	2																	X									X				
	1	X								X								X													
	0		X	X	X	X	X	X	X	X		X	X	X	X	X		X		X	X	X	X	X	X	X		X	X	X
Headache duration (hours)		$\frac{8}{14}$											T						$\frac{7,30}{13}$	$\frac{9}{11}$											

T = all day

Fig. 15.**3** **Headache diary of patient with episodic tension-type headache (ETTH):** about five episodes a month, mild intensity, duration several hours. The menstrual period is highlighted in gray

Fig. 15.**4** Same patient as in Fig. 15.3. The MMPI-2 shows a normal profile in which the D (depression) and Pt (psychasthenia, anxiety index) scales are those with the highest scores (arrows). The STAI shows an increase in the trait anxiety

NAME:	**F. P.**																															
DATE:		24	25	26	27	28	29	30	31	1	2	3	4	5	6	7	8	9	10	11	12	13	14	15	16	17	18	19	20	21	22	23
HEADACHE	5																															
	4																															
	3																															
	2				X							X							X		X			X								
	1			X	X						X											X	X										X
	0	X				X	X	X			X		X	X	X	X	X	X		X					X	X	X	X	X	X	X	
Headache duration (hours)		10/12	13/10	6/10						14/20		6/15							19/23		7/14	18/21	15/17	7/15								6/11

Fig. 15.**5**   Headache diary of a 22-year-old woman with tension-type headache

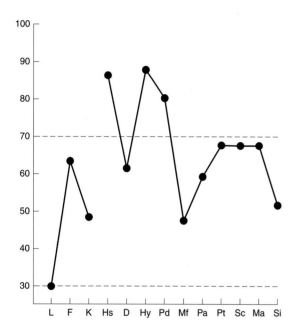

Fig. 15.**6**   Same patients as in Fig. 15.5. The MMPI shows high scores of hypochondria (Hs), hysteria (HY) and psychopathic deviation (Pd)

NAME:	**R. R.**																															
DATE:		20	21	22	23	24	25	26	27	28	29	30	31	1	2	3	4	5	6	7	8	9	10	11	12	13	14	15	16	17	18	19
HEADACHE	5																															
	4																															
	3																															
	2																															
	1																			X												
	0	X	X	X	X	X	X	X	X	X	X	X	X	X	X	X	X	X	X		X	X	X	X	X	X	X	X	X	X	X	X
Headache duration (hours)																				10/12												

Fig. 15.**7**   Same patient as in Figs. 15.3 and 15.4. Remission of symptoms after nondrug treatment

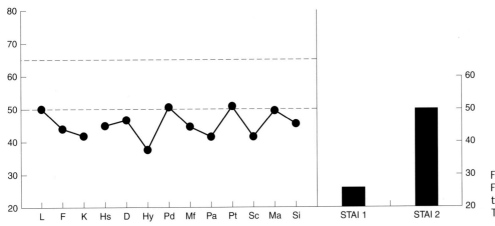

Fig. 15.**8** Same patient as in Fig. 15.7. After MMPI treatment the D and Pt scores decreased. Trait anxiety is also diminished

NAME: **F. P.**																																
DATE:		*1*	*2*	*3*	*4*	*5*	*6*	*7*	*8*	*9*	*10*	*11*	*12*	*13*	*14*	*15*	*16*	*17*	*18*	*19*	*20*	*21*	*22*	*23*	*24*	*25*	*26*	*27*	*28*	*29*	*30*	*31*
HEADACHE	5																																
	4																																
	3																																
	2																						X										
	1																												X				
	0	X	X	X	X	X	X	X	X	X	X	X	X	X	X	X	X	X	X	X	X	X		X	X	X	X	X		X	X	X
Headache duration (hours)																							$\frac{11}{14}$						$\frac{16}{18}$			

Fig. 15.**9** Same patient as in Figs. 15.5 and 15.6. Marked reduction of symptoms after four months of nondrug treatment

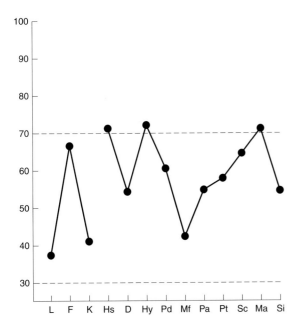

Fig. 15.**10** Same patient as in Fig. 15.9. Improvement of MMPI personality profile after treatment

NAME: D. C.

DATE: JUNE		1	2	3	4	5	6	7	8	9	10	11	12	13	14	15	16	17	18	19	20	21	22	23	24	25	26	27	28	29	30
HEADACHE	5																														
	4																														
	3																														
	2	X	X							X		X								X										X	X
	1			X		X	X	X	X		X		X	X			X	X			X	X		X	X		X				
	0				X										X	X			X				X			X		X			
Headache duration (hours)																															
PAIN	5																														
	4																														
	3																														
	2				X	X							X	X								X									
	1	X	X	X			X	X	X	X	X			X		X	X	X		X					X						
	0														X				X		X		X	X		X	X	X	X	X	
Pain duration (hours)		ALL CRISES LASTED ABOUT ONE HOUR																													

Fig. 15.**11**   Headache and pain diary of 21-year-old woman with CTTH and pain in the cheeks

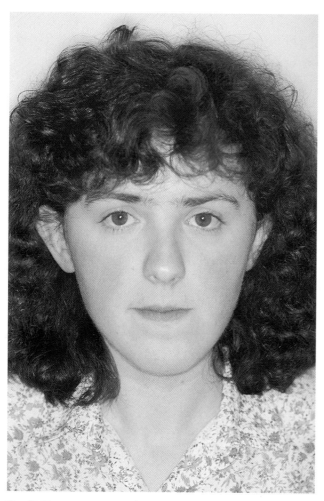

Fig. 15.**12**   Inspection reveals little facial mimic and a mild hypertrophy of the right masseter

Chronic Tension-Type Headache (CTTH). Diagnosis and Therapy

When a tension-type headache becomes chronic, complications tend to occur. The patient often has more or less marked symptoms of anxiety or depression. Signs of muscle hyperparafunction are sometimes very evident. From a clinical and therapeutic standpoint it seems important to make a distinction between patients in whom particular changes in personality are absent or mild and those in whom personality changes of some kind are a distinct feature (see Chapter 8). In the latter case, the degree of the problem and the degree of response to nondrug therapy must be evaluated in order to choose a drug and its dosage.

One patient suffering from CTTH with anxiety and depression implications who responded very well to a nondrug therapy associated with a moderate intake of drugs was a 21-year-old housewife who had a history of frequent headaches on awakening in the morning. The headache had a frontal bilateral location, mild to moderate intensity, was pressing in quality, and lasted about one hour (Fig. 15.**11**). About six years earlier, after experiencing a fright from seeing her mother taken ill, the patient had developed guilt obsessions and psychogenic anorexia. She had been treated with antidepressants and psychotherapy and obtained excellent results. At the time of observation, she reported frequent mood changes, anxiety, palpitations and gastric pain. Her headaches were often associated with a clicking noise at the right TMJ and a bilateral preauricular and cheek pain.

Upon examination, her facial expression appeared rather depressed, with reduced mimic. The right masseter appeared to be slightly hypertrophic (Fig. 15.**12**). Palpation was positive for the right masseter muscle, the external pterygoid and the temporal muscles. The MMPI showed an increase in the scales relative to depression (D), paranoia (Pa), social introversion

(Si) and psychasthenia (Pt). The last-mentioned data, which is a classic indicator of anxiety, was confirmed by the STAI test, which revealed a high level of trait anxiety (Fig. 15.**13**).

Thus, although her past depression had been overcome, she remained in a state of anxiety and mild depression (minor depression), which in turn was one of the factors that induced an intense parafunctional activity, especially at night. This explained her masseter hypertrophy, the occasional clicking noise in the TMJ (see Chapter 3), and the pain in the preauricular and cheek region.

It is therefore reasonable to hypothesize that the psychological factor was, in this case, a variable that acted both directly and indirectly, by means of the muscular parafunction. This is corroborated by the fact that the headache almost always occurred upon awakening.

During an interview it was explained clearly to the patient that the problem was not serious. Since she was recalcitrant to taking antidepressants again, it was agreed that she whould start with the nondrug therapy alone, but it was stressed that she had to carry it out systematically and that the drug therapy to be associated with it could be decided subsequently. A series of biofeedback sessions was started, along with relaxation exercises that the patient carried out assiduously at home. In addition, a maxillary splint was applied at night. The response to the therapy was immediate (Fig. 15.**14**). Since the patient felt reassured psychologically but there were still some symptoms of anxiety, 0.5 mg of chlordemethyldiazepam was prescribed once or twice a day, as needed. Four months later the symptoms had disappeared steadily and the patient was discharged after two further months of observation, with the recommendation to continue doing the relaxation exercises. At the time of discharge the patient reported improved mood and this was confirmed by the results of the psychometric tests that were administered again (Fig. 15.**15**).

A worse case than the previous one is that of a 25-year-old woman, an office worker, who hat CTTH associated with arthropathy. She had had moderate to severe headaches in the frontal location lasting from one hour to all day (Fig. 15.**16**). The pain was for the most part pressing, and only in the moments of most acute pain did it become pulsating. Triggering or aggravating factors were emotions and stress, weather variations, intellectual fatigue, menstrual cycle, and prolonged sleep ("Sunday headache"). There were no autonomic signs and the neurological examination was within the norm. For five months there had been a disk displacement without reduction at the right TMJ. The patient reported frequent epi-

sodes of asthenia, insomnia, anxiety, mood changes, cramps, paresthesia, dorsal pain, palpitations, dizziness, and dysmenorrhea. She also had intense bruxism both day and night.

Upon examination, a reduction in the degree of the mouth opening was observed with a deviation toward the right. Radiography confirmed the reduced excursion of the right condyle resulting from the displaced disk. Palpation was positive for the retrocondylar point, the temporal muscles, and the right lateral pterygoid muscle.

The MMPI revealed the presence of a distinct *hysterical or psychosomatic V* with high scores for the first three scales, which nonetheless showed depression scores that were lower than those of hypochondria and hysteria. The STAI revealed a high level of state and trait anxiety (Fig. 15.**17**).

In this case, too, it seems that the headache problem was linked to certain variables such as repeated and prolonged stressful events affecting the patient, a marked tendency toward daytime and nighttime parafunctions, and probably a personal profile that favored somatization phenomena. The parafunctions in turn caused the articular lesion that created an ulterior source of worry and stress.

The patient underwent manipulation to reduce dislocation of the disk (Mongini, 1996) and an upper splint was applied. This allowed the patient to recover normal mouth mobility but did not in the least affect her headache pattern (Fig. 15.**18**). At this point nondrug therapy was started (biofeedback, relaxation exercises) and the initial response was encouraging (Fig. 15.**18**). One week later the patient was given an evening dose of amitriptyline in drops, starting with a very low dosage (10 mg), which was progressively increased. Since the response was quite satisfactory (Fig. 15.**19**), the maximum dosage was limited to 20 mg/day. This treatment was maintained for six months, during which time the symptoms steadily disappeared, almost entirely (Fig. 15.**20**), and the MMPI profile became completely normal; nonetheless it was interesting to observe that the first three scales, with normal scores, maintained a reciprocal ratio similar to that observed at the beginning of the therapy. The STAI state and trait anxiety scores were considerably lower (Fig. 15.**21**).

As mentioned earlier, in certain cases CTTH may by an epiphenomenon of an accentuated personality problem quite different in nature from those previously described. One of these cases is that of a 39-year-old woman, a factory worker, who in previous years had repeatedly been hospitalized in psychiatric departments for a severe form of endogenous depression and at the time of observation was proceeding with

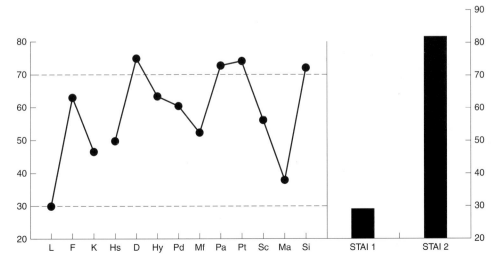

Fig. 15.**13** Increase in numerous MMPI scales. Increased trait anxiety shown by STAI

NAME: D. C.

DATE: JULY

	4	5	6	7	8	9	10	11	12	13	14	15	16	17	18	19	20	21	22	23	24	25	26	27	28	29	30	31	1	2	3
HEADACHE 5																															
4																															
3																															
2																															
1						X		X		X													X	X	X	X	X	X	X	X	X
0	X	X	X	X	X		X		X		X	X	X	X	X	X	X	X	X	X	X	X									
Headache duration (hours)						30'		30'		30'													30'	30'	30'	30'	30'	15'	10'	20'	30'
PAIN 5																															
4																															
3																															
2																															
1																															
0	X	X	X	X	X	X	X	X	X	X	X	X	X	X	X	X	X	X	X	X	X	X	X	X	X	X	X	X	X	X	X
Pain duration (hours)																															

NAME: D. C.

DATE: AUG

	5	6	7	8	9	10	11	12	13	14	15	16	17	18	19	20	21	22	23	24	25	26	27	28	29	30	31	1	2	3	4
HEADACHE 5																															
4																															
3																															
2																															
1																X															
0	X	X	X	X	X	X	X	X	X	X	X	X	X	X	X		X	X	X	X	X	X	X	X	X	X	X	X	X	X	X
Headache duration (hours)																30'															
PAIN 5																															
4																															
3																															
2																															
1																															
0	X	X	X	X	X	X	X	X	X	X	X	X	X	X	X	X	X	X	X	X	X	X	X	X	X	X	X	X	X	X	X
Pain duration (hours)																															

Fig. 15.**14** Symptoms impoved considerably during first month of therapy (**a**) and disappeared during second month (**b**)

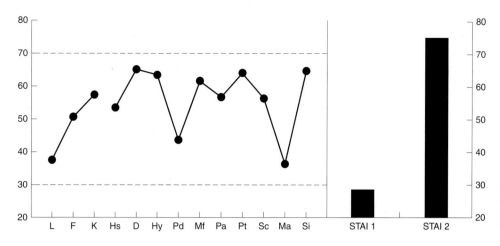

Fig. 15.**15**   Improvement of personality profile shown by psychometric tests administered after therapy

NAME: **M. I.**

DATE: SEPT		1	2	3	4	5	6	7	8	9	10	11	12	13	14	15	16	17	18	19	20	21	22	23	24	25	26	27	28	29	30
HEADACHE	5																														
	4						X									X															
	3							X														X									
	2		X					X			X							X						X	X		X		X		X
	1	X		X			X			X			X			X					X		X					X			
	0	X				X	X					X		X			X		X	X						X					
Headache duration (hours)		3	3	1			4		3	5	4	3		8		3	3		4		12		5	5	4	12		8		4	

Fig. 15.**16**   Headache diary of patient with CTTH and disk displacement without reduction at right TMJ

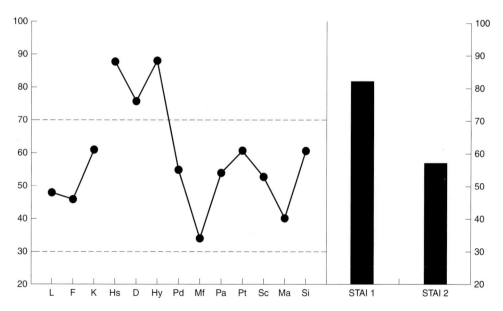

Fig. 15.**17**   Typical *hysterical or conversive V* shown by MMPI. Increased state and trait anxiety shown by STAI

NAME: M. I. (arrow ↓1, arrow ↓2)

DATE: OCT

HEADACHE	1	2	3	4	5	6	7	8	9	10	11	12	13	14	15	16	17	18	19	20	21	22	23	24	25	26	27	28	29	30	31
5																															
4						X							X																		
3					X											X	X														
2				X					X	X				X															X		
1		X					X								X				X				X	X							
0	X		X					X			X	X						X		X	X	X			X	X	X	X		X	X
Headache duration (hours)			3		6	2	2	4		4	3			1	4	3	5	2					2			2	2			2	

Fig. 15.**18**   After manipulation to reduce disk displacement (arrow 1), headache symptoms did not change. There was, however, a partial improvement of the headache at the beginning of the nondrug therapy (arrow 2)

NAME: M. I.

DATE: NOV

HEADACHE	1	2	3	4	5	6	7	8	9	10	11	12	13	14	15	16	17	18	19	20	21	22	23	24	25	26	27	28	29	30
5																														
4																														
3																														
2									X																					
1			X	X								X			X				X					X						
0	X	X			X	X	X	X		X	X		X	X		X	X	X		X	X	X	X		X	X	X	X	X	X
Headache duration (hours)			1	1					3			1					1			1				1						

DRUG INTAKE

AMITRIPTYLINE	X	X	X	X	X	X	X	X	X	X	X	X	X	X	X	X	X	X	X	X	X	X	X	X	X	X	X	X	X	X

Fig. 15.**19**   Remarkable relief from headache after combining low doses of amitriptyline with therapy

---

NAME: M. I.

DATE: MARCH

HEADACHE	1	2	3	4	5	6	7	8	9	10	11	12	13	14	15	16	17	18	19	20	21	22	23	24	25	26	27	28	29	30	31
5																															
4																															
3																															
2																											X				
1										X														X							
0	X	X	X	X	X	X	X	X	X		X	X	X	X	X	X	X	X	X	X	X		X		X	X		X	X	X	X
Headache duration (hours)										1														1		1					

Fig. 15.**20**   Symptoms disappeared almost entirely after six months

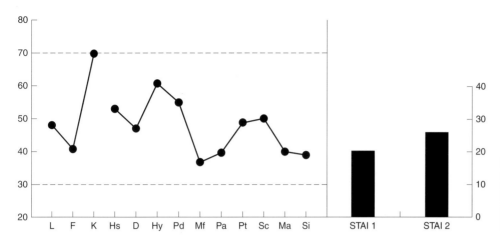

Fig. 15.**21** Psychological tests show clear improvement of profiles. MMPI shows a profile of the first three scales recognizably similar to the before-therapy profile, but scores are now normal

her drug treatment and psychotherapy as an outpatient. About two years earlier the patient started having frequent headaches, mild to severe, located in the periorbital area, and spreading to the frontal, parietal, temporal, and nuchal areas on the right, lasting several hours, heavy or pulsating (the most intense attacks). They were associated with an intense burning pain located in the right cheek area (Figs 15.**22**, 15.**23**). During the most acute headaches, the patient reported moderate lacrimation; other autonomic signs were absent. Changes of weather and stress were the most important triggering factors. The patient often suffered from numerous ailments (Fig. 15.**24**) and complained of intense daytime and nighttime parafunctional activity (Fig. 15.**25**). Also worth noting in the medical history was an elective abortion that had taken place some years earlier.

The neurological examination was negative except for a mild hypoesthesia in the sensory area of the three right trigeminal nerve branches. Palpation revealed a mild tenderness in some cranial and muscular areas. The psychometric tests confirmed the severity of the psychological problem,

with a marked elevation of almost all the MMPI scales and very high levels of anxiety according to the STAI (Fig. 15.**26**). It was therefore a case of CTTH with possibly associated facial pain disorder in a patient with a personality disorder. In this case the parafunctions were an epiphenomenon and there was no relationship between the severity of the pain symptoms and the limited tenderness of the craniofacial musculature.

The patient was treated in conjunction with a psychiatrist, who proceeded with the drug treatment (clomipramine and clopentixol) and psychotherapy. After a few talks with the patient to explain the nature of the pain and its possible causes, a nondrug treatment of biofeedback, relaxation, posture and physical exercises was prescribed along with the application of a protective nighttime splint. The response was positive: the pain in the cheek region disappeared and the headache was considerably attenuated within a few months (Fig. 15.**27**). However, in this case the improvement of the pain was not associated with any change in the personality profile (Fig. 15.**28**).

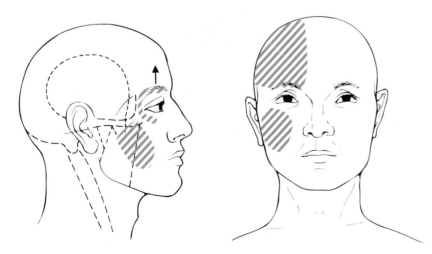

Fig. 15.**22** Pain locations in woman suffering from endogenous depression, CTTH, and burning pain in cheek area

NAME: D. G.

DATE: JAN/FEB	16	17	18	19	20	21	22	23	24	25	26	27	28	29	30	31	1	2	3	4	5	6	7	8	9	10	11	12	13	14	15
HEADACHE 5		X	X	X	X										X	X							X								
4																				X							X				
3						X	X												X		X	X									
2	X								X															X		X					
1										X	X														X						
0								X				X	X	X			X	X										X	X	X	X
Headache duration (hours)	T		1	4	T	T	1		4		T				4	T			4	T	4	5	4	6	4	4	T				
PAIN 5		X	X	X	X										X	X							X								
4																				X											
3						X	X												X		X	X									
2	X								X															X		X	X				
1										X	X														X						
0								X				X	X	X			X	X										X	X	X	X
Pain duration (hours)	2.30	8	8	4	T	T	1								4	8			4	5		6	8	5		4	2				

T = all day

Fig. 15.**23**   Headache and pain diary

Colitis	☒
Gastritis	☒
Kinetosis	☐
Swallowing difficulty	☐
Digestive problems	☐
Anorexia	☐
Bulimia	☒
Anxiety	☒
Phobias	☐
Sleep disorders	☒
Palpitations	☒
Panic attacks	☒
Mood changes	☒
Fainting	☒
Vertigo	☐
Lassitude	☒
Parafunctions	☐
Clonus	☒
Cramps	☒
Paresthesias	☒
Back pain	☒
Urination disturbances	☐
Diarrhea or constipation	☐
Nail fragility	☐
Hair fragility	☐
Circulation disorders	☒
Cold limbs	☒
Frigidity	☐
Vaginism	☐
Frequent depressed moods	☒
Other	☐

Fig. 15.**24**   Complaints reported by the patient

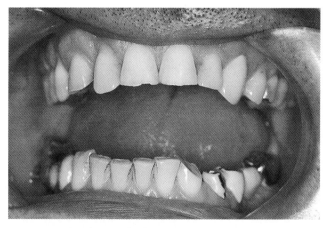

Fig. 15.**25**   The discernible dental abrasion and scalloped tongue edges indicate intense parafunctional activity

Conclusions

As already seen in Chapter 1, the IHS classification indicates a series of possible pathogenic factors of TTH: "oromandibular dysfunction," psychosocial stressors, anxiety, depression, headache as a symptom of hallucination or delirium, muscular stress, and drug abuse. In practice, reference is made to alterations of the function of craniofacial structures (oromandibular dysfunction, muscular stress) on the one hand, and stress and psychiatric problems with varying degrees of severity on the other. However, it can be observed that the factors listed appear for the most part to be subject to a certain

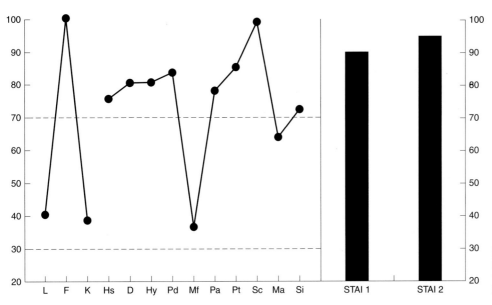

Fig. 15.**26** MMPI confirms the severity of the psychological profile. STAI anxiety scores are very high

NAME: **D. G.**

DATE: MAY/JUNE		4	5	6	7	8	9	10	11	12	13	14	15	16	17	18	19	20	21	22	23	24	25	26	27	28	29	30	31	1	2	3
HEADACHE	5														X							X										
	4																															
	3																															
	2	X																														
	1																															
	0		X	X	X	X	X	X	X	X	X	X	X	X		X	X	X	X	X	X		X	X	X	X	X	X	X	X	X	X
Headache duration (hours)		4													T							4										
PAIN	5																															
	4																															
	3																															
	2	X																														
	1																															
	0																															
Pain duration (hours)		4																														

T A= all day

Fig. 15.**27** Considerable improvement of symptoms four months after starting treatment

shading and interdependence. In some of the patients described above, the psychological component presented a few anxiety traits within an entirely normal personality profile; in other patients, a high index of anxiety and a profile tending toward depression. In the last patient, the characteristics of a distinct personality disorder were revealed. It is also interesting to note that the two variables, headache and psychological problems, improved in a roughly parallel way in most of the patients but not in the last patient, whose personality profile represented the primary problem. On the other hand, in the patients in which the personality profile improved, the im-

provement did note seem to be attributable to the drug treatment alone, which in some cases consisted of particularly small dosages.

Another important observation is that most patients had moderate to severe parafunctional habits, which may induce that the IHS defines a muscular stress. The result can be pain in the craniofacial muscles (causing or worsening the headache), or various signs, more or less severe, of TMJ dysfunction: conditions defined by the IHS classification as oromandibular dysfunction. However, it does not seem correct to hypothesize that an articular dysfunction is a pathogenic factor

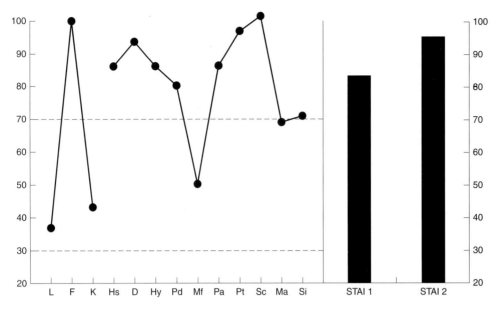

Fig. 15.**28**   The psychometric test profiles of this patient did not improve after treatment

of headache. A seen earlier, in the patient who also had a disk displacement without reduction, management of it did not improve the headache syndrome, which in contrast readily responded to drug and nondrug therapy.

Finally, it should be pointed out that some of the patients described above had sporadic headaches with some migraine characteristics (severe pain, described as throbbing, sometimes accompanied by mild lacrimation) which remitted without the use of antimigraine drugs.

The therapy must therefore be adjusted according to the frequency of TTH (rare episodic, frequent episodic, chronic) and the other characteristics of the patient. Although the nondrug therapy described is almost always advisable both for ETTH and CTTH, the most appropriate drug therapy may vary considerably. Amitriptyline is still the first-choice drug for CTTH. It can be administered in progressively higher dosages (usually not more than 25 mg) once a day in the evening. For patients with marked depression, the dosage should be increased to 75 mg or more a day, divided into two or more doses. If there are serious side effects or scanty response, it is advisable to opt for new-generation nontricyclic antidepressants (such as fluoxetine, paroxetine, venlafaxine, or cytalopram).

References

Andrasik F., Blanchard E.B., Arena J.G., et al., *Psychological functioning in headache sufferers*, Psychosom. Med., 1982, 44 : 171 – 182.

Blanchard E.B., Kirsch C.A., Appelbaum K.A., Jaccard J., *The role of psychopathology in chronic headache: cause or effect?*, Headache, 1989, 29 : 295 – 301.

Blau J.N., *Diagnosing migraine: are the criteria valid or invalid?*, Cephalalgia, 1993, 13 (Suppl. 12):21 – 24.

De Benedittis G., Lorenzetti A. et al., *The role of stressful life events in the onset of chronic primary headache*, Pain, 1990, 40 : 65 – 75.

De Benedittis G., Lorenzetti A., *The role of stressful life events in the persistence of primary headache: major events vs. daily hassles*, Pain, 1992, 51 : 35 – 42.

De Benedittis G., Lorenzetti A., *Minor stressful life events (daily hassles) in chronic primary headache: relationship with MMPI personality patterns*, Headache, 1992, 32 : 330 – 334.

Ellertsen B., Klöve H., *MMPI patterns in chronic muscle pain, tension headache, and migraine*, Cephalalgia, 1987, 7 : 101 – 108.

Hatch J., Moore P., Cyr-Provost M., Boutros N., Seleshi E., and Borcherding S., *The use of electromyography and muscle palpation in the diagnosis of tension-type headache with and without pericranial muscle involvement*, Pain, 1992, 49 : 175 – 178.

International Headache Society, *Classification and diagnostic criteria for headache disorders, cranial neuralgias and facial pain*, Cephalalgia, 1988, 8 (Suppl. 7):19 – 22.

Invernizzi G., Gala C., Sacchetti E., *Life events and headache*, Cephalalgia, 1985, suppl. 2 : 229 – 231.

Jensen R., Rasmussen B.K., Olesen J., *Muscle tenderness and pressure pain threshold in tensiontype headache and migraine*, Pain, 1993, 52 : 193 – 199.

Jensen R., Olesen J., *Initiating mechanisms of experimentally induced tension-type headache*, Cephalalgia, 1996, 16 : 175 – 182.

Kudrow L., Sutkus B.J., *MMPI pattern specificicy in primary headache disorders*, Headache, 1979, 19 : 18 – 24.

Langemark M., Olesen J., *Pericranial tenderness in tension headache*, Cephalalgia, 1987, 7 : 249 – 55.

Michel P., Henry P., Letenneur L., Jogeix M., Corson A., Dartigues J.F., *Diagnostic screen for assessment of the IHS criteria for migraine by general practitioners*, Cephalalgia, 1993, 13 (Suppl. 12):54 – 59.

Mongini F., *ATM e muscolatura cranio-cervico-faciale. Fisiopatologia e terapia*, UTET, Torino, 1996.

Mongini F., Ferla E., Maccagnani C., *MMPI profiles in patients with headache or craniofacial pain a comparative study*, Cephalalgia, 1992, 12 : 91 – 98.

Mongini F., Ibertis F., Ferla E., *Personality characteristics before and after treatment of different head pain syndromes*, Cephalalgia, 1994, 14 : 368 – 73.

Mongini F., Ibertis F., Manfredi A., *Long-term results in patients with disk displacement without reduction treated conservatively*, The Journal of Craniomandibular Practice, 1996, 14 : 301 – 305.

Mongini F., Defilippi N., Negro C., *Chronic daily headache. A clinical and psychological profile before and after treatment*, Headache, 1997, 37 : 83 – 87.

Nattero G., De Lorenzo C., Biale L., Torre E., Ancona M., *Idiopathic headache: relationship to life events*, Headache, 1986, 26 : 503 – 508.

Olesen J., *Some clinical features of the migraine attack. An analysis of 750 patients*, Headache, 1978, 18 : 268 – 271.

Pfaffenrath V., Isler H., *Evaluation of the nosology of chronic tension-type headache*, Cephalalgia, 1993, 13 (Suppl. 12):60 – 62.

Rasmussen B.K., *Migraine and tension-type headache in a general population: psychosocial factors*, Int. J. Epidemiol., 1992, 21 : 1138 – 1143.

Sternbach R.A., Dalessio D.J., Kunzel M., Bowman G.E., *MMPI patterns in common headache disorders*, Headache, 1980, 19 : 311 – 316.

16 Migraine

General Characteristics. Etiological and Triggering Factors

There are two types of migraine: migraine with aura and migraine without aura, depending on whether or not the pain is preceded by premonitory symptoms. As stated in the previous chapter, the diagnostic difference between TTH and migraine is clinical. The IHS classification (1988) proposes the following diagnostic criteria for migraines without aura:

(A) At least five attacks fulfilling (B)–(D).
(B) Headache attacks lasting 4–72 hours (untreated or unsuccessfully treated)
    In children below age 15, attacks may last 2–48 hours.
(C) Headache has at least two of the following characteristics:
    1. Unilateral location
    2. Pulsating quality
    3. Moderate or severe intensity (inhibits or prohibits daily activities)
    4. Aggravation by walking stairs of other similar routine physical activity
(D) During headache at least one of the following:
    1. Nausea and/or vomiting
    2. Photophobia and phonophobia
(E) History, physical and/or neurological examination do not suggest the presence of a condition that can cause a symptomatic headache or, in case of doubt, the latter is excluded by appropriate studies.

In migraines with aura, which are much rarer, the headaches are preceded by a so-called "aura" that is for the most part characterized by vision disorders, both positive (scotomata, fortification spectra) and negative (hemianopsia, scoto-mata, tunnel vision, etc.) (Fig. 16.1). Other manifestations of the aura, though rarer, are paresthesia, aphasia, nausea, and vomiting. According to the IHS classification, these symptoms must be completely reversible and develop gradually within a period longer than four minutes (in some cases two or more symptoms occur successively) and no symptom must last more than 60 minutes. The headache follows the aura with a free interval of no more than 60 minutes (but sometimes it can start before or at the same time as the aura). As seen in Chapters 1 and 15, although the IHS criteria are applicable in a reasonably satisfactory manner in most cases, various authors have made objections and proposals for revision. It has been suggested, for example, that the various accompanying symptoms should be considered individually, rather than grouping them, and to evaluate the severity of each (Iversen et al., 1990; Messinger et al. 1991; Pfaffenrath and Isler, 1993; Michel et al., 1993).

A further problem is that numerous patients have headaches with different characteristics. In these cases there is doubt in the diagnosis whether there are two overlapping pathologies (TTH and migraine) or one pathology causing pain with various aspects. This problem, as we will see in Chapter 17, is connected to the chronic daily headache.

In the etiopathogenesis of migraine, various factors relating to the general systems come into play. First of all, hormonal factors are involved, in the forms of migraine typically connected to phases of the menstrual cycle (menstrual period and ovulation) (see Chapter 7). The migraine without aura may, moreover, be one of the numerous other somatic and behavioral symptoms of the so-called *premenstrual syndrome*.

Vascular and circulatory factors are commonly involved, as shown by studies on blood flow velocity and regional cerebral blood flow before and during migraine attacks and studies on

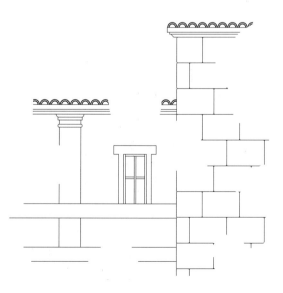

Loss of parts of the image
in the first phase of aura

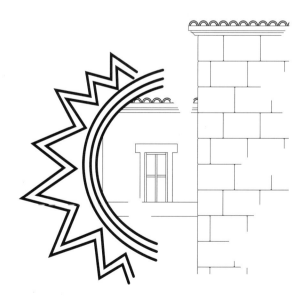

Second phase of aura

Fig. 16.**1** Depiction of **"fortification spectra"** during a migraine aura platelet function in migraine patients (see Chapter 6). The presence of neurological factors is shown by studies on the cortical function, neurotransmitters, endogenous opioids, and reflexes, and the function of the sympathetic system (see Chapter 5).

Finally, the psychological factor is important (see Chapter 8).

Changes in weather, eating habits (chocolate, red wine, matured cheese, preserved meats, nuts, tea, and coffee) can be triggering factors. It is also necessary to consider that local factors, such as muscle contraction and poor posture with alterations of the cervical column, though more frequently involved in other types of headaches, could be an aggravating or triggering factor in some patients.

Since antimigraine drugs belong to numerous categories, as seen in Chapter 12, the correct evaluation of the presence and importance of these factors in various patients is essential in making appropriate therapeutic decisions.

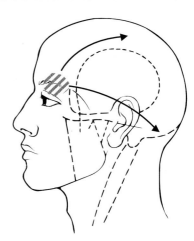

Fig. 16.**2**   Initial location and spreading of headache in a woman suffering from episodic migraine with aura

Migraine with Aura

A typical example of episodic migraine with aura is that of a 20-year-old woman who, for about one year, had headaches in her left periorbital and palpebral area coinciding with her menstrual period; the pain subsequently spread to the vertex and the nucha (Figs. 16.**2**, 16.**3**). The pain was stabbing, of severe intensity, and preceded by scotomata, dizziness and hyperosmia for about 20 minutes. After these symptoms ended, the headache started and lasted from a few hours to two days. During the attack there was an unmistakable presence of accompanying autonomic phenomena: nausea, vomiting, the Horner syndrome, conjunctival hyperemia, pal-

pebral edema lacrimation. There was also photophobia, phonophobia, hyperosmia, intolerance to movement, difficulty in concentrating and frequent amnesia. When the attack was over, intense appetite occurred. There was no family history of migraine. The patient reported suffering from gastritis, dizziness, occasional episodes of fainting and visual disturbances, and a frequent sense of exhaustion. She also reported frequent mood changes, palpitations, a sporadic tendency toward bulimia but not a depressed mood. The MMPI showed a classic hysterical profile (with a *psychosomatic V* and a markedly high level on the hysteria scale): the STAI showed moderate scores of state and trait anxiety (Fig. 16.**4**). Upon inspection, misaligment of the shoulders was observed. The

NAME:	**M. R.**																														
DATE: APR/MAY		28	29	30	1	2	3	4	5	6	7	8	9	10	11	12	13	14	15	16	17	18	19	20	21	22	23	24	25	26	27
HEADACHE	5																												X	X	X
	4			X	X			X																								
	3							X																								
	2							X																								
	1	X	X																								X					
	0				X	X			X	X	X	X	X	X	X	X	X	X	X	X	X	X	X	X	X							
Headache duration (hours)		6	5	5	5			5	4																		4	5	5	4	
PAIN	5																															
	4																						X									
	3							X			X											X	X	X	X							
	2																					X										
	1																		X													
	0	X	X	X	X	X	X		X	X	X		X	X	X	X	X	X	X	X												
Pain duration (hours)							2				1										T	T	T	T							
DRUG INTAKE																																
IBUPROFEN					X	X																			X							

Fig. 16.**3**   Same patient as in Fig. 16.2. Headache and pain diary

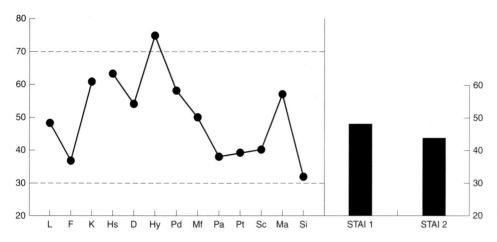

Fig. 16.**4**   Hysteric-type profile shown by MMPI

neurological examination was negative, whereas upon palpation of the cranial muscles, and even more so the cervical muscles, there was tenderness. Blood pressure was within the norm.

Accordingly, the diagnosis was migraine with aura in a patient with signs of occasional CNS dysfunction, with an anxious but not depressed disposition and a personality profile that is common in migraine patients (see Chapter 8). In the intercritical periods there were occasional tension-type headaches. Given the relative infrequency of the migraine attacks (which, however, were of long duration) it was decided to start a symptomatic treatment with 6 mg of sumatriptan subcutaneously to be administered upon first signs of the aura. The usual relaxation and posture correction exercises were also prescribed. The response was extremely favorable insofar as the drug prevented the attack from occurring. Within four months the episodes no longer occurred (Fig. 16.**5**) and the

drug was suspended. The patient complained of moderate symptoms attributable to aura (scotomata and asthenia) during the premenstrual period, but these were not followed by the headaches in spite of the fact that the sumatriptan was no longer being taken. The psychometric tests were administered again and showed an MMPI profile similar to the previous one but with a decrease in the scores of the first three scales, the hysteria score in particular. There was also a significant remission of the state and trait anxiety scores (Fig. 16.**6**). At a check-up three years later, the patient reported having had only three migraine attacks, which were rapidly overcome with 50 mg sumatriptan taken orally.

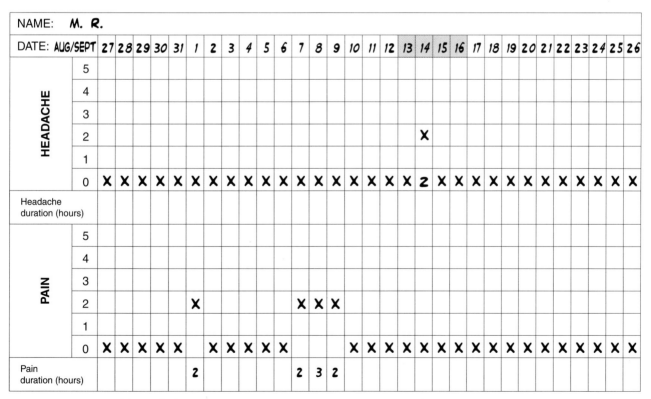

Fig. 16.**5**   Remission of symptoms with sumatriptan as needed and nonpharmacological treatment

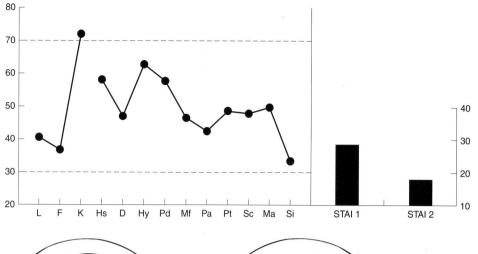

Fig. 16.**6** **Reduction of n numerous MMPI scores and of the STAI indexes after therapy.** The hysteric profile remains at lower levels

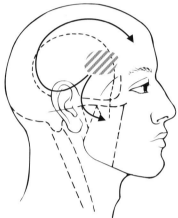
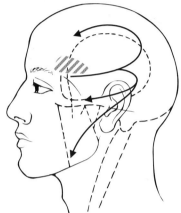

Fig. 16.**7** **Migraine without aura in 38-year old woman.** Initial location and spreading of pain. The attacks were unilateral, alternating on both sides

Migraine without Aura

A case of migraine without aura, clearly connected to the menstrual cycle with an overlapping episodic tension-type headache, was that of a 38-year-old housewife.

The patient had had an extrauterine pregnancy in the past and had undergone nine attempts at artificial insemination without success. As a consequence she suffered from psychophysical prostration. For ten years she had suffered from alternating unilateral headaches in the temporal area which spread throughout the entire hemiface (Fig. 16.**7**). The throbbing pain, of severe intensity, lasting from two to eight hours, was described in her words as "the war of the two worlds" (Fig. 16.**8**). The episodes were accompanied by dramatic vegetative, cardiovascular, sensorial, and intellectual phenomena: intense nausea, occasional vomiting, conjunctival hyperemia and lacrimation, oliguria, perspiration, chills, insomnia, tinnitus, dizziness, scotomata and scintillations, photophobia, phonophobia, hyperosmia, difficulty in concentrating, and memory loss. At the end of the episodes the patient was exhausted, in a state of stupor, and complained of a diffused aching all over the cranium and face. These episodes occurred three to four times a month, mostly during the menstrual or premenstrual and ovulation periods. In the intercritical periods the patient reported a mild, pressing frontal headache that could last all day (Fig. 16.**9**). There were numerous psychosomatic and physical symptoms (Fig. 16.**10**). For several years the patient had been taking five drops of amitriptyline in the evening, 0.5 mg of lorazepam and one tablet of Ergotamine tartrate. She also frequently took painkillers. Her blood pressure was 110/80. The neurological examination showed a mild hyposthenia of the right arm.

1) ☐ Flickering
    ☐ Quivering
    ☐ Pulsing
    ☐ Throbbing
    ☐ Beating
    ☒ Pounding

2) ☒ Jumping
    ☐ Flashing
    ☐ Shooting

3) ☐ Pricking
    ☐ Boring
    ☐ Drilling
    ☐ Stabbing
    ☒ Lancinating

4) ☐ Sharp
    ☐ Cutting
    ☐ Lacerating

5) ☐ Pinching
    ☐ Pressing
    ☐ Gnawing
    ☐ Cramping
    ☒ Crushing

6) ☐ Tugging
    ☐ Pulling
    ☒ Wrenching

7) ☐ Hot
    ☐ Burning
    ☒ Scalding
    ☐ Searing

8) ☐ Tingling
    ☐ Itchy
    ☒ Smarting
    ☐ Stinging

9) ☐ Dull
    ☐ Sore
    ☐ Hurting
    ☒ Aching
    ☐ Heavy

10) ☒ Tender
    ☐ Taut
    ☐ Rasping
    ☐ Splitting

11) ☐ Tiring
    ☐ Exhausting

12) ☒ Sickening
    ☐ Suffocating

13) ☐ Fearful
    ☐ Frightful
    ☒ Terrifying

14) ☒ Punishing
    ☐ Gruelling
    ☐ Cruel

15) ☐ Wretched
    ☒ Binding

16) ☐ Annoying
    ☐ Troublesome
    ☐ Miserable
    ☐ Intense
    ☒ Unbearable

17) ☐ Spreading
    ☒ Radiating
    ☐ Penetrating
    ☐ Piercing

18) ☒ Tight
    ☐ Numb
    ☐ Drawing
    ☐ Squeezing
    ☐ Tearing

19) ☐ Cool
    ☒ Cold
    ☐ Freezing

20) ☐ Nagging
    ☐ Nauseating
    ☒ Agonizing
    ☐ Dreadful
    ☐ Torturing

Fig. 16.**8** The McGill Pain Questionnaire confirms that the pain episodes are experienced dramatically by the patient

NAME: **S. A.**

DATE: AUG/SEPT	9	10	11	12	13	14	15	16	17	18	19	20	21	22	23	24	25	26	27	28	29	30	31	1	2	3	4	5	6	7	8
HEADACHE 5																															
4						X	X					X													X						
3																															X
2													X							X											
1									X						X						X	X	X								
0	X	X	X	X	X			X		X	X			X		X	X	X	X						X	X	X	X	X	X	
Headache duration (hours)						5	3		8			8	5		6					7	7	8	8	8							7
PAIN 5																															
4						X																									
3					X							X																			X
2													X																		
1								X								X				X	X										
0	X	X	X	X						X	X			X	X		X	X	X	X						X	X	X	X	X	
Pain duration (hours)					5	3						8	5																	4	2

DRUG INTAKE

	9	10	11	12	13	14	15	16	17	18	19	20	21	22	23	24	25	26	27	28	29	30	31	1	2	3	4	5	6	7	8
						1						1	1												1						1
ERGOTAMINE TARTRATE	1	1	1	1	1	1	1	1	1	1	1	1	1	1	1	1	1	1	1	1	1	1	1	1	1	1	1	1	1	1	1
LORAZEPAM	½	½	½	½	½	½	½	½	½	½	½	½	½	½	½	½	½	½	½	½	½	½	½	½	½	½	½	½	½	½	½
AMITRIPTYLINE	X	X	X	X	X	X	X	X	X	X	X	X	X	X	X	X	X	X	X	X	X	X	X	X	X	X	X	X	X	X	X

Fig. 16.**9** **Same patient as in Fig. 16.7.** Headache and pain diary

Colitis	[X]	Parafunctions	[ ]
Gastritis	[X]	Clonus	[X]
Kinetosis	[ ]	Cramps	[X]
Swallowing difficulty	[ ]	Paresthesias	[X]
Digestive disorders	[ ]	Back pain	[ ]
Anorexia	[X]	Urination disturbances	[ ]
Bulimia	[ ]	Diarrhea or constipation	[ ]
Anxiety	[X]	Nail fragility	[ ]
Phobias	[X]	Hair fragility	[ ]
Sleep disorders	[X]	Circulation disorders	[X]
Palpitations	[ ]	Cold limbs	[ ]
Panic attacks	[ ]	Frigidity	[ ]
Mood changes	[ ]	Vaginism	[X]
Fainting	[ ]	Frequent depressed moods	[ ]
Vertigo	[ ]	Other	[ ]
Lassitude	[X]		

Fig. 16.**10** Numerous signs and symptoms are present in the current history

Several muscles were painful upon palpation. The MMPI showed a quite abnormal profile with marked elevation of numerous scales, especially in the psychotic area. The STAI showed extremely high state and trait anxiety scores (Fig. 16.**11**).

This was thus a patient in whom all the major etiological factors relating to dysfunction of the general systems seemed to be present to some degree. Cyclical hormonal variations were clearly a triggering factor (the patient had suffered from dysmenorrhea in the past), and there were also signs of occasional alterations of the vascular and nervous systems and a significantly altered psychological profile. Because of the medium-low blood pressure, slow-release ergotamine mesylate was prescribed (one capsule in the morning and one in the evening after meals), as well as the usual exercise program. Improvement was slow and gradual with the episodes decreasing in frequency, intensity, and duration within four months. The tension headaches also diminished (Fig. 16.**12**).

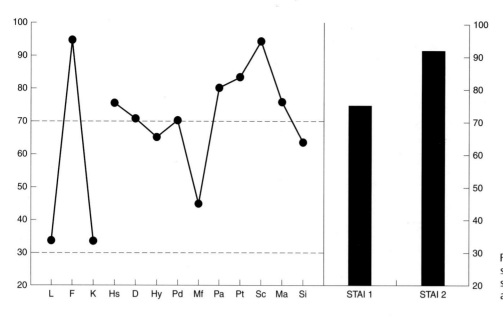

Fig. 16.**11**   Numerous MMPI scales show high scores. STAI shows high state and trait anxiety scores

NAME:	**S. A.**																															
DATE: JAN		2	3	4	5	6	7	8	9	10	11	12	13	14	15	16	17	18	19	20	21	22	23	24	25	26	27	28	29	30	31	1
HEADACHE	5																																
	4																																
	3											X												X	X								
	2					X															X	X											
	1																							X									
	0	X	X	X	X		X	X	X	X		X	X	X	X	X	X	X	X					X	X	X	X	X	X	X	X	X
Headache duration (hours)					3				3						2		2	3	2	2	3											
PAIN	5																																
	4																																
	3																																
	2					X																											
	1																																
	0	X	X	X	X		X	X	X	X	X	X	X	X	X	X	X	X	X	X	X	X	X	X	X	X	X	X	X	X	X	X
Pain duration (hours)						22/1																											
DRUG INTAKE																																	
INDOMETHACIN + PROCLORPERAZINE											1													1								
ERGOTAMINE MESYLATE		2	2	2	2	2	2	2	2	2	2	2	2	2	2	2	2	2	2	2	2	2	2	2	2	2	2	2	2	2	2	2

Fig. 16.**12**   **Symptoms show improvement with use of an ergot derivative.** Diary four months after start of treatment

The MMPI was administered again during this period and showed a moderate decrease in some of the scales and the appearance of a *conversive or hysterical V* (Fig. 16.**13**). At this point the dosage of ergotamine mesylate was first halved (one capsule in the evening), and subsequently interrupted while 100 mg of sumatriptan was prescribed to be taken as needed. At a check-up one year after the beginning of treatment, the patient reported one attack per month (but not every month)

(Fig. 16.**14**), and she was able to manage them satisfactorily by taking sumatriptan orally (50 or 100 mg). A third MMPI showed a significant decrease in the scales that were previously high, with an accentuation of the *conversive V* (Fig. 16.**15**). This is a phenomenon that, as we will see in Chapter 17, is also observed in a certain percentage of patients with daily chronic headaches after treatment. The state anxiety index had also dropped (Fig. 16.**15**).

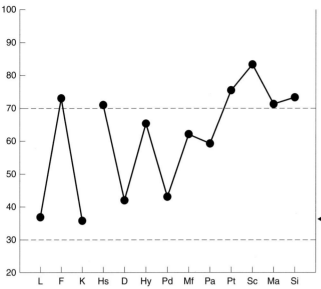

◀ Fig. 16.**13** Partial improvement of MMPI profile in this phase of treatment

Fig. 16.**14** Results appear to be stable one year later
▼

NAME: **S. A.**																																
DATE: AUG		3	4	5	6	7	8	9	10	11	12	13	14	15	16	17	18	19	20	21	22	23	24	25	26	27	28	29	30	31	1	2
HEADACHE	5																																
	4																																
	3																																
	2																X	X															
	1																																
	0	X	X	X	X	X	X	X	X	X	X	X	X	X	X			X	X	X	X	X	X	X	X	X	X	X	X	X	X	X
Headache duration (hours)																	T	3															
PAIN	5																																
	4																																
	3																																
	2																X	X															
	1																																
	0	X	X	X	X	X	X	X	X	X	X	X	X	X	X			X	X	X	X	X	X	X	X	X	X	X	X	X	X	X
Pain duration (hours)																	T	3															

 T = all day

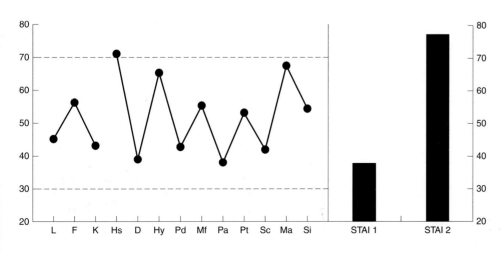

Fig. 16.**15** In this period the MMPI shows a definite improvement of the profile. The remission of state anxiety is notable

In the following case a migraine without aura was overlapped by a chronic tension-type headache. The subject was a 17-year-old woman student who complained of a throbbing headache four or five times a month, mostly during the menstrual or premenstrual period and ovulation, in the right periorbital area, with severe pain lasting four or five hours. The episodes were accompanied by intense nausea, perspiration, feeling cold, chills, hyposomnia, photophobia and difficulty in concentrating; they were followed by sleepiness. During the intercritical periods a mild, pressing, bilateral periorbital headache was frequent and lasted a few hours (Fig. 16.**16**). The patient was hypotensive (blood pressure 110/70) and complained of nail biting, tiredness, anxiety, cramps, and dysmenorrhea, and had experienced a distinctly depressed mood for about a month prior to the first examination. The three *neurotic* scales and the anxiety scale (Psychasthenia, Pt) of the MMPI showed high scores (Fig. 16. **17**). The STAI state anxiety score was high. The neurological examination was negative, whereas upon palpation the temporal muscle was tender. An EEG, from a previous period, showed moderate anomalies in the right temporoparietal area that appeared at the end of the hyperpnea (Fig. 16.**18**).

Several etiopathogenetic factors were probably involved concurrently in this patient's migraine (hormonal, neurological, psychological), while the mood disorder and the muscular parafunction both contributed to the overlapping tension-type headache.

After an explanation to the patient, 50 mg sumatriptan was prescribed to be taken immediately at the onset of the migraine attacks and 10 drops of bromazepam when needed for episodes of anxiety. The nondrug program was also prescribed, as usual in these cases (relaxation and self-control exercises, moderate sporting activity, etc.), which the patient followed scrupulously. Symptoms improved rapidly with an almost complete remission of the migraines and tension headaches within four months (Fig. 16.**19**). The MMPI administered in this period showed a normal personality profile (Fig. 16.**20**). The anxiety scores had also decreased. These findings corresponded with the patient's report of a substantial remission of the psychosomatic symptoms from which she had suffered previously.

The patient described next suffered from migraine without aura but had completely different characteristics. This was a 54-year-old woman factory worker, married, with two pregnancies brought to term, who had been in menopause for about eight years. Since childhood she had suffered from throbbing headaches of moderate to severe intensity in the left temporal and periorbital area, accompanied by palpebral edema, lacrimation, tinnitus, Horner syndrome, and a marked hyperesthesia to noise. Noise could trigger or

NAME:	**B. M.**																														
DATE: JAN/FEB		*15*	*16*	*17*	*18*	*19*	*20*	*21*	*22*	*23*	*24*	*25*	*26*	*27*	*28*	*29*	*30*	*31*	*1*	*2*	*3*	*4*	*5*	*6*	*7*	*8*	*9*	*10*	*11*	*12*	*13*	*14*
HEADACHE	5																															
	4																				X											
	3			X		X	X																									
	2	X	X		X			X													X		X								
	1							X	X	X	X	X	X	X			X	X	X			X				X			
	0										X	X					X			X	X	X		X	X	X
Headache duration (hours)		3	2	3	4	4	5	4	6	2	5	5	5	5	5			3	5	5	4	3		2	5				3		

Fig. 16.**16** Diary of 17-year-old woman suffering from migraine without aura, with intervals of tension-type headaches

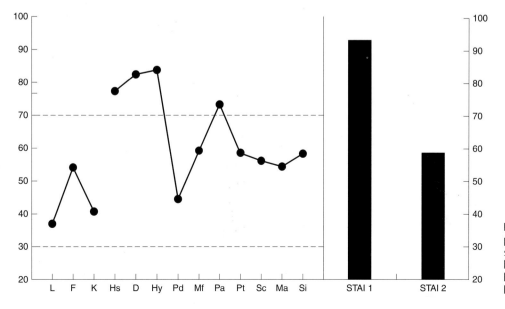

Fig. 16.**17** MMPI of the same patient. Scales 1, 2, and 3 (the so-called "neurotic" scales) are high; scale 7 (anxiety) is also high. State anxiety scores are high

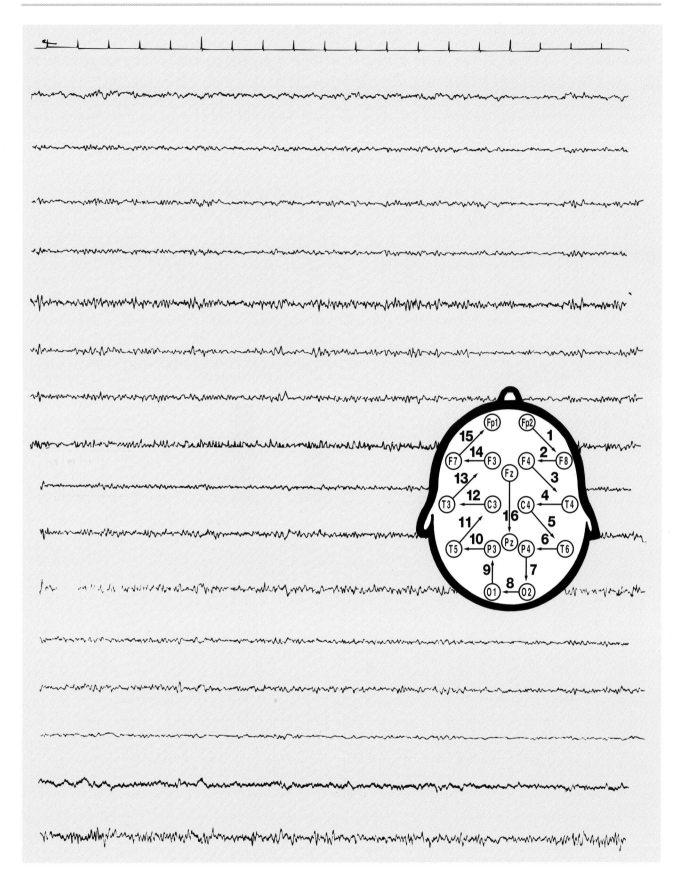

Fig. 16.**18**   Moderate EEG alterations in the right temporoparietal area after hyperpnea

NAME:																																
DATE: JULY		1	2	3	4	5	6	7	8	9	10	11	12	13	14	15	16	17	18	19	20	21	22	23	24	25	26	27	28	29	30	31
HEADACHE	5																															
	4																															
	3																															
	2																															
	1									X							X															
	0	X	X	X	X	X	X	X	X		X	X	X	X	X		X	X	X	X	X	X	X	X	X	X	X	X	X	X	X	X
Headache duration (hours)										2							2															

Fig. 16.**19**   Remission of migraine and tension-type headache after symptomatic drug treatment and nondrug treatment

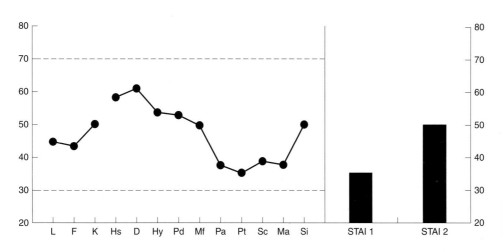

Fig. 16.**20**   Normalization of MMPI profile and state anxiety after therapy

NAME: F. G.																															
DATE: JUNE		1	2	3	4	5	6	7	8	9	10	11	12	13	14	15	16	17	18	19	20	21	22	23	24	25	26	27	28	29	30
HEADACHE	5																														
	4			X	X	X												X			X		X	X		X					
	3										X		X															X			
	2						X	X																	X						
	1													X																	
	0	X	X			X		X		X					X	X	X		X	X	X		X						X	X	X
Headache duration (hours)			3	5	4	4	5	3		8		8	2				4			6		4	7	10	3	3				

Fig. 16.**21**   Headache diary of a 54-year-old woman suffering from migraine with aura with increased frequency of the episodes after menopause

aggravate the attack, along with weather changes and cold. The headaches, initially sporadic, had become more frequent over the years; the frequency had increased, especially after menopause. The headaches lasted from three to four hours to as long as eight hours (Fig. 16.**21**). The patient had almost no psychosomatic symptoms. The neurological examination was negative; palpation was positive only for the left sternocleidomastoid muscle. Blood pressure was high for the minimum (95 mmHg), and relatively normal for the maximum (150 mmHg). MMPI scores were in the norm, though the depression score was rather high, which is inevitable in patients suffering from chronic pain. STAI anxiety scores were not particularly high (Fig. 16.**22**).

In this case there did not seem to be major psychological component. Given the high values of the minimum blood pressure, it was decided to prescribe 20 mg propranolol twice a day, increased, after two weeks to 40 mg twice a day. There were rapid results with a progressive reduction in the

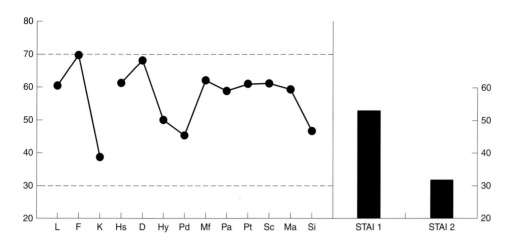

Fig. 16.**22** **MMPI profile with depression score high but still in the norm.** Normal state and trait anxiety scores

NAME:																																	
DATE: AUG		1	2	3	4	5	6	7	8	9	10	11	12	13	14	15	16	17	18	19	20	21	22	23	24	25	26	27	28	29	30	31
HEADACHE	5																																
	4																																
	3																																
	2																		X													
	1																	X											X				
	0	X	X	X	X	X	X	X	X	X	X	X	X	X	X	X	X	X		X	X	X	X	X	X	X	X		X	X	X	X
Headache duration (hours)																		4	2									2				

Fig. 16.**23** Propanolol treatment produced good results

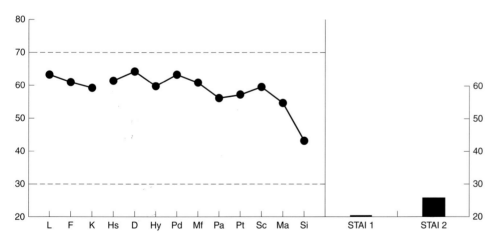

Fig. 16.**24** Mood improvement is confirmed by the decrease of depression (D) score at the MMPI and the abatement of the STAI scores

frequency and severity of the attacks (Fig. 16.23). This improvement understandably affected the patient's mood (Fig. 16.24). The treatment was followed for six months and then gradually withdrawn.

An interesting case of childhood migraine is that of a 10-year-old boy who from the age of five years had suffered from extremely severe migraines, with throbbing pain accompanied by sweating, tachycardia, sleepiness, tremors, and occasional convulsions and fainting. Due to these symptoms the patient had been hospitalized several times in pediatric departments where all the necessary tests were run (including

EEGs and CAT scans): the results were all negative. The prescribed treatment had been 0.5 mg flunarizine in the evening for 30 days, 0.25 mg of pizotyline, and eight drops of dihydroergotamine mesylate. Additionally, the child attended psychological counseling. None of these treatments produced appreciable results.

At the time of observation, the attacks occurred seven or eight days a month, all day (Fig. 16.25). Considering the youth of the patient and the failure of other types of preventive therapy, it was decided to administer 50 mg of 5-hydroxytryptophan twice a day. A decrease in the duration of the attacks

NAME: M. E.																															
DATE: MAR/APR	28	29	30	31	1	2	3	4	5	6	7	8	9	10	11	12	13	14	15	16	17	18	19	20	21	22	23	24	25	26	27
HEADACHE 5					X	X																					X				
4														X																	
3																			X									X			
2																							X								
1	X	X						X	X	X																					
0			X	X			X	X				X	X		X	X	X	X		X	X	X	X	X	X				X	X	X
Headache duration (hours)	T	T			T	T								T					T					T	T	T					

Fig. 16.**25**   Headache diary of 10-year-old child who had been suffering from severe migraine-type attacks for five years

NAME: M. E.																														
DATE: JUNE/JULY	18	19	20	21	22	23	24	25	26	27	28	29	30	1	2	3	4	5	6	7	8	9	10	11	12	13	14	15	16	17
HEADACHE 5																														
4																														
3							X																							
2																											X			
1																														
0	X	X	X	X	X	X		X	X	X	X	X	X	X	X	X	X	X	X	X	X	X	X	X	X	X		X	X	X
Headache duration (hours)							2																				2			

Fig. 16.**26**   Good result two months after treatment with 5-hydroxytryptophan

was observed during the first month of the drug therapy and a significant remission of the symptoms from the second month onward (Fig. 16.**26**). The treatment was continued for six months with the advice to repeat the cycle when needed.

The last case clearly demonstrates the need to evaluate the entire spectrum of possible etiopathogenetic factors, including intake of estroprogestogens for birth control purposes. The cases is that of a 26-year-old woman who had suffered from throbbing headaches unilaterally in the frontal-temporal area (left or right, alternatively) since her menarche. There was a second area of manifestation in the cervical area (Fig. 16.**27**). The pain was severe, lasted four to five hours and was associated with nausea, vomiting, eye pain, dilation of the temporal vessels, hypersomnia, photophobia, phonophobia, hyperosmia, difficulty in concentrating, and memory loss. At the time of the examination the frequency of the attacks was around four to six episodes a month (Fig. 16.**28**). The patient frequently suffered from cramps, colitis, thermoregulation dysfunction, and orthostatic hypotension. Her blood pressure fluctuated from 100/80 in the winter to 80/60 in the summer. The neurological examination and palpation were negative. During the episodes the patient took 20 drops of dipyrone. Additionally, she had been taking birth control pills at a low hormonal dosage for some years. Psychosomatic symptoms were few and the psychometric tests showed data within the norm. Timed-release ergotamine mesylate was prescribed (one capsule in the morning and one in the evening after meals) but during the next two months the symptoms did not improve. The treatment was interrupted and the patient was

then prescribed 5 mg of flunarizine in the evening and 50–100 mg of sumatriptan as needed. In the following month and a half there was a slight decrease in the frequency of the attacks, but subsequently the patient stopped the flunarizine due to an excess of side effects (sleepiness, swollen limbs upon awakening, asthenia) and continued to take sumatriptan as needed. After a few weeks the patient stopped taking her contraceptive pills, which coincided with the complete and lasting remission of the symptoms (Fig. 16.**29**).

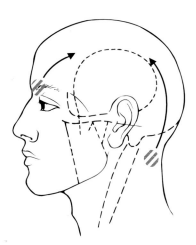

Fig. 16.**27**   Locations of migraine in 26-year-old woman taking contraceptive pills

NAME: G. G.

DATE: OCT

HEADACHE	1	2	3	4	5	6	7	8	9	10	11	12	13	14	15	6	17	18	19	20	21	22	23	24	25	26	27	28	29	30	31
5																															
4	X							X																	X						
3																		X		X											
2													X																		
1																															
0		X	X	X	X	X	X		X	X	X	X		X	X	X	X		X		X	X	X	X		X	X	X	X	X	X
Headache duration (hours)	4							7					4					4		3					3						

DRUG INTAKE

	1	2	3	4	5	6	7	8	9	10	11	12	13	14	15	6	17	18	19	20	21	22	23	24	25	26	27	28	29	30	31
ORAL CONTRACEPTIVE	X	X	X	X	X	X	X	X	X	X	X	X	X	X	X	X	X	X	X	X	X	X	X	X					X	X	X
DIPYRONE								X					X					X		X					X						

Fig. 16.**28**   Same patient as in Fig. 16.27. Headache diary

NAME: G. G.

DATE: MAR

HEADACHE	1	2	3	4	5	6	7	8	9	10	11	12	3	14	15	16	17	18	19	20	21	22	23	24	25	26	27	28	29	30	31
5																															
4																															
3																															
2																															
1																															
0	X	X	X	X	X	X	X	X	X	X	X	X	X	X	X	X	X	X	X	X	X	X	X	X	X	X	X	X	X	X	X
Headache duration (hours)																															

Fig. 16.**29**   Same patient as in Fig. 16.27. Upon suspension of contraceptive treatment, the migraines disappeared completely and permanently

Conclusions

Since migraines can be caused by many different and concurrent etiopathogenetic factors, an appropriate program of therapy must be based on a precise evaluation of their presence and relevance. In this regard, it should be reiterated that there is no first-choice drug for all cases. The pharmacological option must be adjusted on the basis of medical history and clinical examination. Furthermore, as demonstrated by the above cases, migraine patients often have some overlapping tension-type headaches, which can be conveniently treated with nondrug therapy. Nondrug therapy can also be used to support drug therapy for migraine, especially in the cases presenting a clear concurrence of psychological factors, tension in the craniocervical musculature, and head or neck posture problems. The decision to start preventive or symptomatic drug therapy should be based not only on the frequency of migraine but also on the evaluation of the presence of the factors described and the extent of the tension-type headache that may overlap the migraine. In two of the cases described, symptomatic therapy for migraine was prescribed. In one case (migraine with aura), sumatriptan was prescribed as needed,

and this was simply associated with an intense nondrug treatment program (muscle relaxation and posture correction exercises): this entirely eliminated the episodic tension-type headache and almost entirely eliminated the migraine attacks. In the second case of migraine without aura overlapped by a chronic tension-type headache, equally satisfactory results were obtained by combining the symptomatic therapy for migraine with bromazepam as needed and the exercise program. Both patients felt tenderness upon palpation of one or more cranial muscles, both had signs and symptoms of anxiety (a milder case in the first patient and more noticeable, with depressive connotations, in the second patient). Both had high scores on some MMPI scales (with a classic hysterical profile in the first patient) and high STAI scores (especially in the second patient). In both patients the comparison between the starting situation and the result allows us to hypothesize that the supplementary nondrug treatment enhanced symptomatic pharmacological treatment of the migraine attacks.

Analogous considerations can be formulated for another patient suffering from hormone-dependent migraine; in this case, however, it was decided to use a migraine prevention treatment. Since the medical history involved dysmenorrhea and the patient had relatively low blood pressure as well as signs and symptoms of alterations in blood circulation, an ergot derivative was prescribed, associated with the usual nondrug therapy; this route was taken also in consideration of the other disturbances present. In this case too there was a parallel improvement in the headache problem and the mood disorder. In another patient, however, with high minimum blood pressure, no psychosomatic symptoms, and normal MMPI and STAI scores, it was decided to use propranolol as first-choice drug for migraine prevention.

One of the cases described was characterized by the extreme youth of the patient, for whom the selected drug was 5-hydroxytryptophan. This choice was made considering the ineffectiveness of other migraine drugs previously used for the patient.

Finally, the last case clearly indicates the importance of not underestimating the possible impact of other factors such as the intake of oral contraceptives (as in the case described) or particular eating, drinking, or smoking habits.

References

International Headache Society, *Classification and diagnostic criteria for headache disorders, cranial neuralgias and facial pain*, Cephalalgia, 1988, 8 (Suppl. 7):1–96.

Iversen H.K., Langemark M., Andersson P.G., Hansen P.E., Olesen J., *Clinical characteristics of migraine and episodic tension-type headache in relation to old and new diagnostic criteria*, Headache, 1990, 30:514–519.

Messinger H.B., Spierings E.L.H., Vincent A.J.P., *Overlap of migraine and tensiontype headache in the International Headache Society classification*, Cephalalgia, 1991, 11:233–237.

Michel P., Henry P., Letenneur L., Jogeix M., Corson A., Dartigues J.F., *Diagnostic screen for assessment of the IHS criteria for migraine by general practitioners*, Cephalalgia, 1993, 13 (Suppl. 12):54–59.

Pfaffenrath V., Isler H., *Evalutation of the nosology of chronic tension-type headache*, Cephalalgia, 1993, 13(Suppl.12):60–62.

17 Chronic Daily Headache

General Characteristics. Etiopathogenetic Factors

As seen in Chapter 1, in the IHS classification (1988), chronic daily headache (CDH) is not considered a distinct pathology but it is classified as chronic tension-type headache. This, however, creates categorization problems since a certain percentage of patients meet neither chronic tension-type headache criteria nor those for migraines in the IHS classification (Solomon et al., 1992 a, b; Manzoni et al., 1993, 1995; Mongini et al., 1997 b). Consequently, it has been suggested that the IHS criteria be modified to include chronic daily headache. A patient can be considered as suffering from CDH when the headache lasts at least six days a week and has been occurring for a period of at least six months, and when the headache lasts all day or most of the day. CDH is often an evolved form of chronic migraine (Mathew et al., 1982), but it can also develop from a chronic tension-type headache or have a rapidly evolving trend (Silberstein, 1993). Abuse of analgesics can favor the change from episodic migraine to CDH (Mathew, 1982, 1990; Mathew et al., 1987; Saper, 1989; Silberstein and Silberstein, 1992) and can also turn a tension-type headache into CDH (Silberstein, 1993). For the detoxification of these patients, which is easier in a hospital environment, it has been suggested that repeated doses of dihydroergotamine should be administered intravenously in association with antimigraine medications (Silberstein and Silberstein, 1992), or dexamethasone (4 mg a day for two weeks) intramuscularly in association with amitriptyline (50 mg a day for 6 months) (Bonuccelli et al., 1996).

However, the abuse of analgesics is certainly not the only cause of CDH, and not all patients improve after detoxification (Silberstein, 1993). Psychological factors probably play an important role (Kurman et al., 1992; Silberstein, 1993). Mongini et al. (1997 b, c) found that most CDH patients examined by them had both migraine and tension-type headache (TTH) symptoms. Moreover, the anamnestic and clinical data for almost all the patients showed past migraine that had later become CDH. There was also a large predominance of psychosomatic symptoms (colitis, bulimia, anxiety, phobias, palpitations, sleep disorders, etc.). The MMPI showed two characteristic profiles: the *hysterical* profile, in which the first three scales were high but the hypochondria and hysteria scores were higher than the depression score; and the *emotional* profile, with high scores on the *neurotic* scales (especially that of depression), and on one or more of the so-called *psychotic* scales (see Chapter 8).

It is clear that CDH treatment must be adjusted according to the most salient headache trait suffered by the patient, its probable origin (whether it is a transformed migraine or not), and the personality profile of the patient when therapy is undertaken.

Clinical examples

One case of CDH is that of a 22-year-old housewife with a mood disorder, tending toward depression. She had been suffering for four years, more or less constantly, from CDH of mild to moderate intensity (Fig. 17.1), pressing in quality, located bilaterally in the occipital and nuchal area. Weather changes, passive smoke and stress were aggravating factors. There were no autonomic symptoms. The patient reported frequent gastritis, asthenia, insomnia, bulimia, mood changes, claustrophobia, panic attacks, dizziness, palpitations, onychophagia (Fig. 17.2). She also complained of a frequently depressed mood in relation to family problems. As a result of her bulimic tendencies she had gained about 10 kg in a couple of years. She had suffered from intense daytime and nighttime bruxism and for some time previously had been experiencing partial block of the mouth opening movement. Her facial expression appeared constantly sad (Fig. 17.3) and palpation of the entire craniofacial and cervical musculature caused extreme pain.

The MMPI scores were not excessively high on any of the scales but they showed a tendency toward depression with high scores of hypochondria (Hs) and depression (D) and low scores of self-esteem (Mf) and hypomania (Ma) (Fig. 17.4). In

NAME: L. E.

DATE:	1	2	3	4	5	6	7	8	9	10	11	12	13	14	15	16	17	18	19	20	21	22	23	24	25	26	27	28	29	30	31
PAIN 5																															
4																															
3		X										X						X													
2			X						X	X																X					
1	X				X	X	X	X			X		X	X	X	X			X	X	X		X	X	X		X	X	X	X	X
0																															
Pain duration (hours)	4	12	12	12	12	12	12	12	12	12	12	3	6	12	12	12	12	12	12	12	12	12	12	12	12	12	12	12	12	12	12

Fig. 17.**1** Headache diary of a young woman with CDH

Colitis	☐
Gastritis	☒
Kinetosis	☐
Swallowing difficulty	☐
Digestive problems	☐
Anorexia	☐
Bulimia	☒
Anxiety	☒
Phobias	☒
Sleep disorders	☒
Palpitations	☒
Panic attacks	☒
Mood changes	☒
Fainting	☐
Vertigo	☒
Lassitude	☒
Parafunctions	☒
Clonus	☐
Cramps	☐
Paresthesias	☐
Back pain	☐
Urination disturbances	☐
Diarrhea or constipation	☐
Nail fragility	☒
Hair fragility	☐
Circulation disorders	☐
Cold limbs	☒
Frigidity	☐
Vaginism	☐
Frequent depressed moods	☒
Other	☐

Fig. 17.**2**   The patient had several symptoms suggestive of the presence of a mood dysfunction

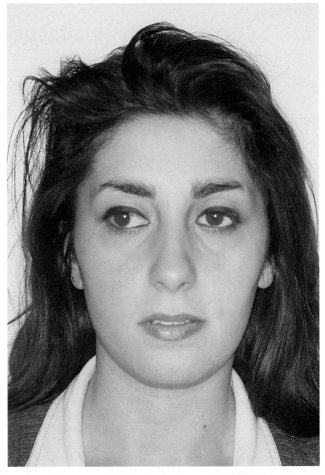

Fig. 17.**3**   The patient had a clearly depressed facial expression and her eyes shifted

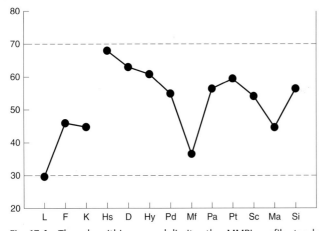

Fig. 17.**4**   Though within normal limits, the MMPI profile tends toward depression

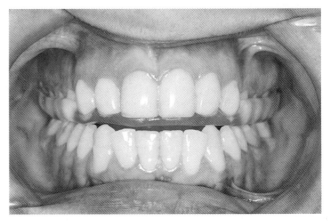

Fig. 17.**5**   Application of splint as an aid against nighttime parafunction

the past the patient had suffered from occasional migraine episodes.

This was therefore a case in which a past episodic migraine was overlapped by a TTH gradually but rapidly evolved into a CDH. Underlying the problem was a latent depression caused or aggravated by a prolonged period of stress. This situation in turn induced significant muscular parafunctions (bruxism, onychophagia, etc.) resulting in aching of all the craniocervical muscles and an initial TMJ problem (a displaced articular disk).

After a throrough discussion with the patient regarding her problem and the ways to manage it, the following therapy was prescribed: low doses of amitriptyline and perphenazine (20 mg amitriptyline and 4 mg of perphenazine divided into two daily doses), 50 mg alprazolam as needed (in case of severe anxiety or panic attacks), a series of biofeedback sessions, relaxation exercises, and physical exercise daily. The articular problem was easily managed by applying a splint, initially both day and night and subsequently only at night (Fig. 17.**5**).

NAME:	L. E.																														
DATE:	1	2	3	4	5	6	7	8	9	10	11	12	13	14	15	16	17	18	19	20	21	22	23	24	25	26	27	28	29	30	31
PAIN 5																															
4																															
3													X																	X	
2								X											X							X		X			
1																															
0	X	X	X	X	X	X	X		X	X	X	X		X	X	X	X	X		X	X	X	X	X		X	X				X
Pain duration (hours)								12					12						5							12				12	12

Fig. 17.**6** Symptoms improve after drug and nondrug treatment

The response was almost immediate and quite satisfactory, with a gradual and progressive reduction in the number of days with headache until they became sporadic within three months (Fig. 17.**6**). In parallel, the psychosomatic symptoms present before treatment diminished, the mood improved considerably (Fig. 17.**7**), and the patient returned to her ideal weight without dieting. Palpation showed that muscle soreness had decreased notably. The MMPI administered in this period showed a significant change from the pre-treatment profile, with a drop in the depression and psychopathic deviation scores (Pd) and an increase in the self-esteem (Mf) and hypomania (Ma) scores (Fig. 17.**8**). Higher Ma scores within the norm indicate an improvement in mood and the capacity for taking initiative.

After six months, the dosage of amitriptyline and perphenazine was halved and was totally suspended after another four months. The patient was nonetheless urged to continue with the prescribed exercise program. A year later, a check-up indicated the situation appeared to be stable.

The next example of CDH has characteristics that are radically different from the previous case. This is the case of a 24-year-old woman, a university graduate working in a rather exacting office job. From menarche, ten years previously, the patient had started to suffer from headaches almost every day, of average intensity, throbbing or pressing, and all over the head. Later, this situation was overlapped by occasional intense throbbing headaches in the right parietal-temporal area, lasting about 24 hours, and accompanied by nausea, vomiting, hyperesthesia to light and noise, and a sensation of cold (Fig. 17.**9**). Menstrual periods and stress were triggering or aggravating factors. During these episodes, the patient took several different painkillers but to little or no avail. She complained of dysmenorrhea, fragility of nails and hair, back pain, frequent anxiety and mood changes, vaginismus, and orthostatic hypotension (Fig. 17.**10**); in addition she smoked 40 cigarettes a day. She had undergone several tests in the past

Fig. 17.**7** The facial expression confirms improvement in mood

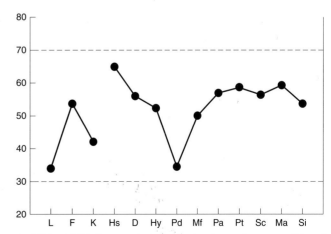

Fig. 17.**8** MMPI shows a decrease in the depression score (D) and psychopathic deviation (Pd) score and a rise in the Mf (self-esteem) and Ma (initiative) scores

NAME: **S. M.**																																
DATE:		1	2	3	4	5	6	7	8	9	10	11	12	13	14	15	16	17	18	19	20	21	22	23	24	25	26	27	28	29	30
PAIN	5							X																								
	4					X		X										X														
	3				X					X																			X	X		
	2	X		X													X															
	1		X		X					X		X	X	X	X	X			X	X	X	X	X	X	X	X	X				X
	0																															
Pain duration (hours)		12	6	12	6	18	18	6	6	6	12	12	12	12	12	12	12	8	12	12	12	12	12	12	12	12	12	12	12	12	12
DRUG INTAKE																																
DIPYRONE						X	X	X	X									X														

Fig. 17.**9** **Headache diary in a second young patient with CDH.** This patient had various attacks with severe intensity and throbbing pain

Colitis	☒
Gastritis	☐
Kinetosis	☐
Swallowing difficulty	☐
Digestive problems	☐
Anorexia	☐
Bulimia	☐
Anxiety	☐
Phobias	☐
Sleep disorders	☐
Palpitations	☒
Panic attacks	☐
Mood changes	☐
Fainting	☐
Vertigo	☐
Lassitude	☐
Parafunctions	☐
Clonus	☐
Cramps	☐
Paresthesias	☐
Back pain	☒
Urination disturbances	☐
Diarrhea or constipation	☐
Nail fragility	☒
Hair fragility	☒
Circulation disorders	☐
Cold limbs	☐
Frigidity	☐
Vaginism	☒
Frequent depressed moods	☐
Other: Dysmenorrhea	☒
Orthostatic hypotension	☒

Fig. 17.**10** This patient, too, had numerous concurrent disturbances, suggestive for anxiety and hormonal disorders

(cranial radiography, cranial CAT scan, EEG, hemochrome and hematological examinations, etc.) and all the results were within the norm. She had also undergone a period of treatment with amitriptyline and flunarizine, but these drugs were ineffective.

Her blood pressure was low (105/70 mmHg), the neurological examination was negative, and palpation of the craniocervical muscles caused intense pain. The MMPI

showed scores within the norm but they pointed to a definite hysterical profile, depression scores very low, hypochondria and hysteria scores relatively high. Moreover, unlike the previous patient, this patient's self-esteem (Mf) and hypomania (Ma) scores were medium to high (Fig. 17.**11**). The STAI showed high state anxiety. The subject was therefore hypotensive, anxious but not depressed, with true migraine episodes overlapping the CDH, and showed signs of hormonal dysfunction (occasional dysmenorrhea, nail and hair fragility). Given this clinical situation it was decided to prescribe slow-release ergotamine mesylate preparations, 5 mg in the morning and 5 mg in the evening, in addition to the daily relaxation exercises. The symptoms clearly improved in three months, but the migraine episodes remained, coinciding with the menstrual period, and the patient took sumatriptan to overcome them (Fig. 17.**12**). At this point the ergotamine was halved for a week and then suspended. After four further months the patient was practically asymptomatic. Even the pain upon palpation of the musculature had disappeared and the menstrual cramps had diminished. The MMPI showed a psychological profile that was similar to the initial one with a considerable increase in the self-esteem scores (Fig. 17.**13**).

The following case is a typical example of a CDH that had rapidly evolved from an episodic migraine as a result of drug abuse. The case is that of a 32-year-old housewife who had

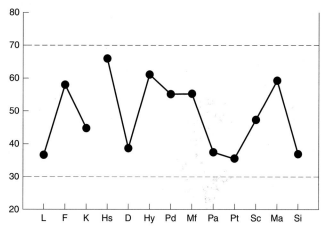

Fig. 17.**11** MMPI shows a *hysterical* profile with low depression scores (D)

NAME: S. M.																																
DATE:		1	2	3	4	5	6	7	8	9	10	11	12	13	14	15	16	17	18	19	20	21	22	23	24	25	26	27	28	29	30	31
PAIN	5																																
	4																																
	3																	X															
	2															X	X																
	1	X						X							X																		
	0		X	X	X	X	X		X	X	X	X	X	X					X	X	X	X	X	X	X	X	X	X	X	X	X	X	X
Pain duration (hours)		2						3							2	3	3	2															
DRUG INTAKE																																	
SUMATRIPTAN																X	X	X															

Fig. 17.**12** Symptoms improve after treatment

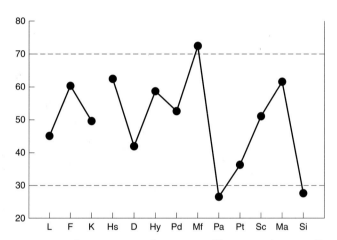

Fig. 17.**13** After treatment, the MMPI profile remained essentially unchanged except for a notable increase in the self-esteem score (Mf)

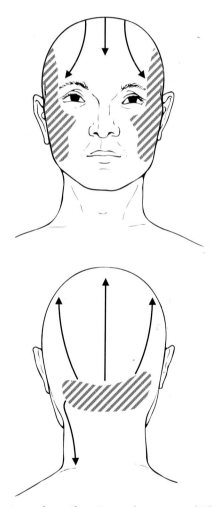

Fig. 17.**14** Area of manifestation and areas to which headache spread in a 32-year-old woman suffering from CDH due to the abuse of medication

given birth to a child two years prior. There was a family history positive for migraine (father and mother). For several years the patient had been suffering from migraine episodes once a month and 18 months before observation the episodes became more frequent (they had progressively become daily), lasted longer (for most of the day), and were more intense. The headache started in the left occipital area and spread forward toward the face and down to the cervical area, more on the left (Fig. 17.**14**); it was pressing or throbbing (when more intense), and accompanied by nausea during the acute moments. At the time of observation she was having mild to moderate headache upon awakening that became progressively worse throughout the day, to the point of stabbing pain (Figs. 17.**15**, 17.**16**). Over time she had been treated at various clinics with strong doses of NSAIDs, amitriptyline, benzodiazepines, levosulpiride, and pizoriline but to no avail. She reported obtaining some relief from taking a preparation based on propyphenazone which she had been taking in large doses for some time (up to 19–20 tablets a day) (Fig. 17.**15**). She had suffered from postpartum depression in the period immediately before the symptoms had worsened. She also reported an extremely tense relationship with her mother-in-law. She had numerous psychosomatic symptoms as well as constipa-

tion, fragile nails and hair, occasional tinnitus, back pain, and cold hands and feet (Fig. 17.**17**). The neurological examination showed a positive Romberg sign and hypoesthesia of sensory distribution of the three branches of the left trigeminal nerve. She also had a frontal and sagittal posture problem (Fig. 17.**18**)

NAME:	**M. N.**																														
DATE: MAR/APR		*21*	*22*	*23*	*24*	*25*	*26*	*27*	*28*	*29*	*30*	*31*	*1*	*2*	*3*	*4*	*5*	*6*	*7*	*8*	*9*	*10*	*11*	*12*	*13*	*14*	*15*	*16*	*17*	*18*	*19*	*20*
HEADACHE	5	X	X	X	X	X	X	X	X	X	X	X	X	X	X	X	X	X	X	X	X	X	X	X	X	X	X	X	X	X	X	X
	4	↑	↑	X	↑	X	↑	X	X	X	X	↑	X	X	X	X	X	↑	↑	X	X	↑	X	X	↑	X	X	X	X	X	X	↑
	3	X	X		X		X					X							X	X		X			X							X
	2																															
	1																															
	0																															
Headache duration (hours)		T	T	T	T	T	T	T	T	T	T	T	T	T	T	T	T	T	T	T	T	T	T	T	T	T	T	T	T	T	T	T
													DRUG INTAKE																			
PROPYPHENAZONE		*10*	*8*	*6*	*10*	*6*	*12*	*12*	*8*	*10*	*10*	*12*	*11*	*10*	*12*	*12*	*12*	*12*	*12*	*14*	*6*	*8*	*10*	*4*	*12*	*10*	*10*	*12*	*6*	*10*	*12*	*12*

Fig. 17.**15**   **Headache diary of the patient.** Headache was present every morning, moderate to severe, and reached very acute levels in the early afternoon. Note the amount of analgesic medications taken daily

and a mild hypertrophy of the masseters (Fig. 17.**19**). Palpation of the sternocleidomastoid muscle was extremely painful and caused pain referred to the occipital region (Fig. 17.**20**). The MMPI-2 showed high scores for hypochondria, depression (which was the highest of all scales), psychopathic deviation and psychasthenia (Fig. 17.**21**). The content scales showed high scores of anxiety, obsession, depression and anger (Fig. 17.**22**). STAI showed a very high level of state and trait anxiety (Fig. 17.**21**). This was therefore a case of a migraine transformed into a CDH triggered or favoured by drug abuse and mood disorder. Moreover, the muscular hyperparafunction, along with the posture problems, caused aching in the cervical muscles with pain referred to the area where the headache occurred.

The problem was discussed with the patient and she was reassured that it was resolvable, at least for the most part, but that it would require drug and nondrug treatment to be adhered to scrupulously, including interruption of the propyphenazone. The patient left this meeting encouraged. She had been horrified at the prospect of suffering in this way for her whole life. A biofeedback program was started, along with relaxation exercises, posture correction exercises and moderate physical exercise. Additionally, she was given 10 mg amitriptyline and 2 mg perphenazine in the morning and 25 mg amitriptyline and 2 mg perphenazine in the evening. The

propyphenazone dosage was decreased to one – two tablets a day and entirely suspended after a month. After one month the patient reported a reduction in the duration of the headaches (from 8 – 14 hours a day to 2 – 4 hours a day), which occurred only toward the evening (Fig. 17.**23**). She was then advised to divide the evening dose in half and take the first half in the late afternoon.

The last case presented here seems to correspond to the rapidly developing CDH described by Silberstein (1993). It is

Worst pain imaginable

X

No pain

Fig. 17.**16**   The severity of the pain is confirmed by the VAS (**a**) and by the McGill Pain Questionnaire (**b**)

1) □ Flickering
    □ Quivering
    □ Pulsing
    □ Throbbing
    □ Beating
    □ Pounding

2) □ Jumping
    □ Flashing
    □ Shooting

3) □ Pricking
    □ Boring
    □ Drilling
    ☒ Stabbing
    □ Lancinating

4) □ Sharp
    □ Cutting
    ☒ Lacerating

5) □ Pinching
    □ Pressing
    □ Gnawing
    □ Cramping
    ☒ Crushing

6) □ Tugging
    □ Pulling
    □ Wrenching

7) □ Hot
    □ Burning
    □ Scalding
    □ Searing

8) □ Tingling
    □ Itchy
    □ Smarting
    ☒ Stinging

9) □ Dull
    □ Sore
    □ Hurting
    □ Aching
    ☒ Heavy

10) □ Tender
    □ Taut
    □ Rasping
    □ Splitting

11) □ Tiring
    ☒ Exhausting

12) □ Sickening
    ☒ Suffocating

13) □ Fearful
    ☒ Frightful
    □ Terrifying

14) □ Punishing
    □ Gruelling
    □ Cruel

15) □ Wretched
    □ Binding

16) □ Annoying
    □ Troublesome
    □ Miserable
    □ Intense
    ☒ Unbearable

17) □ Spreading
    □ Radiating
    ☒ Penetrating
    □ Piercing

18) ☒ Tight
    □ Numb
    □ Drawing
    □ Squeezing
    □ Tearing

19) □ Cool
    □ Cold
    □ Freezing

20) □ Nagging
    □ Nauseating
    □ Agonizing
    □ Dreadful
    ☒ Torturing

Colitis	☐
Gastritis	☒
Kinetosis	☐
Swallowing difficulty	☐
Digestive problems	☐
Anorexia	☒
Bulimia	☒
Anxiety	☒
Phobias	☐
Sleep disorders	☒
Palpitations	☒
Panic attacks	☒
Mood changes	☒
Fainting	☐
Vertigo	☒
Lassitude	☒
Parafunctions	☒
Clonus	☐
Cramps	☐
Paresthesias	☒
Back pain	☒
Urination disturbances	☒
Diarrhea or constipation	☒
Nail fragility	☒
Hair fragility	☒
Circulation disorders	☐
Cold limbs	☒
Frigidity	☒
Vaginism	☒
Frequent depressed moods	☒
Other	☐

Fig. 17.**17** The patient complained of numerous disturbances, predominantly psychosomatic

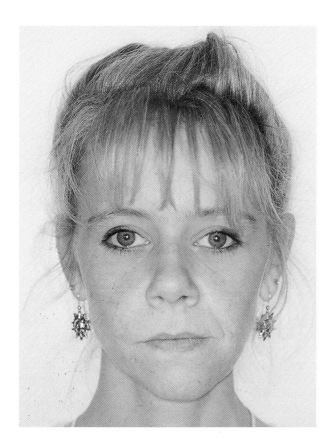

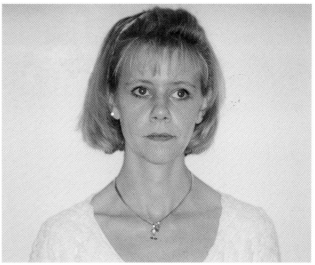

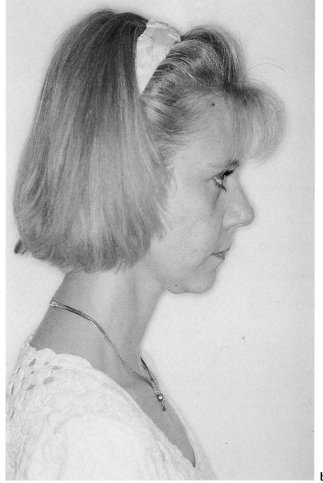

Fig. 17.**18** A posture disturbance can be observed on the frontal plane (unevenness of shoulders) (**a**) and the sagittal (**b**)

◄ Fig. 17.**19** There is a slight hypertrophy of the masseters. The contraction of the sternocleidomastoidei muscles can be seen

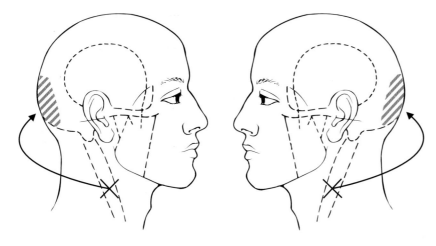

Fig. 17.**20** Palpation of the sternocleidomastoid muscles causes a pain referred in the occipital area

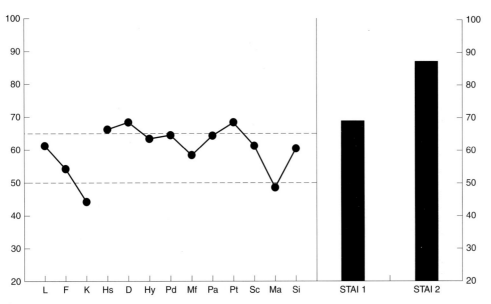

Fig. 17.**21** Several MMPI-2 scales are high, as are STAI anxiety scores

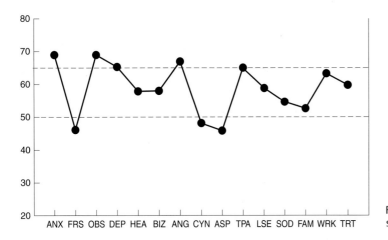

Fig. 17.**22** High anxiety (ANX), Obsessions (OBS), Depression (DEP), and anger (ANG) in the MMPI-2 content scales

the case of a 38-year-old married woman, an office worker, with a three-year old son. Suddenly, seven years before consultation, in a period of her life that was not particularly stressful, she had suffered from a pressing headache located in the left temple. From that time on, the headache was constant, mild with exacerbations during the premenstrual and menstrual period, during which the pain spread until it was in proximity to the eye socket (Figs. 17.**24**, 17.**25**). Other aggra-

vating factors were intellectual fatigue and moving the head into a supine position. She also reported having enjoyed a period of improvement during her pregnancy. There were no autonomic symptoms. Unlike the patients previously described, there was a remarkable absence of psychosomatic symptoms, except for lassitude, frigidity and vaginismus. The patient had been hospitalized on two different occasions in a neurology department where all the routine tests had been

NAME: M. N.																														
DATE: APR/MAY	22	23	24	25	26	27	28	29	30	1	2	3	4	5	6	7	8	9	10	11	12	13	14	15	16	17	18	19	20	21
HEADACHE 5	X	X	X	X	X	X	X		X		X	X	X	X	X		X	X	X				X			X				
4	X	X	X	X	X	X	X				X	X	X	X	X	X	X	X	X	X	X	X	X		X			X	X	
3	X	X				X	X										X					X	X	X		X	X	X	X	X
2	↑	↑																												X
1																														
0	X	X	X	X	X	X	X	X	X	X	X	X	X	X	X	X	X	X	X	X	X	X	X	X	X	X	X	X	X	X
Headache duration (hours)	HEADACHE AT 0 LEVEL UNTIL 3 PM. THEN STARTS AND INCREASES GRADUALLY																													
	DRUG INTAKE																													
PROPYPHENAZONE	4	3	4	2	3	3	3		2	3	3	3	2	3	2	3	4	4	3	3	2	2	1	1	1	2	1	1	2	2

Fig. 17.**23** Partial improvement of the symptoms after a month. The headache appears only in the late afternoon

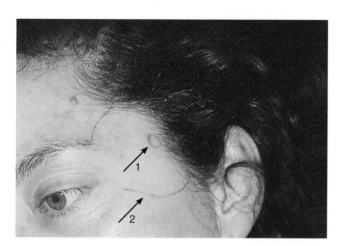

Fig. 17.**24** Initial location (1) and area of subsequent spreading (2) of the pain in 38-year-old woman with CDH with sudden onset

performed and the results were normal. Ergotamine tartrate, pizotyline, amitriptyline, hydroxytryptophan, autogenic training, acupuncture, splint, and infiltration of botulin toxin into the left temporal muscle had all been attempted. None of these treatments had produced any significant results. Only inhalation of nascent oxygen had been partially effective during acute attacks. The neurological examination was negative. The usual signs of muscular parafunction were present and the left temporal muscle ached intensely upon palpation of the preauricular and supraauricular areas. The headache worsened during palpation of these areas. The MMPI-2 showed a clearly *hysterical* profile (Fig. 17.**26**).

This was therefore a case of uncertain etiology. Amitriptyline was prescribed, limited to only 6–8 mg in the evening, considering that there were no connotations of depression, but the patient had reported side effects with previous intakes of this drug. TENS sessions, applied to the left temporal area, and biofeedback sessions were begun. In the following months there was an attenuation of the acute attacks while the basic symptoms remained unchanged. The patient enjoyed a remarkable but fleeting improvement (with disappearance of the symptoms for five days), which she attributed to the fact that she had changed eyeglass frames but which also corresponded to a brief vacation period that was particularly relaxing (Fig. 17.**27**). During a subsequent visit, an anesthetic infiltration was made into the aching point of the left temple muscle, followed by the application of the TENS in the same location. Since the patient reported a decrease of pain, she was advised to apply the TENS apparatus (which she had purchased in the meantime) for several hours a day. However, this gave her only temporary relief and the case remained unresolved.

NAME: Z. M.																															
DATE: FEBRUARY	1	2	3	4	5	6	7	8	9	10	11	12	13	14	15	16	17	18	19	20	21	22	23	24	25	26	27	28			
HEADACHE 5																															
4																X				X											
3																↑				↑											
2	X	X	X	X	X	X	X	X	X	X	X	X	X	X	X	X	X	X	X	X	X	X	X	X	X	X	X	X			
1																															
0																															
Headache duration (hours)	T	T	T	T	T	T	T	T	T	T	T	T	T	T	T	T	T	T	T	T	T	T	T	T	T	T	T	T			

Fig. 17.**25** Patient's headache diary

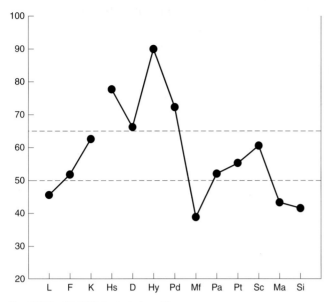

Fig. 17.**26**   MMPI-2 *hysterical* profile

Conclusions

As already seen in the chapter on migraine, the CDH therapy program must be based on an aggregated evaluation of various clinical parameters and can therefore be quite different from one case to the next. The cases described exemplify this variety of therapeutic options.

In the first case, the depressive disorder was the predominant etiopathogenetic element and its management resolved the headache problem as well as the set of accompanying symptoms. Once again it should be reiterated that a tailored drug and nondrug treatment program can produce much more satisfactory results for these patients than a mere administration of drugs (see Chapter 14). This is also true for mood disorders per se and for the consequences induced by them (hyperparafunction of the craniofacial and cervical musculature).

In the second case, in contrast, there were no depressive symptoms, whereas there were the connotations of a hormone-dependent migraine. The patient also suffered from orthostatic hypotension and previous treatments with amitriptyline were ineffective. These were the considerations that led to the choice of drug therapy with ergotamine mesylate for a relatively short period, associated with the usual nondrug treatment program.

The third case, more similar to the first, was aggravated by the abuse of medications and a more severe mood disorder. Moreover, unlike most CDH cases, the patient reported daily periods of extremely intense headaches. Here the cognitive aspect of the therapy was particularly effective. After an initial biofeedback session, to which the patient responded particularly well, it was easier to speak with her about the nature of her problems and possible ways to manage them. The enthusiasm and rigor with which the patient followed the nondrug treatment made it possible to limit the dosage of the drugs and obtain good results relatively easily in a case that seemed complex at first sight.

The last case described is the most difficult one to interpret because of the apparent absence in the medical history of a triggering event in the face of a symptomatology with sudden onset, and the relative paucity of signs or symptoms that might lead to identification of definite etiopathogenetic factors. Considering the failure of the various therapies the patient had undergone in the past, and given the presence of a pain clearly located in the limited area of the temporal muscle, local physical therapy was chosen for the case. Unfortunately, not even this therapy brought about significant results.

References

Bonuccelli U., Nuti A., Lucetti C., Pavese N., Dell'Agnello G., Muratorio A., *Amitriptyline and dexamethasone combined treatment in drug-induced headache*, Cephalalgia, 1996, 16(3):198–200.

International Headache Society, *Classification and diagnostic criteri for headache disorders, cranial neurolgias and facial pain*, Cephalalgia, 1988, 8(Suppl. 7):1–96.

Kurman R.G., Hursey K.G., Mathew N.T., *Assessment of chronic refractory headache: the role of the MMPI-2*, Headache, 1992, 32:432–435.

Manzoni G.C., Micieli G., Granella F., Martignoni F., Malferrari G., Nappi G., *Daily chronic headache: classification and clinical features. Observations on 250 patients*, Cephalalgia, 1987, 7 (Suppl. 6):169–170.

Manzoni G.C., Zanferrari C., Sandrini G. et al., *Inability to classify all the cronic daily headache subtypes by IHS criteria*, Cephalalgia, 1993, 13 (Suppl. 13):12.

Manzoni G.C., Granella F., Sandrini G., Cavallini A., Zanferrari C., Nappi G., *Classification of chronic daily headache by International Headache Society criteria: limits and new proposals*, Cephalalgia, 1995, 15:37–43.

Mathew N.T., *Drug-induced headache*, Neurol. Clin., 1990, 8:903–912.

Mathew N.T., Stubits E., Nigam M.P., *Transformation of episodic migraine into daily headache: analysis of factors*, Headache, 1982, 22:66–68.

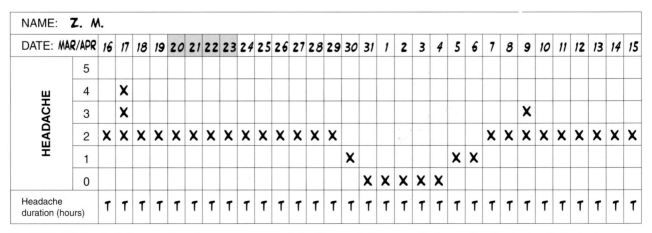

Fig. 17.**27**   **Brief period of regression of symptoms connected with uncertain causes.** Further explanation is given in the text

Mathew N.T., Reuveni U., Perez F., *Transformed or evolutive migraine*, Headache, 1987, 27 : 102 – 106.

Mongini F., Defilippi N., Negro C., *Chronic daily headache. A clinical and psychological profile before and after treatment*, Headache, 1997 a, 37 : 83 – 87.

Mongini F., Ibertis F., Bava M., Negro C., *A psychological profile of migraine in women*, Cephalalgia, 1997 b, 17 : 260.

Mongini F., Bava M., Defilippi N., Ibertis F., *Chronic daily headache. A clinical and psychological profile*, Cephalalgia, 1997 c, 17 : 364.

Saper J.R., *Chronic headache syndromes*, Neurol. Clin., 1989, 7 : 387 – 412.

Silberstein S.D., *Tension-type and chronic daily headache*, Neurology, 1993, 43 : 1644 – 1649.

Silberstein S.D., Silberstein J.R., *Chronic daily headache: long-term prognosis following inpatient treatment with repetitive IV DHE*, Headache, 1992, 32 : 439 – 445.

Solomon S., Lipton R.B., Newman L.C., *Clinical features of chronic daily headache*, Headache, 1992 a, 32 : 325 – 329.

Solomon S., Lipton R.B., Newman L.C., *Evaluation of chronic daily headache – comparison to criteria for chronic tension-type headache*, Cephalalgia, 1992 b, 12 : 365 – 368.

18 Cluster Headache and Chronic Paroxysmal Hemicrania

General Characteristics

Cluster headaches and chronic paroxysmal hemicrania have been recognized only in the recent past as autonomous forms of primary headache (group 3 in the IHS classification).

Cluster headaches were once placed, along with migraine, in the same group as "migraine-type headaches" (Ad Hoc Committee on Classification of Headache, 1962). In the past, syndromes with characteristics that practically overlap with what was later called cluster headache (CH) have been described under various eponyms (Kunkle et al., 1952). This definition was selected to highlight the typical clustering of the attacks in periods that last from a minimum of one week to a maximum of one year (however, it is more common to see them last from one to three months).

Chronic paroxysmal hemicrania (CPH) is a nosological entity described by Sjaastad and Dale (1976). These authors have used the term *hemicrania* to underline the fact that in this form of headache the pain is always unilateral. This is also one of the salient characteristics of CH, whereas for migraine with or without aura it occurs frequently but does not necessarily occur at all.

CH and CPH have some common characteristics such as unilaterality and location of pain, and an abundance of accompanying autonomic phenomena, but differ in others such as duration and frequency of attacks, a different degree of prevalence in the two sexes, a different response to drugs, and in particular to indomethacin, which is effective in CPH but not in CH.

Cluster Headaches

According to the IHS classification, for a diagnosis of CH there must be at least five attacks with the following characteristics:

- The pain is intensely severe, unilateral, located in the orbital, supraorbital and/or temporal area, and lasts from 15 to 180 minutes.
- The headache is associated with at least one of the following symptoms: conjunctival injection; lacrimation, nasal congestion, rhinorrhea, forhead and facial sweating, miosis, ptosis, eyelid edema.

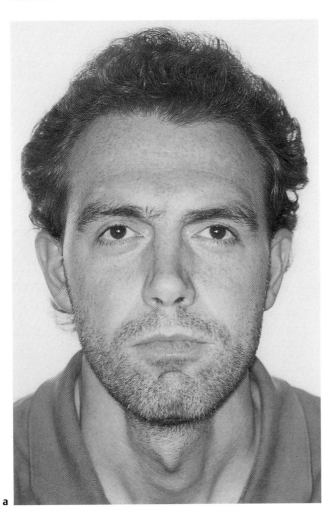
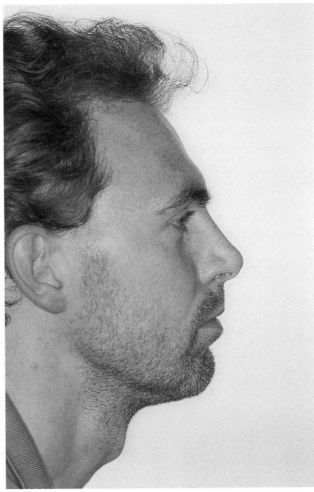

a b

Fig. 18.**1** Slight *leonine* aspect with marked brow and zygomatic arches in a patient suffering from cluster headaches

- The frequency of the attacks is between one attack every two days and eight attacks a day.

It must also be possible to exclude the possibility that the headache is associated or closely related to a cranial trauma, vascular, endocranial, metabolic or infective pathologies. The intake of or withdrawal from exogenous substances must also be excluded.

CH rarely presents a positive family history (Kudrow, 1980; Nappi and Manzoni, 1990) and it definitely predominates in males (Sutherland and Eady, 1972; Kudrow, 1980; Andersson, 1985; Krabbe, 1986; Manzoni et al., 1988; Nappi and Manzoni, 1990).

Certain physical traits were found with a significant frequency in patients with CH: a wide cranium, deep furrows, a *leonine* appearance with a protruding brow (Graham, 1972) (Fig. 18.**1**), and hazel eyes.

As stated, the pain is extremely intense (thus the term *suicide headache* has been coined) and it is associated with severe local and general autonomic signs. During the attack the patient experiences a deep state of agitation and, unlike the migraine patient, prefers to keep in motion. Many CH patients are heavy drinkers and smokers (Graham, 1972; Kudrow, 1980). Alterations of the CNS and hormonal dysfunctions are among the possible etiopathogenetic factors (see Chapters 5 and 7). It is also possible, as we shall see, that local irritants could favor the onset of attacks in predisposed patients.

There are two types of CH: episodic and chronic. The episodic form has active periods alternating with periods of remission. The active periods can have a frequency that varies from two or more per year to one every two or more years. They typically tend to reoccur at regular intervals. The duration of the active periods is extremely variable: from seven days to a year (without treatment) according to the IHS. In the chronic forms, however, this temporal pattern is altered and the remission phases, for the most part, last less than 14 days, while the prolonged ones are absent for at least one year (Fig. 18.**2**).

The differential diagnosis is essentially from CPH (see below), SUNCT (see Chapter 20), and temporal arteritis. It should also be noted that sometimes CH can start with a pain that seemingly originates in the teeth.

Temporal arteritis (or Horton arteritis) is a serious illness that occurs mostly in the elderly and is characterized by a head pain, unilateral or bilateral, that follows a period of malaise, weakness, poor appetite, and aching all over the body. Extremely important is the marked increase in the erythrocyte sedimentation rate, which is not found in cluster headaches. Moreover, upon inspection one observes a tortuosity and thickening of the temporal artery. It should,

however, be taken into consideration that the migraine patient can have a dilated temporal artery (Fig. 18.**3**). The biopsy is decisive as it shows, in the case of temporal arteritis, the presence of inflammatory alterations with giant cells. In the presence of this disease, it is extremely important to reach a diagnosis promptly and to administer cortisone-based drugs. If this is not done, serious and irreversible complications, such as blindness and cerebral ischemia, occur.

The most widely used drugs in the treatment of CH are ergotamine tartrate, cortisone derivatives, lithium, verapamil and new-generation serotonin agonists (see Chapter 12). In practice, verapamil and sumatriptan are currently first-choice drugs for prevention and symptomatic treatments, respectively.

One case of CH is that of a 29-year-old man, an office worker, who for ten years complained of headaches occurring in the periorbital area, extending to the right parietal, temporal, and genial areas (Fig. 18.**4**). These attacks, initially occasional, had become progressively more frequent (at the time of observation the frequency was almost daily) (Fig. 18.**5**). They also manifested a typical seasonal trend with active periods of approximately 4–5 months during the spring and at the beginning of the summer every year. The duration of the attacks was around 2–3 hours and the pain, pulsating in quality, could become excruciating (Figs. 18.**5**, 18.**6**), with an abundance of accompanying phenomena: nausea, perspiration, conjunctival hyperemia, lacrimation, the Horner

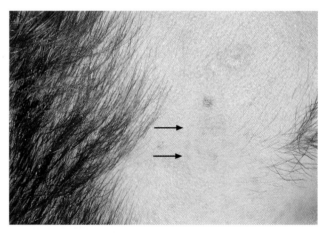

Fig. 18.**3**   Dilated temporal artery (arrows) in migraine patient

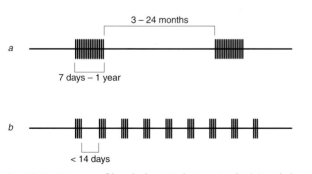

Fig. 18.**2**   Diagram of headache attacks in episodic (**a**) and chronic (**b**) (cluster) headache

3 – 24 months

7 days – 1 year

< 14 days

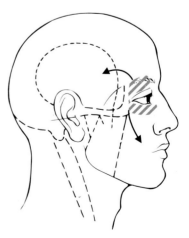

Fig. 18.**4   Twenty-nine-year-old man with cluster headaches.** Areas of origin and spreading of pain

NAME:	**D. G.**																															
DATE:		1	2	3	4	5	6	7	8	9	10	11	12	13	14	15	16	17	18	19	20	21	22	23	24	25	26	27	28	29	30	31
HEADACHE	5		X					X									X									X						
	4	X		X		X			X	X				X	X				X		X	X						X			X	X
	3										X		X							X			X				X					
	2																															
	1				X		X					X					X				X											
	0																		X								X			X		
Headache duration (hours)		2	3	2		2		3	2	2		1		1	2	2	2			2		2	2	2	2	2½		2	2		3	2

Fig. 18.**5**   Patient's headache diary

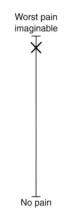

syndrome, rhinorrhea, pale face, dilation of temporal blood vessels, and photophobia.

Some attacks occurred in the night. After the attacks there was intense prostration and aching in the right hemiface. In the past the patient had been treated with carbamezapine (unsuccessfully) and Cafergot (which was partially useful in overcoming the single attacks but did not prevent the onset of successive attacks). A subsequent treatment with flunarizine, 5 mg in the evening, was followed by a period of remission lasting about one year.

The patient was a moderate smoker, normotensive, with quite a few psychosomatic symptoms as well as other types of symptoms (Fig. 18.**7**). The neurological examination was

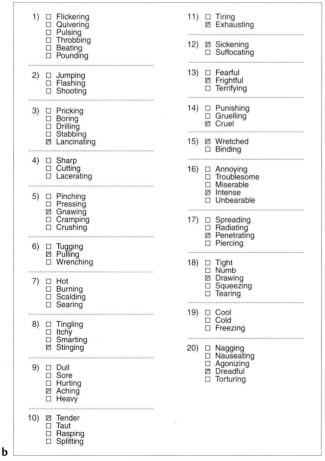

Fig. 18.**6**   Severity of pain is confirmed by the VAS (**a**) and the McGill Pain Questionnaire (**b**)

Fig. 18.**7**   The patient's complaints

within the norm as was the EEG. Palpation of the temporal muscle and right external pterygoid bone was painful. Skull radiography showed a moderately thickened theca (Fig. 18.**8**). The MMPI showed a tendency toward a *hysterical* profile, though the scores were within the norm (except that for hypochondria) (Fig. 18.**9**).

Slow-release verapamil tablets (120 mg) were prescribed to be taken once in the evening, and this gradually reduced the frequency of the attacks until they disappeared entirely within about 20 days (Fig. 18.**10**). After a year the patient complained of the reccurrence of a few attacks in milder form, which were readily overcome by taking verapamil for 20 days.

The following case presented different characteristics: a 51-year-old man, a financial consultant, who had complained of tension-type headaches in the frontal area since he was a boy, concomitantly with stressing events. These episodes gradually diminished over time until they entirely disappeared. Four years before observation, after a period of tension due to work-related issues, he had started to complain of headaches located at the top of the head and spreading to the periorbital and supraorbital area and, subsequently, to the lower part of the face. These attacks were always on the right side (Fig. 18.**11**) and were preceded by intense yawning. The pain was very intense, pulsating and associated with intense lacrimation and conjunctival hyperemia, nausea, itchy eyes, a sensation of heat, and facial pallor. The attacks lasted from 30 minutes to two hours. From the beginning the frequency had been one attack every one or two days. There was, however, a period of complete remission for seven months. At the time of observation, the attacks had been present for about a year and a half and occurred once a day or once every two days. Moreover, two attacks a day sometimes occurred, especially during the weekend (Fig. 18.**12**). Alcohol and stress were aggravating factors, as was resting at the weekend. He had been taking ergotamine in drops during the attacks for some considerable time and had had partial success. Inhalation of nascent oxygen was also somewhat effective. In addition, he took propranolol in cycles (40 mg) to avoid excessive rises in blood pressure (which aggravated the symptoms). A series of acupuncture sessions had produced only fleeting comfort.

The patient was a heavy smoker (40 cigarettes a day), a moderate drinker of wine and liquor, and reported suffering

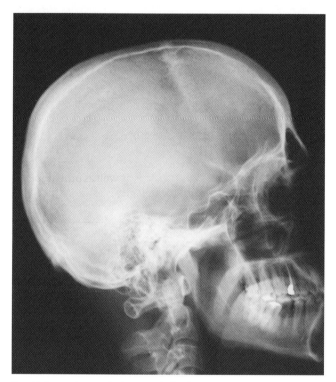

Fig. 18.**8**   Radiograph shows a slight thickening of the cranial bone

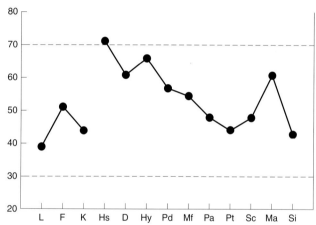

Fig. 18.**9**   MMPI hypochondria score (Hs) is high and a tendency toward a *conversive V* is observed

NAME:																																
DATE:		1	2	3	4	5	6	7	8	9	10	11	12	13	14	15	16	17	18	19	20	21	22	23	24	25	26	27	28	29	30	31
HEADACHE	5																																
	4	X	X																														
	3			X			X				X																						
	2														X		X									X							
	1				X			X											X			X								X			
	0					X			X	X			X	X	X		X	X		X		X	X	X			X	X	X	X		X	X
Headache duration (hours)		2	2	1			2				1				1				1				2	10						1			
												DRUG INTAKE																					
VERAPAMIL		X	X	X	X	X	X	X	X	X	X	X	X	X	X	X	X	X	X	X	X	X	X	X	X	X	X	X	X	X	X	X	X

Fig. 18.**10**   Improvement of symptoms with verapamil

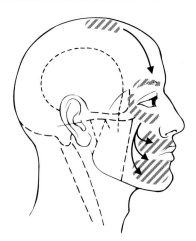

Fig. 18.**11**   **Fifty-one-year-old man with cluster headache.** Points of origin and spreading of pain are shown

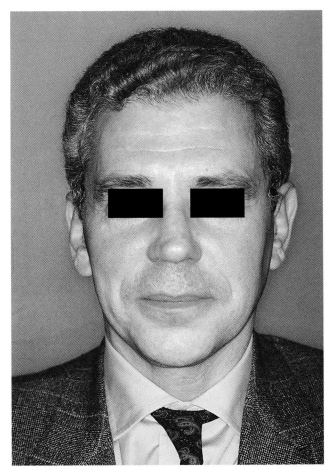

Fig. 18.**13**   Some features of the patient's face are among those described as typical of patients with CH

frequently from asthenia, insomnia, anxiety, colitis, and palpitations. His blood pressure was slightly raised (150 maximum/85–90 minimum). Upon inspection his face showed some of the traits described as typical of CH patients: protruding brow, deep furrows (Fig. 18.**13**), and hazel eyes. Neurological examination and muscle palpation were negative. Thermography showed the presence of areas of hypothermia corresponding to the naso-orbital corner and right nose wing (Fig. 18.**14**). According to some authors (Drummond and Lance, 1984; Kudrow, 1985; Mongini et al., 1990), this is a relatively frequent finding in patients with CH. The MMPI gave a high score for depression (Fig. 18.**15**).

Sumatriptan taken during the attacks did not provide any benefit. Before establishing a preventive pharmacological regime, the patient, who wore a dental prosthesis on a osteus implant (Fig. 18.**16a**), consulted a dentist, on his own initiative, and insisted that the implant be removed. Its removal (Fig. 18.**16b**) was followed, within about 20 days, by the almost total disappearance of the symptoms. At a check-up five years later, the patient reported that the situation had remained stable during that whole time, except for occasional much milder attacks (once every two or three months), especially under stress, which he readily managed with dihydroergotamine drops.

NAME: **N. L.**																															
DATE: DEC/JAN	21	22	23	24	25	26	27	28	29	30	31	1	2	3	4	5	6	7	8	9	10	11	12	13	14	15	16	17	18	19	20
HAEDACHE — 5																					X										
HAEDACHE — 4				X			X	X	X								X							X				X			
HAEDACHE — 3		X			X					X	X												X						X		
HAEDACHE — 2																															
HAEDACHE — 1																															
HAEDACHE — 0	X		X		X	X		X				X	X	X	X		X	X	X			X			X	X	X			X	X
Time of occurrence of headache	22	21		23 / 15	23		22 / 15	17													20		21	15	22			22	15		
Headache duration (hours)		30'		30'	1		30'	2	1												30'			2	30'	2			1	30'	
DRUG INTAKE																															
DIHYROERGOTAMINE		15		15	15		15	15													15		15	15				15	15		
					15		15																								
CAFERGOT																							1		2						

Fig. 18.**12**   **Patient's headache diary.** As well as pain level and duration, the time of day at which each attack occurred is indicated

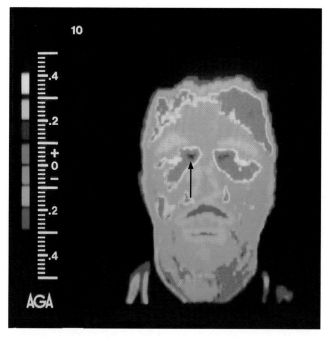
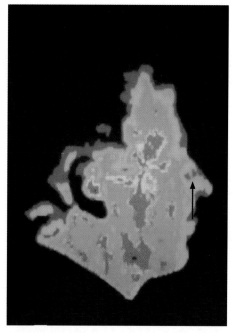

Fig. 18.**14**   Thermography shows an area of hypothermia corresponding to the naso-orbital angle and the right nose wing (arrows)

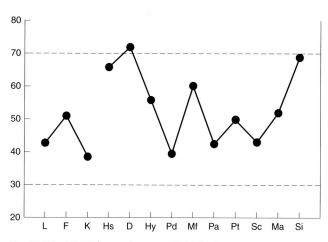

Fig. 18.**15**   MMPI depression score (D) is high

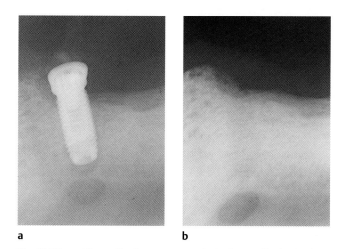

Fig. 18.**16**   **a** The patient wore an endosteal mandibular inplant. **b** When it was removed the symptoms disappeared

Chronic Paroxysmal Hemicrania

The most salient characteristics of CPH, as described in the IHS classification are as follows:

- The pain is severe, unilateral, located in the orbital, supraorbital and/or temporal areas, always on the same side.
- Its duration varies from 2 to 45 minutes and the frequency of the attacks (whether daytime or nighttime) is more than five per day in more than half of the time.
- These attacks are associated with one or more of the following signs on the pain side: conjunctival injection, lacrimation, nasal congestion, rhinorrhea, ptosis, eyelid edema.
- CPH responds quite well to intake of indomethacin (Sjaastad, 1987).

A typical case of CPH is that of a 35-year-old woman, a medical doctor, who reported the first pain attacks nine years before observation. Pain was burning and perforating, located at the left hemiface and spreading to the neck (Fig. 18. **17**). It lasted about 20 minutes and could appear several times during the day. These symptoms continued for about two years (with some remissions for about two months) and then disappeared for four years. The attacks subsequently reappeared, gradually becoming more frequent and intense. At various times aspirin, propranolol, verapamil, flunarizine, bromocriptine, steroids and lithium had been prescribed. None of these drugs, which are typically indicated for migraine or CL, had been successful.

At the time of examination, pain attacks occurred almost every day (or night) with a frequency variable from two or three to more than 10 times per day (Fig. 18.**18**). Stress and fatigue were aggravating factors. The attacks were accompanied by many autonomic symptoms and by sensory dysfunction, including conjunctival and nasal congestion, lacrimation (Fig. 18.**19**), rhinorrhea, diarrhea, polyuria, sweating, Horner syndrome, photophobia, phonophobia, and dysosmia. After each attack the patient felt very prostrated and experienced nausea and shivering. She also reported frequent

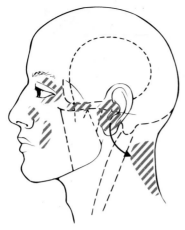

Fig. 18.17 Thirty-five year-old woman with chronic paroxysmal headache. Points of origin and spreading of pain

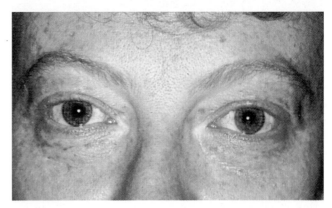

Fig. 18.**19** Congestion and lacrimation of left eye during the attack

NAME: C. S.

DATE:		1	2	3	4	5	6	7	8	9	10	11	12	13	14	15	16	17	18	19	20	21	22	23	24	25	26	27	28	29	30
HEADACHE	5																														
	4				↑		↑	↑	↑	↑																					↑
	3					↑						X	X	X	X	X															
	2	X	X	X	X	X	X	X	X	X							X	X	X		X									X	X
	1	X	X	X							X									X			X	X							
	0																														
Number of attacks during day/night		3	3	1	1/4	1/5	2/5	2/5	3/4	2/5	5/0	2/0	1/3	2/3	2/4	2/3	1/2	2/3	3/3	3/2	2/2		2/1	2/0		3	2	2	2		3
DRUG INTAKE																															
NAPROXEN			½	½	1	1	1	1	1	1	½	½	1	1	1	1	1	1	½	½	½	½	½	1	½		½	½			½
ASPIRIN		1																													

DATE:		1	2	3	4	5	6	7	8	9	10	11	12	13	14	15	16	17	18	19	20	21	22	23	24	25	26	27	28	29	30	31
HEADACHE	5																															
	4																															
	3	X				X																										
	2		X				X			X	X	X			X	X		X	X		X	X	X	X		X			X			X
	1																															X
	0																															
Number of attacks during day/night		1/1	1	1	1		1	1	2		2	1	2			1	1	2	1	2/1	1	1		3/1	2/3	4/3	2/3	3/5	3/5	3/5		2/3
DRUG INTAKE																															
NAPROXEN			½	½	1		1		½	½		½	½	½		½	½				½	½	½	½	½	½	½	½	½	½	½	½
ASPIRIN		½											½																			
DIAZEPAM									X	X	X	X	X	X		X	X	X	X	X	X	X	X	X	X	X	X	X	X	X	X	X

Fig. 18.**18 Headache diary.** Note the large numer of daytime and nighttime attacks

fatigue, anxiety, palpitations, orthostatic hypotension, and frequent and severe tooth grinding.

Indeed, her facial expression was one of suffering. Left temporal muscle hypertrophy was noted on inspection (Fig. 18.**20**). Muscle palpation was positive on the left side for the lateral pterygoid, the temporal, the trapezius and the nuchal muscles. There was a grating noise of the left TMJ during opening and closing movements. MMPI hysteria score was above 70. On thermography, a hypothermic zone was observed on the left fronto-orbital region and the nose wing (Fig. 18.**21**).

The patient was given indomethacin, 25 mg once a day, initially, gradually increasing to three times a day after a month. Improvement was quite rapid (Fig. 18.**22**). The usual treatment (biofeedback, relaxation exercise, nighttime splint) was also applied against parafunction and improved the muscle tension and the neck pain. One month later the patient gradually reduced the intake of the indomethacin to 50 mg and then to 25 mg a day. The intake was completely interrupted after four months, when the patient felt well (Fig. 18.**23**). She remained symptom-free for about six months, after which she had a recurrence of the attacks and started the use of indomethacin again for approximately one month. In the following three years, the patient's health remained good overall, and she was able to control her condition with short cycles of indomethacin (keeping doses to 25 mg per day). The patient reported that, as the symptoms improved, there was also a regularization of the menstrual cycle, previously very irregular.

Conclusions

CH and CPH are rarer than the other forms of primary headaches (tension-type headache and migraine). This, along with the fact that they have some characteristics in common and also in common with other pathologies, exposes them more frequently to diagnostic errors. Nonetheless, a thorough analysis of the history and clinical data allows us to reach a correct differential diagnosis between CH and CHP and between these and migraine, trigeminal neuralgia, and SUNCT. This is clearly very important for therapeutic purposes be-

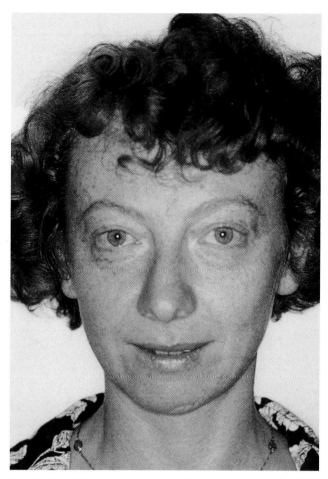

Fig. 18.**20**   Suffering look on patient's face. Note hypertrophy of left temporal muscle

cause, as seen earlier, drugs that are effective for some of these pathologies (e.g. indomethacin or carbamezapine) are not effective for others.

An important element to consider once a correct diagnosis is made is the presence of risk factors or irritating factors. Determining and eliminating these can increase the effective-

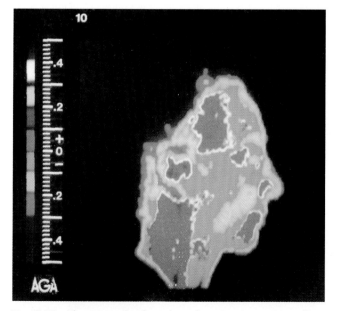

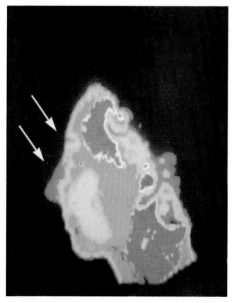

Fig. 18.**21**   Thermography shows hypothermic area corresponding to the left frontal-orbital region and the left nose wing (arrows)

NAME: **C. S.**

DATE:	1	2	3	4	5	6	7	8	9	10	11	12	13	14	15	16	17	18	19	20	21	22	23	24	25	26	27	28	29	30	31
HEADACHE 5																															
4																															
3											X		X																		
2								X								X	X														
1																															
0																															
Number of attacks during day/night								1/0			1/0		1/0			1/0	1/0	1/0													

DRUG INTAKE

| INDOMETHACIN | 50 | 50 | 50 | 50 | 50 | 50 | 50 | 50 | 50 | 50 | 50 | 50 | 25 | 25 | 25 | 25 | 25 | 25 | 25 | 25 | 25 | 25 | 25 | 25 | 25 | 25 | 25 | 25 | 25 | 25 | 25 |

Fig. 18.**22**   Considerable improvement of symptoms after drug therapy (indomethacin) and nondrug therapy

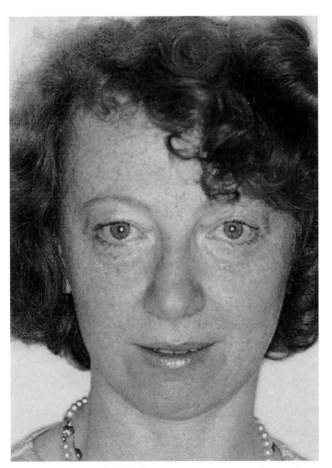

Fig. 18.**23**   Improvement is confirmed by patient's facial expression

ness of the drug therapy and, in some cases, as seen earlier, re-solve the problem entirely.

Finally, to evaluate the effectiveness of the therapy it is necessary to take into account the tendency of CH, and to a certain degree of CPH, to be cyclical. This is important so that the passage from an active period to a remission phase, which can be part of the natural history of the disease, is not inter-preted as therapeutic success. To this end, check-ups at long intervals are useful.

References

Ad Hoc Committee on Classification of Headache: classification of head-ache, JAMA, 1962, 178 : 717 – 718.

Andersson P.G., *Migraine in patients with cluster headache*, Cephalalgia, 1985, 5 : 11 – 16.

Drummond P.D., Lance J.W., *Thermographic changes in cluster headache*, Neurology, 1984, 34 : 1292 – 1298.

Graham J.R., *Cluster headache*, Headache, 1972, 11 : 175 – 185.

International Headache Society, *Classification and diagnostic criteria for headache disorders, cranial neuralgias and facial pain*, Cephalalgia, 1988, 8 (Suppl. 7):1 – 96.

Krabbe A.A., *Cluster headache: a review*, Acta Neurol. Scand., 1986, 74 : 1 – 9.

Kudrow L., *Cluster headache. Mechanisms and management*, New York, Oxford University Press, 1980.

Kudrow L., *A distinctive facial thermographic pattern in cluster headache – the "chai" sign*, Headache, 1985, 25 : 33 – 36.

Kunkle E.C., Pfeiffer J.R., Wilhoit W.M., Hamrich L.W., *Recurrent brief headaches in "cluster" pattern*, Trans. Am. Neurol. Assoc., 1952, 77 : 240 – 243.

Manzoni G.C., Micieli G., Granella F., Martignoni E., Farina S., Nappi G., *Cluster headache in women: clinical findings and relationship with re-productive life*, Cephalalgia, 1988, 8 : 37 – 44.

Mongini F., Caselli C., Macrì V., Tetti C., *Thermographic findings in cranio-facial pain*, Headache, 1990, 30 : 497 – 504.

Nappi G., Manzoni G.C., *Manuale delle cefalee*, Cluster Press, Milan, 1990.

Sjaastad O., *Chronic paroxysmal hemicrania: clinical aspects and contro-versies*, in: Blau J.N. (ed.), *Migraine. Clinical, therapeutic, conceptual and research aspects*, Chapman and Hall Medical, London, 1987, 135 – 152.

Sjaastad O., Dale I., *A new (?) clinical headache entity "chronic paroxysmal hemicrania"*, Acta Neurol. Scand., 1976, 54 : 140 – 159.

Sutherland J.M., Eadie M.J., *Cluster headache*, Res. Clin. Stud. Headache, 1972, 3 : 92 – 125.

19 Primary Headache Variants and Other Clinical Features

Introduction

The clinical cases described in Chapters 15 – 18 include the overwhelming majority of commonly observed headaches. However, difficulties in diagnosis can arise due to the presence of syndromes with aspects that are partly similar to and partly different from the syndromes already described. In some patients these syndromes may be the only clinical problem, whereas in others they might alternate with the more usual ones described earlier.

On the other hand, although the triggering or aggravating factors of migraine and headaches in general are numerous and diverse, some headaches have been classified separately because they are typically caused by the intake of certain foods or substances, or by particular stimuli; they therefore deserve a brief, separate description.

Migraine Variants

The IHS classification codes *migraine without aura* (Table 19.**1**, point 1.1) without further distinction, whereas *migraine with aura* (1.2) is divided into six subgroups. Another five types of migraine are successively listed in points 1.3 – 1.7 (Table 19.**1**).

The migraine aura must not last longer than 60 minutes, according to the classification criteria (in most cases it lasts less than 30 minutes). However, in a minority of patients this criterion is not fulfilled and at least one of the aura symptoms lasts longer than the stated period. In those cases the term *migraine with prolonged aura* (1.2.2) is used. If neuroimaging shows a cerebral ischemic lesion, the definition proposed is *migrainous infarction* (1.6.2).

In other variants the aura is characterized by the onset, fleeting or prolonged, of a hemiparesis *(familial hemiplegic migraine,* 1.2.3) or symptoms that originate in the brain stem or the occipital lobes *(basilar migraine,*1.2.4, also known as *Bickerstaff migraine)* (Bickerstaff, 1961, 1986).

The *migraine aura without headache* (1.2.5), also known as the *decapitated migraine* or *migraine without migraine,* defines migraine attacks that occur with the aura only, not followed by headache. Patients with these types of attacks are less frequent than those in which the migraine aura without headache alternates with migraine attacks with the typical aura.

The following case is a good example of the last-mentioned type and demonstrates the variability of the aura symptoms with signs of involvement of the cortical areas outside the visual cortex. The case is that of a 22-year-old woman, a university student, who reported the onset a year before observation of an initial attack characterized by vision disturbances typical of the migraine aura with *fortification spectra* vision, blurred vision and blind areas in the visual field. In addition to these symptoms was an *autopoagnosia* of the hands: in other words, the patient reported observing her hands and perceiving them as "not hers." These symptoms lasted for about 30 minutes and when they terminated, an extremely severe pulsating headache occurred in the frontal area and lasted about one hour. In the next 12 months the patient had complained of another three episodes identical to the first. Moreover, these episodes alternated with more frequent episodes of autopoagnosia of the hands not followed by headache. The patient also had frequent tension-type headache and showed the typical signs of parafunction (Fig. 19.**1**). She was prescribed 50 mg of sumatriptan orally, to be taken at the onset of the aura, and, after a biofeedback session, relaxation exercises daily, which she carried out diligently. At a check-up six months later she reported that neither the penomenon of autopoagnosia nor the migraines had recurred and the tension-type headaches had also totally disappeared.

The other types of migraine in the IHS classification are as follows:

The *ophthalmoplegic migraine* (1.3), characterized by repeated migraine attacks associated with the paresis of one or more oculomotor nerves in absence of intracranial lesions.

The *retinal migraine* (1.4), with concomitant mono-ocular scotoma or amaurosis lasting less than one hour.

The *periodic infancy syndromes* may be precursors of the migraine or associated with the migraine (1.5), divided into *benign paroxysmal vertigo of childhood* (brief attacks of vertigo affecting otherwise healthy children) and *alternating hemiplegia of childhood.*

The *migraine complications* (1.6) are the *migrainous state* (1.6.1) with migraine attacks that last over 72 hours without intervals or with intervals shorter than four hours and the *migrainous infarction* (1.6.2), mentioned above.

Finally, under point 1.7 we find the *migraine disorders that do not fulfil the previous criteria.* However, as seen in Chapters 1 and 17, according to some authors, headaches that can be classified under this heading or *under tension-type headache not fulfilling previous criteria* are not rare.

Table 19.**1** Classification of migraine and its variants according to the I. H. S.

1. Migraine

1.1	Migraine without aura
1.2	Migraine with aura
	1.2.1 Migraine with typical aura
	1.2.2 Migraine with prolonged aura
	1.2.3 Familial hemiplegic migraine
	1.2.4 Basilar migraine
	1.2.5 Migraine aura without headache
	1.2.6 Migraine with acute onset aura
1.3	Ophthalmoplegic migraine
1.4	Retinal migraine
1.5	Childhood periodic syndromes that may be precursors to or associated with migraine
	1.5.1 Benign paroxysmal vertigo of childhood
	1.5.2 Alternative hemiplegia of childhood
1.6	Complications of migraine
	1.6.1 Status migrainosus
	1.6.2 Migrainous infarction
1.7	Migrainous disorder not fulfilling above criteria

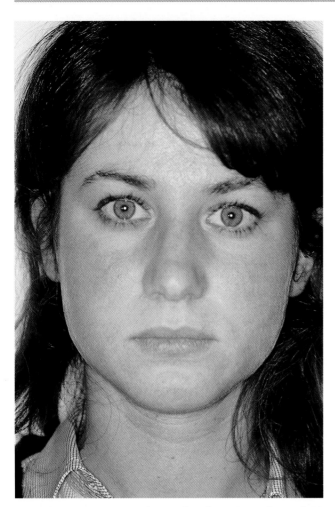

Fig. 19.**1**   Young woman with episodes of migraine with aura (with *fortification spectra* vision and *autopoagnosia* of her hands) **alternating with aura without headache.** She also had tension-type headaches. A marked hypertrophy of the masseters due to daytime and nighttime parafunction can be seen

Variants of Cluster Headache and Chronic Paroxysmal Hemicrania

The *cluster tic syndrome* is a variant of the cluster headache, of which a few dozen cases have been described (Hornabrook, 1964; Eadie, 1966; Lance and Antony, 1971; Green and Apfelbaum, 1978; Diamond et al., 1984; Solomon et al., 1985; Watson and Evans, 1985; Klimek, 1987; Hannerz, 1993; Alberca and Ochoa, 1994). It is characterized by two types of pain. One type has all the characteristics of the pain attacks of trigeminal neuralgia: severe pain of brief duration, located in the region of the second and/or third branch of the trigeminal nerve (see Chapter 20); the second type has the characteristics of cluster headache described in the Chapter 18. The two components of pain occur separately or overlap, depending on the patient or the period of illness. Although some authors (Kunkle, 1982; Diamond et al., 1984; Solomon et al., 1985) suggest that they are two overlapping pathologies, it is for the most part considered that the occurrence of the two types of pain together is not chance and therefore that the cluster tic syndrome is a distinct pathology. This is also supported by the fact that preventive treatment with drugs that are effective for cluster headache are ineffective for the cluster tic syndrome, whereas some relief can be obtained from carbamezapine, associated, if necessary, with steroids intramuscularly (Alberca and Ochoa, 1994).

A case of chronic paroxysmal hemicrania associated with neuralgic type pain was described by Hannerz (1993) and the eponym *chronic paroxysmal hemicrania-tic* (CPH-tic) was proposed. The patient presented a bilateral constriction of the upper ophthalmic veins.

The following case is one of a probable migraine variant associated with other problems. One year before observation the patient, a 35-year-old housewife whose mother suffered from migraines, had complained of a severe pulsating headache in the frontotemporal area accompanied by a sense of motor impediment in the right facial muscles, orbital tumefaction, and a very marked eyelid ptosis. Subsequently she suffered from bouts of stabbing pain lasting 5–6 seconds in the right periorbital region associated with lacrimation, ptosis, and nasal obstruction. These symptoms persisted several minutes after disappearance of the pain. In the period of observation, the bouts occurred about once an hour during the day. Some attacks occurred in the night. They could be triggered by tactile stimuli at the orbital corner and nose wing, by chewing, and by eye movements. During the intercritical periods, the patient complained of a sense of pain and constant stiffening of the right hemiface (Fig. 19.**2**): the pain was particularly acute in the auricular region. The patient suffered from a sense of overall and constant fatigue and numerous psychosomatic disturbances (Fig. 19.**3**). Neurological examination, CAT scans, brain MRI and angiography were negative. Mouth and head movements were seriously limited (Fig. 19.**4**), upon palpation all craniofacial muscles were tender (especially on the right side). An MRI of the TMJ with

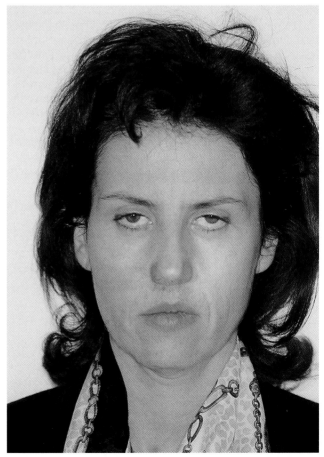

Fig. 19.**2   Thirty-five-year-old woman with severe facial pain syndrome** (possible CPH variant overlapping muscle contraction and pain). There is also palpebral ptosis and a stiffening of the entire right half of the face

Colitis	☒
Gastritis	☒
Kinetosis	☐
Swallowing difficulty	☒
Digestive problems	☒
Anorexia	☒
Bulimia	☐
Anxiety	☒
Phobias	☒
Sleep disorders	☒
Palpitations	☒
Panic attacks	☒
Mood changes	☒
Fainting	☒
Vertigo	☐
Lassitude	☒
Parafunctions	☐
Clonus	☐
Cramps	☒
Paresthesias	☒
Back pain	☒
Urination disturbances	☐
Diarrhea or constipation	☒
Nail fragility	☐
Hair fragility	☒
Circulation disorders	☒
Cold limbs	☒
Frigidity	☐
Vaginism	☐
Frequent depressed moods	☐
Other	☐

Fig. 19.**3**　The patient's complaints

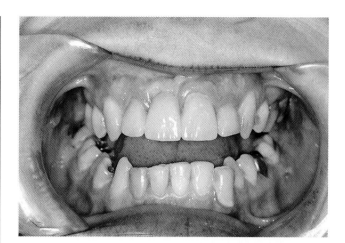

Fig. 19.**4**　Mouth opening movement is extremely reduced

closed and open mouth made it possible to exclude the coexistence of a displaced disk as the cause of the limitation in opening (Fig. 19.**5**). The MMPI-2 scores were all high except for self-esteem (Mf). The STAI showed maximal state and trait anxiety scores (Fig. 19.**6**). The patient had previously been treated with methylprednisone for 30 days, with gradually decreasing doses (starting with 25 mg a day), inhalation of nascent oxygen, carbamezapine 200 mg three times a day, ergotamine, sumatriptan, and NSAIDs, but without relief.

The case was therefore difficult to interpret. Some aspects pointed to SUNCT, an acronym defining a rare neurological pathology in the region of the first branch of the trigeminal nerve accompanied by autonomic symptoms and caused by tactile stimuli (see Chapter 20). Other aspects seemed to be those of a migraine variant (it had all started after a severe headache lasting several days) or a CPH variant. This last hypothesis was considered in light of the following factors: sex, location, the co-occurrence of autonomic symptoms; however, the fact that the attacks were sometimes caused by tactile stimuli and were of very short duration did not point to CPH. In any case, other problems certainly overlapped to justify such a host of symptoms: a marked mood dysfunction and an intense overall myogenic pain. This last symptom was presumably due to a chronic state of muscle contraction that also caused severe limitations in mandibular movements.

Indomethacin was prescribed (increased gradually to 125 mg a day divided into five doses) associated with antidepressants (ademetionine 200 mg twice a day and amitrip-

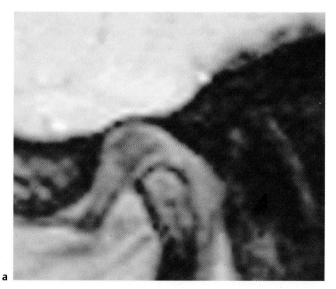

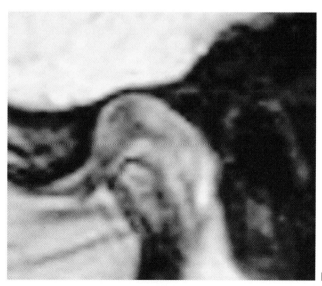

Fig. 19.**5**　The articular MRI with mouth closed (**a**) and open (**b**) shows a normal positioning of the articular disk (arrows), which rules out the possibility that the limited mandibular movements have an arthrogenic origin

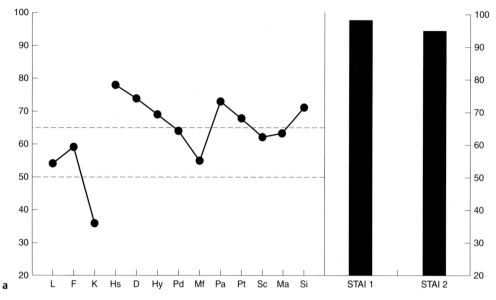

a

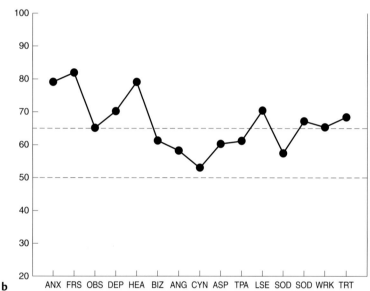

b

Fig. 19.**6** The MMPI-2 shows that almost all the clinical scores are very high (**a**) as are the content scores (**b**). The STAI test shows remarkably high state and trait anxiety scores (**a**)

tyline associated with perphenazine in increasing doses). The neuralgic-type attacks became less frequent (three or four a day) and mood improved slightly. The pain in the intercritical period remained unchanged. The response to indomethacin, though only partial, it would seem to point to a CPH variant.

Other Clinical Pictures

Under point 8 of the IHS classification is *headache associated with substances or their withdrawal* (Table 19.**2**). Some of these are associated with particular eating habits such as: *nitrite/ nitrate-induced headache* (8.1.1), also called the *hot dog headache; monosodium glutamate-induced headache* (8.1.2), the *Chinese restaurant syndrome;* and *alcohol-induced headache* (8.1.4). As mentioned in Chapter 17, the abuse of drugs (ergotamine, analgesics) can cause headache and, in particular, can be one of the factors that transform a migraine into a chronic daily headache. Chapter 16 presented a case typically associated with the use of contraceptives.

Among the headaches associated with particular stimuli are the benign cough headache and those related to sexual activity. They are coded in the IHS classification under the head-

ing *Miscellaneous headaches unassociated with structural lesions* (point 4) (Table 19.**3**).

The *benign cough headache* (4.4) is characterized by headaches of short duration (usually less than one minute), of bilateral location, triggered by coughing. It is a rather rare form of headache that can be treated satisfactorily with indomethacin.

One case of cough headache, anomalous in the duration of the attacks, is that of a 53-year-old woman, a teacher, who two years before observation complained of a pain after coughing, originating in the nuchal region and spreading to the temples and the upper dental arch. The pain was excruciating for a few minutes, and remained severe for the entire day. From that time the attacks recurred with the same characteristics each time she coughed, which she obviously tried her best to avoid doing. Her blood pressure was 150/ 105. Neurological examination, brain MRI and other routine examinations were negative. Indomethacin was prescribed, 25 mg to be taken orally twice a day. After just one week of taking the drug, the symptoms disappeared completely. At a check-up two years later the patient was still symptom-free.

Headache associated with sexual activity (4.6) is characterized by the progressive or explosive manifestation of head-

Table 19.**2** Classification of headaches caused by exogenous substances or their withdrawal

8. Headache associated with substances or their withdrawal

8.1 Headache induced by acute substance use or exposure
    8.1.1 Nitrate/nitrite–induced headache
    8.1.2 Monosodium glutamate–induced headache
    8.1.3 Carbon monoxide–induced headache
    8.1.4 Alcohol–induced headache
    8.1.5 Other substances

8.2 Headache induced by chronic substance use or exposure
    8.2.1 Ergotamine–induced headache
    8.2.2 Analgesics abuse headache
    8.2.3 Other substances

8.3 Headache from substance withdrawal (acute use)
    8.3.1 Alcohol withdrawal headache (hangover)
    8.3.2 Other substances

8.4 Headache from substance withdrawal (chronic use)
    8.4.1 Ergotamine withdrawal headache
    8.4.2 Caffeine withdrawal headache
    8.4.3 Narcotics abstinence headache
    8.4.4 Other substances

8.5 Headache associated with substances but with uncertain mechanism
    8.5.1 Birth control pills or estrogens
    8.5.2 Other substances

Table 19.**3** Classification of headaches not associated with structural lesions

4. Miscellaneous headaches unassociated with structural lesions

4.1 Idiopathic stabbing headache

4.2 External compression headache

4.3 Cold stimulus headache
    4.3.1 External application of a cold stimulus
    4.3.2 Ingestion of a cold stimulus

4.4 Benign cough headache

4.5 Benign exertional headache

4.6 Headache associated with sexual activity
    4.6.1 Dull type
    4.6.2 Explosive type
    4.6.3 Postural type

ache coinciding with sexual intercourse. This type of headache can also be treated with indomethacin. Both the cough headache and the headache associated with sexual activity are found in both sexes.

References

Alberca R., Ochoa J.J., *Cluster tic syndrome*, Neurology, 1994, 44:996–999.

Bickerstaff E.R.: *Basilar artery migraine*, Lancet, 1961, 1:15–17.

Bickerstaff E.R.: *Basilar artery migraine*. In: Clifford Rose F. (ed.), *Handbook of Clinical Neurology*, vol. 4 (48), Headache, Elsevier, Amsterdam, 1986, 135–140.

Diamond S., Freitag F.G., Cohen J.S., *Cluster headache with trigeminal neuralgia*, Postgrad Med., 1984, 75:165–172.

Eadie M.J., Sutherland J.M., *Migrainous neuralgia*, Med. J. Aust., 1966, 1:1053–1057.

Green M., Apfelbaum R.I., *Cluster-tic syndrome*, Headache, 1978, 18:112.

Hannerz J., *Trigeminal neuralgia with chronic paroxysmal hemicrania: the CPH-tic syndrome*, Cephalalgia, 1993, 13:361–364.

Hornabrook R.W., *Migrainous neuralgia*, NZ Med. J., 1964, 66:774–779.

International Headache Society, *Classification and diagnostic criteria for headache disorders, cranial neuralgias and facial pain*, Cephalalgia, 1988, 8 (Suppl. 7):1–96.

Klimek A., *Cluster-tic syndrome*, Cephalalgia, 1987, 7:161–162.

Kunkle E.C., *Clues in the tempos of cluster headache*, Headache, 1982, 22:158–91.

Lance J.W., Anthony M., *Migrainous neuralgia or cluster headache?*, J. Neurol. Sci., 1971, 13:401–414.

Solomon S., Apfelbaum R.I., Guglielmo K.M., *The clustertic syndrome and its surgical therapy*, Cephalalgia, 1985, 5:83–89.

Watson P., Evans R., *Cluster-tic syndrome*, Headache, 1985, 25:123–126.

Part IV Diagnosis and Therapy of Facial Pain

20 Neuropathic Facial Pain

Trigeminal Neuralgia

Trigeminal neuralgia (12.2 in the IHS classification) (Table 20.1) (also called tic doloureux in the past), is a pathology characterized by attacks of lancinating facial pain. There is a distinction between the idiopathic form (12.2.1) and the symptomatic form (12.2.2): in the latter the pain is caused by a demonstrable structural lesion. The diagnostic criteria supplied by the IHS for the idiopathic form are the following:

(A) Paroxysmal pain attacks last from a few seconds to less than two minutes.
(B) Pain has at least four of the following characteristics:
1. Distribution along one or more branches of the trigeminal nerve.
2. Sudden, intense, sharp, superficial, stabbing or burning in quality.
3. Pain intensity severe.
4. Precipitation from trigger areas, or by certain daily activities such eating, talking, washing the face or cleaning the teeth.
5. Between paroxisms the patients is entirely asymptomatic.

(C) There are no neurological deficits.
(D) Attacks are stereotyped in the individual patient.
(E) The medical history, clinical examination and laboratory tests when necessary, exclude the presence of other causes of facial pain.

The affected regions are mostly the second and/or third branches of the trigeminal nerve. In much rarer cases the first branch is affected. The attacks can occur many times a day and normally no pain occurs in the intercritical periods. The pain often produces facial muscle spasms on the affected side (Fig. 20.1). However, these spasms occur only in the critical phase and should be distinguished from dystonic phenomena and persistent muscle spasms, which can occur alone or concomitantly with myogenic pain from muscle contraction (see Chapter 21).

As the pathology evolves, especially in elderly patients, trigeminal neuralgia traits may be less typical and thus justify doubts as to their nosological placement. The intensity and duration of the pain attacks can be variable (from moderate to

Table 20.1 Classification of facial neuropathic pain according to the I.H.S.

12. Cranial neuralgies, nerve trunk pain and deafferentation pain

12.1 Persistent (in contrast to ticlike) pain of cranial nerve origin
    12.1.1 Compression or distortion of cranial nerves and second or third cervical roots
    12.1.2 Demyelination of cranial nerves
        12.1.2.1 Optic neuritis (retrobulbar neuritis)
    12.1.3 Infarction of cranial nerves
        12.1.3.1 Diabetic neuritis
    12.1.4 Inflammation of cranial nerves
        12.1.4.1 Herpes zoster
        12.1.4.2 Chronic postherpetic neuralgia
    12.1.5 Tolosa–Hunt syndrome
    12.1.6 Neck–tongue syndrome
    12.1.7 Other causes of persistent pain of cranial nerve origin

12.2 Trigeminal neuralgia
    12.2.1 Idiopathic trigeminal neuralgia
    12.2.2 Symptomatic trigeminal neuralgia
        12.2.2.1 Compression of trigeminal root or ganglion
        12.2.2.2 Central lesions

12.3 Glossopharyngeal neuralgia
    12.3.1 Idiopathic glossopharyngeal neuralgia
    12.3.2 Symptomatic glossopharyngeal neuralgia

12.4 Nervus intermedius neuralgia

12.5 Superior laryngeal neuralgia

12.6 Occipital neuralgia

12.7 Central causes of head and facial pain other than tic douloureux
    12.7.1 Anaesthesia dolorosa
    12.7.2 Thalamic pain
12.8 Facial pain not fulfilling criteria in groups 11 or 12

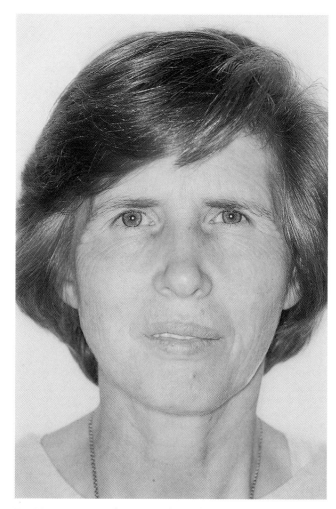

Fig. 20.1 Patient with trigeminal neuralgia of the second and third left branches associated with moderate spasms in the perioral musculature on the same side

severe, from seconds to minutes) and some painful sensations can persist even during the intercritical periods. In some cases there are signs of hyperemia in the affected area during the critical (Fig. 20.2) or intercritical periods (Fig. 20. 3).

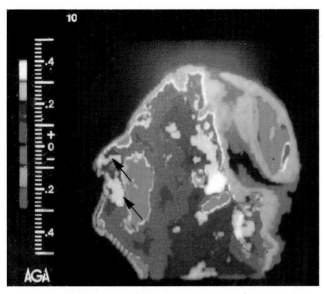

Fig. 20.**2** **Female patient suffering from neuralgia of the second and third branches of the trigeminal nerve.** During the neuralgic attack, thermography shows the appearance of two notably hyperthermic areas at the base of the nose and lip corner (arrows)

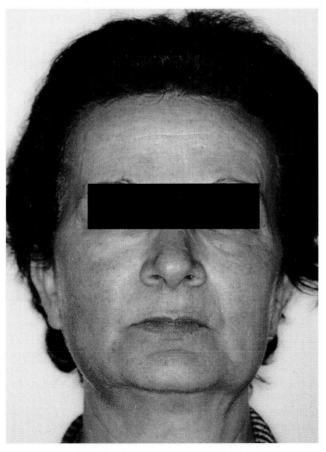

Fig. 20.**3** **A 52-year-old woman with trigeminal neuralgia of the second and third right branches.** Redness of affected areas of the face can be seen

When trigeminal neuralgia occurs in its typical form, the diagnosis is easy. There may, however, be differential diagnosis problems with chronic paroxysmal hemicrania (CPH) and, especially in chronic cases, with somatoform facial pain disorder.

As seen in Chapter 18, CPH pain attacks last longer (from 2 to 45 minutes) and, unlike trigeminal neuralgia, are associated with significant signs of involvement of the autonomic system. Moreover, CPH responds to indomethacin, which is totally ineffective in trigeminal neuralgia.

In somatoform pain disorder (see Chapter 23), the pain is variable in quality, intensity, and location. It is rarely very intense, often being described as a nuisance, and does not coincide with the sensory distribution areas of the trigeminal nerve. On the other hand, in neuralgia the pain is stereotyped and never exceeds the median line (except in rare cases in which the neuralgia is bilateral).

Numerous drugs are used to treat trigeminal neuralgia. Generally they develop a GABAergic activity, and some of them are commonly used in the treatment of epilepsy.

The first-choice drug is still carbamazepine, taken in doses varying from 400 to 800 mg or more per day. As seen in Chapter 12, this drug has numerous side effects (nausea, drowsiness, skin reactions, etc.) and requires a regular control of the blood formula due to the potential depressive action on hematopoiesis.

Other drugs that can be used as an alternative to carbamezapine are baclofen, sodium valproate, lamotrigine and gabapentin. Sodium valproate is used at an average daily dose varying from 800 to 1600 mg, to be reached gradually. It must be prescribed for periods limited to two or three months with monitoring of the hepatic function. With lamotrigine, the initial dose should be 50 mg on the first day and increased by 50 mg/day in separate dosages of 50 mg each until the minimum effective dosage is reached (between 150 and 400 mg). This drug probably has fewer side effects than carbamezapine (Meldrum, 1993). The initial dose of gabapentin is usually 300 mg/day, which should be gradually increased to 900–1200 mg/day or more, as needed.

In chronic cases, especially if overlapped by anxiety symptoms and myogenic pain, it can be effective to prescribe bromazepam, though this particular benzodiazepine is not normally considered as a drug for treating trigeminal neuralgia.

Clonazepam must also be considered. It is a benzodiazepine with anticonvulsive properties, particularly indicated for cases of persistent neuropathic pain (see below), but in cases of slight response to other drugs it can be used either alone or in combination, even in cases of trigeminal neuralgia, at a dose of 0.5 mg/day in a single dose in the evening or half the dose twice a day, increasing if necessary up to the minimum effective dose (a maximum of 2 mg/day).

Response to these drugs is highly unpredictable and it is virtually impossible to establish in advance which will be the most effective. A reasonable sequence of drug choice might indicate carbamezapine as the first choice and then, if results are poor, lamotrigine, baclofen, or sodium valproate. Bromazepam could be considered as a third choice. However, in chronic patients with a significant anxiety level, bromazepam could be the first choice, either alone or combined with another anticonvulsant drug.

In chronic cases with the persistence of some pain in the intercritical period, clonazepam, taken alone or with another drug, may be effective.

Likewise, the efficacy of nondrug therapy such as lasers or TENS (see Chapter 13) is highly unpredictable. While in most cases nondrug therapy has little or no effect, in some cases it can be notably effective, especially TENS.

Two cases that were successfully resolved with a treatment alternative to carbamezapine are discussed. A particularly complex case of trigeminal neuralgia with a traumatic basis is that of a 47-year-old man, a mason, who four months before observation had fractured his left zygomatic bone in falling from scaffolding. He was hospitalized in a maxillofacial surgery department and a metal plate was inserted to support the fracture. About one month after the operation he suffered from attacks of intense burning and stabbing pain in the region of the second branch of the left trigeminal nerve (zygomatic arch and upper lip). These attacks were caused by tactile stimulation in the genial region and nose wing, and by chewing and cheek movements. They were associated with slight spasm of the left cheek and eyelid muscles (Fig. 20.**4**). In the intercritical period, paresthesias (tingling) were almost constantly present in the same region. Removal of the supporting splint had no effect. The patient had previously been treated with carbamezapine 200 mg twice a day and phenobarbital 50 mg in the evening, with only partial and fleeting effect.

Clonazepam 0.5 mg was prescribed twice a day. At a later check-up the patient reported an initial improvement with a partial relapse after a few days. The drug was then increased to 0.5 mg three times a day. Since the patient reported that his depressed mood tended to worsen the emotional component of the disturbance, he was also prescribed amitriptyline drops, 20 mg twice a day. In addition, upon the advice of an otologist, the patient underwent a cycle of anesthetic blocks

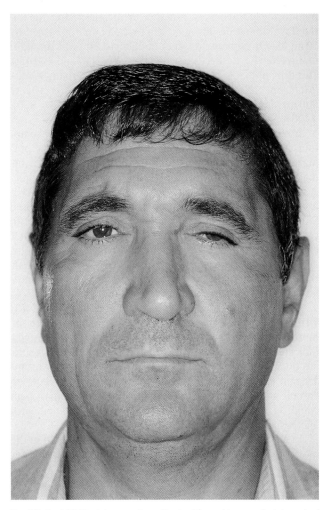

Fig. 20.**4**   Mild facial spasm in patient with posttraumatic trigeminal neuralgic pain

in the sphenopalatine ganglion region with tampons soaked in procaine 10% and betamethasone 4 mg applied to the nasal choanae. The symptoms improved notably and the paroxysmal pain evoked by tactile stimulations disappeared. However, intermittent sensations of paresthesia persisted. After three months of taking clonazepam, the dose was reduced to 50 mg twice a day. Since this reduction coincided with a partial relapse of the symptoms, the previous regime was quickly resumed. The situation improved again and remained stable in the subsequent months. The clonazepam dose was again progressively reduced after three more months, this time without consequences. At a later check-up the acute attacks had disappeared, whereas sensations of hypoesthesia and paresthesia persisted in a smaller area than before.

Another case of combined drug therapy is that of a 34-year-old woman who six months before observation had complained of a sudden manifestation of lancinating pain attacks in the region of the second and third branch of the right trigeminal nerve. These attacks were initially very frequent (10–15 times or more a day); they lasted from a few seconds to a maximum of 30 seconds and were triggered by mild tactile stimulation in the genial area or the nose wing or by tongue movements that involved contact between the tongue and the internal wall of the right check. The patient was prescribed carbamezapine at relatively high doses (1000 mg/day, divided into three dosages). The effect was good; the attacks were virtually eliminated but tended to relapse as soon as the patient reduced the dose of the drug. Because the drug produced side effects (nausea, drowsiness) and she had been taking it for a long time, the problem in this case was to find a substitute drug that would at least make it possible to reduce the dose of carbamezapine. Bromazepam drops were prescribed, 1 mg twice a day, and the dose of carbamezapine was to be reduced gradually. After a TENS session with electrodes applied to correspond to the foramina of the second and third trigeminal branches, the patient reported an improvement of the symptoms lasting several hours. Consequently, á series of sessions was prescribed. The result was initially very satisfactory, but after one month there was a partial relapse of the symptoms. She was then prescribed 0.25 mg clonazepam in the evening in association with the TENS sessions. The situation improved again and remained stable with a regime of 400 mg carbamezapine, 1 mg bromazepam twice a day, and 0.25 mg clonazepam.

Other Neuralgias. SUNCT

Idiopathic glossopharyngeal neuralgia (12.3.1 in the IHS classification) is a pathology characterized by acute pain attacks located unilaterally in the glossopharyngeal nerve distribution region and sometimes also in the auricular and pharyngeal branches of the vagal nerve (the rear part of the tongue, the tonsillar fossa, the pharynx, the area under the mandibular angle, the ear). All the other pain characteristics are identical to those of trigeminal neuralgia: the pain is strictly unilateral, extremely intense, stabbing or burning; it is stereotyped, lasts from a few seconds to under two minutes and can be precipitated by stimulating the trigger points, swallowing, coughing, phonation, or yawning. The therapy is the same as that for trigeminal neuralgia.

An anomalous case of neuralgia primarily affecting the region of the glossopharyngeal nerve is that of a 27-year-old woman who had suffered for about ten years from neuralgic pain attacks at the root and right rear edge of her tongue, sometimes extended to the mandibular corner. The attacks were triggered by tongue movements, phonation, swallowing, and chewing and had become progressively more frequent. The patient had been treated with carbamezapine at increasing doses (up to 800 mg/day) in intermittent cycles of 6 – 8 months. The drug was notable effective at the beginning of treatment but its effect diminished progressively and at the time of observation the patient suffered from very frequent attacks (15 – 20 or more per day) with the persistence of aching and paresthesias in the intercritical periods. Consequently, she was in a severe state of anxiety and prostration. A marked tenderness on palpation of most of her craniofacial muscles was associated. She was tentatively prescribed bromazepam drops, 1.5 mg twice a day. The symptoms gradually improved and almost totally disappeared within a month. The patient was still symptom-free at a check-up two years later.

Occipital neuralgia (12.6) is characterized by pain with analogous characteristics but situated in the distribution region of the large or small occipital nerve. Palpation of the nerve at the point of emergence from the skull is intensely painful and the symptoms can be temporarily eliminated by anesthetic blocades of the nerve. This situation must be differentiated from pain referred to the occipital area as a result of alterations of the antlantoaxial or upper zygoapophyseal joints. It must also be distinguished from occipital pain caused by the presence of trigger points or tender points of the cervical muscles (see Chapter 21).

The term SUNCT is an acronym (shortlasting unilateral neuralgiform pain with conjunctival injection and tearing) indicating a rare condition characterized by attacks of intense pain, usually in the orbital or periorbital region, lasting from 30 to 120 seconds, and accompanied by conjunctival hyperemia, lacrimation, and rhinorrhea. This pathology was reported for the first time in 1978 (Sjaastad et al, 1978) and since then various cases have been described (more frequently in males) (Sjaastad et al., 1989, 1991; Bouhasira et al., 1994; Pareja et al., 1994, 1996 a, b). The frequency of the attacks can vary from one or two a day to 30 or more an hour. They can be precipitated by slight tactile stimulation. Little or no benefit is obtained from the intake of indomethacin, ergotamine, or carbamezapine. The taxonomy of the syndrome is still uncertain: the pain appears to be neurogenic, but vascular factors also seem to be involved. Some characteristics are those of trigeminal neuralgia, but the conspicuous presence of auto-

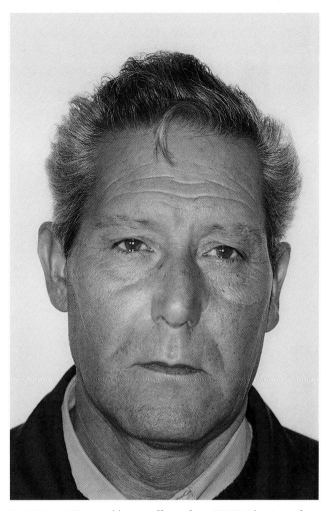

Fig. 20.**5**　A 52-year-old man suffering from SUNCT. The signs of autonomic concurrence can be seen on the right eye

nomic signs is more indicative of a migraine disturbance (Sjaastad and Kruszewski, 1992; Sjaastad et al., 1997; Pareja and Sjaastad, 1997). Cases of SUNCT associated with vascular malformations of the encephalic stem have been described (Bussone et al., 1991; Morales et al., 1994; De Benedittis, 1996).

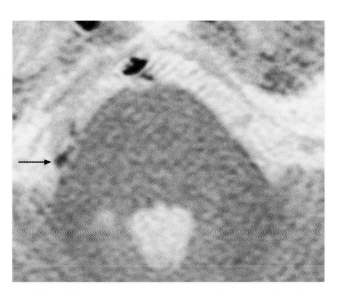

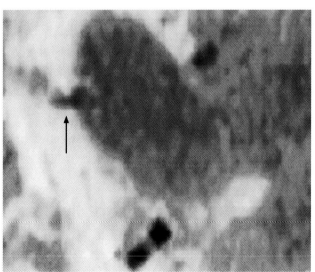

Fig. 20.**6**　MRI with volumetric acquisition of the origin of the V nerve shows the contact between the nerve and a blood vessel (possibly cerebellar) (arrows). **a** Horizontal section. **b** Sagittal section

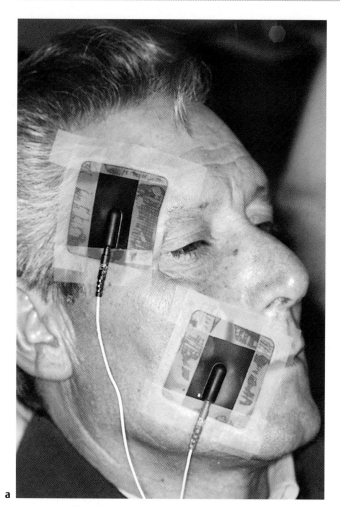
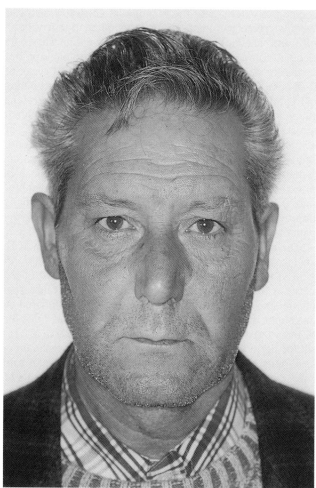

Fig. 20.**7**   After a TENS session (**a**) there is a partial and temporary improvement of the symptoms (**b**)

A probable case of SUNCT is that of a 52-year-old man, without headache precedents, who suffered from unilateral pain attacks in the right periorbital region. The attacks lasted from 60 to 120 seconds, they reached a maximum intensity after 10 seconds, and their frequency was about 30 per day. They were accompanied by a host of autonomic signs with conjunctival injection, lacrimation, edema, and eyelid ptosis (Fig. 20.**5**). The neurological examination was negative. MRI with volumetric acquisition of the origin of the trigeminal nerve showed a contact between the nerve and a blood vessel (possibly cerebellar) (Fig. 20.**6**). We must, however, consider this finding cautiously because it can sometimes be observed in symptom-free subjects. Treatments with carbamezapine (800 mg/day for three months), sumatriptan as needed, indomethacin (75 mg/day for 15 days) and various analgesics were totally ineffective. Partial and temporary comfort (for a few hours) with an abatement of the pain and the autonomic signs during the attacks was sometimes observed after application of TENS in the supraorbital and infraorbital region (Fig. 20.**7**).

Persistent Neuropathic Facial Pain

In other cases, neuropathic facial pain is more persistent and, often, less intense than neuralgic pain. It can be located in the gums and/or lips and cheek. It is frequently described as a burning pain. The differential diagnosis should be placed essentially with the somatoform pain disorder and the *burning*

mouth syndrome (Chapter 23), although it differs from them in that the neuropathic pain has stereotypical characteristics and conforms to the region of innervation of a sensory nerve. First-choice drugs are amitriptyline and clonazepam in increasing doses up to the minimum effective dose (generally not more than 50 mg divided into one or two daily dosages for amitriptyline and 2 mg divided into two or more daily dosages for clonazepam). In certain cases the two drugs can be used simultaneously. Good results against neuropathic pain were also reported with gabapentin, starting with 300 mg/day and gradually increasing to 900–1200 mg/day or more.

The next case describes neuropathic pain in the oral cavity, although various etiopathogenetic factors seem to be concurrent. The patient is a 69-year-old woman with latent diabetes, who for about eight years had complained of virtually constant burning pain in the gums of the left hemimandible, overlapped by a bothersome sense of a persistent salty taste in her mouth. Because of these symptoms the patient had undergone, without benefit, the removal of teeth, which left her totally edentulous (Fig. 20.**8**). She also had a gingival flap lifted for exploration. She reported intolerance of smells (especially perfumes), which, according to her, aggravated the symptoms notably. The symptoms also worsened under stress and when her blood glucose levels increased. In the past she had been treated for depression and reported that some years earlier the symptoms had worsened in a period in which she had also lost a lot of hair. She suffered from anxiety, palpitations, gastritis, sleep disorders, frequent fatigue, and depressed mood. The pain was therefore presumably neuropathic (because it was always lo-

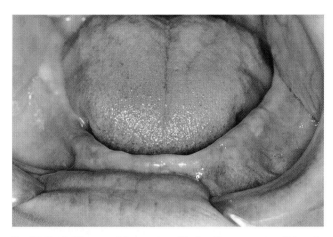

Fig. 20.**8**   **A 69-year-old woman suffering from neuropathic pain in the left mandible.** Due to her symptoms she had all her teeth removed. The gingival mucosa has a normal appearance

cated along the third trigeminal branch distribution and accentuated by particular stimulation) and perhaps favored by the latent diabetes. However, stressors also seemed to have a triggering or aggravating effect. Amitriptyline in drops were prescribed, two doses a day, 20 mg in the morning and 30 mg in the evening. The symptoms diminished considerably but there were fluctuating relapses.

In other cases, neuropathic facial pain takes on some of the characteristics of *sympathetically maintained pain.* Signs of circulatory alterations can be observed in the painful area (with palor or, more often, redness), dryness or sweating, dermographism, and fluctuating swellings (Fig. 20.**9**). In these cases it may be useful to prescribe, in addition to other drugs, slow-release clonidine patches (see Chapter 12). This treatment is naturally contraindicated in hypotensive patients.

A case of neuropathic pain with sympathetically maintained pain was seen in a 44-year-old woman, moderately hypertensive (blood pressure 150–100), who had suffered for about two years from a pain that originated in the left subauricular region and gradually spread to the genial, zygomatic, and temporal regions. Sometimes it extended to the area of the third lower molar. It was a constant burning and sometimes stabbing pain, often accompanied by redness and swelling in the subauricular and preauricular areas. Since she also had an intense, pulsating headache in the temporal region twice a month with nausea and vomiting, a cluster headache had previously been hypothesized and she was treated with cortisone derivatives, dihydroergotamine, propranolol, and inhalation of nascent oxygen, without any benefit. Nor did local anesthetic infiltrations produce any appreciable effect. The patient reported having had periods of depression, especially after a pregnancy (19 years earlier) and after the accidental death of her father five years earlier. She had numerous symptoms, some psychosomatic and some indicative of circulation disorders (Fig. 20.**10**). The neurological examination was negative. The MMPI-2 showed high scores on several "psychotic" scales (Fig. 20.**11**). This was therefore a relatively

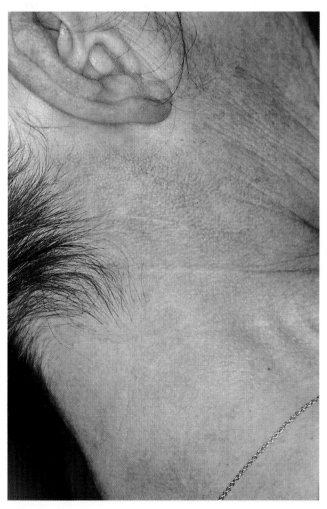

Fig. 20.**9**   Area of redness and fluctuating swelling in a patient with probable sympathetically maintained pain

Colitis	☐
Gastritis	☐
Kinetosis	☐
Swallowing difficulty	☐
Digestive problems	☐
Anorexia	☐
Bulimia	☒
Anxiety	☒
Phobias	☒
Sleep disorders	☒
Palpitations	☒
Panic attacks	☒
Mood changes	☒
Fainting	☐
Vertigo	☒
Lassitude	☒
Parafunctions	☒
Clonus	☐
Cramps	☐
Paresthesias	☒
Back pain	☒
Urination disturbances	☐
Diarrhea or constipation	☐
Nail fragility	☐
Hair fragility	☐
Circulation disorders	☒
Cold limbs	☒
Frigidity	☐
Vaginism	☐
Frequent depressed moods	☒
Other	☐

Fig. 20.**10**   **Patient with a multifactorial facial pain syndrome.** Numerous disturbances are present, some psychosomatic and some indicating circulating problems

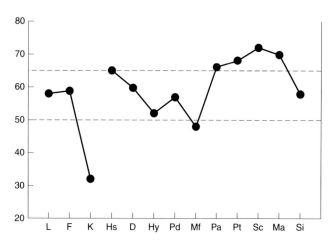

Fig. 20.**11**   The same patients as in Fig. 20.10. The MMPI shows high scores in the *psychotic* **scales**

References

Bogetto F., Maina G., Ferro G., Carbone M., Gandolfo S., *Psychiatric co-morbidity in patients with burning mouth syndrome (BMS)*. Psychosomatic Medicine, 1998, 60: 378 – 385.

Bouhasira D., Attal N., Esteve M., Chauvin M., *"SUNCT" syndrome. A case of transformation from trigeminal neuralgia?*, Cephalalgia, 1994, 14: 168 – 170.

Bussone G., Leone M., Dalla Volta G., Strada L., Gasparotti R., Di Monda V., *Shortlasting unilateral neuralgiform headache attaks with tearing and conjunctival injection: the first "symptomatic" case?*, Cephalalgia, 1991, 11: 123 – 127.

De Benedittis G., *SUNCT syndrome associated with cavernous angioma of the brain stem*, Cephalalgia, 1996, 16: 503 – 506.

International Headache Society, *Classification and diagnostic criteria for headache disorders, cranial neuralgias and facial pain*, Cephalalgia, 1988, 8 (Suppl. 7):1 – 96.

Meldrum B.S., *Pharmacology and mechanisms of action of lamotrigine*, in: Reynolds E.M., *Lamotriginem—a new advance in the treatment of epilepsy*. RSMS international congress and symposium series no. 204. London: Royal Society of Medicine Services, London, 1993.

Morales F., Mostacero E., Marta J., Sanchez S., *Vascular malformation of the cerebellopontine angle associated with "SUNCT" syndrome*, Cephalalgia, 1994, 14: 301 – 302.

Pareja J.A., Sjaastad O., *SUNCT syndrome in the female*, Headache, 1994, 34: 217 – 220.

Pareja J.A., Shen J.M., Kruszewski P., Caballero V., Pamo M., Sjaastad O., *SUNCT syndrome: duration, frequency, and temporal distribution of attacks*, Headache, 1996 a, 36: 161 – 165.

Pareja J.A., Caballero V., Sjaastad O., *SUNCT syndrome, statuslike pattern*, Headache, 1996 b, 36: 622 – 624.

Pareja J.A., Sjaastad O., *SUNCT syndrome. A clinical review*, Headache, 1997, 37: 195 – 202.

Sjaastad O., Russel D., Hørven I., Bunæs U., *Multiple neuralgiform, unilateral headache attacks associated with conjunctival injection and appearing in cluster. A nosological problem*, Proceedings of the Scandinavian Migrain Society, 1978, 31.

Sjaastad O., Saunte C., Salvesen R. et al., *Shortlasting unilateral neuralgiform headache attacks with conjunctival injection, tearing, sweating, and rhinorrhea*, Cephalalgia, 1989, 9: 147 – 156.

Sjaastad O., Zhao J.M., Kruszewski P., Stovner L.J., *Shortlasting unilateral neuralgiform headache attacks with conjunctival injection, tearing, etc. (SUNCT): III. Another Norwegian case*, Headache, 1991, 31: 175 – 7.

Sjaastad O., Kruszewski P., *Trigeminal neuralgia and "SUNCT" syndrome: similarities and differences in the clinical pictures. An overview*, Funct. Neurol., 1992, 7: 103 – 107.

Sjaastad O., Pareja J.A., Zukerman E., Jansen J., Kruszewski P., *Trigeminal neuralgia. Clinical manifestations of first division involvement*, Headache, 1997, 37: 346 – 357.

complex case in which a mood disorder was associated with facial pain that was presumably neuropathic with an autonomic component and concomitant episodic migraine.

Paroxetine (20 mg in the morning) and amitriptyline drops (20 mg in the evening) were prescribed. There was notable improvement of mood and an abatement of the headache symptoms. However, the burning pain, swelling and pain in the dental area persisted. Slow-release clonidine patches were prescribed and they eliminated the pain. Periodic headaches occurred, accompanied by intense lacrimation and palpebral ptosis, which were advantageously managed, considering the high minimum blood pressure value, with propranolol (200 mg twice a day for three months).

21 Myogenic Cervicofacial Pain

General Principles

Myogenic pain located in the cervical and/or craniofacial region is common, which is understandable if we consider that two local etiological factors, both highly prevalent in the population, can cause it: muscle hyperparafunctions and posture disorders of the skull, neck, and shoulders (see Chapters 3 and 4) and, as mentioned in Chapter 8, anxiety and/or depression can accentuate neuromuscular dysfunction.

Myogenic pain often has fluctuating duration and intensity, with alternating periods of acuteness and remission. Moreover, the patient frequently reports the persistence of slight pain or discomfort during the intercritical periods. Pain location can vary from one patient to the next and within the same patient, occurring sometimes in the preauricular and cheek area, and sometimes in the nuchal and cervical area. The pain can start at a given site and spread to the adjacent areas during the periods of maximal intensity. There are several possible triggering or aggravating factors: stress or situations that require intense concentration, meteorological changes or certain weather conditions (cold, humidity, wind), sports involving prolonges isometric contractions, and so on.

It is usually easy to diagnose myogenic pain from the history, clinical data, inspection for signs of muscular hyperparafunction, and/or posture alterations, and muscle palpation (see Chapter 10). If the pain is located in the preauricular and buccal region, the differential diagnosis is with the arthrogenic pain of the TMJ. Some diagnostic difficulty could arise when pain is accompanied by tonic–clonic spasms or contractions of the muscles (see below).

Therapy aims at reducing muscle contraction both by acting directly on the muscles and by removing or reducing the causes that originate such contraction. Physical therapy can be applied to the contracted muscle (TENS sessions, heat applications, cold sprays, stretching maneuvers, etc., as mentioned in Chapter 13), using topical medications (slow-releasing NAID applications) or general drug administration (muscle relaxants, see Chapter 12). If there is intense parafunctional activity, biofeedback sessions will be prescribed along with relaxation exercises and training in self-control of the degree of contraction of the craniocervical muscles.

However, as already mentioned in other contexts (especially for tension-type headache), it is important to remember that, in the presence of muscle hyperparafunction producing myogenic pain, there is a fundamental difference between the case of a person under stress but with a completely normal personality profile and that of a patient with a mood dysfunction of varying degrees of severity. While in the former case it is sufficient to apply the forms of therapy mentioned, in the latter case the psychological problem must also properly treated.

Myogenic Facial Pain Associated with Mouth Movement Limitation

Limited mouth movements are a frequent symptom accompanying myogenic pain originating from the elevator muscles (especially the masseter). This limitation is a consequence of muscle contraction caused by parafunctional habits. Sometimes in these cases the pain is erroneously attributed to a TMJ problem because various craniofacial muscles have pain projection areas that include the preauricular region.

Generally the differential diagnosis between myogenic and arthrogenic facial pain is easy (see Chapter 11). An extremely typical characteristic that differentiates myogenic from articular pain is that myogenic pain is rarely aggravated by normal mastication. It can, however, be aggravated by chewing particularly hard foods, because the elevator muscles are subjected to a more intense and prolonged contraction (with a greater amount of isometric contraction) (see Chapter 3). Normal chewing, on the other hand, is rhythmic, alternating between contraction and decontraction, which is why patients not infrequently report some pain relief while chewing. Upon inspection, there are signs of muscular hyperparafunction: unilateral or bilateral hypertrophy of the elevator muscles, dental abrasion, and scalloped tongue margins (see Chapter 10). Opening and lateral movements of the mouth might be limited. However, the restriction of opening movements can be overcome gradually by applying a gradual and constant finger pressure on the jaws (Fig. 11.**6**). It may be useful to apply a cold spray locally before starting to apply pressure. The limitation of lateral movements is in most cases symmetrical on both sides. An important discriminating factor in the history is whether onset was gradual or sudden: in the case of myogenic pain it is gradual (over a period a few hours or days) and in the case of articular disorder with a displaced disk it is usually sudden. Palpation of the muscles involved causes intense pain in most cases. Often *tender points* may be identified by palpation; these should be distinguished from *trigger points*. The latter are characterized by nodules or contraction bands which, when palpated, cause not only local pain but a local contractile response and referred pain in typical distant sites (see Chapter 3).

Two cases of myogenic facial pain associated with limited mouth opening in patients with different emotional components will be described. The first case is that of a 22-year-old woman, a university graduate, who had been complaining for about two years of a widespread bilateral buccal pain with a fluctuating trend, which had become more frequent over time. The pain was associated with a sense of constriction during mouth opening, which movement was limited (Fig. 21.**1**), and an occasional bilateral articular clicking sound. The symptoms worsened with cold, damp weather and with stress. A hypertrophy of the masseter and temporal muscles, especially on the right (Fig. 21.**2**), a marked abrasion of the upper right central incisor, and scalloped tongue edges (Fig. 21.**1**) were observed upon inspection. When the patient was asked to perform lateral movements of the mouth with her teeth touching, it was evident that the abrasion was caused by an accentuated grinding movement on the right side at night (Fig. 21.**3**). Palpation of the elevator muscles (masseters and temporal) and of the lateral pterygoid muscle caused intense pain.

The symptoms had started when the young woman had returned home after a gratifying period of study out of town.

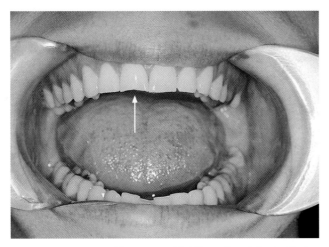

Fig. 21.**1** **A 22-year-old woman with bilateral genial pain.** Limitation of mouth opening, scalloped tongue edges and a marked abrasion of the upper central and right incisors (arrow) can be seen

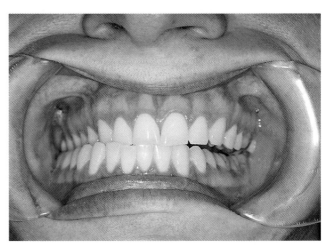

Fig. 21.**3** Grinding movement at night causing the dental abrasion shown in Fig. 21.**1**

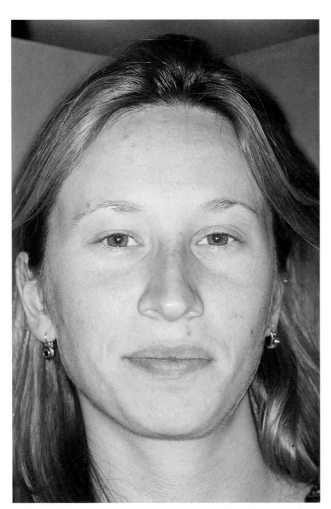

Fig. 21.**2** Hypertrophy of masseter and temporal muscles, especially on the right

She reported a slightly tense relationship with her father. Otherwise, she was an intelligent and enterprising woman who had no particular symptoms related to anxiety or depression. After the causes of her disturbances had been explained to her, the therapy prescribed was biofeedback, relaxation exercises to be done at home, and the regular practice of some

form of sport. The patient diligently followed this therapy and the symptoms disappeared within 20 days.

The second case is that of a 27-year-old woman, a university student who, 15 days before observation, had suffered a left TMJ condyle luxation at opening, which had regressed spontaneously within a short time. Nevertheless, a severe mouth opening limitation had occurred (with maximum opening capacity limited to 7–8 mm) (Fig. 21.**4**), together with complete abolition of the lateral movements and stabbing pain in the left buccal region. A marked hypertrophy of her masseter muscles was observed (Fig. 21.**5**) and in this case too palpation of the elevator muscles and the lateral pterygoid muscle was very painful.

The patient reported having suffered from depression in the past and, under stress, she had episodes of hypoparesthesia in the left hemiface, which at times spread to the entire left half of the body. She reported numerous psychosomatic symptoms (Fig. 21.**6**) and was in an evident state of anxiety and prostration. This was also because she had been diagnosed with a severe lesion of the TMJ which would probably require surgery. The anxiety and depression were confirmed by the MMPI and the STAI (Fig. 21.**7**).

History and clinical data pointed to a myogenic problem even though a concurrent disk displacement could not be entirely ruled out. Given the extremely reduced degree of open-

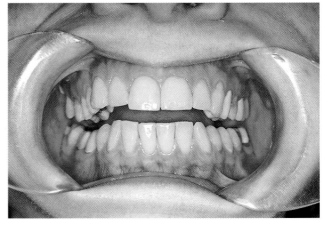

Fig. 21.**4** A 27-year-old woman with a severe limitation of the mouth opening movement

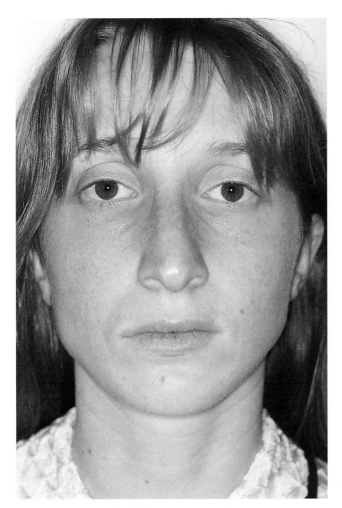

Fig. 21.**5**   Hypertrophy of the masseter muscles

Colitis	☒
Gastritis	☐
Kinetosis	☒
Swallowing difficulty	☐
Digestive problems	☐
Anorexia	☐
Bulimia	☒
Anxiety	☒
Phobias	☒
Sleep disorders	☒
Palpitations	☒
Panic attacks	☒
Mood changes	☒
Fainting	☒
Vertigo	☒
Lassitude	☐
Parafunctions	☒
Clonus	☒
Cramps	☐
Paresthesias	☒
Back pain	☒
Urination disturbances	☐
Diarrhea or constipation	☒
Nail fragility	☒
Hair fragility	☒
Circulation disorders	☐
Cold limbs	☒
Frigidity	☐
Vaginism	☐
Frequent depressed moods	☒
Other	☐

Fig. 21.**6**   Complaints reported by the patient

ing, the severe aching of every movement, and the psychological situation of the patient, it was decided to temporarily postpone any examination of joint visualization. The patient was first of all reassured and informed that there was no need for surgery in any case. She underwent a TENS session with the electrodes applied corresponding to the masseters, and this was followed by a biofeedback session. Relaxation exer-

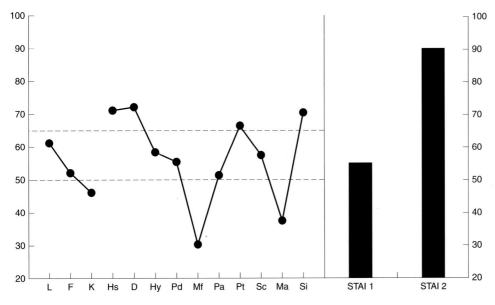

Fig. 21.**7**   MMPI-2 scores regarding hypochondria, depression, anxiety, and social introversion are high. STAI shows high state and trait anxiety levels

cises were prescribed, along with hot packs, the practice of sporting activity, and tablets of 10 mg amitriptyline and 2 mg perfenanzine, starting with half a tablet in the evening and increasing the dose gradually every three or four days up to half a tablet in the morning and one in the evening. At a check-up 15 days later, mouth opening had already improved (Fig. 21.**8**) and there were no signs of articular disfunction, so further in-

vestigation in that direction was deferred. Within two months there was an almost total remission of the symptoms. The pain had practically disappeared and mouth movements were normal (Fig. 21.**9**). The patient also reported the reduction or disappearance of most of the psychosomatic symptoms (Fig. 21.**10**) and her mood improvement was confirmed by the normal MMPI and STAI scores (Fig. 21.**11**).

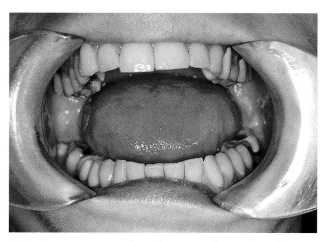

Fig. 21.**8**   Improvement of mouth opening after 15 days of therapy

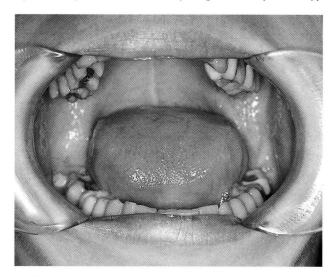

Fig. 21.**9**   Normalization of mouth opening at end of therapy

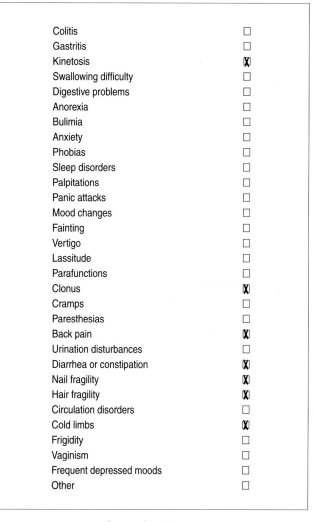

Colitis	☐
Gastritis	☐
Kinetosis	☒
Swallowing difficulty	☐
Digestive problems	☐
Anorexia	☐
Bulimia	☐
Anxiety	☐
Phobias	☐
Sleep disorders	☐
Palpitations	☐
Panic attacks	☐
Mood changes	☐
Fainting	☐
Vertigo	☐
Lassitude	☐
Parafunctions	☐
Clonus	☒
Cramps	☐
Paresthesias	☐
Back pain	☒
Urination disturbances	☐
Diarrhea or constipation	☒
Nail fragility	☒
Hair fragility	☒
Circulation disorders	☐
Cold limbs	☒
Frigidity	☐
Vaginism	☐
Frequent depressed moods	☐
Other	☐

Fig. 21.**10**   Remission of most disturbances previously reported by patient (see Fig. 21.**6**)

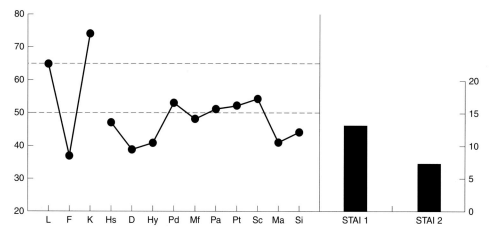

Fig. 21.**11**   MMPI and STAI show improvement of personality profile

Myogenic Craniocervical Pain

Cervical myogenic pain is favored by posture problems. Especially in young patients, it can occur without any lesions whatsoever to the cervical vertebrae, though it is common to find a partial or total loss of cervical lordosis to which a scoliotic posture of the spine can sometimes be associated (see Chapter 4). On the other hand, the coexistence of a neuromuscular and postural problem is frequent, and this explains why the myogenic pain can originate in the face (often in the cheek) and spread during the acute phases to the neck and shoulders on one or both sides. Trigger points and, to a greater extent, tender points are quite common in the long craniocervical muscles (the sternocleidomastoid and trapezius in particular) (Figs. 3.**33** – 3.**36**). It should be pointed out, however, that after a whiplash trauma, pain originating in a zygoapophyseal joint between the cervical vertebrae can be observed (with characteristics very similar to the trigger points) (Aprill et al., 1990; Aprill and Bogduk, 1992; Bogduk and Aprill, 1993) (see Chapter 3). Moreover, the presence of vertebrae alterations can be associated with neuromuscular alterations and complicate the overall symptom picture (Figs. 21.**12**, 21.**13**).

A case presenting characteristics that are often observed is that of a 20-year-old woman, a university student, who had suffered for about six years from pain in the cervical and nuchal region, spreading to the shoulders and back (Fig. 21.**14**). The pain was virtually continuous (Fig. 21.**15**), pressing, and of moderate or medium intensity except for rare episodes of acute pain. Aggravating factors were stress and sitting down for long periods. Upon inspection, the shoulders were somewhat uneven, with he right shoulder higher than the left, a slight twist of the head toward the right and contraction of the long muscles of the neck, especially the left sternocleidomastoid (Fig. 21.**16**). The postural defect was confirmed by the cervical radiograph in front–rear projection (Fig. 21.**17**). Palpation of the sternocleidomastoid and trapezius muscles was painful. The patient suffered occasionally from colitis and thermoregulation dysfunction but apart from that she reported no particular psychosomatic disturbances.

An intense physical therapy program was prescribed: TENS, cold spray on points of maximum aching, mild cervical traction and posture exercises to be performed several times a day (see Chapter 13). Tizanidine was also prescribed, 2 mg in the morning and 3 mg in the evening for three months. Improvement was slow and gradual, with a significant reduction in the intensity and frequency of the pain within eight months

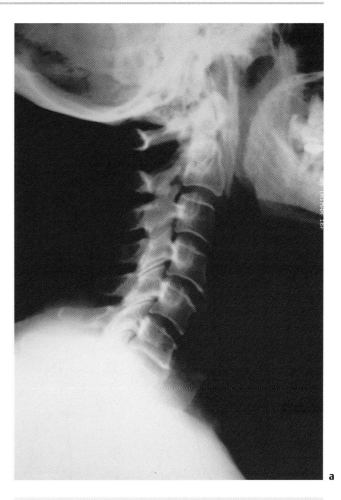

a

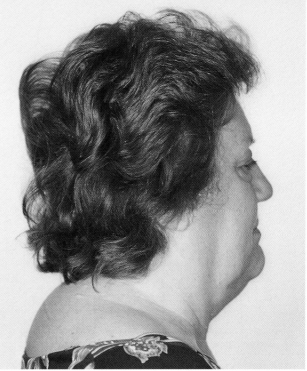

b

Fig. 21.**13**   Same case as in Fig. 21.**12**. In this patient an alteration of the cervical column (**a**) overlaps with a resulting severe posture disorder (**b**)

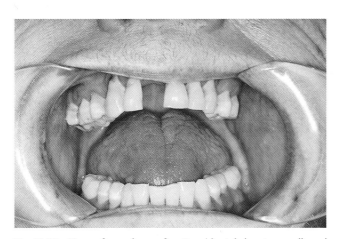

Fig. 21.**12**   Signs of muscle parafunction (dental abrasion, scalloped tongue) in woman with diffused and constant craniofacial pain

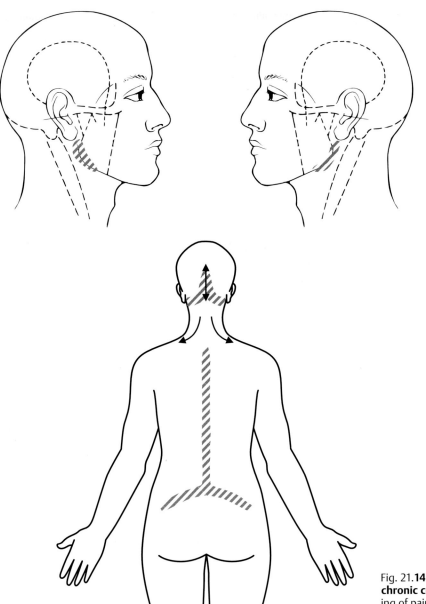

Fig. 21.14   A 22-year-old patient suffering from chronic cerviconuchal pain. Primary sites and spreading of pain

NAME: I. D.																																			
DATE: MAY			6	7	8	9	10	11	12	13	14	15	16	17	18	19	20	21	22	23	24	25	26	27	28	29	30	31	1	2	3	4	5
PAIN	5																																	
	4																				X	X												
	3								X	X		X	X																				
	2			X		X	X	X	X				X		X								X		X	X	X		X	X		X		
	1		X		X					X							X	X	X			X				X			X		X		X
	0															X																		
Pain duration (hours)			T	3	T	5	7	T	7	10	4	T	2	5	5	T		T	T	T	3	1	4	T	6	T	5	T	T	T	T	3	T

Fig. 21.**15**   Pain diary of the patient

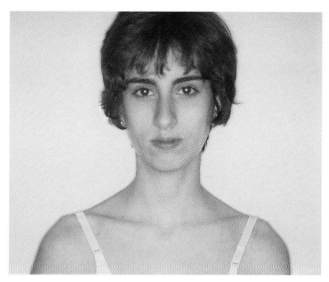

Fig. 21.**16**   A posture defect can be observed with hyperactivity of the cervical muscles

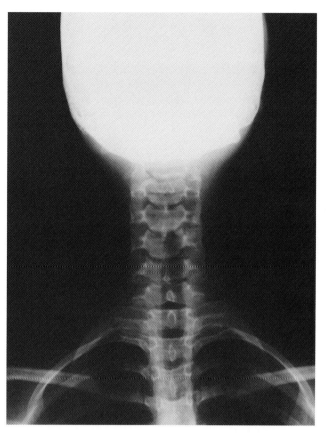

Fig. 21.**17**   Cervical radiograph shows a moderate scoliosis

(Fig. 21.**18**). On discharge, the patient was recommended to continue the posture exercises indefinitely.

A much more severe case of myogenic cervicofacial pain associated with a wide range of symptoms is that of a 21-year-old woman, a university student, whose problems had started a year and a half earlier, after a period of intense and prolonged stress (she was intelligent and headstrong and, when she was still at school, she had been not only the best student but also the only woman in her class). At that time she had started to suffer from pangs of intense pain in the right occipitonuchal and cervical region (Fig. 21.**19**) lasting from seconds to minutes, with frequency varying from one to two or three attacks per hour (increasing in the afternoon) and permanent marked aching in the intercritical period. The pain was associated with severe subjective vertigo with a sensation of falling to the ground (although this did not occur). The symptoms worsened concomitantly with orthodontic treatment.

The patient reported frequently waking up fatigued with marked aching in the right half of the body. She also suffered from drowsiness, thermoregulation dysfunction, anxiety, panic attacks, cramps, paresthesia of hands and feet, back pain, hair loss, and dysmenorrhea. She was acrophobic and experienced a morbid and disquieting sense of attraction to "the Void." At the neurological examination it was impossible for her to remain standing during the sensitized Romberg test. Other alterations were not found. The EEG was spiky but without any slowing or signs of focality.

Upon inspection, a marked postural problem was noted both on the frontal plane, and the sagittal plane (Fig. 21.**20**). Typical signs of parafunction were also evident: hypertrophy of the elevator muscles (Fig. 21.**21**) and scalloped tongue edges (Fig. 21.**22**). Opening of the mouth was 38 mm without pain and 42 mm with pain at the cheeks. Palpation of all the craniocervical muscles on the right caused distinct pain. The cervical radiography showed the loss of the cervical curve with a tendency to its inversion (Fig. 21.**23**). The MMPI showed a typical *conversive V* with high hypochondria and hysteria scores (Fig. 21.**24**).

NAME: I. D.																																
DATE: MAR		1	2	3	4	5	6	7	8	9	10	11	12	13	14	15	16	17	18	19	20	21	22	23	24	25	26	27	28	29	30	31
PAIN	5																																
	4																																
	3																X																
	2					X			X	X								X									X	X	X	X	X	X	
	1	X	X	X	X	X	X		X	X			X	X	X	X		X	X	X	X	X	X	X	X								
	0																																
Pain duration (hours)		T	T	T	T	T	T	T	T	T	T	T	T	T	T	T	T	T	T	T	T	T	T	T	T	T	T	T	T	T	T	T	T

Fig. 21.**18**   Considerable improvement of symptoms after eight months, but with a residue of virtually constant but moderate aching

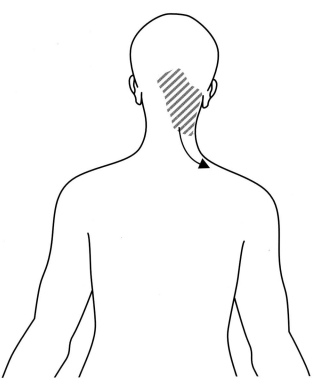

Fig. 21.**19**   A 21-year-old woman with pangs of intense nuchal pain spreading to right cervical region

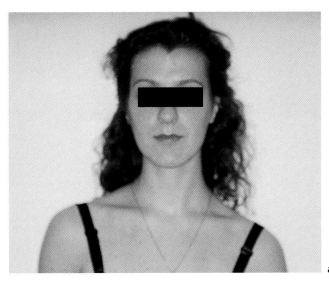

a

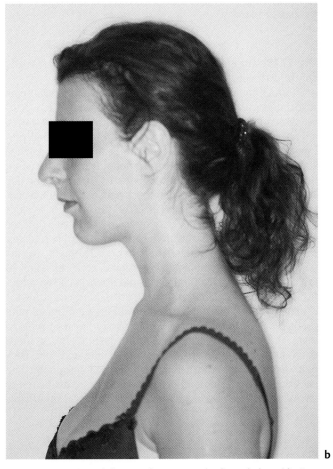

b

Fig. 21.**20**   Posture defect can be seen on the frontal plane (distinct unevenness of shoulders) (**a**) and sagittal plane (head falling forward) (**b**)

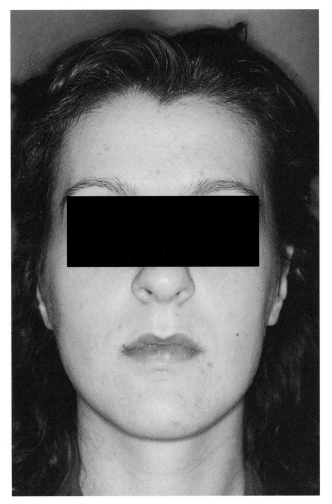

Fig. 21.**21**   Hypertrophy of masseter and temporal muscles

This was thus a case of myogenic pain in the cerviconuchal region aggravated by the posture problem and parafunctional habits, the latter causing fatigue and, consequently, pain to muscles already predisposed to fatigue and pain by the postural deviation. This explained the prevalence of pain on one side. However, unlike the case described above, in this case there was a distinct psychological component, at least an anxiety disorder, which required treatment as such. Another important characteristic was the history of an exacerbation of

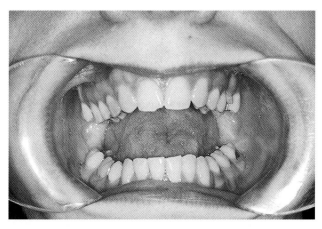

Fig. 21.**22** Scalloped tongue edges

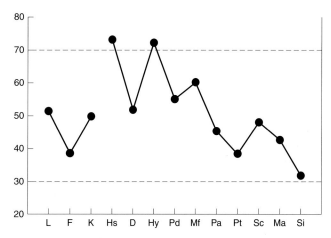

Fig. 21.**24** MMPI hypochondria (Hs) and hysteria (Hy) scores are high with a *conversive V*

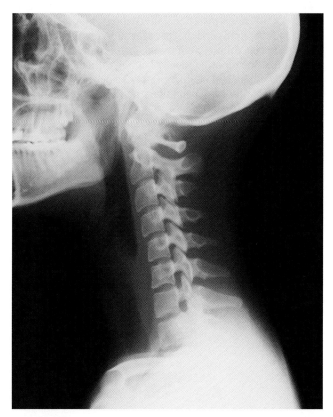

Fig. 21.**23** Cervical radiogram shows curve inversion tendency

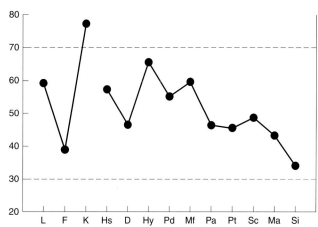

Fig. 21.**25** **Normalization of the MMPI profile after therapy.** A *conversive V* remains but with normal scores on the various scales

the symptoms concomitantly with a particularly invasive dental treatment.

The nondrug therapy prescribed was a series of biofeedback sessions, anesthetic injections of the tender points of the long muscles of the neck, mild cervical traction, relaxation and posture exercises daily, and regular swimming. The drug therapy was alprazolam 0.25 mg ($^1/_2$ tablet) bromazepam 0.5 mg in drops, ademetionine 200 mg, all in two doses, morning and evening. There was a gradual improvement in the following months, although there were a few relapses of symptoms related to stressful events. Six months after the beginning of therapy, attacks of vertigo and acute pain episodes had virtually disappeared and the spontaneous pain and tenderness at palpation were substantially reduced. Mood had improved with a significant remission of the anxiety symptoms. After one year, during which the patient had proceeded with the exercise program and the drug therapy continued (except

for brief periods) at half the original dosage, a check-up was conducted and the situation appeared to have stabilized. This was confirmed by the MMPI and the STAI test, conducted again at that time (Fig. 21.**25**).

Myogenic Pain Associated with Tonic-Clonic Spasms or Contractions

Myogenic pain, especially if chronic and intense, can in certain cases be associated with dystonic or spastic phenomena and/or episodes of tonic–clonic contraction that can create problems in differential diagnosis. There even may be doubt whether it is a case of epiphenomen of the primary neuromuscular disturbance or true overlapping pathologies (dystonia, focal epilepsy, etc.). Naturally, these situations should be distinguished from brief spastic contractions which, as seen in Chapter 20, can be evoked by neuralgic pain in facial muscles on the affected side. In fact, facial spasms may result from various neurological disturbances–alterations in the processes of the central nervous system (Delwaide and Oliver, 1987; Playford et al., 1992), tumors located in the brain stem (Lipkin et al., 1987; Levin and Lee, 1987), dysplasia of the temporal bone (Benecke, 1993)–or they may be sequelae of a facial palsy (Biglan et al., 1988; Kawai, 1989).

It is nonetheless relatively frequent to find spastic phenomena in patients with chronic and intense muscle pain resulting from marked neuromuscular dysfunction. These spasms and contractions can occur in the muscles subject to parafunction or in adjacent muscle groups.

Blepharospasms are commonly observed, characterized by intermittent or sustained lowering of the eyelids by involuntary contraction of the orbicular muscle (Fig. 21.**26**). In other patients, spasms and dyskinesia of the labial (Fig. 21.**27**), lingual (Fig. 21.**28**) or facial (Fig. 21.**29**) muscles may be observed.

Besides the extremely marked parafunctional habits, in these patients there is usually a prominent psychological factor as well (mood disorders and sometimes personality disorders); it is therefore advisable to treat the neuromuscular and psychological problem and evaluate whether to combine other therapies generally prescribed for dystonia (such as infiltration of botulinum A toxin) immediately or later.

Two complex cases will be described in which acute myogenic pain was associated with marked dyskinesias. The first case is that of a 29-year-old woman who started to suffer from facial pain five years before observation, after the extraction of a molar tooth. The pain was moderate to severe, located in both cheeks but more intense on the left. During those five years the patient was subjected to a sequence of dental treatments that were entirely inappropriate and unjustified, with tooth grinding and orthodontic movement. These treatments

caused a severe alteration of her dental contact (Fig. 21.**30**). The symptoms worsened progressively and after two years she had tonic–clonic contraction of the left masseter which spread to the orofacial and cervical regions on the same side (Fig. 21.**31**). At the time of observation, these phenomena occurred with a frequency varying from five to more than 20 times an hour but did not occur at night. The duration of the attacks varied from one minute to several minutes. The patient reported that she could provoke the motor phenomena at will and, to some extent, postpone the onset. Furthermore, she felt a compulsion to provoke them. After each episode of facial pain, always acute, the pain diminished for a brief period, though it remained at moderate to severe levels.

In the course of previous consultations, the patient had been offered local infiltrations of botulinum A toxin or, as an alternative, a neuroleptic drug (pimozid) orally. She had refused both treatments. She had dropped out of university and was in an evident state of anxiety and depression. She suffered from sleep disorders, alternating bulimia and anorexia, claustrophobia and the fear of "going crazy," paresthesia of the limbs, colitis, abdominal pain, palpitations, and vaginismus. She reported having been a "difficult" child with bizarre ideas. She had been very close to her father, who had recently died. She took painkillers daily in large quantities, but obtained no relief from them.

The neurological examination was negative, whereas palpation of the entire craniocervicofacial musculature caused

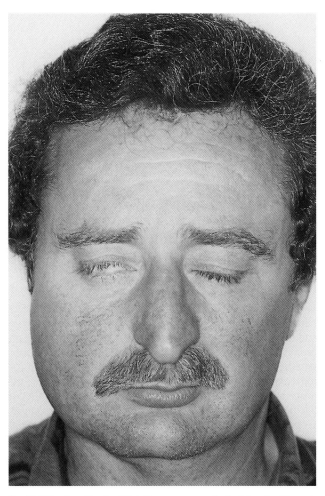

Fig. 21.**26   A patient with intense myogenic facial pain.** There is an extremely marked hypertrophy of the right masseter and frequent blepharospasm

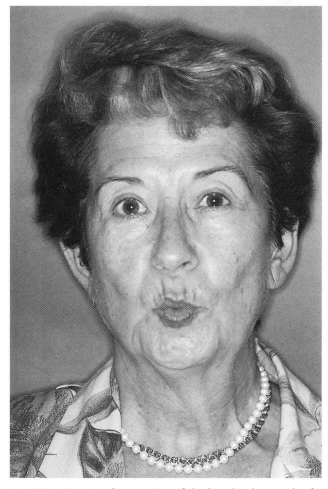

Fig. 21.**27**   Occasional contraction of the lip orbicular muscle of a patient with myogenic facial pain

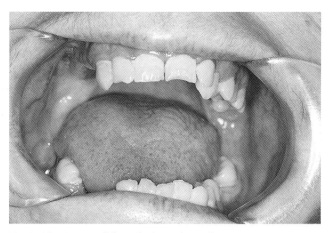

Fig. 21.**28**   Spasm of the right lingual muscles

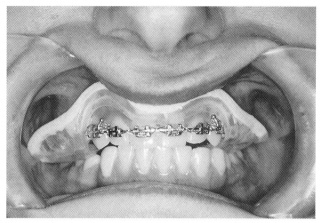

Fig. 21.**30**   **A patient with severe myogenic pain and spasms of orofacial musculature.** After a series of incongruous dental treatments, tooth contact is completely altered and the patient requires a type of brace in her mouth

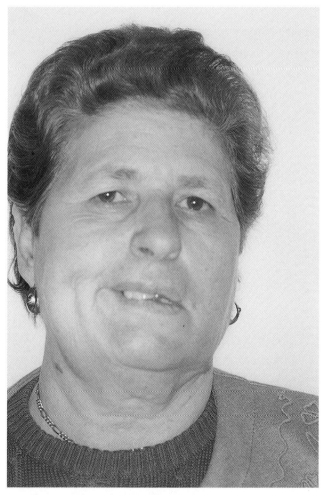

Fig. 21.**29**   Spasm of the orofacial muscles

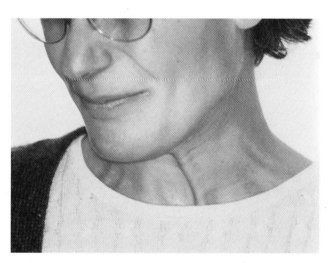

Fig. 21.**31**   **Same patient as in Fig. 21.30.** Tonic-clonic contraction of masseter with spreading to orofacial and cervical region

intense pain. Moreover, palpation of certain muscle spots triggered the motor attacks.

Both the MMPI and the STAI showed very high scores. In particular, the MMPI depression and schizophrenia scores were extremely high (Fig. 21.32).

This was therefore a case in which the intense and prolonged contraction of the craniofacial muscles occurred in a patient with a marked psychological disturbance; a triggering

and aggravating factor had been the inappropriate and invasive dental treatment. The characteristics of the motor phenomena and the possibility, within limits, to plan them, excluded the hypothesis of dystonia. Nor did the hypothesis of a tic seem appropriate. The psychological problem as a primary factor and the concomitance of other somatic disturbances made it plausible to define the case as *pain disorder as a somatoform disorder* (see Chapter 23). However, in this case the major source of pain was muscular, which is why it is being reported in this chapter.

Amitriptyline was prescribed at incremental doses up to 150 mg/day in three doses, and 0.50 mg alprazolam twice a day. The patient was also placed on a psychotherapy program and intensive nondrug therapy was prescribed: biofeedback (to which she responded very positively), relaxation exercises and moderate sports (swimming). Subsequently, there were periods of distinct improvement alternating with relapses of the episodes of pain and motor impediment in the lower limbs. Nevertheless, two years later the contraction episodes had become much less frequent, mood had improved and the psychosomatic symptoms had subsided. The patient was able to go back to university.

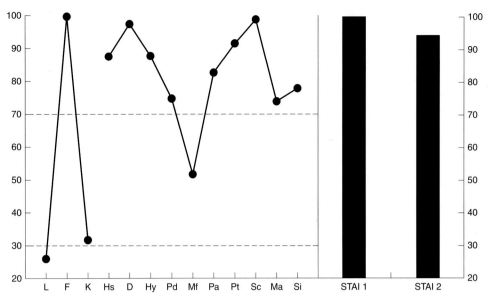

Fig. 21.**32** **Same patient as in Fig. 21.30.** MMPI and STAI scores confirm presence of a marked personality disorder

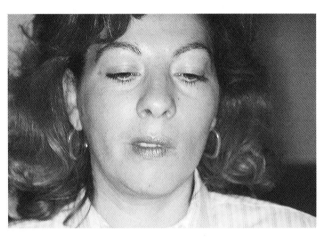

Fig. 21.**33** A 32-year-old woman suffering from attacks of tonic-clonic contractions in the right perioral and buccal regions

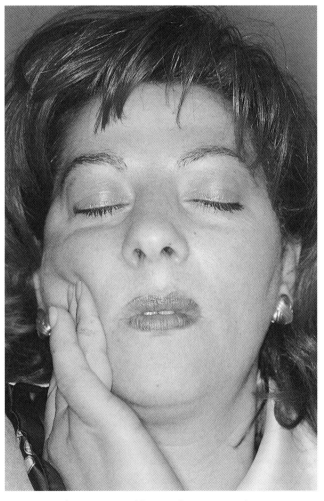

Fig. 21.**34** The patient is able to reduce or stop the contractions with digital pressure on the cheek

The second case is that of a 32-year-old woman who for eight years had suffered from tonic – clonic contractions in the perioral and right buccal regions (Fig. 21.**33**). The symptoms had started during a pregnancy and varied over time in intensity, duration, and frequency, with more acute periods in spring and autumn. The patient was hospitalized, diagnosed with focal epilepsy, and prescribed treatment with anticonvulsive drugs. At the time of observation, she was taking carbamezapine 400 mg and clonazepam 3 mg three times a day. The attacks were extremely frequent (about one every three minutes) and lasted from 30 to 60 seconds. It is interesting to note that the patient could often interrupt the attack with digital pressure applied to the buccal region (Fig. 21.**34**). The neurological examination was negative and so were the EEG (Fig. 21.**35**) and the evoked potentials. There was a trigger point on the right masseter, which upon palpation caused a sharp pain locally and in the hemiface and could trigger the motor attack.

While the patient continued with the drug therapy, a series of anesthetic infiltrations were applied to the trigger point. There was a distinct reduction and subsequent disappearance of the episodes for the next ten months, during which the dose of carbamezapine was halved.

Later she had alternating relapses and improvements. During the relapses the dosage of carbamezapine was increased. Three years later, during a particularly severe attack, the patient was again hospitalized. EEG conducted on this occasion showed the presence of focal spikes and waves in the

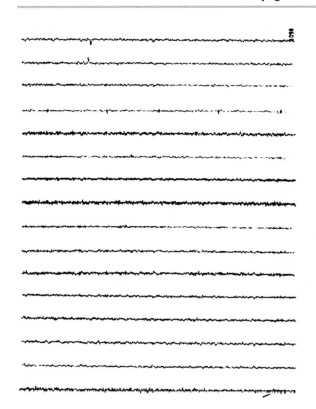

Fig. 21.**35**   Normal EEG result

left centrotemporal region (Fig. 21.**36**). Intensive treatment with anticonvulsant drugs was prescribed and a check-up a few days later showed that these alterations had almost entirely disappeared (Fig. 21.**37**).

Unlike the patient described previously, it seems that this patient had two coexistent pathologies: a focal epilepsy and a local myogenic problem (evidenced by the trigger point and the response to anesthetic infiltration). It is possible that this problem, overlapping an epileptogenic focus, acted as a triggering or aggravating factor of episodes of the tonic–clonic contraction.

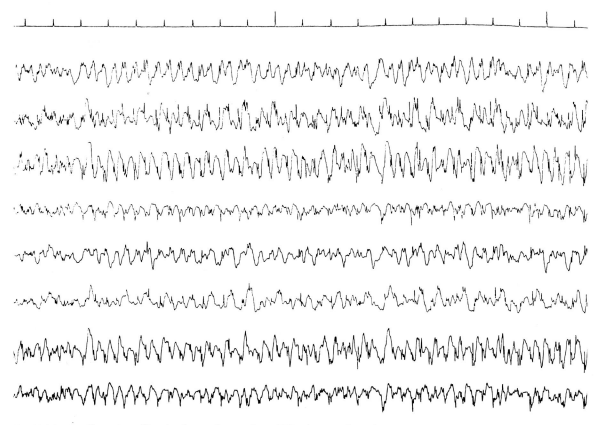

Fig. 21.**36**   Manifestation of focal spikes and waves in an EEG taken at a later time

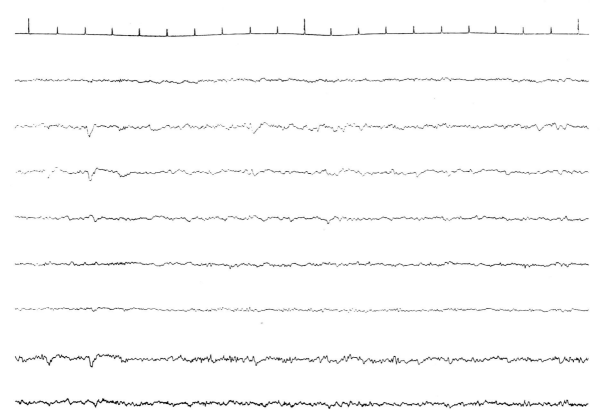

Fig. 21.**37**   Improvement of EEG result after a few days of therapy with anticonvulsive drugs

References

Aprill C., Dwyer A., Bogduk N., *Cervical zygapophyseal joint pain patterns, II., A clinical evaluation*, Spine, 1990, 15 : 458 – 461.

Aprill C., Bogduk N., *The prevalence of cervical zygapophysial joint pain: a first approximation*, Spine, 1992, 17 : 744 – 747.

Benecke J.E. Jr., *Facial nerve dysfunction in osteopetrosis*, Laryngoscope, 1993, 103 : 494 – 497.

Biglan A.W., May M., Bowers R.A., *Management of facial spasm with Clostridium botulinum toxin, type A (Oculinum)*, Arch. Otolaryngol. Neck Surg., 1988, 114 : 1407 – 1412.

Bogduk N., Aprill C., *On the nature of neck pain, discography and cervical zygapophysial joint blocks*, Pain, 1993, 54 : 213 – 217.

Delwaide P.J., Oliver E., *Pathophysiological aspects of spasticity in man*, in: Benencke R., Conrad B., Marsden C.D. (eds.), Academic Press, London, 1987, 153 – 196.

Kawai M., *Sequelae and transient sequelae-like symptoms in Bell's palsy*, Nippon Jibiinkoka Gakkai Kaiho, Tokyo, 1989, 92 : 88 – 92.

Levin J.M., Lee J.E., *Hemifacial spasm due to cerebellopontine angle lipoma: case report*, Neurology, 1987, 37 : 337 – 339.

Lipkin A.F., Coker N.J., Jenkins H.A., Alford B.R., *Intracranial and intratemporal facial neuroma*, Otolaryngol. Head Neck Surg., 1987, 96 : 71 – 79.

Playford E.D., Pasingham R.E., Marsden C.D., Brooks D.J., *Abnormal activation of striatum and dorsolateral prefrontal cortex in dystonia [abstract]*, Neurology, 1992, 42 (Suppl. 3):377.

22 Arthrogenous Facial Pain

General Principles

Temporomandibular joint (TMJ) lesions induce pain by activating the auriculotemporal nerve nociceptors in the joint capsule and retrodiskal attachment.

TMJ pathology may a consequence of genetic, congenital, or acquired factors. TMJ morphofunctional alterations resulting from nonmacrotraumatic, nontumoral, and noninfectious events are essentially disk displacement, disk compression, and TMJ arthrosis.

Disk displacement is the TMJ disorder most frequently observed. As we have seen (see Chapters 3 and 4), it is a consequence of anatomic and functional alterations between the mandibular condyle and disk. In the great majority of cases, disk displacement occurs ahead of and medial to the condyle.

Disk displacement produces a sprain or tearing of the posterior attachment and the disk–condyle attachments. The displacement may be partial, if the posterior sector of the disk is ahead of the superior condylar pole, or may be total if this sector is displaced ahead of the anterior condyle border. A distinction is made between disk displacement with and without reduction.

In *disk displacement with reduction* the disk–condyle relationship is altered at closed mouth but becomes normal when the mouth is fully opened. With the mouth closed, the disk is in most of the cases located ahead of and medially respect to the condyle. During mouth opening, the tension of the elastic fibers of the posterior attachment overcomes the resistance opposed by the condyle and the articular eminence, which are in closer than normal reciprocal position, and the disk is suddenly drawn backwards (Fig. 22.**1**). This produces a typical "clicking noise." During mouth closure, the disk is again displaced ahead of the condyle with a second "reciprocal click."

Disk displacement with reduction may be followed by *disk displacement without reduction*. In this situation, the disk does not acquire its normal position at open mouth but stays displaced during all opening movements (Fig. 22.**2**); the opening movement is consequently restricted and deviated toward the lesion side. Obviously, no clicking noise occurs. In disk displacement without reduction, the lesions of the posterior attachment and of the disk–condyle attachments are aggravated. With time, disk deformities and perforation may follow (Fig. 22.**3**), together with adhesions between the superior aspect of the disk and the glenoid fossa (Figs. 22.**4**, 22.**5**). TMJ arthrosis may eventually follow (see later).

In other cases, alterations of the disk–condyle relationship occur mainly along the vertical plane, with upward condyle displacement and resulting increase of the compressive forces on the disk, which is not displaced, at least at first (Fig. 22.**6**). This may be the consequence of partial edentulousness or dental attrition due to severe parafunction. In this case also, TMJ arthrosis may eventually follow.

Arthrosis is a noninflammatory, primarily degenerative process leading to typical soft-tissue and hard-tissue alterations. As the process worsens, macroscopic morphological changes occur, including loss of substance and interruptions of the articular surface, which becomes progressively more irregular; in addition the underlying tissues become altered by formation of horizontal and vertical fissures. This produces thinning of the articular cartilage with denudation of the underlying bone (Fig. 22.**7**). These changes are then visible radiologically (Fig. 22.**8**).

An inflammatory process may overlap arthrotic degeneration in the synovium (synovitis), in the capsule (capsulitis) and/or in the posterior attachment (retrodiskitis). Such aseptic inflammation may occur as a reaction to a tissue lesion or to disk displacement (Fig. 22.**9**).

The diagnosis of TMJ dysfunction is based on data from the history and the clinical and radiographic examinations. Of the anamnestic data, those relating to the onset and evolution of

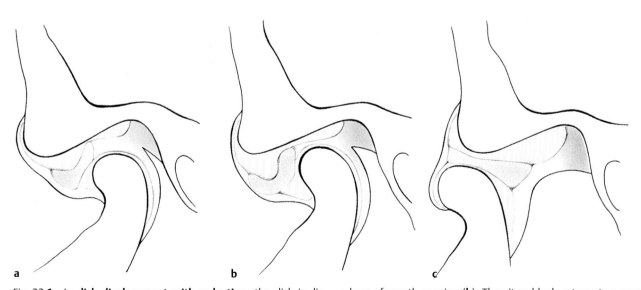

a   b   c

Fig. 22.**1** In **disk displacement with reduction,** the disk is displaced ahead of the condyle at closed mouth (**a**) and during a first phase of mouth opening (**b**). Then it suddenly returns to a normal position (**c**), producing a characteristic clicking noise

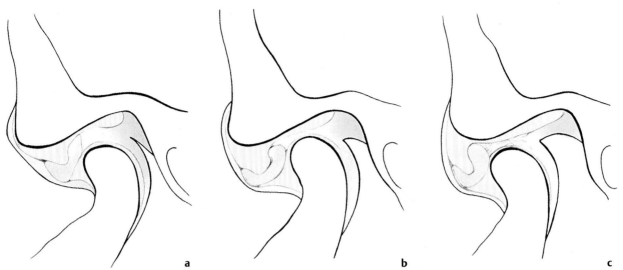

Fig. 22.2 In disk displacement without reduction, the disk is displaced ahead of the condyle at closed mouth (**a**) and during moderate (**b**) and maximal (**c**) mouth opening. The opening movement is consequently restricted

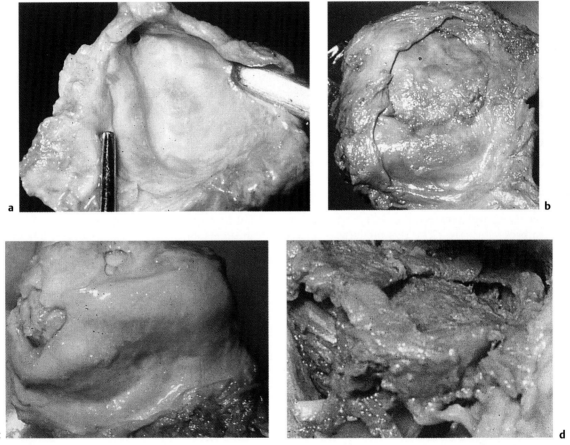

Fig. 22.3 Autopsy specimens with disk deformity (**a**) and perforations (**b–d**) resulting from disk displacement. (Courtesy of I. Grunert, University of Innsbruck.)

joint noises, pain worsening during mastication of normal or hard food and occurrence of a sudden mouth opening impediment are particularly important. The more relevant clinical findings are jaw movement limitation and/or alterations; pain at palpation of the articular points and, in particular, of the retrocondylar aspect at open mouth (Fig. 10.**18**); and joint noises. In disk displacement with reduction, a characteristic clicking noise occurs during mouth opening: this noise disap-

pears if the opening movement is performed after closing into a protruded position, because, by doing this, the patient keeps the disk in the correct position. On conventional radiography performed at closed mouth, if a structural factor is present (see Chapter 4) there may be evidence of asymmetrical condyle position, the condyle of the lesion side being positioned more posteriorly. At open mouth, a normal condylar excursion is observed bilaterally. In cases consequent on neuro-

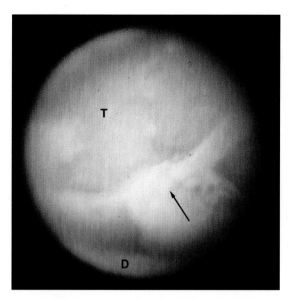

Fig. 22.**4** **Arthroscopic view of a TMJ upper compartment.** Areas of adesion (arrow) are observed between the disk (D) and the articular tuber (T). (Courtesy of Dr. R. Romagnoli and F. Secco, University of Turin)

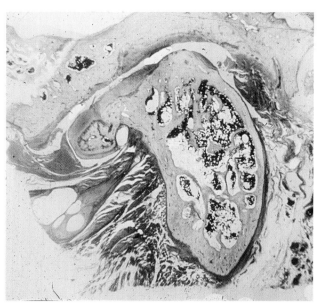

Fig. 22.**7** Extensive TMJ arthrotic lesion with destruction of the disk and of a great part of the articular cartilage (Courtesy of Professor G. Steinhard, Erlangen)

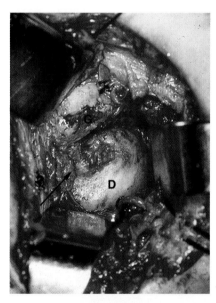

Fig. 22.**5** **Open surgery of the TMJ:** ares of adhesion (arrow) between the disk (D) and the glenoid fossa (G). (Courtesy of Professor F. Mela, University of Turin)

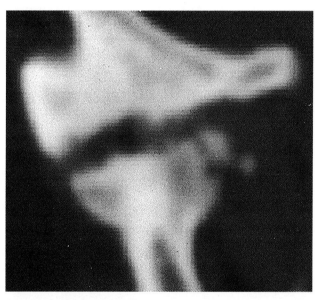

Fig. 22.**8** **TMJ tomography;** coronal view. A severe arthrotic degeneration of the condyle and the glenoid fossa is observed

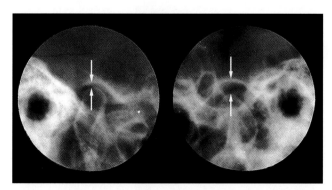

Fig. 22.**6** **TMJ radiography in a case of right disk compression.** Note the definite ipsilateral joint space reduction (arrows)

muscular dysfunction (see Chapter 3), no specific radiographic signs are detected. Only MRI shows a disk displaced ahead of the condyle at closed mouth and in normal position at open mouth. However, MRI is totally unnecessary for a correct diagnosis.

In disk displacement without reduction, typically the disappearance of a joint click coincides with a sudden limitation of mouth opening. Moreover, during mouth opening a deviation toward the lesion side is observed (Fig. 22.**10**) (which is not observed in case of movement impediment due to myogenous pain). MRI shows the disk displaced ahead of the condyle at closed and open mouth (Fig. 22.**11**). Conventional radiography at open mouth shows a definite reduction of condyle excursion on the lesion side with respect to the opposite side (Fig. 22.**12**).

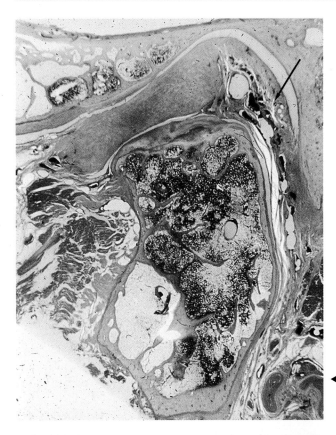

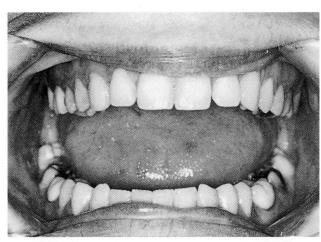

Fig. 22.**10   A woman of 21 years of age with disk displacement without reduction of the right TMJ.** On inspection, a typical limitation of mouth opening with deviation towards the lesion side is visible

◀ Fig. 22.**9   TMJ section with posterior condyle displacement.** Inflammatory signs with congestion and edema are observed in the posterior attachment (arrow). (Courtesy of Professor G. Steinhard, Erlangen, Germany)

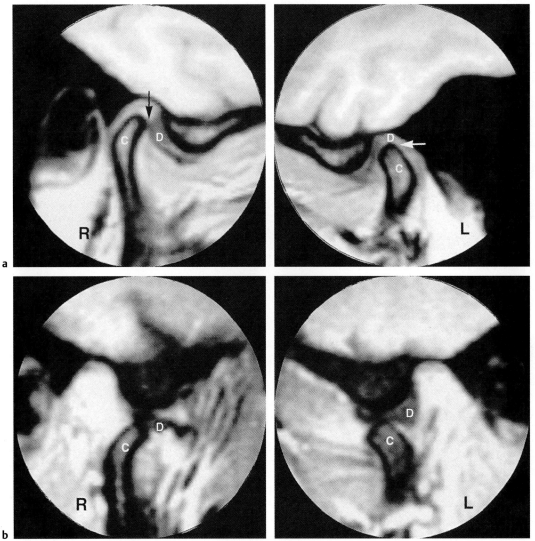

Fig. 22.**11   Same patient as in Fig. 22.10. MRI of the TMJ in sagittal section.** At closed mouth (**a**) the disk of the right TMJ (R) is located forward of the condyle (C). The arrows indicate the posterior margins of the disc (D). At open mouth (**b**) the right disk stays forward of the condyle, whereas on the left the disk–condlye relationship is normal

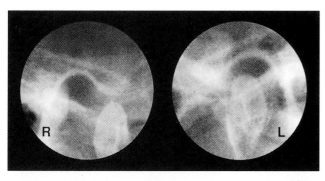

Fig. 22 .**12** **Disk displacement without reduction of the left TMJ** (L). Note the different degree of excursion of the condyles at open mouth: almost normal for the right condyle (R), extremely limited for the left condyle (L)

In disk compression, the joint noise tends to be more similar to crepitation and there is usually radiological evidence of intra-articular space restriction (Fig. 22.**6**).

In joint arthrotic degeneration, crepitation (or a rubbing or "sandy" noise) is present during all opening and closing movements and is practically pathognomonic. On radiography, changes in shape of the hard tissues are observed, in conjunction with interruptions of the bony articular surface (Fig. 22.**8**).

The treatment of TMJ dysfunctions aims to remove the neuromuscular and/or structural factors of dysfunction. For the neuromuscular factor the treatment plan is practically identical to what has been described for tension-type headache and myogenous pain (see Chapter 13). If a structural factor is present, an orthopedic splint will be applied to keep the

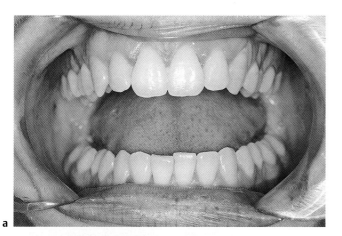

mandible in the correct position. For disk displacement without reduction, a mandibular manipulation will be performed first, to reestablish more appropriate condyle–disk relations (Fig. 14.**2**). Physical treatment and traction exercises will be programmed to encourage healing of the joint lesion (see Chapter 13).

Clinical Examples

A case of alternating disk displacement with and without reduction is given by a 30-year-old woman, a geologist, who for 10 years complained of episodes of mouth opening limitation and a sensation of locking of the left TMJ. These episodes were short in duration and resolved spontaneously. One year before observation, there was an acute and prolonged lock with acute pain at the left joint, which was resolved after several hours with a forced opening movement. From that time, opening was restricted and deviated to the left. However, the patient could overcome this movement impediment by applying digital pressue on the left TMJ during mouth opening (Fig. 22.**13**).

The patient complained of gastralgia, anxiety, acrophobia, palpitations, panic attacks, mood changes, and occasional depressed mood. Moreover, she reported intense day and night parafunctions. The left TMJ was painful during extended mouth movements and mastication. A further aggravating factor was her habitual face-down sleeping position.

On inspection, jaw opening was 18 mm with deviation toward the left (Fig. 22.**13 a**). However, when the patient applied digital pressure on the joint, opening was 40 mm without deviation (Fig. 22.**13 b, c**). The left masseter was slightly hypertrophic (Fig. 22.**14**). Dental arches were normal (Fig. 22.**15**). Palpation was positive for the left retroarticular point and for the lateral pterygoid, temporal, and masseter muscles. In particular, the left masseter was extremely painful at palpation.

MRI confirmed the presence of a disk displacement at closed and open mouth (Fig. 22.**16**).

The case in question was one of disk displacement without reduction, occasional at first and then permanent, which the patient could overcome with digital pressure. The etiological factor was neuromuscular (parafunctions) in a patient with some degree of anxiety.

An orthopedic appliance was applied to the upper jaw to keep the mandible in a position in which proper condyle–disk relationships were assured, and biofeedback and TENS sessions were programmed with application of electrodes on

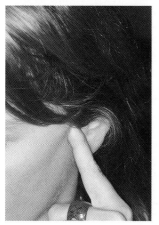

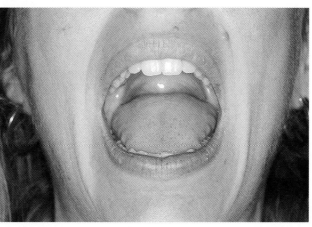

Fig. 22.**13** Restriction and deviation of the mouth opening movement (**a**) as a consequence of disk displacement without reduction of the left TMJ that the patient can resolve by applying digital pressure on the left TMJ (**b, c**)

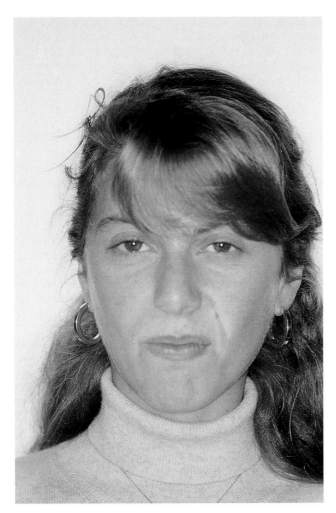

Fig. 22.**14**   A slight hypertrophy of the left masseter is visible

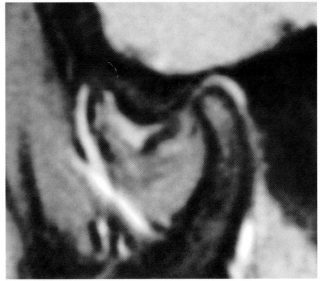

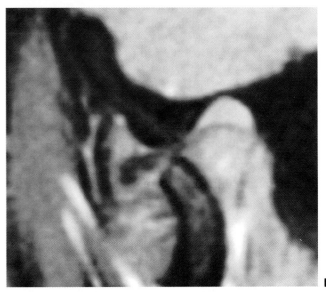

Fig. 22.**16**   MRI shows a displaced disk at closed (**a**) and open (**b**) mouth

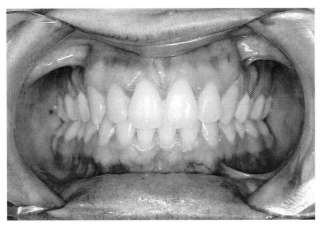

Fig. 22.**15**   The perfect condition of the dental arches confirms that the etiology is neuromuscular in this case

the masseter muscles. Relaxation, traction, and counter-resistance exercises were also prescribed. Amitriptyline 10 mg and perphenazine 2 mg were administered at night. Complete recovery and perfect joint function occurred within three months. The patient was recommended to continue the relaxation exercises and to wear the splint during the night.

A case of traumatic etiology is that of a 20-year-old boy who suffered a trauma on the chin six months before observation. He subsequently developed a left TMJ click, occasionally followed by periods of articular lock that resolved spontaneously. After two months, however, the lock was permanent. On inspection, mouth opening was limited with leftward deviation (Fig. 22.**17**). Palpation was negative except for the left retrocondylar point. The diagnosis of disk displacement without reduction which was already reasonably indicated was confirmed by MRI (Fig. 22.**18**). The patient was instructed to perform joint traction exercises repetitively to facilitate the manipulation for disk displacement reduction. However, when he came to consultation again 15 days later, disk displacement was now "with reduction" and the patient showed a normal opening range and a left TMJ click. An orthopedic splint was placed in the mouth (Fig. 22.**19**) and the click disappeared. Four months later, TMJ function was perfect and the mouth range of movement was normal (Fig. 22.**20**): consequently, the splint was removed. Full healing was confirmed by MRI (Fig. 22.**21**).

The following case is of a chronic disk displacement without reduction with aggravation of the joint lesion and initial arthrotic degeneration. The patient was a 23-year-old woman, an office employee, who two years before consulta-

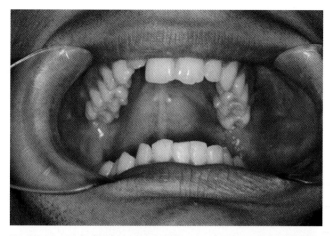

Fig. 22.17   Disk displacement without reduction of the left TMJ consequent on macrotrauma. The opening movement is restricted and deviated to the left

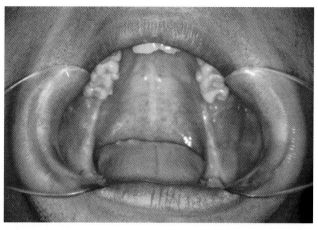

Fig. 22.**20**   Mouth opening after reduction of the disk displacement

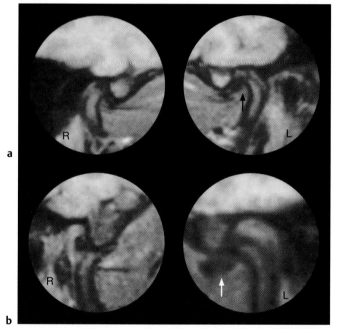

Fig. 22.**18**   Same patient as in Fig. 22.**17**. **MRI of the joint.** Both at closed (**a**) and open (**b**) mouth the disk of the left TMJ (arrows in L) is displaced ahead of the condyle. On the right (R) the disk has a normal position at closed and open mouth

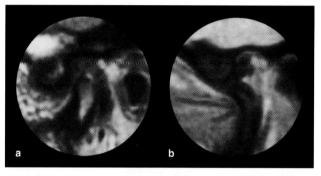

Fig. 22.**21**   MRI of the left TMJ at closed (**a**) and open (**b**) mouth confirms that at the end of treatment the disk is positioned normally

tion, after the extraction of three wisdom teeth, suffered a sudden limitation of mouth opening with pain at the left TMJ during mouth movements and mastication. On inspection, mouth opening was 30 mm with leftward deviation (Fig. 22.**22**). Palpation of the retrocondylar point was painful and on radiography there was no left condyle translation at open mouth (Fig. 22.**23**). Tomography showed an arthrotic lesion of the left condylar head (Fig. 22.**24**).

The patient reported intense tooth bruxing at night with pronounced aching in the cheek area upon awakening. Moreover, she reported suffering from tension-type headache if she slept longer during the weekend.

The case was one of a chronic disk displacement without reduction whose etiologic factor was neuromuscular and in which a degenerative arthrotic process had started. Mandibular manipulation was performed with success, a splint was applied in conjunction with an intense program of physical therapy (TENS and laser sessions), and relaxation and joint traction exercises. A soft diet was also prescribed for some months. Articular function was completely restored after three months (Figs. 22.**25**, 22.**26**) and at that time the splint was removed during the day.

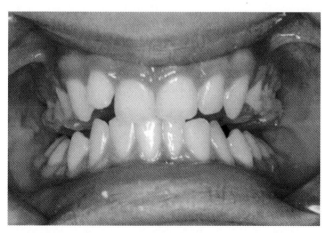

Fig. 22.**19**   An orthopedic splint is applied

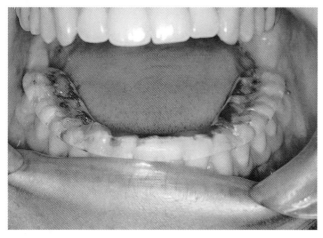

Fig. 22.**22** **Chronic disk displacement without reduction of the left TMJ.** Mouth opening is limited and deviated to the left. An inappropriate splint had previously been inserted in the patient's mouth

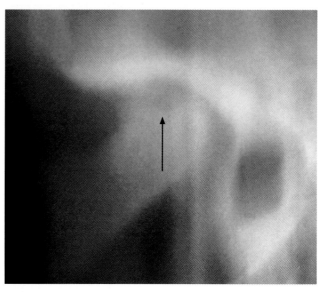

Fig. 22.**24**   Tomography shows an arthrotic lesion of the left condylar head (arrow)

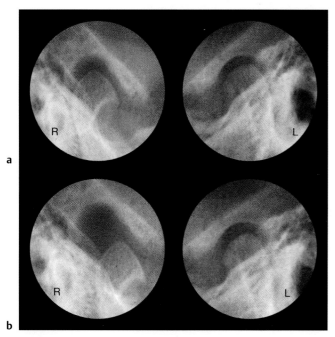

Fig. 22.**23**   Radiography at open mouth (**b**) shows no left condyle translation

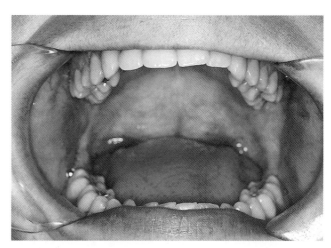

Fig. 22.**25**   At the end of treatment, good articular function is restored

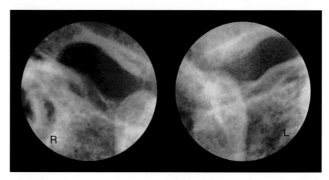

Fig. 22.**26**   Open mouth radiography confirms improvement of function

23 Psychogenic Facial Pain

General Principles

As stated in Chapter 1, psychogenic pain develops in the absence of potentially dangerous peripheral stimuli or intrinsic damages to the nervous system. It is important to emphasize that psychogenic pain is just as "real" as that caused by lesions or a pathological somatic condition. As such, it should be clearly distinguished from simulated pain (e.g. to support a claim for damages) and the expression of simulated pain, associated with personality disorders, known as *malingering*.

The IASP classification of chronic pain (1994) makes reference to *pain of psychological origin* and distinguishes between muscle tension pain; delusional or hallucinatory pain; hysterical, conversion, or hypochondriacal pain; and pain associated with depression. Clearly, psychogenic pain belongs to the last four categories, while the first category is muscle pain (nociceptive) resulting from muscle hyperparafunction, which can in turn be one of the effects of a psychological problem (see Chapters 1, 3, and 8). Patients suffering from psychogenic facial pain often have associated myogenic pain (see below).

A term that was once used frequently to define psychogenic facial pain, especially by neurologists, was *atypical facial pain*. This term, which was initially in the IHS classification (1988), was replaced in the latest edition by *facial pain not fulfilling criteria of previously described groups* (code 12.8) (see Chapter 1).

For a more precise categorization of these syndromes, it is advisable to make reference to the *Diagnostic and Statistical Manual of Mental Disorders* (DSM-IV) (American Psychiatric Association, 1994). These syndromes may reasonably be considered as *somatoform disorders* as defined by the DSM-IV. The principal characteristic of these disorders is the "presence of physical symptoms that suggest a general medical condition (hence the term somatoform) and are not fully explained by a general medical condition, by the direct effects of a substance, or by another mental disorder." In particular, these conditions can be grouped in the somatoform disorders defined as pain disorder. This disorder is characterized by pain as "the predominant focus of clinical attention. In addition, psychological factors are judged to have an important role in its onset, severity, exacerbation or maintenance." The other categories of somatoform disorder according to the DSM-IV are the somatization disorder; the conversion disorder; hypochondriasis; and the body dysmorphic disorder.

In the context of psychogenic facial pain that is the focal point of clinical attention, it seems appropriate to make reference to a *facial pain disorder* as a *somatoform disorder*. Facial pain can be also present in the other somatoform disorder categories mentioned above.

In the facial pain disorder the pain is either continuous or present for most of the day, and is variable in intensity and quality (sometimes described as burning, other times as a sense of swelling, strain, etc.). The site is also mutable: the pain can start as a sense of localized gingival burning and then spread or move to a buccal site. Other times it starts in the zygomatic region, unilaterally or bilaterally, and then spreads to a broader area of the face and/or neck. In any case, the site of pain distribution is always anarchical in relation to the territory of distribution of the sensitive nerves. Inevitably, patients complain of a plethora of psychosomatic symptoms and the psychometric tests show results that are outside the norm (see Chapter 8).

In other cases, facial pain is only one aspect of a multisymptomatic disorder characterized by pain with multiple locations, and gastrointestinal, sexual, and pseudoneurological symptoms. In this case, the category psychogenic facial pain in *somatization disorder* is the most appropriate. If, on the other hand, the pain is associated with a sensory or motor deficit that simulates a pathology of the nervous system, it will be considered a *conversion disorder*. Cases in which the predominant caracteristic is fear of a serious illness, generated by the patient's incorrect interpretation of his on her symptoms, are coded as *hypochondriasis* associated with psychogenic facial pain. Finally, if the pain is associated with a serious preoccupation with a slight or totally imagined aesthetic alteration, it will be considered psychogenic facial pain in *body dysmorphic disorder*.

Naturally, the treatment must aim to manage the psychological problem, with drug therapy and/or psychotherapy, as the basis of the disorder. However, this does not mean that these patients cannot benefit from other forms of palliative treatment to recondition muscle function, especially if there is concurrent myogenic pain.

Facial Pain Disorder

Patients with facial pain disorder are among those who most often run the risk of being subjected to various inappropriate therapies, often dental work, more or less invasive, that have no effect except to aggravate the symptoms. Such aggravation is also due to false expectations and the wasting of large sums of money.

The histories of these patients often contain a dramatic event or trauma that coincides with the initial manifestation of the symptoms.

A characteristic example is that of a 53-year-old woman, a housewife, who had been suffering for ten years from constant pain in the bilateral preauricular and buccal region associated with back pain on the right side (Fig. 23.1). The patient reported having had a troubled life: she had brought two pregnancies to term and had had one miscarriage and four abortions. Five years after the birth of her second daughter (18 years before observation), she was abandoned by her husband. Ten years earlier she had lost her job and undergone whiplash in a car accident; lastly, three years earlier her daughter had had both her legs amputated after being hit by a train.

The patient reported having suffered from severe depressive disorders in different periods (especially after her first pregnancy and then as a result of the events described). A problem similar to that noted upon observation had already occurred when she was abandoned by her husband. At that time the patient had suffered from a sudden pain in her face and difficulty in moving her mouth. The problem had gradu-

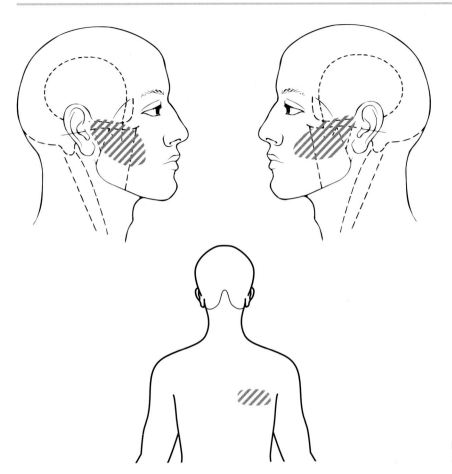

Fig. 23.**1**   Sites of persistent chronic pain in a 53-year-old woman

ally disappeared within one year. The pain had also occurred ten years earlier, when she lost her job, it was practically impossible for her to move her mouth and there was also a considerable phonation impediment frequently associated with a lip tremor.

The patient had been subjected, to no avail, to a series of dental treatments involving the extraction of most of her teeth and the application of upper and lower prostheses. There had been several attempts to modify these prostheses, but the results were unsatisfactory (Fig. 23.**2**).

At the time of observation, the pain persisted continuously; it was of moderate intensity, described as an extremely bothersome sense of tension. It was associated with a marked limitation of mouth movements and a deviation to the right when opening (Fig. 23.**3**).

The patient suffered from numerous symptoms, predominantly psychosomatic (Fig. 23.**4**). She also reported frequent episodes of amnesia and loss of spatial orientation. She was extremely worried and saddened by the precarious state of her mouth, which she perceived as seriously compromised both esthetically and functionally. As a result of this state of mind, she had avoided looking in the mirror for about a year and a half.

At the neurological examination, the Romberg test was positive: she fell backwards from a standing position with her eyes closed. Her balance improved if she concentrated her at-

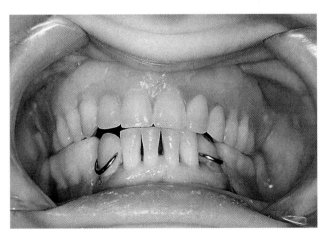

Fig. 23.**2**   After inappropriate dental treatment, the patient's oral cavity is in extremely poor condition. This problem deeply distreessed the patient

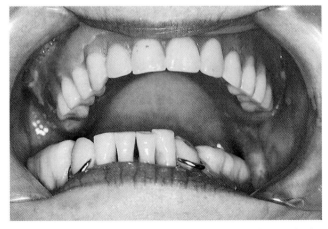

Fig. 23.**3**   Mouth opening movement is limited and severely deviated to the right

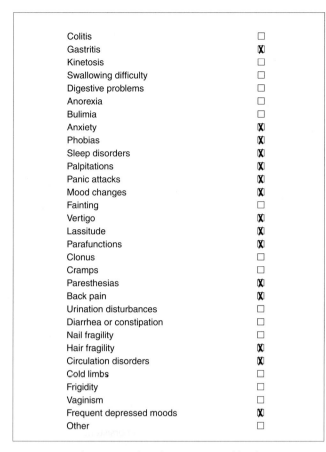

Colitis	☐
Gastritis	☒
Kinetosis	☐
Swallowing difficulty	☐
Digestive problems	☐
Anorexia	☐
Bulimia	☐
Anxiety	☒
Phobias	☒
Sleep disorders	☒
Palpitations	☒
Panic attacks	☒
Mood changes	☒
Fainting	☐
Vertigo	☒
Lassitude	☒
Parafunctions	☒
Clonus	☐
Cramps	☐
Paresthesias	☒
Back pain	☒
Urination disturbances	☐
Diarrhea or constipation	☐
Nail fragility	☐
Hair fragility	☒
Circulation disorders	☒
Cold limbs	☐
Frigidity	☐
Vaginism	☐
Frequent depressed moods	☒
Other	☐

Fig. 23.**4** Psychosomatic disturbances reported by the patient

tention on the task of guessing a number being traced on her forehead with a finger (the "psychogenic" Romberg sign). There was slight hyposthenia in her right leg. Palpation was moderately positive for the mandibular foramen, the retrocondylar point, the internal pterygoid muscle bilaterally, and the right masseter and sternocleidomastoid muscle.

The MMPI confirmed the presence of a personality disorder with very high scores on all the scales except Mf (self-esteem) and Ma (hypomania). The state and trait anxiety scores were at the maximum levels (Fig. 23.**5**).

For a long time the patient had been taking large doses of benzodiazepines during the day and before going to sleep. She nevertheless suffered from severe insomnia.

This was therefore a case of facial pain disorder in a patient with a significant mood disorder. Moderate myogenic pain was associated but was not so severe as to account for the entirety of symptoms, in particular the limitation of mouth movements, which could resemble an arthrogenic problem. It was also characteristic that the deteriorated situation of the oral cavity produced a tendency in the patient to focus her attention on that area, inducing an avoidance behavior (the avoiding of mirrors).

The patient's problems were discussed with her in the course of a long talk, after which drug therapy was started with paroxetine in one morning dose (10 mg for two weeks and then 20 mg), initially maintaining the administration of lorazepam 2.5 mg tablets ($^1/_2$ a tablet in the afternoon and $^1/_2$ in the evening). In addition, an intensive nondrug therapy program was prescribed (biofeedback, relaxation exercises, physical exercises, etc.). Articular traction exercises and opening/closing of the mouth in front of a mirror were also prescribed. There was gradual improvement, but there were a few relapses coinciding with particularly stressful times. The facial pain diminished considerably and the degree of mouth opening increased progressively, with a simultaneous decrease of the mandibular deviation toward the right (Fig. 23.**6a**). This confirmed that there was no articular component among the patient's symptoms.

Eight months later, the pain had virtually disappeared and the mouth opening had normalized (Fig. 23.**6b**). There was a distinct improvement of the well-being and the patient was referred to a dentist for proper rehabilitation of her oral cavity (Fig. 23.**7**). This had a positive effect on the patient's mood and eliminated the mirror avoidance. It should be noted, however, that it would have been wrong to send the patient to the dentist before the facial pain disorder had been cured.

The next case is a further example of facial pain disorder. A 37-year-old woman, divorced, with a good level of education, in the process of looking for a job, had suffered for about seven years from a sensation of moderate "burning" and "swelling" in the right infraorbital and buccal region (Fig. 23.**8**). These symptoms were occasionally associated with prickling paresthesias. About two years after the symptoms began, they diminished to minimum levels for 2–3 years and then re-

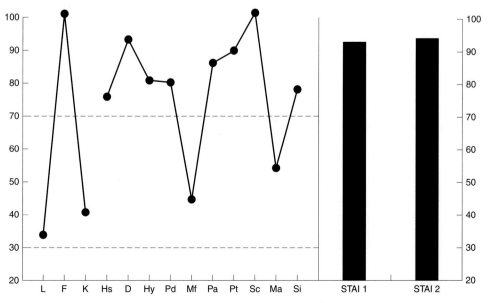

Fig. 23.**5** Notably high MMPI scores and high state and trait anxiety scores

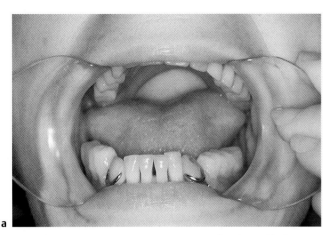
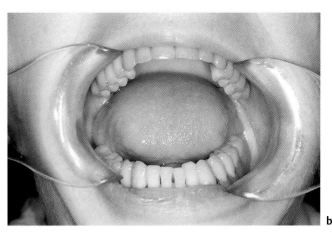

Fig. 23.**6**   Reduction (**a**) and disappearance (**b**) of mandibular movement impediment during therapy

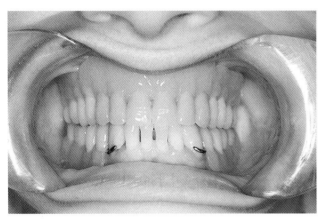

Fig. 23.**7**   After improvement of symptoms, the patient was referred to a dentist for a rehabilitation of the oral cavity

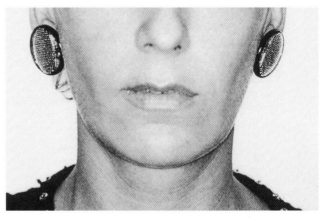

Fig. 23.**9**   Upon inspection, a slight swelling of the right cheek is noted

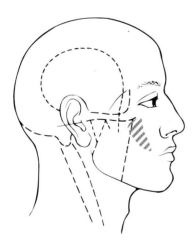

Fig. 23.**8**   Site of burning and swelling sensation, virtually continuous, in a 37-year-old woman

turned to the previous levels. At the time of observation, these disturbances were constant and were described as extremely "frustrating." The patient maintained that the whole problem had started after dental work in the superior right quadrant of the dental arch and since then she had requested the opinion and intervention of several odontologists. She had also undergone allergy tests to determine whether any of the products used in the dental work might be the cause of the symptoms,

but without success. In addition, a flap of the maxillary mucosa was lifted to explore the underlying bone, which turned out to be entirely normal.

The physiological history included an abortion immediately before the symptoms had begun. This event was remembered by the patient as "extremely stressing" and was followed by recurring horrifying dreams.

Upon inspection, there was a slight tumefaction of the right cheek (Fig. 23.**9**). This sign was corroborated by thermography, which indicated the presence of a hyperthermal area corresponding to the symptomatic region (Fig. 23. **10**). There was no pain upon palpation of the cranial points or the muscles. The MMPI personality profile indicated a severe form of depression with a tendency toward autistic fantasies (Fig. 23.**11**). State and trait anxiety evels were also very high.

During the discussion with the patient regarding her problems, she initially flatly denied the possibility that a psychological factor might have been the origin of her disturbances, after which she suddenly and dramatically accepted the hypothesis and the resulting treatment plan. She was treated with amitriptyline (10 mg twice a day), perfenazine (2 mg twice a day) and clotiazepam (10 mg) and was referred for psychotherapy. Within three months the symptoms had practically disappeared. This improvement was confirmed by normalization of the thermographic test (Fig. 23.**12**). However, the personality profile shown by the MMPI remained similar to the initial one. At a check-up three years later, the improvement of the pain symptoms proved to be stable.

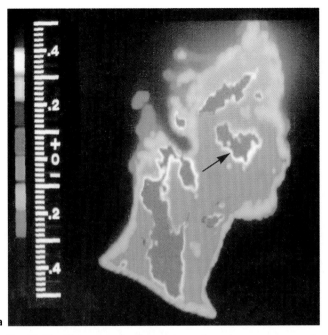
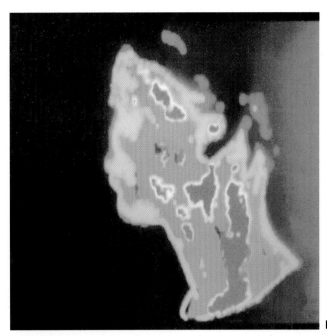

Fig. 23.**10**   Thermography shows a hyperthermic area corresponding to the symptomatic area (arrow)

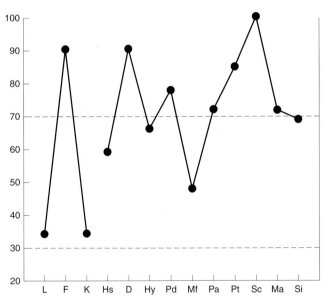

Fig. 23.**11**   The MMPI shows a severe form of depression with a tendency to autistic fantasies (Sc)

Psychogenic Facial Pain in Somatization Disorder

In other cases, pain is not only in the face but has multiple and variable locations and is associated with various types of symptoms (gastrointestinal, sexual, pseudoneurological, etc.). An example of these *somatization disorders* is the case of a 48-year-old man who seven years before observation, after a severe disappointment related to work, had developed various disturbances with progressive severity that induced him to quit work and request early retirement.

Initially he had pharyngitis, followed by esophagitis, with excessive salivation and chills all over his body. These symptoms remitted but frequent and brief episodes of burning pain in the pharynx and left arm remained. Two years later, the

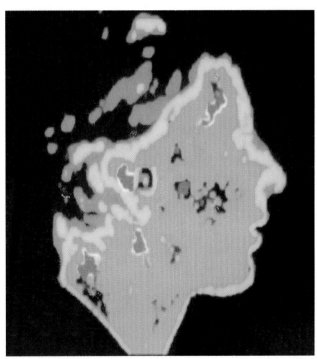

Fig. 23.**12**   After drug therapy and psychotherapy, thermography confirms improvement of the symptoms by showing disappearance of the hyperthermic area

symptoms had worsened due to the manifestation of an intense sensation of throat constriction and being pulled to the left while walking. The pain had spread to the nuchal and retroauricular region. After various types of treatment, brain MRI and a CAT scan were performed and revealed microfoci of subcortical damage. The patient was transferred to a neurology ward to be tested for a demyelination disease. He underwent a lumbar puncture for cerebrospinal fluid extraction after which, according to the patient, an excruciating burning-stabbing type of pain appeared in his left hemiface and the left side of the body, associated with accommodation disturbances. These symptoms worsened progressively and resulted in a left hemiparesis that kept the patient in bed for about one year. During this period he consulted specialists of various kinds and was subjected to diverse and clearly inappropriate treatments: vaccines and antiviral preparations, homeopathic cures, and others. He then left the bed and began wandering abroad to private clinics of doubtful reliability. The patient was convinced that he was suffering from an autoimmune disease and every subjective symptom was, according to him, proof of it. He also believed that movement was an aggravating factor and therefore spent his days at home in a state of semiimmobility.

At the time of observation, the patient reported that the pain was virtually continuous in the left hemiface with occasional diffusion to the left side of the body (in the form of neuralgic attacks). More rarely, the pain appeared on the right side (whereupon it disappeared from the left side) (Fig. 23.**13**). This pain was experienced dramatically by the patient (Fig. 23.**14**) and was associated with dysphagia and

difficulty in swallowing, esophageal pain, occasional disturbances of visual accommodation, and back pain. His gait was cautious, he took small steps, and his degree of facial expression was reduced. He lived with his parents in an ambivalent relationship and refused to entertain any hypothesis of a psychological factor in his illness.

Upon clinical analysis, the neurological examination was negative except for a mild sign of pronation of the right hand. Palpation of the muscles and cranial points created no pain whatsoever.

It was prudently explained to the patient that a full investigation was necessary and that psychological tests were a part of that investigation, that it was standard procedure regardless of the type of problem being treated. The MMPI was administered and showed high scores for the first three *neurotic* scales (hypochondria, depression, hysteria) with a tendency toward a *conversive V* (Fig. 23.**15**). The Pd scores (psychopathic deviation) were high. The STAI showed high state and trait anxiety scores. The MMPI profile was shown to the

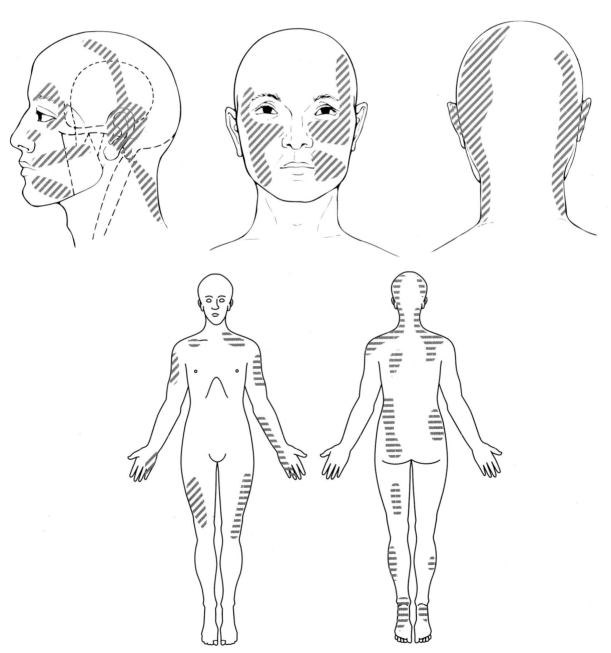

Fig. 23.**13**   Pain sites in 48-year-old man with somatization disorder

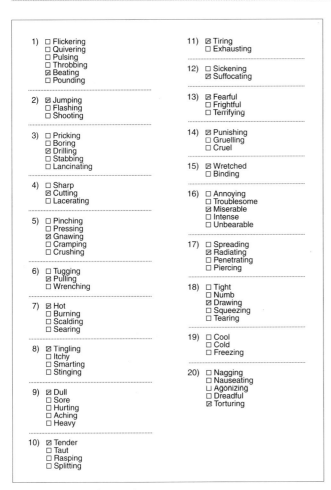

Fig. 23.**14** The McGill Pain Questionnaire shows an intense affective participation in the pain

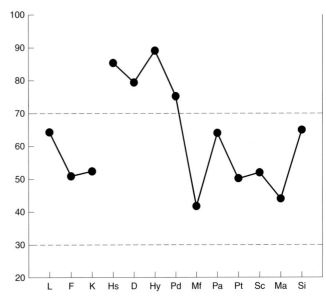

Fig. 23.**15** MMPI shows notably high scores on *neurotic* scales with a *conversive* V

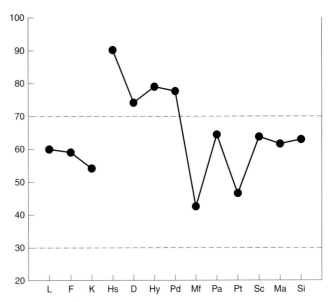

Fig. 23.**16** Slight reduction in depression (D) and hysteria (Hs) scores during treatment

patient and explained to him in mild terms. He was also shown iconographic material of similar cases. He was therefore persuaded that, even in the face of a hypothetical organic neurological and muscle disorder, it was useful to manage the "psychological" aspect as well. Therefore he was initially prescribed 200 mg tablets of ademetionine, twice a day, essentially to create more compliance than would otherwise presumably have been obtained from another antidepressant. Since the patient explicitly refused the idea of psychotherapy with a specialist, long talks were held with him during which it was attempted to refocus his attention on his work (art photography). In the meantime he was prescribed posture exercises and mild physical activity.

Two months later it was possible to replace the morning tablet of ademetionine with fluoxetine 20 mg. During the following observation period (about nine months in duration), there was an improvement in mood. Upon inspection, his face appeared to be more expressive, his gait was totally normalized, and, according to his father, he went for walks and seemed to have regained some interest in his previous activity. An MMPI administered again at this point showed a slight decline in the depression and hysteria scores, while the hypochondria score had remained the same (Fig. 23.**16**). The STAI showed that the anxiety scores were lower. Nevertheless, although the patient admitted there had been some improvement, he was still convinced that he had an incurable disease and did not go back to work.

Facial Pain in Conversion Disorder

In other cases, facial pain is associated with a deficit of sensitivity or motility that simulates a nervous system pathology. It is therefore psychogenic facial pain as an epiphenomenon of a *conversion disorder*.

An exemplary case of this situation is that of a 28-year-old housewife who, ten months before observation, had suffered from progressive phonation disturbances associated with an evident facial asymmetry, including a lowering of the right corner of the mouth. About 15 days after these symptoms appeared, she began to suffer from a more or less constant pain in the right buccal region; it was a dull pain, but from time to time lancinating, associated with a limitation in mandibular movements. She previously had an oral splint inserted, on the erroneous assumption that her problem was a TMJ intracapsular disorder.

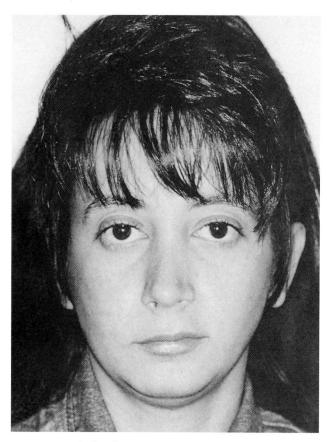 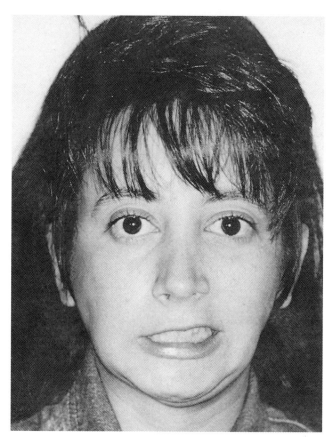

Fig. 23.**17**   Right facial nerve palsy occurring simultaneously with phonation disturbances in a 28-year-old woman

An interesting item in the family history was that her father was hypertensive and had recently suffered from a cerebral ictus with a resulting facial–brachial–crural hemiparesis, from which he had recovered satisfactorily.

The patient reported having suffered several times from depression in the past.

About a year and a half before onset of the symptoms, she had undergone plastic surgery on her nose, but was extremely disappointed with the results, which produced considerable psychological prostration. Ten months before the symptoms appeared, she had brought her first pregnancy to term.

She reported suffering from digestive difficulties, fatigue, anxiety, agoraphobia, claustrophobia, vertigo, episodes of tachycardia, gastritis, nail and hair fragility, and menstruation disturbances. Her current symptoms worsened under stress.

Blood pressure and hematological examinations were normal. Neurological examination was positive for the Romberg test and revealed a palsy of the right facial nerve (Fig. 23.**17**). This palsy was of the central type as it did not involve the upper branch of the nerve (Fig. 23.**18**). She also had a mandibular deviation to the left during the opening movement, which was limited to 33 mm (Fig. 23.**19**). Palpation of the muscles was painful bilaterally for the temporal, lateral pterygoid, and neck muscles. A slight clicking noise could be heard at the left TMJ, but articular radiography produced normal findings.

The acute onset of neurological symptoms in a young women justifies suspicion of a demyelination disease. Other neurological problems to be considered were a vascular accident or a tumor. A CAT scan was performed and the result was normal. On the other hand, numerous considerations suggested the possibility that the problem might be conversive in nature: the past hemiplegia of her father, the start of the prob-

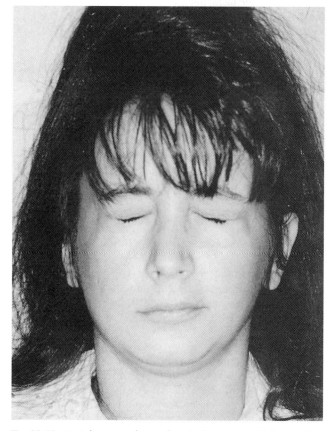

Fig. 23.**18**   Facial nerve palsy is of central type since it does not involve the superior branch of the nerve

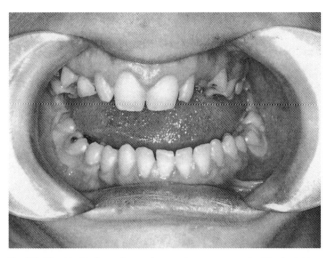

Fig. 23.**19** Limitation of mouth opening movement with deviation to the left had led to an erroneous diagnosis of TMJ lesion

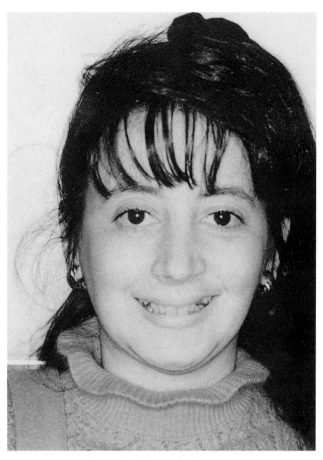

Fig. 23.**21** Paralysis of the facial nerve disappears after treatment with amitriptyline, clotiazepam, and psychotherapy

lem after potentially stressing events (plastic surgery and pregnancy); the number of psychosomatic symptoms reported by the patient; the worsening of the symptoms under stress (including the facial nerve palsy). The MMPI showed a high degree of depression and social introversion (Fig. 23.**20**). Trait anxiety scores were also extremely high. The patient was put on a waiting list for brain MRI, including the brain stem, and in the meantime drug therapy was started with amitriptyline (30 mg twice a day) and clotiazepam (10 mg in the morning). The patient also started a biofeedback program.

Two months later, the pain symptoms had diminished considerably. The facial palsy had also receded notably. At this stage, while the drug therapy continued, the patient was referred to a psychiatrist for psychotherapy sessions for six months. At the end of that period, the patient was virtually without pain, and the signs of facial palsy had disappeared (Fig. 23.**21**). The patient also reported a distinct improvement in her well-being and mood and a marked reduction of all the psychosomatic complaints. The personality profile of the MMPI and the trait anxiety scores had almost completely nor-

malized (Fig. 23.**22**). Upon inspection, the mandibular movements were normal (Fig. 23.**23**), which confirmed in this case that the intracapsular lesion of the TMJ diagnosed in the past had actually been simulated by another pathology.

The next case is also a quite characteristic example of craniofacial pain associated with a somatization disorder. It is the case of an 18-year-old girl who had been suffering for a long period from gait disturbances, with the frequent tendency to lose her balance leftward. That symptom had recently worsened. About two months before observation she experienced episodes of pain and paresthesia (with a prickling sensation) on the right hemiface, along with a sense of "stiffness" on the left corner of the mouth and the left eyelid. From that time, the mouth opening movements tended to deviate leftward. The pain attacks were of sudden onset, lasted about one hour, and were pulsating. The pain could migrate from the forehead to the temporal, occipital, and parietal areas and it was accompanied by intense lacrimation of the left eye, salivation, sweating, tachycardia, and motor impediment in the left half of the body. Moreover, the patient reported that her eyesight and hearing capacities were reduced on the left. A few days before observation she had suffered some episodes of loss of consciousness for a few seconds, followed by a brief period of spatial–temporal disorientation.

The family and remote pathological history were of little significance, but the patient pointed out that she had a conflicting relationship with her family and her partner. She complained of tingling in her limbs, vertigo, palpitations, colitis, gastritis, peripheral circulation disturbances, and fragility of the nails and hair.

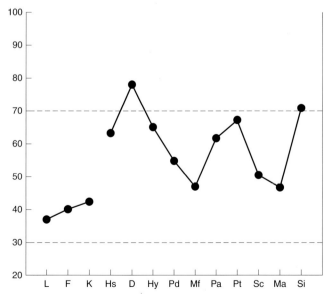

Fig. 23.**20** The MMPI reveals high scores for depression (D) and social introversion (Si)

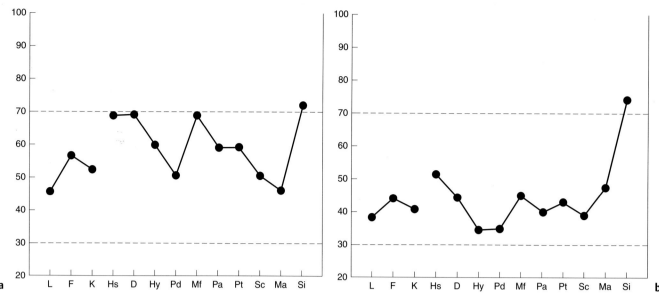

Fig. 23.**22**   Improvement (**a**) and subsequent disappearance (**b**) of depression at MMPI after treatment

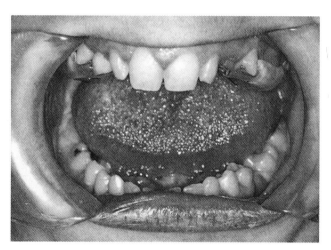

Fig. 23.**23**   Normalization of mouth opening after recovery

Neurological examination revealed numerous positive signs: it was almost impossible for her to stand straight with her eyes closed (due to the tendency to fall leftward) and there was a distinct deviation toward the left during the index-finger test. There was also a hypoesthesia of the three left branches of the trigeminal nerve, a slight paresis of the inferior left branch of the facial nerve, and a slight hypoacusia on the left. Moreover, hyposthenia of the right arm (Fig. 23.**24**) and the lower limbs was detected, and the index finger-to-nose test showed dysmetria (Fig. 23.**25**). The Lhermitte sign was also present (a pain like an electrical shock along the spinal column while passively flexing the head forward). Abdominal reflexes were present.

Opening of the mouth was limited and presented a marked leftward deviation (Fig. 23.**26**). Palpation of the cranial points and the muscles evoked moderate to severe pain in all the palpation points on the left, but not in the ones on the right.

The facial pain attacks reported by the patient could be attributed to migraine, though some characteristics (such as pain migration) were atypical. On the other hand, the sudden onset of multifocal neurological symptoms pointed once again to the possibility of a demyelination disease. The patient was hospitalized in the Neurological Clinic of the University of

Turin, where, beside the routine tests (hematological, radiography of the thorax, ECG, etc.), the following examinations were conducted: EEG, cerebrospinal fluid examination, evoked potentials, and brain and brain stem MRI. All results were normal. The vestibular tests conducted during the oto-

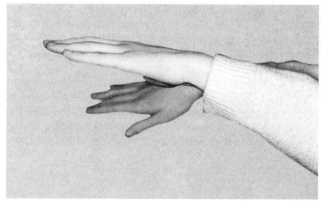

Fig. 23.**24   Conversion disorder in an 18-year-old woman.** Hypoasthenia of right arm

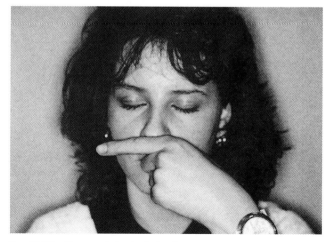

Fig. 23.**25**   Dysmetria in the index finger-to-nose test

logical examination, and the TMJ radiographs, were also normal. The MMPI scores were very high for the three neurotic scales, with a tendency toward a conversive V. All the other scales were within normal limits (Fig. 23.**27**).

Since all laboratory tests were negative, a conversion disorder was conjectured, possibly associated with a muscle contraction pain of the craniofacial muscles on the left (which ached considerably upon awakening in the morning).

The patient was referred to a psychiatrist for treatment and was reexamined at intervals of about six months for two and a half years. During this period, a progressive and significant improvement of all the symptoms was observed. At the last check-up, some neurological symptoms were still present (Romberg test positive, deviation of the index fingers) but all the others had either disappeared or were notably diminished (Fig. 23.**28**). The facial pain and headache had almost entirely

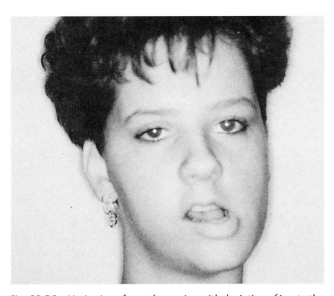

Fig. 23.**26** Limitation of mouth opening with deviation of jaw to the left

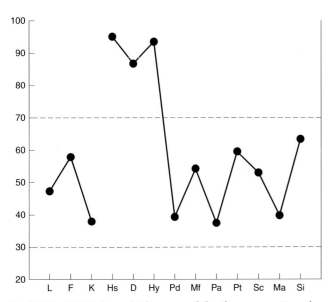

Fig. 23.**27** **MMPI shows high scores of the three neurotic scales with tendency toward** *conversive V.* Normal scores of psychotic scales

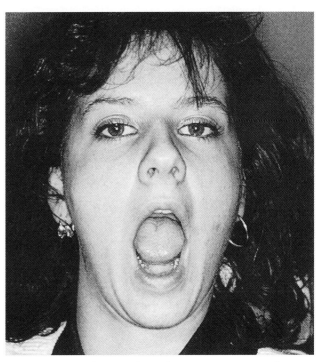

Fig. 23.**28** Normalization of mouth opening movement after psychiatric treatment

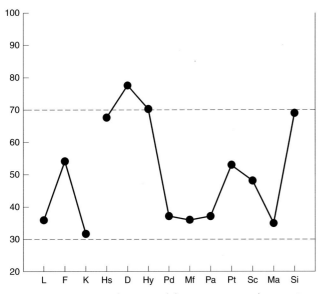

a

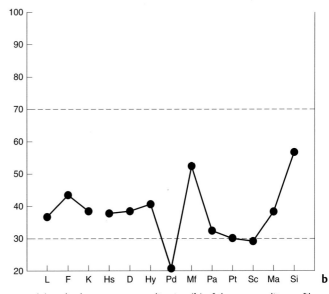

b

Fig. 23.**29** MMPI test administered during treatment shows an improvement (**a**) and subsequent normalization (**b**) of the personality profile

disappeared. The patient reported a distinct improvement in her mood. This improvement was confirmed by the MMPI results (Fig. 23.**29**) and the reduction in the trait anxiety level.

Facial Pain and Hypochondriasis

Psychogenic facial pain is rather frequently accompanied by hypochondriacal ideas. In some cases, however, the fear that the pain is a symptom of a serious illness (especially a tumor), inasmuch as it is an invasive and obsessive fear, represents the salient feature of the pathology.

This was the case with a 58-year-old housewife, married, without children and with an excellent relationship with her husband. Eight years earlier, after an invasive prosthetic treatment with the capping of numerous teeth, she had begun to complain of a diffused bilateral pressing pain in her cheeks, neck and shoulders and a burning pain in the parietal area bilaterally and at the vertex of the head (Fig. 23.**30**). These symptoms were associated with a marked sense of exhaustion and diffused pain in her limbs. These disturbances, in spite of various types of treatment, had remained practically unchanged until observation, and they were associated with the deepening conviction that they were the result of a tumoral process. For this reason, the patient had subjected herself over time to a long series of clinical examinations, radiography, and laboratory tests, all of which had negative results. The idea had nevertheless by then become obsessive and practically never left her. Consequently, the quality of her life declined, much more than was due to the pain itself. The patient, who was wealthy, had gradually ceased social relationships and was also reluctant leave her own home to go on vacation with her husband.

She reported numerous psychosomatic symptoms (Fig. 23.**31**). The neurological examination showed a positive

Colitis	☐
Gastritis	☐
Kinetosis	☐
Swallowing difficulty	☐
Digestive problems	☐
Anorexia	☐
Bulimia	☒
Anxiety	☒
Phobias	☐
Sleep disorders	☒
Palpitations	☒
Panic attacks	☒
Mood changes	☒
Fainting	☐
Vertigo	☐
Lassitude	☒
Parafunctions	☒
Clonus	☐
Cramps	☐
Paresthesias	☒
Back pain	☒
Urination disturbances	☐
Diarrhea or constipation	☐
Nail fragility	☐
Hair fragility	☐
Circulation disorders	☐
Cold limbs	☒
Frigidity	☐
Vaginism	☐
Frequent depressed moods	☒
Other	☐

Fig. 23.**31**   Disturbances reported by the patient

Romberg test and hyposthenia in all four limbs. Due to daytime and nighttime grinding of the teeth, there was conspicuous abrasion of the teeth, both the natural and artificial ones (Fig. 23.**32**). This had also facilitated the drop of the corners of her lips, which emphasized the patient's depressed expression (Fig. 23.**33**). The cranial muscles were not particularly tender upon palpation, whereas all the neck muscles were. The cervical radiograph showed a loss of lordosis with arthrotic lesions on some vertebrae (Fig. 23.**34**).

The mood was clearly depressed: the patient felt a sense of shame in admitting it because, as she herself stated, "there was no reason to be sad." She had the same attitude about her fear of having cancer. During the consultations she could not overcome the compulsion to seek reassurance in this regard, though she obtained only temporary relief from such reassurance.

The MMPI indicated a distinctly depressed profile (profile 1, 2, 3, 7) with high scores for the first three scales, depression in particular, and for psychasthenia (Fig. 23.**35**). The STAI demonstrated extremely high state and trait anxiety scores.

This patient required a long clarifying talk before starting therapy. She gratefully accepted the explanations and proposals for therapy, which consisted of 20 mg paroxetine once in the morning and 10 mg zolpidem when needed for insomnia. At the same time, a series of biofeedback sessions was

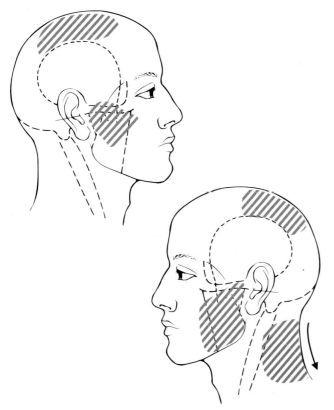

Fig. 23.**30**   Pain site in a 58-year-old hypochondriac woman

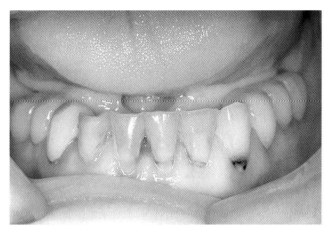

Fig. 23.**32** Notable dental abrasion, especially on the right, as a result of parafunction

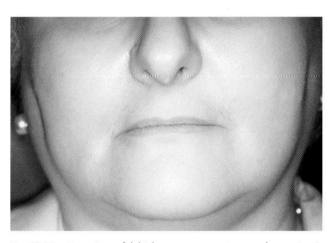

Fig. 23.**33** Drooping of labial corners accentuates the patient's depressed facial expression

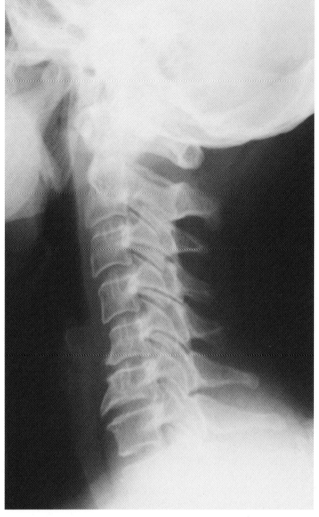

Fig. 23.**34 Loss of cervical lordosis and arthrotic lesions on some vertebrae.** This, in addition to muscle contraction, could facilitate the cervical myogenic pain suffered by the patient

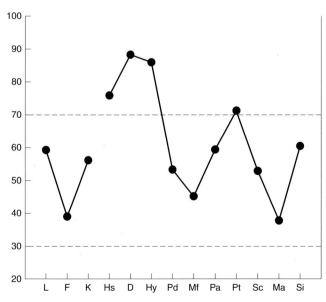

Fig. 23.**35 MMPI reveals typical depressed provile with high scores for scales 1, 2, 3, and 7.** The depression score (D) is the highest

started and the usual relaxation exercises were prescribed. At every consultation a conversation, sometimes prolonged, was held with the patient, the topics of which centered on the frequency with which depression occurs in the general population; the fact that depression is not the patient's fault any more than an organic disturbance of any kind is the patient's fault; the fact that depression can often be managed in a relatively simple way; and that the initial therapeutic difficulties are born of a certain degree of subconscious resistance by the patient to treatment. As regards the obsession, rational phrases ("all the exams are negative," "if it were a tumor you would be dead by now") were less effective than the question "Well, if I tell you there is no tumor, will you trust me?"

In the following six months there was a progressive improvement of the symptoms, both the pain (with a progressive abatement and eventually the complete disappearance of the facial pain) and the psychosomatic disturbances, with the elimination of palpitations and panic attacks. The mood and sleeping patterns improved and the obsessive ideas diminished significantly.

The MMPI was administered again and showed a normalization of the scores, with a steep drop in the depression score and a psychosomatic V that was within the norm (Fig. 23.**36**). The anxiety scores had also partially decreased.

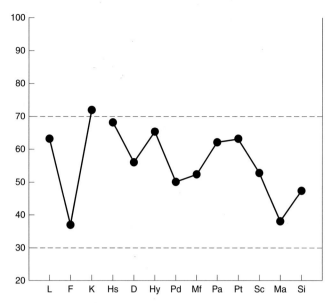

Fig. 23.**36 Notable improvement of personality profile is revealed by the MMPI after therapy.** Note that now the highest score, though within normal limits, is hypochondria (Hs)

Body Dysmorphic Disorder

Pain is sometimes associated with a serious preoccupation with an aesthetic alteration, either slight or entirely imagined, often perceived as progressive. These cases are coded as psychogenic facial pain in *body dysmorphic disorder.*

A clear case of this disorder is that of a 39-year-old woman, married, a psychologist by profession. Two and a half years earlier, after experiencing a facial trauma (a rubber ball hurled by her young son had hit her in the left buccal and mandibular region), she had started to complain of various mutable symptoms characterized by swelling in the right periorbital area, pain in the right preauricular area with subsequent extension to the upper right dental hemiarch. Later a pain also appeared in the right temporal, nuchal, and cervical region (Fig. 23.**37**). The patient was alarmed by the conviction that a tumefaction was forming in the right zygomatic region associated with a hollowing of the right cheek, which, according to her, she had not had previously. She claimed that these morphological al-

terations were progressive and attributed them to some local organic alteration triggered by the trauma. To "prove" her belief, she exhibited a series of photographs taken in periods prior to the trauma. She had stopped working and started traveling to various cities to consult specialists of various types (internists, maxillofacial surgeons, dental surgeons, physiotherapists, etc.). She had undergone a long series of clinical examinations and radiography and several dental splints had been placed in her mouth (Fig. 23.**38**). These therapies had no effect except that of iatrogenically altering her dental contact (Fig. 23.**39**).

The patient reported having suffered from bulimia during her adolescence. She also reported asthenia, fatigued awakening, anxiety and a constantly depressed mood. She took diazepam drops (2 – 3 mg/day). At the neurological examination there was instability in the sensitized Romberg test, though nothing else was notable. Upon inspection, her facial expression was depressed and it seemed evident that the dysmorphism indicated by the patient was a simple physiognomic trait (Fig. 23. **40**). Mouth movements were normal. The sternocleidomastoid and trapezius muscles appeared notably contracted (Fig. 23.**40**). Palpation on the right side was positive for some cranial points (supraorbital, infraorbital, retrocondylar), the craniomandibular muscles (external and internal pterygoid, masseter, temporal), and especially for the sternocleidomastoid and trapezius, where trigger points causing

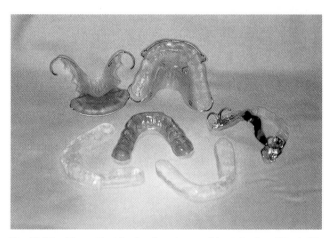

Fig. 23.**38**   The patient had various types of dental splints fitted: this doggedness worsened her situation

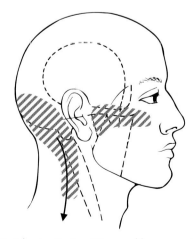

Fig. 23.**37**   Facial pain site in a 37-year-old woman with body dysmorphic disorder

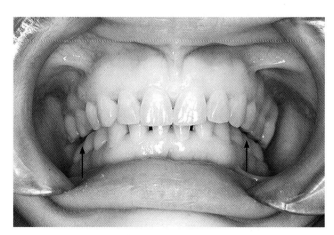

Fig. 23.**39**   As a result of inappropriate treatments (see Fig. 23.**38**), the patient's posterior teeth were not in contact (arrows); this naturally accentuated the patient's discomfort

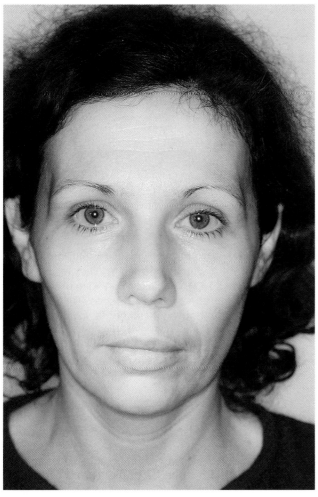

Fig. 23.**40**   The patient did not recognize her drawn face with protruding cheekbones as her own and was convinced it was the consequence of a dysmorphic process in progress

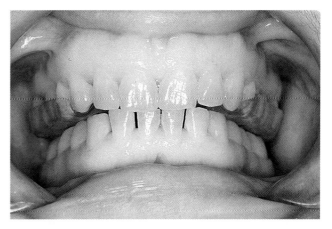

Fig. 23.**42**   Application of a jaw splint to compensate for the alteration of dental contact induced iatrogenically

pain referred to the forehead were found. The TMJ radiographs were normal, whereas the cervical ones showed a slight reduction of lordosis.

The MMPI personality profile was markedly depressive, with high scores on some *psychotic* scales. The STAI indicated extremely high state and trait anxiety scores (Fig. 23.**41**).

The case was thus that of a patient with a body dysmorphic dirsorder and facial pain that was presumably myogenic and psychogenic. The first problem was getting the patient to accept the diagnosis and therapy. In fact, she insisted that more tests be conducted, even histological examinations to ascertain the nature of the process that, in her opinion, was causing a deteriorating dysmorphism for which she was seeking a remedy. The patient's profession, instead of facilitating the task, complicated it in some ways.

During a long and tranquil discussion, since she refused to take a new-generation antidepressant, it was agreed that she would take amitriptyline at low dosages (30 mg a day divided into to three doses), and tizanidine, 4 mg in the evening. A parallel therapy was also prescribed, consisting of anesthetic infiltrations, cold spray on the trigger points, cervical traction, and biofeedback along with the usual exercise program to be followed at home. A maxillary splint was put in to obviate the erroneous dental contact induced iatrogenically (Fig. 23.**42**). After about one month, during which the pain symptoms improved somewhat (though the patient was unwilling to acknowledge this, fearing that doing so would shift attention from the dysmorphism problem), the drug therapy was adjusted to amitriptyline associated with perfenazine in progressively increasing dosages up to 25 mg amitriptyline and 2 mg perfenazine twice a day. In the following four months, there was further improvement: the facial pain disappeared

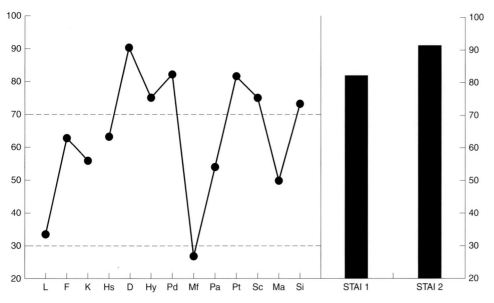

Fig. 23.**41   Significantly high scores on most of the MMPI scales.** High state and trait anxiety scores

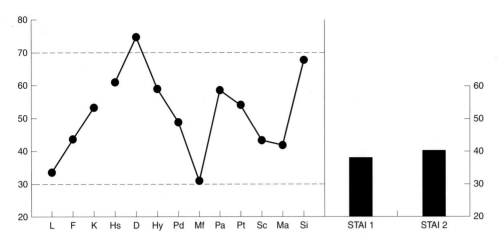

Fig. 23.**43**   Distinct improvement of MMPI profile and anxiety scores after treatment

and the cervical pain diminished. The well-being had improved notably and the patient then agreed to take an antidepressant of more recent generation. She was prescribed paroxetine (20 mg in the morning) and zolpidem when needed for occasional insomnia (difficulty falling asleep) and continued the nondrug therapy. The patient went back to work and the impact was much less traumatic than she had feared. Although she did not specifically admit it, she realized that she no longer felt that she was a victim of dysmorphism. The tests were administered again in that period and showed considerable improvement in the personality profile: only the

depression score was still high, though significantly lower than it was at the beginning of therapy. The anxiety scores were normal (Fig. 23.**43**). The facial expression of the patient also confirmed the improvement of mood (Fig. 23.**44**). The drug therapy was continued for another six months.

The Burning Mouth Syndrome

The burning mouth syndrome, also known as "glossalgia" or "oral dysesthesia", is characterized by a burning sensation in the oral cavity in the absence of clinical signs to justify it. The pain is almost always bilateral and often occurs in more than one site, with an inclination for distal areas (Table 23.**1**). The pain does not seem to be neuropathic because it does not conform to the areas of distribution of the sensory nerves. The syndrome is more frequent in women, particularly in postmenopausal women (Grushka, 1987; Van der Waal, 1990; Sharav, 1994; Zakrzewska, 1995). A large percentage of subjects have other local disturbances associated with it: dryness

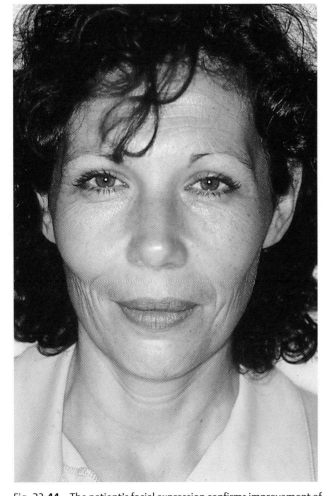

Fig. 23.**44**   The patient's facial expression confirms improvement of mood

Table 23.**1**   Prevalence of sites of burning pain in a group of patients suffering from the "burning mouth" syndrome

Site	Prevalence (%) (n = 72)
Tongue	
Tip	78
Anterior two–thirds	58
Ventral	17
Posterior third	11
Floor of mouth	13
Hard palate	
Anterior third	49
Posterior two–thirds	26
Soft palate	6
Oropharynx	13
Lower lip	
Mucosa	49
Cutaneous portion	24
Upper lip	
Mucosa	39
Cutaneous portion	18
Alveolar ridges	
Lower	25
Upper	24
Buccal mucosa	14

From Grushka, 1987, with modifications

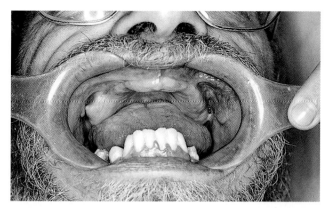

Fig. 23.**45** **"Burning mouth" syndrome in a 55-year-old man.** The pain was located in the gingiva of the upper jaw and the patient was subjected to the extraction of all his upper teeth. The symptoms, which had worsened progressively after tooth extraction, disappeared after four months of taking amitriptyline

of the mouth, dysgeusia, and taste alterations. Moreover, these subjects suffer more frequently than healthy subjects of the same age and sex from sleep disorders, irritability, and depressive mood (Grushka, 1987). As stated above, upon inspection of the oral cavity there are no alterations of the mucosa in the area affected by the phenomenon.

Many etiological factors have been suspected: a deficiency of iron, vitamin B_{12} or other vitamins of the B group, folates, and zinc, and diabetes. In reality, none of these hypotheses has been supported by controlled studies. A more solid hypothesis seems to be that alterations of the immune system might be a causal or predisposing factor in a certain percentage of subjects (Grushka, 1987). Several authors have emphasized the prevalence of psychological problems in patients suffering from this syndrome (Grushka, 1987; Van der Ploeg et al.,

1987; Van der Waal, 1990). In particular, Van der Ploeg et al. (1987) found a greater prevalence of anxiety, depression, and neurotic tendencies in affected subjects than in control subjects. This does not entitle us to conclude that the psychological factor is necessarily an etiological factor of the burning mouth syndrome, since these psychological alterations are commonly observed in patients suffering from chronic pain. Nonetheless, anecdotal observations (Mongini, 1996) as well as controlled studies (Bogetto et al., 1998) indicate that treatment with antidepressants is often effective in relieving the symptoms (Fig. 23.**45**). It is therefore possible that the pain is, for the most part at least, psychogenic.

References

American Psychiatric Association (DSM-IV), *Diagnostic and statistical manual of mental disorders*, 4 th ed., Washington, 1994.

Bogetto F., Maina G., Ferro G., Carbone M., Gandolfo S., *Psychiatric comorbidity in patients with burning mouth syndrome (BMS)*, Psychosomatic Medicine, 1998, 60 : 378 – 385.

Grushka M., *Clinical features of burning mouth syndrome*, Oral Surg. Oral Med. Oral Pathol., 1987, 63 : 30 – 36.

International Association for the Study of Pain, *Classification of chronic pain: descriptions of chronic pain syndromes and definitions of pain terms*, 2 d ed. IASP Press, Seattle, 1994.

International Headache Society, *Classification and diagnostic criteria for headache disorders, cranial neuralgias and facial pain*, Cephalalgia, 1988, 8 (Suppl. 7):1 – 96.

Mongini F., *ATM e Muscolatura cranio-cervico-faciale. Fisiopatologia e Terapia*, Utet, Torino, 1996.

Sharav Y., *Orofacial pain*, in: Wall P.D., Melzack R. (ed.), *Textbook of pain*, Churchill Livingstone, Edinburgh, 1994, 563 – 582.

Van der Ploeg H.M., Van der Wal N., Eijkman M.A.J., Van der Waal I., *Psychological aspects of patients with burning mouth syndrome*, Oral Surg. Oral Med. Oral Pathol., 1987, 63 : 664 – 668.

Van der Waal I., *The burning mouth syndrome*, Munksgaard, Copenhagen, 1990, 5 – 90.

Zakrzewska J.M., *The burning mouth syndrome remains an enigma*, Pain, 1995, 62 : 253 – 257.

24 Facial Pain and Headache

General Principles

As we have seen, patients who suffer primarily from headache may also have frequent pain attacks, mostly myogenic, in various regions, especially the cheeks and/or cervical area. Conversely, patients with facial pain may suffer from headaches. The case is quite different when both pain pathologies are manifested to such extent that they represent problems of equal severity.

All types of facial pain described in the previous chapters can be accompanied by chronic headache. Nor is it rare to find that, in addition to headache, the patient suffers from more than one type of facial pain. These cases are mostly chronic and involve depression. Even if depression is not the primary etiological factor (because the depression itself may be caused by the chronic pain), it must be attentively evaluated and treated. However, the complexity of the problems creates numerous triggering or aggravating factors and therefore the therapy program must be modulated very carefully. In fact, it is precisely with this type of patients that it is easy for physicians to be biased by their own specialty and to give priority to one aspect of the problem and neglect other aspects.

Both drug and nondrug therapies are always prescribed to treat these cases. Moreover, the drug therapy usually includes various types of drugs. Sometimes there can be a conflict between the various needs, so that the duration and sequence of the different treatments require careful evaluation. For example, the application of an orthopedic jaw splint to manage a TMJ problem can be perceived as extremely invasive by a patient with a severe mood disorder and, as a result, aggravate a psychogenic pain caused by that disorder. When prescribing drugs, there may be doubts about which ones to choose, as in the case of some antimigraine drugs contraindicated for patients with depression (see Chapter 12).

Facial Pain and Chronic Tension Headache

A case of facial pain overlapped by a severe tension-type headache is that of a 54-year-old married woman, a retired factory worker, normotensive, without children, whose medical history was unusual and rather bizarre. Twelve years before observation she had a sudden and intense attack of bilateral tinnitus (a "whistling noise") immediately followed by severe vertigo. She was diagnosed as suffering from Menière syndrome and treated with antivertigo drugs, which caused a partial regression of the symptoms. However, after a few months the symptoms began to be associated with a severe anxiety disorder with obsessive–phobic characteristics and avoidance behavior. The patient had developed a phobia of all noise, even if it was not loud (e.g. someone nearby blowing his nose, the television, etc.). The burglar alarm of a home nearby had triggered a dramatic panic attack that made her flee from her house. This was also partly due to a hyperacusia from which she also suffered. Four years before observation, she had had a relapse of the episodes of intense vertigo for which she was hospitalized for a while. The patient had long suffered occasionally from headaches and cervicofacial pain. Three

years before observation, these problems had become daily. The pain was located in the bilateral preauricular and buccal region and the right retrocervical region. She also had a pressing pain in her right shoulder (Fig. 24.1) that was exacerbated by movement and cold, damp weather. The headache was located in the right frontal–orbital–parietal region (Fig. 24.1), had differing characteristics (sometimes pulsating, other times pressing), and its frequency was daily. There were no autonomic symptoms. Both these pains daily reached moderate to severe intensity for all or most of the day (Fig. 24.2) and were always present in a mild form. In the previous three years, the patient had suffered from prolonged periods of severe depression. At the time of observation, she reported a tinnitus of varying pitch (rustle-whistle) constantly on the right and occasionally on the left. Moreover, she had a large number of other disturbances (Fig. 24.3) and reported, in addition to the phobia of noises, frequent ideas of ruin. She had been taking benzodiazepines and NSAIDs every day for a long time.

At the neurological examination, a paresis of the sixth cranial nerve on the right and a hypoesthesia of the first and second branches of the right trigeminal were found. A mild hyposthenia of the upper limbs and the right lower limb was also observed. It is interesting to note that the patient had no problems standing straight with her eyes closed. Upon inspection, her shoulders were uneven (the right shoulder was on a lower plane). There were the usual signs of parafunction (notable dental abrasion, scalloped tongue edges, etc.) in addition to an evident habit of frequent nibbling of the lower lip (Fig. 24.4). Palpation caused pain in the bilateral retrocondylar region and most of the facial and cervical muscles. Lastly, during mouth opening movements, repeated clicking noises of the left TMJ were heard. The degree of opening, however, was normal. Radiography of the spinal column showed a severe thoracolumbar scoliosis. The brain CAT scans and MRI performed previously were within the norm.

The MMPI showed extremely high levels of hypochondria, depression and hysteria. Psychasthenia and social introversion were also notably high. State and trait anxiety levels were near the maximum (Fig. 24.5).

The patient's problems could therefore be summarized as follows: a severe mood disorder with depression and high anxiety level with specific phobia and avoidance behavior; myogenic, and probably to some degree psychogenic, cervicofacial pain; chronic tension-type headache; and a mild TMJ problem on the left side resulting from the parafunction. The tinnitus and hyperacusia were probably a residue of the Menière syndrome.

A cycle of ademetionine, 200 mg i.m., was prescribed for 20 days and fluoxetine 20 mg in the morning. Since the patient reported a worsening of the anxiety, the fluoxetine was replaced after ten days with 10 mg amitriptyline and 2 mg perfenazine twice a day, plus trazodone drops, 30 mg in the evening. The patient also took lorazepam 1 mg tablets during the day as needed. A series of biofeedback sessions was begun in addition to an intensive program for treating the cervical pain: anesthetic infiltrations and laser therapy at the painful points, mild cervical traction, posture exercises. Re-

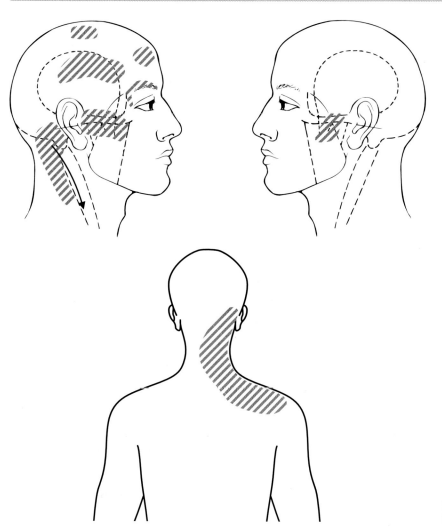

Fig. 24.**1**   Site of facial pain and chronic tension-type headache in a 54-year-old woman

NAME: P. R.

DATE: NOV/DEC		14	15	16	17	18	19	20	21	22	23	24	25	26	27	28	29	30	1	2	3	4	5	6	7	8	9	10	11	12	13
HEADACHE	5																														
	4					X	X	X	X	X					X			X		X	X	X		X						X	
	3	X		X							X	X	X			X	X		X				X		X	X	X	X	X		X
	2		X		X									X																	
	1																														
	0																														
Headache duration (hours)		3	4	6	12	10	10	12	4	4	8	6	10	10	6	4	10	6	13	8	6	12	12	12	7	7	12	12	12	9	12
PAIN	5																														
	4		●	●			●	●				△	△●				●	●	●	●		●	●			●		●		●	●
	3	●	△		●	●		△	△	△	●				△	△●			△	△	△●	△	△	△	▲	△	△	△	●	△	△
	2	△		△	△	△	△		●	●		●		●	●		△	△						●			●		△		
	1																														
	0																														
Pain duration (hours)		6	5	8	12	12	12	12	10	12	12	10	10	10	10	10	12	12	13	12	8	12	12	12	8	12	12	12	12	12	12

△ = Shoulder pain

● = Cervical pain

Fig. 24.**2**   Headache and pain diary

Colitis	☐	Back pain	☐
Gastritis	☒	Urination disturbances	☐
Kinetosis	☐	Diarrhea or constipation	☐
Swallowing difficulty	☐	Nail fragility	☒
Digestive problems	☐	Hair fragility	☒
Anorexia	☐	Circulation disorders	☐
Bulimia	☒	Cold limbs	☒
Anxiety	☒	Frigidity	☒
Phobias	☒	Vaginism	☒
Sleep disorders	☒	Frequent depressed moods	☒
Palpitations	☒	Visual disturbances	☒
Panic attacks	☒	Orthostatic hypotension	☒
Mood changes	☒	Other	☐
Fainting	☐		
Vertigo	☒		
Lassitude	☒		
Parafunctions	☒		
Clonus	☒		
Cramps	☐		
Paresthesias	☒		

Fig. 24.**3**   Accompanying symptoms reported by the patient

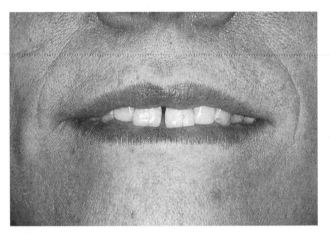

Fig. 24.**4**   Signs of parafunction, including nibbling of the lower lip, were observed in this patient

sponse was gradual, with a partial alleviation of the symptoms after the second month of therapy (Fig. 24.**6**). After three months, the trazodone was interrupted while the combination of amitriptyline and perfenazine was continued. Since the patient complained of insomnia, triazolam 0.125 mg was also prescribed before going to bed. The nondrug treatment continued unchanged. The headache and facial pain continued to improve gradually. Six months after therapy was started, the pains persisted but had notably abated (Fig. 24.**7**). The patient reported a considerable improvement of mood to the point that she could plan trips with her husband, something which she had not done for many years. The MMPI, repeated in this period, showed an improvement in the profile, though the scores of the first three scales continued to be high. The depression and hysteria scores had decreased significantly. The anxiety scores had regressed, though they remained medium-high (Fig. 24.**8**).

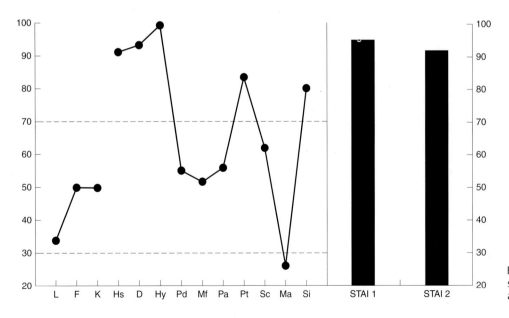

Fig. 24.**5**   Extreme elevation of several MMPI scales and state and trait anxiety scores

NAME: P. R.

DATE: FEB

		1	2	3	4	5	6	7	8	9	10	11	12	13	14	15	16	17	18	19	20	21	22	23	24	25	26	27	28		
HEADACHE	5																														
	4						X																								
	3	X	X			X		X	X					X	X		X	X	X		X										
	2			X	X					X	X	X	X			X	X					X		X	X		X	X	X	X		
	1																								X						
	0																														
Headache duration (hours)		12	12	12	12	12	12	12	12	12	12	12	12	12	12	12	12	12	12	12	12	12	12	12	12	12	12	12	12		
PAIN	5																														
	4	●	●			●	●																								
	3	△		●	△	△	△	●	●	●	●	●	●	●	●	●	●	●	●	●	●										
	2		△	△	●△			△	△	△	△	△	△	△	△	△	△	△	△	△	△	●			●	●	●	●	●		
	1																					△	●	●	△	△	△	△	△		
	0																						△	△							
Pain duration (hours)		12	12	12	12	12	12	12	12	12	12	12	12	12	12	12	12	12	12	12	12	12	12	12	12	12	12	12	12		
DRUG INTAKE																															
LORAZEPAM		1	1					1	1	1	1	1	1	1	1	1	1	1	1	1	1	1	1	1	1	1	1	1	1		
AMITRIPTYLINE + PERPHENAZINE		2	2	2	2	2	2	2	2	2	2	2	2	2	2	2	2	2	2	2	2	2	2	2	2	2	2	2	2		
TRAZODONE		X	X	X	X	X	X	X	X	X	X	X	X	X	X	X	X	X	X	X	X	X	X	X	X	X	X	X	X		

a

NAME: P. R.

DATE: MAR

		1	2	3	4	5	6	7	8	9	10	11	12	13	14	15	16	17	18	19	20	21	22	23	24	25	26	27	28	29	30	31
HEADACHE	5																															
	4																															
	3			X					X		X	X			X	X	X			X	X								X			
	2	X	X		X	X	X	X		X				X	X			X	X	X			X	X	X	X						
	1																										X	X		X	X	X
	0																															
Headache duration (hours)		12	12	12	12	12	12	12	12	12	12	12	12	12	12	12	12	12	12	12	12	12	12	12	12	12	12	12	12	12	12	12
PAIN	5																															
	4																															
	3	●	●	●	●	●	●	●	△	△	●	●	●	●	●	●	●	●	●	●												
	2	△	△	△	△	△	△		●	●	△	△	△	△	△	△	△	△	△	△	●	●	●	●	●	●	●	●	●	●	●	●
	1																				△	△	△	△	△	△	△	△	△	△	△	△
	0																															
Pain duration (hours)		12	12	12	12	12	12	12	12	12	12	12	12	12	12	12	12	12	12	12	12	12	12	12	12	12	12	12	12	12	12	12
DRUG INTAKE																																
LORAZEPAM		1	1	1	1	1	1	1	1	1	1	1	1	1	1	1	1	1	1	1	1	1	1									
AMITRIPTYLINE + PERPHENAZINE		2	2	2	2	2	2	2	2	2	2	2	2	2	2	2	2	2	2	2	2	2	2	2	2	2	2	2	2	2	2	2

b

△ = Shoulder pain   ● = Cervical pain

Fig. 24.**6** Slow but gradual improvement of symptoms after two (**a**) and three (**b**) months of therapy

NAME: P. R.

DATE: JUNE	1	2	3	4	5	6	7	8	9	10	11	12	13	14	15	16	17	18	19	20	21	22	23	24	25	26	27	28	29	30
HEADACHE 5																														
HEADACHE 4																		X												
HEADACHE 3																	X							X			X			
HEADACHE 2			X	X						X	X	X	X	X	X	X			X	X		X	X		X	X				
HEADACHE 1	X	X			X	X	X	X	X																					
HEADACHE 0																					X							X	X	X
Headache duration (hours)	6	6	12	12	6	8	8	12	6	6	6	12	8	8	8	8	10	4	8	8		6	6	6	8	6	6			
PAIN 5																														
PAIN 4																														
PAIN 3																	•	•						•						
PAIN 2			•	•			•	•	•	•	•	•	•	•	•	•			•	•	•	•	•		•	•	•			
PAIN 1	•	•	△		•	•	•	△	△	△	△	△	△	△	△	△	△	△	△	△	△	△	△	△	△	△	△			
PAIN 0	△	△		△	△	△	△																							
Pain duration (hours)	6	6	12	12	12	8	8	12	12	12	12	8	8	8	8	8	10	10	12	8	8	6	8	8	8	8	6	6		

DRUG INTAKE

	1	2	3	4	5	6	7	8	9	10	11	12	13	14	15	16	17	18	19	20	21	22	23	24	25	26	27	28	29	30
TRIAZOLAM	1	1	1	1	1	1	1	1	1	1	1	1	1	1	1	1	1	1	1	1	1	1	1	1	1	1	1			
AMITRIPTYLINE + PERPHENAZINE	2	2	2	2	2	2	2	2	2	2	2	2	2	2	2	2	2	2	2	2	2	2	2	2	2	2	2			

△ = Shoulder pain

● = Cervical pain

Fig. 24.**7**   Considerable improvement of symptoms six months after start of treatment

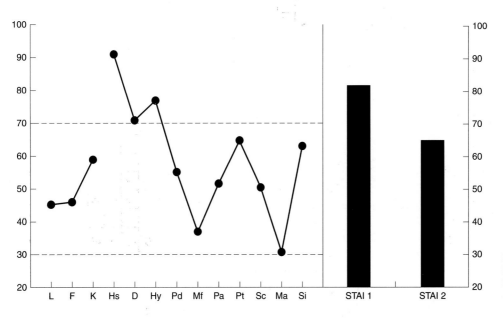

Fig. 24.**8**   Improvement of the MMPI personality profile and alleviation of the trait anxiety (see Fig. 24.**5**)

Facial Pain and Transformed Migraine

The next case is that of a patient with an arthrogenic and myogenic pain overlapping a migraine that had progressively changed from episodic to chronic until it became a daily chronic headache. The patient was a 33-year-old woman, a factory worker, married, with three children. She had been suffering from a stabbing pain in her right TMJ, exacerbated by pronounced mouth movements and chewing and associated with a clicking noise on the same side. A pressing pain in the bilateral zygomatic, buccal, and cervical region, as well as a back pain, developed later (Fig. 24.9) and appeared three or four times a week for several hours. The patient had suffered from intense migraines since she was a young girl. These attacks had

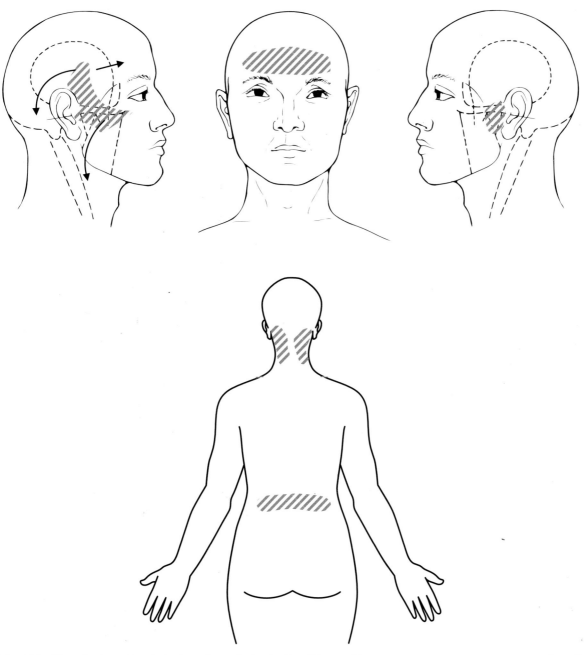

Fig. 24.**9** Sites of pain and headache (transformed migraine) in a 33-year-old woman

been occasional (once or twice a month) until a year before observation, when they became progressively more severe and frequent, occurring almost every day. They were located in the frontal region, more intense on the right, and lasted six hours or more. The pain was pulsating and intense and the attacks were accompanied by intense nausea and lacrimation. In the intercritical period there was a constant and pressing pain all over the head (Fig. 24.**10**). Aggravating factors were stress and prolonged sleep during the weekend.

The patient reported a large number of accompanying disturbances (Fig. 24.**11**). Besides those that were clearly psychosomatic, there were others indicating the possibility of hormonal and circulation disorders (dysmenorrhea, fragile nails and hair, intense paresthesias in the lower limbs, problems with circulation of the extremities, dizziness). Neurological examination was negative, except for a mild hyposthenia of the lower right limb. Inspection revealed a marked defect in the posture of the neck and shoulders (Fig. 24.**12**). Some teeth

were missing, others were in poor condition. The mouth opening movement was limited to 22 mm without pain and 32 mm with accentuated pain in the TMJ and buccal region. There was no deviation of the mandible to either side (Fig. 24.**13**). Palpation of the cranial points was markedly positive for the lateral pole and retrocondylar point bilaterally; palpation of all the craniocervicofacial muscles caused intense pain. Upon auscultation, a moderate crepitating noise was heard at the right TMJ during mouth opening and closing movements.

TMJ radiographs, with the mouth closed, showed a reduced articular space bilaterally and, with the mouth open, a marked limitation of the movement of both condyles (Fig. 24.**14**). Cervical radiography confirmed a moderate posture problem (Fig. 24.**15**).

The MMPI showed an extremely high *hysterical or conversive V.* State anxiety was within the normal limits, whereas trait anxiety was high (Fig. 24.**16**).

NAME: **P. A.**																															
DATE: MAY/JUNE	5	6	7	8	9	10	11	12	13	14	15	16	17	18	19	20	21	22	23	24	25	26	27	28	29	30	31	1	2	3	4
HEADACHE — 5																															
4						X	X	X	X			X									X								X	X	X
3	X	X	X	X						X	X						X			X		X	X		X		X				
2					X								X		X	X		X	X					X		X					
1														X																	
0																															
Headache duration (hours)	10	12	12	10	9	10	10	T	10	12	12	10	T	T	T	T	12	T	T	10	10	T	T	T	10	12	10	12	10	9	10

Fig. 24.**10**   Headache diary

Colitis	☒
Gastritis	☒
Kinetosis	☐
Swallowing difficulty	☐
Digestive problems	☐
Anorexia	☐
Bulimia	☒
Anxiety	☒
Phobias	☒
Sleep disorders	☒
Palpitations	☐
Panic attacks	☒
Mood changes	☒
Fainting	☐
Vertigo	☒
Lassitude	☒
Parafunctions	☐
Clonus	☐
Cramps	☒
Paresthesias	☒
Back pain	☒
Urination disturbances	☐
Diarrhea or constipation	☐
Nail fragility	☒
Hair fragility	☒
Circulation disorders	☒
Cold limbs	☒
Frigidity	☐
Vaginism	☐
Frequent depressed moods	☒
Urticaria	☒
Dysmenorrhea	☒
Other	☐

Fig. 24.**11**   The patient reported numerous disturbances, both psychosomatic and indicative of hormonal and circulation disorders

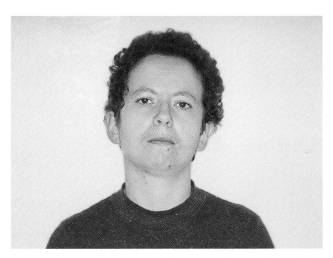

Fig. 24.**12**   Inspection revealed a posture defect in the shoulders and neck

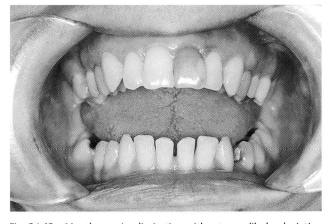

Fig. 24.**13**   Mouth opening limitation without mandibular deviation

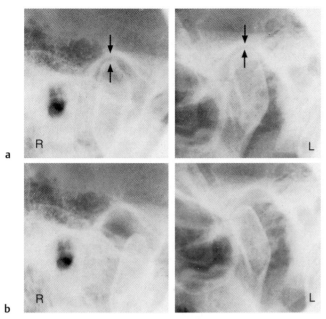

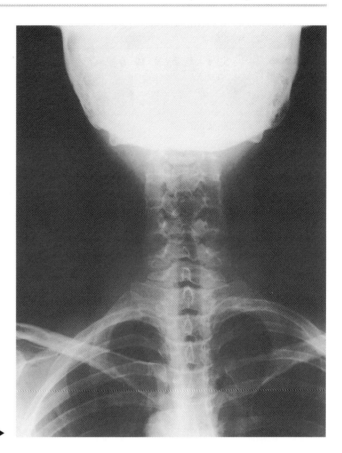

Fig. 24.**14**   **TMJ radiographs** at closed mouth (**a**) show a narrow vertical articular space (arrows). Those at open mouth (**b**) show a limited translating movement of both condyles

Fig. 24.**15**   The cervical radiographs show a moderate scoliosis   ▶

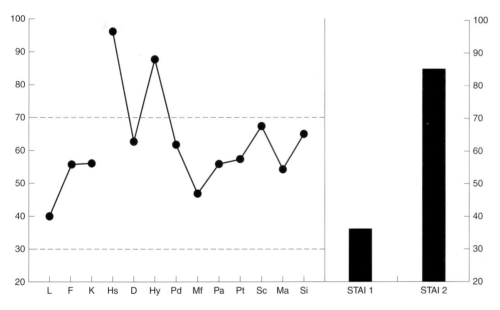

Fig. 24.**16**   The MMPI shows a marked *hysterical or conversive V.* The STAI shows very high trait anxiety

The patient therefore had more than one problem. She had an intracapsular alteration of the TMJ, to a more advanced degree on the right as a result of disk compression. This was shown by some of the clinical results (pain upon palpation of the articular points, worsening of the pain during mastication, articular noise) and radiological results. The alteration was most probably caused by a neuromuscular factor (daytime and nighttime parafunction) and a structural factor (deteriorated situation of the oral cavity with disk compression in closed mouth position). The relative pain component was obviously arthrogenic and it was overlapped by myogenic facial pain (exacerbated by palpation of the elevator muscles of the

mandible) and cervical pain (exacerbated by palpation of the neck muscles). Furthermore, the patient had all the characteristics of a transformed migraine, including the hysterical trait revealed by the MMPI, which is found in a considerable number of patients suffering from migraine transformed into chronic daily headache (Mongini et al., 1997 a, b).

An orthopedic jaw splint was applied, slightly raised bilaterally in the rear section to obtain a moderate downward distraction of the articular condyles (Fig. 24.**17**). The patient was initially instructed to wear the splint only if it did not cause her discomfort or accentuate parafunction and muscle pain. There was no problem, because she reported feeling re-

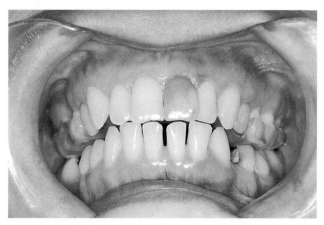

Fig. 24.**17** Application of the jaw splint, with rear section slightly raised for condylar distraction

lief when using the splint and therefore kept it in place 24 hours a day, even during meals. Amitriptyline drops, 10 mg in the morning and 20 mg in the evening, were prescribed.

A biofeedback program was started and regular relaxation exercises and gymnastics were prescribed. Within three months, there was a progressive and marked alleviation of the symptoms, with a considerable regression of the articular, facial, and cervical pain and a reduction in the frequency of the headache to two attacks per week, which the patient resolved partially with an analgesic (Fig. 24.**18**). The drug and nondrug therapy was continued and the patient was instructed to increase her daily exercises over the next five months, after which only a mild headache lasting a few hours, four or five times a month, remained, along with one or two attacks typical of migraine coinciding to her menstrual period. In other words, the problem had regressed to become the episodic migraine that the patient had suffered from since she was a child, in addition to a mild episodic tension-type headache. For the migraine attacks she was prescribed sumatriptan, 50 mg as needed, which effectively eliminated the attacks. In the meantime, the TMJ, facial, and cervical pain had disappeared almost permanently. The crepitating noise at the right TMJ had also disappeared and the mouth opening movement had almost normalized (Fig. 24.**19**). The situation was kept under control in the next few months and, since it had improved further (Figs. 24.**20**, 24.**21**), it was decided to gradually eliminate the intake of amitriptyline and insist on the need to continue with the exercises indefinitely. The MMPI administered 16 months after the start of therapy showed a normali-

NAME: **P. A.**																																
DATE: JULY		*1*	*2*	*3*	*4*	*5*	*6*	*7*	*8*	*9*	*10*	*11*	*12*	*13*	*14*	*15*	*16*	*17*	*18*	*19*	*20*	*21*	*22*	*23*	*24*	*25*	*26*	*27*	*28*	*29*	*30*	*31*
HEADACHE	5																																
	4									X																							
	3																																X
	2													X																			
	1	X			X			X	X	X								X	X												X		
	0		X	X		X	X				X	X	X		X	X	X		X		X	X	X	X	X	X	X	X	X		X		
Headache duration (hours)		3			2					2								1		2										2		3
DRUG INTAKE																																	
PROPYPHENAZONE										X																							
AMITRIPTYLINE		X	X	X	X	X	X	X	X	X	X	X	X	X	X	X	X	X	X	X	X	X	X	X	X	X	X	X	X	X	X	X	X

Fig. 24.**18** Symptom improvement three months after start of therapy

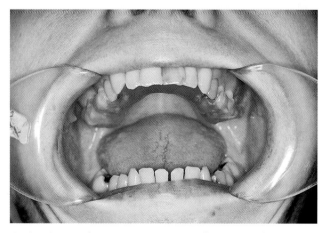

Fig. 24.**19** Mouth opening movement is almost normal

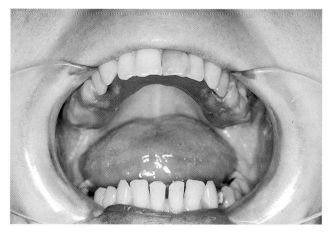

Fig. 24.**20** Further improvement of mouth opening movement

NAME: **P. A.**																															
DATE: AUG		2	3	4	5	6	7	8	9	10	11	12	13	14	15	16	17	18	19	20	21	22	23	24	25	26	27	28	29	30	31
HEADACHE	5																															
	4																															
	3																						X									
	2																							X								
	1		X																	X												
	0	X		X	X	X	X	X	X	X	X	X	X	X	X	X	X	X	X		X	X				X	X	X	X	X	X	X
Headache duration (hours)		2																					2	2								
DRUG INTAKE																																
SUMATRIPTAN																							X									

Fig. 24.**21** Headache diary at end of treatment

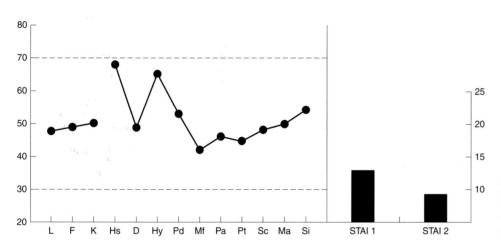

Fig. 24.**22** Improvement of personality profile according to the MMPI and abatement of state and trait anxiety scores at end of treatment

zation of her profile, which remained of the hysterical type but had normal hypochondria, depression, and hysteria scores (Fig. 24.**22**). This is a frequent result in patients successfully treated for chronic daily headache (Mongini et al., 1997 a) (see Chapter 8). The STAI showed very low state and trait anxiety scores (Fig. 24.**22**).

References

Mongini F., Defilippi N., Negro C., *Chronic daily headache. A clinical and psychological profile before and after treatment*, Headache, 1997 a, 37 : 83 – 87.

Mongini F., Bava M., Defilippi N., Ibertis F., *Chronic daily headache. A clinical and psychological profile*, Cephalalgia, 1997 b, 17 : 364, (abs.).

Index

Note: 'vs' indicates the differentiation of two conditions.